MOTIVATION

MOTIVATION

A Biosocial and Cognitive Integration
of Motivation and Emotion

Eva Dreikurs Ferguson
Southern Illinois University Edwardsville

with a chapter contribution by
Beth Eva Ferguson Wee
Tulane University

New York   Oxford
OXFORD UNIVERSITY PRESS
2000

Oxford University Press

Oxford   New York
Athens   Auckland   Bangkok   Bogotá   Buenos Aires   Calcutta
Cape Town   Chennai   Dar es Salaam   Delhi   Florence   Hong Kong   Istanbul
Karachi   Kuala Lumpur   Madrid   Melbourne   Mexico City   Mumbai
Nairobi   Paris   São Paulo   Singapore   Taipei   Tokyo   Toronto   Warsaw

and associated companies in
Berlin   Ibadan

Copyright © 2000 by Oxford University Press, Inc.

Published by Oxford University Press, Inc.,
198 Madison Avenue, New York, New York, 10016
http://www.oup-usa.org

Library of Congress Cataloging-in-Publication Data

Ferguson, Eva Dreikurs.
    Motivation : a biosocial and cognitive integration of motivation
and emotion / Eva Dreikurs Ferguson ; with chapter contribution by
Beth Eva Ferguson Wee.
        p.   cm.
    ISBN-13: 978-0-19-506866-5 (alk. paper)
    ISBN 0-19-506866-1 (alk. paper)
    1. Motivation (Psychology)   2. Emotions.   I. Wee, Beth Eva
Ferguson.   II. Title.
BF503.F46   2000
153.8—dc21   99-25805
                                                        CIP

Printing (last digit): 9 8 7 6 5 4 3

Printed in the United States of America
on acid-free paper

*This book is dedicated to Rudolf Dreikurs, who was the first to stimu-
late my inquiry into the topic of motivation; Bill Linden, whose incredible patience and support enabled the writing to proceed; and Beth Eva
Ferguson Wee, who as daughter and colleague contributed to this book
in ways too numerous to cite.*

Contents

Preface   xv

CHAPTER 1   INTRODUCTION: WHAT IS MOTIVATION?   1

Historical Considerations   1

Understanding Motivation Helps to Explain Behavior   1
Will, Drive, Instinct, and Motivation   2
Motivation Is an Intervening Variable   3
Motivation Is Energizing and Directional   4
Variability and Stability   4

Summary   6

CHAPTER 2   HOW DO WE STUDY MOTIVATION?   7

Definitions: How Do You Define Motivation?   7

Defining a Construct   7
Operational Definitions   9

The Relationship Between Motivation and Other Variables   10

Motivation Leads to Action   10
How Do Rewards and Incentives Become Motivation?   11

Summary   12

CHAPTER 3   AROUSAL: THE ENERGIZING AND INTENSITY ASPECT OF MOTIVATION   14

The Construct of Arousal   14

Defining and Measuring Arousal   14
The Reticular Activating System   15
Physiological Measurements   18

Arousal Has Many Aspects   19

Situational Specificity and Response Stereotypy   19
State Versus Trait: Arousal Compared with Arousability   20
Tense Compared with Energetic Arousal   21

Arousal—Performance Relationships   23

Motor Activity and Arousal   23
Inverted-U Function and the "Yerkes-Dodson Law"   26

Summary   29

CHAPTER 4 BIOLOGICAL RHYTHMS AND SLEEP *by Beth Eva Ferguson Wee* **30**

Relationship of Biological Rhythms to Motivation 30
Biological Rhythms 30
Introduction 30
Biological Rhythms Versus Biorhythms 31
Measuring Circadian Rhythms 32
Seasonal Rhythms 38
Nonphotic Factors that Influence the Circadian System 38
Control of Biological Rhythms 40
The Mammalian Biological Clock 40
Multiple Oscillators Within the Circadian System 41
Melatonin 42
Advantages of Biological Timekeeping 44
Effects of Disrupting Biological Rhythms 45
Seasonal Affective Disorder and Phototherapy 45
"Jet Lag" 47
Sleep 48
Stages of Sleep 48
Why Do We Sleep? 51
Relationship of Sleep to Circadian Rhythms 52
Effects of Aging on Biological Rhythms and Sleep 54
Summary 56

CHAPTER 5 TIME OF DAY, ALERTNESS, AND PERFORMANCE **58**

Variables of Importance in Addition to Time of Day 59
Time Since Sleeping 59
Prior Activity 59
Stimulation and Goals 60
Are There Several Rhythms? 61
Sleep Compared with Temperature Rhythms 61
Alertness-Sleepiness 62
Performance Varies with Alertness and Time of Day 64
Performance and Alertness 64
Different Tasks Show Different Effects 65
Time of Day, Shift Work, and Mood 68
Shift Work 68
Mood Changes 70
Personality Characteristics and "Morningness" Versus "Eveningness" 75
Morningness-Eveningness 75
Extraversion, Impulsiveness, and Morningness-Eveningness 76
Summary 79

CHAPTER 6 EMOTION AND MOOD: I. PROBLEMS OF DEFINITION AND MEASUREMENT **81**

How Are Motivation and Emotion Different? 81
Emotion and Motivation: Duration and Congruence 81
Situational Variables and Goals 82

Definitions and Classifications of Emotion   82
   Historical Considerations   83
   Categories, Classification of Basic Emotions, and Face Muscle Movement   85
   Intensity and Arousal of Emotions   90
Emotion and Everyday Life   91
   Dimensions of Emotions   92
   Person-Environment Relationships   95
   How Can Emotions Be Changed?   99
Emotion, Mood, and Affect   100
   Are Emotion, Mood, and Affect Different?   100
   Pleasantness-Unpleasantness: Dimensions Are Different from Categories   101
Emotion and Opponent Processes   102
   Opponent Process Theory   102
   Test of the Opponent Process Theory   102
Summary   103

CHAPTER 7   EMOTION AND MOOD: II. COGNITION AND
INFORMATION PROCESSING   106
Complexity of Emotion and Cognition   106
   Multiple Targets at a Given Moment   106
   Developmental Factors and the Question of Blends Versus Pure Emotions   107
   An Ecological Perspective   108
   Long-term Versus Short-term Targets   109
Emotion and Mood Have a Reciprocal Relationship with Cognition   110
   What Kinds of Cognitions Relate to Emotion?   110
   Bower's Studies of Emotion and Mood   111
Emotion and Information Processing   113
   Are Emotion and Cognition One or Two Separate Systems?   113
   Computer-based Perspectives   114
   Emotion as a Node in an Associative Network   114
   Emotional States Regulate Allocation of Capacity   119
   State-dependent Effects   120
   Are There Additional Issues?   121
Approach and Withdrawal   121
   Emotion and Cerebral Asymmetry   121
   Visual Recognition of Emotional Stimuli   125
Summary   127

CHAPTER 8   HUNGER AND THIRST: BIOLOGICAL AND
CULTURAL PROCESSES   129
Biological Processes and the Regulation of Energy in Hunger   129
   Problems of Definition: Motivational States Versus Consummatory Responses   129
   Consummatory, Appetitive, and Instrumental Responses   129
   Consummatory Responses and Subjective Descriptions   130
   Concepts and Terms   130
   Primary Versus Secondary   130
   Homeostasis, Negative Feedback, and Feedforward Regulation   131
   Short-term Versus Long-term Regulation   132

Hunger and Satiety, Onset and Cessation of Eating: The Role of the Central
    Nervous System   133
    The Role of the Lateral Hypothalamus   133
    The Role of the Ventromedial Hypothalamus   136
    The Role of the Caudal Brainstem   136
Hunger and Satiety, Onset and Cessation of Eating: The Role of
    Peripheral Sites   138
    The Autonomic Nervous System   138
    Cholecystokinin (CCK)   139
The Role of Glucose, Insulin, and Lipids in Onset and Offset of Eating   139
    Glucose   139
    Insulin   140
    Lipids   141

Biological Processes in Thirst and Fluid Level Regulation   143
    Different Kinds of Thirst and Definitions   143
    Osmoreceptors, Vasopressin, and the Lateral Hypothalamus   145
    Salt Appetite   146
    Drinking, Drinking Offset, and Nonprimary Factors   147
The Role of Culture and Learning in Hunger and Eating   149
    Taste and Appetite   149
    Culture   149
    Learned Aversions   150
    Appetite and Appetizing   152
    Weight Maintenance and Eating Disorders   155
    Cues, Obesity, and Eating Restraint   155
    Anorexia, Bulimia, and Obesity: Disorders and Disease   160
    Is There an Ideal Figure and an Ideal Weight?   163
Effects of Hunger, Thirst, and Glucose on Responding and
    Information Processing   166
    The Directional Effects of Hunger and Thirst   166
    Sensitivity to Cues   166
    The Interactive Effects of Hunger and Food   169
    Information Processing and Learning in Nonhuman Animals   173
    Human Information Processing   173
    Effects of Sweets and Hunger on Measures of Memory   177
    Sugar Can Enhance Memory Performance   177
    Event-related Brain Potentials and Memory Performance   179
Summary   180

CHAPTER 9 REWARDS, INCENTIVES, AND GOALS: ADDICTIVE PROCESSES,
    EXTRINSIC INCENTIVES, AND INTRINSIC MOTIVATION   183
General Theoretical Issues   183
    In What Ways Has the Effect of Reward Been Studied?   183
    Instrumental and Operant Conditioning: A Brief Historical Overview   183
    Praise as a Verbal Reinforcer   186
    Reward Variables That Affect Learning and Performance   187
    Unlearned and Conditioned Rewards and Motivations   187
    Delay and Magnitude of Reward   189

Brain Stimulation, Reward Systems, and Drug Abuse   190
  Reward Systems   191
  Addiction and Substance Abuse   192
Intrinsic Motivation, Extrinsic Incentives, and Achievement Motivation   198
  Incentive and Incentive Motivation   198
    Intrinsic Motivation and External Rewards   199
    Does Intrinsic Motivation Decrease with Extrinsic Rewards?   199
    Additional Perspectives   206
  Incentives, Success and Failure, and the Achievement Motive   208
    Achievement Motivation Theory: McClelland and Atkinson   209
    Expectancy-Value Theory and Success and Failure   212
Summary   214

CHAPTER 10   GOALS AND SUCCESS-FAILURE BELIEFS   217

Goals, Level of Aspiration, and Level of Expectation   217
  The Work of Kurt Lewin and Colleagues   217
  Other Research on Level of Aspiration and Level of Expectation   218
Individual Differences in Goal Setting   222
  Goal Setting and the Achievement Motive   222
  Dweck: Performance Goals Versus Learning Goals   222
  Other Goal-Expectancy Approaches   224
Beliefs Regarding Success (Versus Failure) and Reinforcement   226
  Beliefs About Success and Failure on Tasks and Self-Efficacy   226
  Locus of Control of Reinforcement   227
Goals and Performance Attainment   230
  Locke and Goal-setting Theory   230
  Research by Others on Goal Setting and Goal Striving   231
Summary   233

CHAPTER 11   AGGRESSION AND ANGER: ATTRIBUTION, MASTERY, POWER, COMPETITION   235

Attribution and Achievement   235
  Weiner and Attribution Theory   236
  Other Research Approaches   237
Anger   239
  Anger in Everyday Life   240
  Measurement of Anger   246
Hostility, Anger, and Type A Personality   247
  Hostility   247
  Type A Personality and Coronary Heart Disease   248
Summary   250

CHAPTER 12   AGGRESSION, POWER, AND MASTERY   252

What Is Meant by Aggression?   252
  The Motivational Aspects of Aggression   252

The Frustration-Aggression Hypothesis   254
Aggression in Animals   255
  Is There an Aggression Drive?   255
  Conspecific Aggression   255
  Situational Variables   258
  Interspecies Aggressive Behavior   259
Brain Areas and Hormones   260
  Brain Areas   260
  Hormones   261
Self-Interest Versus Collective Interest: Competition and
Human Aggression   264
  Self-Interest Versus Collective Interest   264
  Sports and Games   265
  Culture   268
Human Aggression: Power, Arousal, and Learning   270
  Power   270
  Arousal and Learning   274
Machiavellianism, Mastery, and Assertiveness   276
  Machiavellianism   276
  Mastery   277
  Assertiveness   277
Summary   279

CHAPTER 13 FEAR AND ANXIETY   281

General Considerations   281
Early Experimental Work   282
  Escape and Avoidance Conditioning Studies of Fear and Anxiety   282
  Punishment, Fear, and Anxiety   284
  Learned Helplessness and Flooding   285
Contemporary Research in Fear Learning   286
  Psychobiological Findings   286
  Human Conditioning Studies   290
  Social Variables Involved in Fear Learning   292
Anxiety, Individual Differences, Cognition, and Coping   293
  State and Trait Anxiety   294
  Cognition and Coping   297
Summary   300

CHAPTER 14 SEX, GENDER, AND LOVE   301

Hormonal Effects, Sexual Dimorphism, and Sexual Motivation   302
  Gonadal Steroid Hormones   302
  Social Animals: Prairie Voles and Spotted Hyenas   304
  Human Studies   306
Gender   309
  The Importance of Gender   309
  Gender Identity, Gender Schema, and Gender Differences   310

Love   316
    Parent-Child Love   316
    Peer Relationships and Friendship   319
    Romantic Love and Adult Love Relationships   321
Summary   324

References   327
Author Index   377
Subject Index   388

Preface

The topic of motivation continues to have great fascination for lay persons and students. For many years it was a major topic of interest for psychologists, but for about 2 decades only a few of us devoted our writing and research to this topic. I would ask graduate students and new faculty about concepts in motivation that were important only a few years earlier, and they would indicate neither interest nor knowledge. Motivation courses that had been held in high regard at one time in major psychology programs were gradually phased out, and many universities no longer taught courses in motivation. At the time that the rat was replaced by the computer as the model for research, motivation was replaced by cognition.

Happily for many of us, motivation found its way back into mainstream psychology. Cold cognition gave way to, if not hot, at least warm cognition. Many psychological processes were better understood if studied from a motivational approach. People and animals are motivated, and their motivation affects countless cognitions, emotions, and actions.

The present book seeks to bring to advanced undergraduate and graduate students a broad overview of the field of motivation. Although written as a textbook, it is also intended for professionals who want to know more about motivation. This book was written to show how motivation relates to cognitive, biological, and social issues. Emotions are given prominence in the book, because emotion is closely interwoven with motivation. The literature on rewards and incentives is provided to show the close relationship between reinforcement and motivation. Biological rhythms bear on motivation, be-

cause during some times we are much more alert and lively than at other times. The breadth of topics covered in the book reflects the ways motivation is relevant to many aspects of contemporary psychology. A large research literature has accumulated on topics bearing on motivation, and that literature is presented to help the reader understand motivation from the point of view of contemporary scientific psychology.

The book serves as a textbook for seminar courses on motivation, and it can be used in an experimental psychology course. Many experiments are presented in detail, and the book includes basic issues of design and methodology. Because the book provides information in depth on a variety of issues, it can be used also as supplementary reading for courses on cognition and biological as well as social psychology.

Many people have contributed to this book, some in direct ways and others through inspiration. To my father, Rudolf Dreikurs, goes the largest debt of gratitude. Since my earliest childhood he instilled in me an eagerness to learn about and understand motivation and behavior. His enormous enthusiasm about the ways psychology, especially Adlerian psychology, can help improve the quality of human life led him to be an outstanding teacher and writer as well as practitioner, and many of us reap the benefits of his wisdoms.

Some of my mentors and colleagues over the years have given me invaluable insights and guidance, and these have left traces in the way I conceptualize problems and consider implications. Although their views in many ways differ from my own, their wisdoms remain. They may not wish me to claim them in this light, but I nevertheless do acknowledge the impact made on my thinking by Benton J. Underwood and Janet Taylor Spence.

Special gratitude goes to my home university, Southern Illinois University Edwardsville, for research support, sabbatical leaves, library help, and many other institutional and departmental supports that permitted this book to come to fruition. To the Psychology Department at the University of California at Berkeley goes a special heartfelt thanks. Colleagues there gave me hours of their time in intense intellectual exchanges and in comments on specific chapters of the book. I sought to put many of their ideas and wisdoms into my writing.

When I teach, here or abroad, my students always add to my understanding. This book is written for students, but it is the contributions from stu-

dents that helped to guide how my ideas were formulated. To Nancy Johnson Sullivan goes a warmly felt gratitude for helping me through the final stages of manuscript preparation. Finally, it is the enrichment brought from loved ones that gives the vitality needed to complete the writing of a book. To Bill, Beth, Bruce, Linda, Rodney, Ryan, Alex, Kirsten, Nicole, Eric, Adam, Karen, Dan, Kathleen, and Jim go my warmest thanks for countless expressions of support and hours of shared love. To Bruce, Beth, and Linda go my deepest gratitude and appreciation for the incredible help given with family crises and obligations, which permitted my continued writing. To Bill goes my heartfelt tribute for the long periods of neglect endured with kindness during the many months of research and writing.

E. D. F.

MOTIVATION

CHAPTER 1

Introduction: What Is Motivation?

The term *motivation* is used in everyday language and with many meanings. The term also has technical meanings when used by psychologists. As will be evident throughout this book, the scientific study of motivation can be quite complex.

Motivation refers to an *internal process* that pushes or pulls the individual, and the push or pull relates to some *external event*. For example, in everyday language one might say, "she is driven by the motivation to succeed in her job," and this links the internal motivation or drive to the work place. Another expression, such as "what motivates me is the desire to please my parents," refers to an internal process (desire) to achieve an outcome involving other persons. These statements use the language of motivation (*drive, desire*) and they are *goal oriented* (success at work, pleasing one's parents). Another expression might be, "boy, I sure am starved—I haven't had a bite to eat since breakfast." Here the internal process (*hunger*) does not refer to an outcome or goal but instead relates to the past, in terms of the length of time since one last ate. The scientific study of motivation deals both with past events (*antecedent conditions*) and with anticipated outcomes (*goals*), and these are discussed throughout the book. Many expressions have been used to refer to the internal process of motivation, such as "want," "will," "need," "wish," and "seek." The present book examines these from the viewpoint of scientific psychology and research findings.

HISTORICAL CONSIDERATIONS

Understanding Motivation Helps to Explain Behavior

Concepts in contemporary psychology can be understood better when their meaning is considered from a historical perspective (Danziger, 1997; Hergenhahn, 1997; Thorne & Henley, 1997). Like other major psychological concepts, motivation has had many meanings in the history of psychology. The significance and meaning of the concept of motivation reflect the theoretical perspectives and current empirical knowledge at a given time in that history.

Since ancient times, humans have sought to explain and understand why people and animals behave the way they do, and they have observed complex patterns of behavior. In everyday life one notices that people are sometimes angry and sometimes fearful, sometimes energetic and sometimes lethargic. To ancient as well as to modern observers, animals and humans can appear to act in unpredictable fashions (Berndt & Berndt, 1952). From the earliest days of existence, humans have sought to understand themselves and the experienced world, which included plants, animals, stars, seasons, weather, rocks, and terrain as well as the actions and reactions of people. Tribal groups recognized that human actions vary, and beliefs in natural as well as supernatural forces have been used to explain such variation and to provide a sense of order in a changing world (Simpson, 1951).

The development of philosophy and rational thought (Wertheimer, 1987) led the move away from animism (belief that all objects are inhabited by animal spirits) and vitalism (belief that all things have an immaterial life force) as explanations of human variability. Science in the nineteenth century and the impact of Darwin provided many concepts that remain incorporated in modern psychology. Although the earliest laboratories in the new discipline of psychology focused on the structure of "mind" and studied *emotion and feeling* (Titchener, 1896/1921; Wundt, 1910), they did not yet focus on the more dynamic, action-oriented concept of motivation. By the 1920s, however, motivation was a major concept in psychology.

Will, Drive, Instinct, and Motivation

Early psychologists were concerned with topics that are now called "motivation," but they used different terms. For example, the famous psychologist William James (1890) placed great emphasis on the concept of *will.* He argued for the importance of *will* and *habits.* Will allowed for alteration in behavior or for doing actions in unfavorable circumstances, whereas habit allowed for establishing a routine or continuity in actions. Some processes and actions come with ease when highly practiced, and he advocated that people should develop such automatic-like responses or habits. However, people are confronted with new circumstances for which the prior habits are inadequate, and thus individuals also require internal processes for meeting new events and crises. *Will* involves choices, decision making, and thought, and James considered will to provide the force either to maintain desirable tendencies when these are challenged or to make new ones. The cognitive construct of "will" was compatible with James' psychology, because at the turn of the 20th century psychology concerned itself with the study of the mind. Only gradually psychology turned toward the study of behavior of humans and nonhuman animals. That change in psychology also brought forth new terms.

The decades after the early writings of James brought many changes in psychology. The Functionalists and later the Behaviorists showed the importance of observing adaptive actions (Kendler,

1987), and during that period the word "drive" was often used for the study of motivation. Woodworth (1918; Woodworth & Schlosberg, 1954) formulated a stimulus-organism-response (S-O-R) model, which proposed that an organism (O) behaves in an environment, and stimulus (S) events describe the way the environment impinges on the organism. The organism, in giving a response (R), makes a behavioral output. In the S-O-R model, motivation was a key variable inside the organism (O).

By 1920 the new discipline of psychology utilized the concept of motivation, but its meaning and how it related to theory was far from uniform. Some theorists used the term *drive,* because that term seemed congruent with a scientific perspective. Woodworth (1918) advocated this term and he conceptualized it to mean a mechanical process, in the way a *machine is driven* by some motive power. Freud also used the term drive, but he conceptualized it in a different way than did Woodworth. Freud (1915/1959) considered it from the perspective of biological energy, in which an *animal is driven* by primitive biological forces. The German word *Trieb,* which is a translation of "drive," refers to this "driven" quality.

In the way both Woodworth and Freud used the term, drive emphasized a *dynamic* quality. That is, humans and animals are not static. They change and adapt. They respond to an environment, they modify an environment, and they have internal (organismic) forces that move the individual in time and space. These internal forces are powerful and necessary. However, a large difference existed in the way that Woodworth viewed drive within a mechanistic, machine sense, and the way Freud viewed drive within an evolutionary, biological sense.

The Construct of Motivation.   A *construct* refers to a hypothesized internal event that is not directly observed but is tied theoretically and empirically to observable, external events. The construct of motivation fits into the scientific approach within psychology, and it helps to explain variations in human behavior. In Europe, Freud, Adler, and the various psychodynamic theorists who formed the beginnings of modern psychiatry placed major importance on the construct of motivation (Cofer & Appley, 1964). In America, the Functionalists and

Behaviorists gave the concept of motivation a core role in the new discipline of psychology (Kendler, 1987).

Around the time that drive was used to describe motivation, another term was introduced by McDougall (1923), *instinct,* and this term also came into favor to refer to motivational processes. "Instinct" tended to refer to inborn characteristics, but later McDougall employed it to refer to more changeable biological tendencies (Kendler, 1987). Psychologists have used "instinct" in many other ways than the meaning given by McDougall, and in contemporary writings by animal behaviorists, the term is used to describe not only motivational processes but a large variety of inborn tendencies. Moreover, from the early 1970s many psychologists have rejected using both drive and instinct, viewing humans as more cognitive and complex than an animal or a machine. The term instinct implied a biologically preprogrammed tendency (Tinbergen, 1952) that minimizes the role of modifiability through learning and experience, and psychologists increasingly recognized that human and animal behavior changes as a function of experience from the time of infancy. For this reason, "instinct" did not appear to be as appropriate a construct as "motivation" to account for modifiability (plasticity) in humans as well as animals.

Evaluating the Terms.   From a historical perspective, it is useful to consider why the terms *drive* and *instinct* had been adopted by the earlier psychologists and also why they were rejected by later psychologists. The early 20th-century psychologists rejected the term *will* because it implied free will and lack of determinism. In the process of developing psychology with its own identity, independent of philosophy and the study of "mind," psychologists in the early 20th century had sought deterministic causes of behavior. Terms such as drive and instinct were compatible with the early psychologists' scientific endeavors. The terms did not capture the full meaning of motivation, but they represented an important move away from a prior influence, and they did capture more of the meaning of motivation than was evident in the writings of earlier psychologists. The move by people like Woodworth (1918) and McDougall (1923) was

against the early figure in American psychology, William James, and against his use of the term will. Because emphases in psychology continuously change, many of the emphases of James have reappeared, and the emphases of Behaviorism declined by the early 1970s.

For some time, the study of motivation was diminished in favor of the study of cognitive processes. Following the "cognitive revolution" in psychology and the impact of computer models of cognition, psychology became the *science of mind and behavior,* and less research attention was given to the dynamic aspects of behavior than had occurred in the first half of the 20th century. Nevertheless, motivation continues to be a major topic of study with regard to animals and humans, and the contemporary perspectives include neurophysiological, cognitive, and a wide array of social and cultural variables.

Common characteristics can be identified for the construct of motivation throughout the first hundred years that psychology existed as an independent discipline. Thus it is useful to ask, what key characteristics can be said to exist for the construct of motivation, regardless of what term seems most appropriate at any historical point?

Motivation Is an Intervening Variable

Early in psychology motivation was identified as an internal process inside the "O," or organism. In contemporary psychology we speak of these internal events within the individual as *intervening variables,* following the work of Tolman (1922, 1932) and Hull (1943, 1951). Psychologists study many intervening variables. Well-known examples are personality, attitudes, intelligence, and memory. A great deal of psychology is devoted to events that are internal to the individual. The psychologist makes inferences about these internal processes from observation of overt behavior, with all intervening variables tied empirically to observable events.

Major categories of intervening variables that relate to but can be distinguished from motivation are *cognitions* (which include beliefs, thought, decision making, problem solving, expectancy, attitudes, schemata), *learning and memory* (based on multitudes of experiences in the course of one's life), and *biologically preprogrammed tendencies* (that involve species characteristics as well as individual maturational and genetic dispositions and potentialities). Emotions are also intervening variables that are related to but, according to many theorists, different from motivation (Kuhl & Kraska, 1989; Lazarus, 1991). In addition to intervening variables, many variables *external* to the individual influence behavior. These are *stimuli* of all kinds present in the environment, and *rewards* or other *consequences* that are outcomes of actions. To separate out motivation from all of these other variables, the focus for the study of motivation is on those internal processes that provide the energizing and direction of behavior.

Motivation Is Energizing and Directional

Motivation refers to a *dynamic* internal process. At any given moment that process can involve change or variability. When motivation is described as a momentary dynamic process it is called a motivational "state." Motivation can also refer to a predisposition regarding dynamic action tendencies, and this is called a motivational "trait." The study of motivational dispositions or traits tends to emphasize the differences between individuals, whereas the study of motivational states tends to emphasize differences in momentary dynamics of action. Motivational variation is evident in two possible ways, that is, in terms of quantity or intensity, and in terms of quality or kind. Variability in intensity involves an increase or decrease in energy mobilization (being keyed up versus being lethargic) and in the *amount* of effort that is expended in action. "Intensity" refers to how strong or weak the motivation is. Variability in quality or kind leads to selective *direction for action*, that is, in what specific way or toward what goal the action is directed. "Kind" refers to the type of motivation, such as hunger compared with thirst.

The *energizing* aspect can vary from extreme lethargy to intense alertness and responsiveness. For example, when we first wake up in the morning most of us are not full of pep and vigor. We tend to walk and talk slowly and act drowsy. The amount of energy we exert for work or even for play is fairly low compared with the amount an hour or two later. This illustrates the energizing aspect of the dynamic

nature of motivation. A change in alertness and responsiveness occurs at various hours of the day or when circumstances change at a given time of day. Under high energy compared with low energy or alertness we increase our effort and *amount* of response output.

A number of terms have been used to describe this energizing aspect of motivation: *arousal* (Anderson, 1990; Brehm & Self, 1989; Revelle, Anderson, & Humphreys, 1987; Thayer, 1989); *activation* (Duffy, 1962; Malmo, 1959; Thayer, 1970); *dynamogenic tension* (Courts, 1942), and *energy mobilization* (Duffy, 1951). Arousal is related to specific patterns of brain activity (Munk, Roelfsema, Konig, Engel, & Singer, 1996; Steriade, 1996; Steriade, McCormick, & Sejnowski, 1993) and is very important when one considers the activation or energizing state of an animal or human.

The *directional* aspect of motivation does not refer to the quantitative aspect but, instead, to the qualitative aspect of our actions and tendencies. The directional aspect of motivation pertains to the variation in the kinds of goals or antecedents to which the individual responds. For example, if a student has not eaten for many hours while studying, the student may walk a long distance to obtain food but not exert much energy to meet a friend to go to a movie. On the other hand, if that person has studied a long time and also eaten a filling meal, but has not recently interacted with the friend or had recreational activity, the student may walk a long distance to meet the friend to go to a movie. The different goals and circumstances lead to a different direction in actions, strivings, or attention. This second major aspect of the dynamic nature of motivation provides *direction* to the variety of actions we are likely to display under different circumstances and internal states.

Variability and Stability

Variation. Variation in action can be at the individual and momentary level, with the behavior of an individual differing on various occasions and in different circumstances. Variation also occurs at the interindividual and interspecies level, with differences in behavior occurring between individuals and also between species. Although much of the study of motivation focuses on the variability of internal states and overt behavior for a given individual, the research literature in the field of motivation investigates all three types of variation: between *circumstances* (momentary and situational variation for any given individual), between *individuals* (the study of individual differences), and between *species* (the study of species-specific characteristics).

Everyday events serve as an illustration. Suppose Mrs. Smith and her young son are taking their dog for a walk on a sunny spring day. They are standing near a bench at a playground near their house. They see a neighbor who also is walking with her dog coming toward their location. Mrs. Smith smiles at the neighbor and moves with a friendly gesture toward her. The small boy runs away with a yell, and the dog lurches toward the other woman's pet. Analyzing the motivations, we could guess that the friendly approach and gesture by Mrs. Smith is due to an affiliative motivation (wanting to affiliate, to be with peers). In contrast, her son may be motivated by fear (an avoidance motivation, seeking to escape from danger), and their dog's attack may be due to territoriality (wanting to protect one's turf). This small vignette illustrates motivation and how behavior of the three main characters changed with altered *circumstances* (the neighbor and her dog coming into their area of the playground), and it illustrates a difference between *individuals* (between the mother and son), and between *species* (the dog displaying species-specific characteristics that are not the same as those of the humans).

Other motivations could have been operating in the above example. When one only observes overt behavior without knowing the antecedent events or the individuals' cognitions, one can only identify motivations with considerable uncertainty. However, the *energizing* of behavior was evident by the increased activity shown by Mrs. Smith, her son, and their dog when the neighbor and her dog appeared on the scene. Also the *directionality* of behavior was evident by the qualitative differences in the way all three acted and by the apparently different goals toward which the behaviors were directed: Mrs. Smith moved (in a friendly way) toward the neighbor, her dog moved (in an aggressive way) toward the neighbor's dog, and the boy moved

away from all of them. Motivation as an intervening variable was evident, but one cannot be certain what the specific motivations were within Mrs. Smith, her son, and their dog. Had one known the antecedent events better, one might have identified quite different kinds of motivation. For example, if the neighbor had promised to return the $100 she owed Mrs. Smith the next time they met, we would not assume that Mrs. Smith's actions reflected primarily affiliative motivation!

Stability. Although motivation is largely studied in terms of its variability, an individual's motivational state may persist for a considerable time, and a motivational disposition is likely to remain for many years. Motivational states have been described by two terms, borrowed from descriptions of physiological reactions (Malmo, 1965, 1975). The term *phasic* refers to brief reactions or excitations, and the word *tonic* refers to sustained levels of excitation. For example, if a woman is quietly reading and sees a bug crossing the page, she may get excited and dispose of the bug. If this passes in a short time and her previous moderate level of excitation is resumed, this illustrates a phasic motivation increase. A tonic heightened motivation would be evident if the woman were tense the total time she is reading, perhaps for hours. This may be because she fears that her house is bug-infested or, unrelated to bugs, she is waiting for a telephone call.

Both these examples show the energizing aspects of a motivational *state*. The active state of motivation contrasts to a predisposing latent tendency to become motivated, a *trait*. Traits are stable characteristics. They may last the whole lifetime of the individual. Psychologists study traits of all kinds, and many do not pertain directly to motivation. For example, "honesty" is a trait but is not usually described as a motivational variable. In contrast, trait anxiety does have motivational characteristics. A person may be predisposed to become anxious under a wide range of circumstances, and this anxiety would be a motivational trait. Because this person will be calm many times, in spite of his or her predisposition to become anxious, the person with *high trait anxiety* nevertheless may be in a *low state anxiety* in especially calming circumstances. The study of motivation includes both tonic as well as phasic motivational processes, and trait as well as state motivations.

The study of motivation focuses on *dynamic* characteristics, and these differ from other kinds of psychological variables. For example, learning and memory are important topics in psychology, but they are different intervening variables and not motivation. Events and behavior that are learned may not always be readily remembered, but psychologists make the assumption that learning involves a relatively permanent process (Houston, 1991). Long-term memory is presumed to last for a long time in the life of an individual (Ellis & Hunt, 1989). A study of learning and memory is likely to emphasize conditions of practice or of information encoding and retrieval, and the person's or animal's motivation may not be considered. The following illustrates one way of differentiating learning from motivation. If a student fails an examination because she or he did not learn the material, this is different from failing because of a state of anxiety that occurs even though the student has learned the material. Anxiety can lead to worrisome thoughts that interfere with the ability to give correct answers. The first case reflects insufficient learning and the second case reflects an intense inappropriate motivation.

Because much of what one learns refers to facts or movements and does not deal directly with issues of motivation, the distinction between motivation and learning is useful. Learning that Brazil is in South America or to put in the clutch when shifting gears in certain types of cars illustrates the learning of facts or movements. However, some kinds of learning involve motivation, like learning to be anxious or to be achievement oriented. Many studies have shown that learning and memory influence motivation and, in turn, motivation influences learning and memory (Karniol & Ross, 1996).

SUMMARY

Motivation is a *dynamic* internal process that energizes and directs actions and action tendencies. Motivation pushes or pulls the individual. Environ-

mental antecedents and goals provide sources of motivation.

Motivation is a *construct,* not directly observable but tied theoretically and empirically to observable, external events. Motivation, like the constructs of learning, memory, and personality, is an *intervening variable,* which means an event or process that occurs within the individual.

In former years, *drive* and *instinct* were terms used to denote processes that today are assumed to be motivational. Other terms, like *will,* emphasized more cognitive components that today are also subsumed under the topic of motivation.

Motivation varies in amount (quantity, intensity), which is described by words like more and less, high and low. The *energizing* aspect of motivation deals with this intensity (quantitative) characteristic and refers to the fact that when one is highly motivated one is more alert and responsive and exerts more effort in actions. Tension is increased. Terms like *arousal, activation,* and *energy mobilization* all refer to this dimension of motivation.

Motivation also varies in type (quality in contrast to quantity). The *directional* aspect of motivation deals with this selective (qualitative) characteristic and refers to the fact that when one is motivated, a specific kind or type of motivation is usually involved. This leads to selective actions, strivings, or attention, like eating when hungry and drinking when thirsty, or running away from a stimulus when fearful.

Motivation varies according to circumstances, between individuals, and between species. Different circumstances lead to differences in motivation (in kind and amount) within an individual, and various individuals in identical circumstances will not have the same motivation (in kind as well as amount). Just as differences in motivation occur between individuals, so do differences occur between species. The motivation psychologist studies all these variations.

Motivation that is active at any given moment is called a *state.* This contrasts to a motivational *trait,* which is a tendency to be motivated in a selective way, even though one may not be actively motivated in that way at a given moment. Brief bursts of motivation are called *phasic* and are distinguished from a quite long-lasting *tonic* level of motivation.

CHAPTER 2

How Do We Study Motivation?

A number of issues arise when we consider doing a study of motivation. For example, how do we define it? How do we measure it? Should we study motivation in the real world, often called a field study, or should we study it in the laboratory? We have already considered that motivation differs from learning and memory, but we still need to consider a number of other variables that either do or do not bear on the study of motivation.

DEFINITIONS: HOW DO YOU DEFINE MOTIVATION?

Chapter 1 described a construct as being tied theoretically and empirically to observable, external events. In the present chapter we shall consider how to accomplish this.

Defining a Construct

Problems can arise when a construct is defined. Valuable help toward resolving some of these problems was provided by Underwood (1957).

Stimulus Definitions. One way to make an empirical connection is by means of a *stimulus definition.* By this is meant that a condition is created or a stimulus is presented that presumably induces a motivational state within an individual. Consider an experiment in which six persons went without eating for 12 hours and another six persons were asked to eat a big meal within the hour before they came to the experimental session. Then the two groups were compared on their performance on a word-

recognition task. The food deprivation (12 hours without eating) compared with food satiation (eating just before the experimental session) constituted the *stimulus definition* of hunger motivation. The experimenter created a condition prior to the testing that induced the hunger motivation in the subjects. One condition induced a low amount of motivation (the satiation condition) and the other induced a high amount (the deprivation condition).

The two conditions make up the *independent variable,* and the *intervening variable* is the hunger (high or low amount). The *dependent* variable is the performance measure, of how well or poorly the subjects performed on a word-recognition task. Such a study has been done (e.g., Erwin & Ferguson, 1979) and, as one might expect, the hungry subjects performed significantly better than did the satiated subjects.

Response Definitions. One can also define intervening variables solely on the basis of a *response definition.* One can study hunger by the kinds of responses an individual makes. The definition of the construct (hunger) would not be related to antecedent events, but instead would rely on the way subjects react in a particular way assumed to relate to hunger. Eating rate can be a good response measure to define the construct. For 40 persons who just got their food in the student cafeteria, one can observe how fast they are eating. The 6 who are observed to eat the fastest ("gobbled up" their food) and the 6 who are observed to eat the slowest ("dawdled" with their food) could be stopped and asked to be in the word-recognition experiment. In this way a high hunger level is defined by fast eating rate and a low hunger level is defined by a slow eating rate. Without knowing *why* they "gobbled" or "dawdled," and without knowing when they last ate, one still can select subjects solely on the basis of some relevant behavior.

Response definitions of motivation are used commonly in everyday life, even though people are not always aware of this. Examples include looking at the expression on a person's face and inferring that the person is in a state of anxiety, or seeing the neighbor's child intently building a complex construction with blocks and inferring that the child is high in achievement motivation. We explain others' motivation to ourselves without asking about the antecedent conditions. Just observing the way people walk, talk, make gestures or facial expressions, we infer and, without our being aware of it, define their internal states.

The previous illustration of the cafeteria shows that this may be a very impractical approach for certain types of studies. One is not likely to get people with high hunger levels to stop their eating and go to an experimental word-recognition session, so for practical reasons an eating measure is not recommended for a response definition of hunger. One can, however, go to a psychology class and ask for volunteers for an experiment and give the volunteers a set of questions, among which are items that ask about subjective ratings of hunger. Those persons who rate themselves as very hungry can be selected and compared with persons who rate themselves as satiated and not at all hungry. The two groups can then be tested in the word-recognition experiment. Hunger as a construct would have been *response defined* on the basis of hunger ratings. As with other response definitions, one does not know why these ratings were made. One would not know how long a time elapsed since the subjects ate a meal, but nevertheless one can select subjects merely by their responses.

Defining intervening variables by self-made ratings or other tests is a common method in psychology. Variables like personality and intelligence are *response defined* by scores on relevant tests, and in motivation research, questionnaires are very fre-

quently used. To study the construct of anxiety, for instance, the use of questionnaires based on self-ratings is common practice (e.g., Spielberger, Gorsuch, & Lushene, 1970) even though other types of response definitions are possible, such as the observation of clinical signs of anxiety.

Advantages and Disadvantages of Response Definitions. With response definitions one observes and measures but one cannot tell *why* the responses occurred. Considering the previous examples again, it could be that a number of the fast-eating individuals in the cafeteria had a time pressure of hurrying to go to the next class. Their eating rate would not reflect great hunger, in the sense of self-ratings or in terms of a long interval since their last meal. It would reflect time-pressure tension rather than hunger motivation. Likewise, the neighbor's child, intently building a complex construction with blocks, may have had a motivation akin to affiliation (seeking to please parents and other family members, or seeking to entice them to come over and play) rather than a motivation of achievement (seeking to attain success by one's own efforts).

Often one can gauge what the motivation is by observing a longer sequence of actions. After observing all the actions, later one can pinpoint more clearly what type of motivation had occurred. In the above examples, for instance, upon finishing eating, the people in the cafeteria might run off to a class or sit contentedly. Thus the observer could conclude more readily which motivation had been represented by the hasty eating. Waiting for the end of a sequence to understand the nature of a motivational state can prove to be a problem for a response definition, however. For example, the persons in the cafeteria would be far less hungry once they completed their meal. The response definition of fast eaters being the hungry subjects would be no longer suitable for assigning subjects to the experiment.

Although valuable, response definitions can lead to difficulties. Response definitions are used when, for ethical or practical reasons, a *stimulus definition* cannot be employed. Researchers cannot create high levels of fear or anxiety as motivating conditions in humans. In other cases, such as in achievement motivation, it is not practicable to develop motivational dispositions that require many years of specific parental and educational training. Thus, in spite of difficulties with their use, response definitions play a major role in motivation research.

Using Both Response and Stimulus Definitions Together. There are times when a response definition is preferable and other times when a stimulus definition is more useful. Because each type has limitations, Underwood (1957) described the advantages of a third type, the *stimulus-response* definition. It provides more rigor because it includes both the antecedent manipulations (stimulus events) and the relevant responses. This is illustrated in animal studies of hunger. Bolles (1967) found that defining hunger solely on the basis of length of time since last eating did not yield as reliable data as when hunger was defined both in terms of hours of food deprivation (stimulus definition) and the body's responses in terms of amount of body weight loss (response definition). Such a stimulus-response approach is useful.

The variable of food-deprivation time was found to relate to the variable of percentage of weight loss in a logarithmic and curvilinear way. Bolles (1965) found that one can estimate the percentage of weight loss on the basis of the hours of deprivation, and under normal circumstances, hours of food deprivation can be inferred from the amount of weight the animal lost. Clearly, a stimulus-response definition would permit the identification of animals that were sick and losing weight abnormally. A definition of hunger based on both a specified amount of weight loss and a specified length of time since last eating would permit the experimenter to eliminate animals whose weight loss was due to factors other than the specified deprivation. Equally, a stimulus-response definition would eliminate obese animals that did have the specified food deprivation but did not have the required weight loss.

Studies with humans also benefit by the use of a stimulus-response rather than only a stimulus or only a response definition of motivation. Suppose one studied incentive motivation and used a stimulus definition. The high-incentive motivation sub-

jects would be told they will receive $100 for very fast performance and the low-incentive motivation subjects would be told they will receive 10¢ for very fast performance. The *experimenter* has defined the conditions as high versus low incentive motivation, but if the subjects did not believe what they were told, the stimulus definition alone would be quite inadequate. In contrast, a *stimulus-response* definition can be used that includes two components, *inducing* the condition, and *selecting* only those subjects who gave self-ratings that showed they appropriately believed their condition. This stimulus-response definition is useful because instructions regarding the incentive combined with subjects' self-rating of beliefs would more appropriately define the motivation.

Even when the definition is clearly made, many problems may still arise, but at least a major source of difficulty can be avoided when the definition of motivation is well thought out and the procedures are clearly stated.

Operational Definitions

An *operational definition* means clearly defining a variable in terms of procedures or operations. As already discussed, motivation can be defined in terms of procedures used to induce the motivation (the stimulus definition), in terms of measured responses that presumably reflect the motivation (the response definition), or by using both types of procedures (the stimulus-response definition). All of these involve explicit procedures or operations. These procedures need to be *reliable,* which means that one can replicate or repeat the procedure (the methods are replicable). Thus, the self-reports subjects give cannot be at a whimsical or chance level, and if observers' ratings are used, the interobserver reliability needs to be high. Although operational definitions need to be *reliable,* another question is whether they are *valid.* Two response measures of anxiety may be reliable, for example, but only after many years of research may the investigator know which one is more valid, in that it better represents the anxiety construct.

Validity is defined with respect to some external

criterion. *Face validity* is a commonly used type of validity, which means that the construct is presumed to have certain characteristics and the stimulus events that induce it and the response measures that define it also have these characteristics. Rate of eating as a response measure of hunger has face validity, in that it is a common experience to eat fast when hungry and to "play with one's food" or slowly "pick at" the food when not hungry. Validity involves conceptual as well as operational factors. Theorists differ in the meanings given to various terms. For example, the term *anxiety* had specific meanings within Freudian theory (Freud, 1920/1938), which differed conceptually from the meaning of anxiety within achievement motivation theory (Atkinson, 1964). One needs to relate a given motivation term to the theoretical underpinnings of a particular study. Although *procedural* clarity is essential for operational definitions, this does not assure *conceptual* clarity.

THE RELATIONSHIP BETWEEN MOTIVATION AND OTHER VARIABLES

Many variables are closely related to motivation, and several later chapters will discuss these. Examples of such variables are constructs of emotion, incentives, intentions, goals, rewards, and cognitions. Controversy exists regarding how these constructs relate to motivation. Various theorists advocate different kinds of relationships. The viewpoint in the present book is that *motivation energizes and directs and leads to action.* When a goal or an incentive energizes and directs and leads to action, it functions as a source of motivation. However, not all goals or incentives do so. Likewise, cognitions can lead to strivings representing motivation, but not all cognitions do so. Considerable controversy exists regarding the relationship between emotion and motivation, and different theoretical perspectives will be considered in later chapters.

Motivation Leads to Action

How emotions and cognitions (attitudes, beliefs) energize, direct, and lead to action is still debated. One type of distinction was made by William

James, between cognitions that move a person to action versus those that don't necessarily do so. James (1890) distinguished the term *will* from *wish*, a wish being an idea or fantasy that need not translate into action. James contrasted "will" and "wish" by the fact that willing leads to action, whereas wishing refers to a preference or liking that remains passive. He pointed out that one may wish to get out of bed on a cold morning, all the while remaining under the warm covers, and this differs from the resolve that one will get up and get out of bed.

Emotion and the James-Lange Theory. Some writers consider emotion to lead to action (Franken, 1994; Malmo, 1975). However, for William James the construct of "emotion" was a conscious state that *followed* the awareness of visceral activity or muscular action. Whereas "will" consciously *led* to action, for James an emotion consciously *followed* internal or outward activity. For James and for Carl Lange, after whom the James-Lange theory of emotion is named, emotion is different from what one would identify as motivation. Textbooks that give examples of the James-Lange theory of emotion (e.g., Zimbardo & Weber, 1994, p. 318), cite words used by James (1890, p. 450): "We feel sorry because we cry, angry because we strike." This perspective is controversial today. In support of James' view that emotions *follow* actions, some contemporary researchers have shown that when facial muscles are moved in specific ways these movements lead to specific emotions (Ekman, 1984, 1992c, 1994). In contrast, others (e.g., Izard, 1994a, 1994b) propose that emotion is related to motivation and that both lead to action.

Goals and Intentions. Some writers consider emotion as preparation for action insofar as visceral and autonomic nervous system activity occurs, which energizes the individual. Not all theories of emotion relate emotion to an outcome or a goal, however. The language of emotion uses such statements as "I am angry" or "I am happy," and they lack a goal that follows as outcome of the emotion. The language of motivation, in contrast, tends to relate to outcomes. "I am motivated to do well in school" or "I seek to do excellent work in my job" are goal-oriented statements commonly used in the language of motivation. Although the expression "I am hungry" is less clearly linked to a goal, food seeking and food consumption are implied. Thus, "hunger" has the characteristics of motivation more than does a state of emotion like "happiness."

Animal researchers have referred to the "goal box" as the place toward which an animal learns to run in a maze (Kimble, 1961), and in that context "goal" is a concrete site. For humans a goal may be equally concrete, but it need not be. When the student is motivated to "do well in school" or the worker seeks to do "excellent work," the goal is symbolic or abstract. It may be translated into concrete outcomes, such as obtaining a "straight A" record in school, and it may involve a specific place such as a restaurant in a specific location, but typically human motivation involves more symbolic goals.

Intentions refer to goals. Words like "purpose," "intent," and "goal" are largely interchangeable. Motivation involves not only the internal state but also the goal or intent of that state. When James referred to being "angry because we strike, afraid because we tremble" (James, 1890, p. 450), the language of the emotion focused on an action that preceded the emotion, and no goal was identified. Contemporary conceptualizations of emotion also relate emotions to antecedent events (Bower, 1994; Frijda, 1994). Often the conceptualizations do not identify goals for the emotions.

Some theorists do emphasize the goal-directed nature of emotions, but these are exceptions. Writers who advance the theory of Alfred Adler (1927/1959), like Dreikurs, state that "it is the function of emotion to make us forceful in our intentions and goals" (Dreikurs, 1982, p. 214). Like Malmo (1975), Dreikurs' view is that emotion mobilizes us to action. Moreover, Adlerians consider all action purposive (directed toward goals), and emotion is defined according to the strivings set by the motivating property of goals. This goal-directed conceptualization of emotion is a theoretical perspective that differs from most contemporary views of emotion.

Although *emotions* are not defined as goal directed by most writers, *motivation* is generally considered to be directed toward goals. A goal-oriented motivational statement would be "I aim to hug you," in contrast to the emotional expression of "I love you." The specificity of goals provides action outcomes and directionality to motivation.

How Do Rewards and Incentives Become Motivation?

A goal is "in the here and now" as a cognitive representation of a future event. It is an anticipation that *precedes an action*. This contrasts with a *reward* that occurs *after an action*. The student who is motivated to attain a grade of "A" may take appropriate action (studying) and then receive the anticipated "A." The grade that follows the action is called a reward. If for some reason the student were to pursue the incorrect action, like studying the wrong material or studying while being inebriated, the anticipated goal and the actual outcome are likely to be different. Instead of the anticipated "A," the actual grade might be "C." Rewards are usually described as reflecting a positive quality, of something one wants or seeks, but negative outcomes also exist, of events one strives to avoid. The word "incentive" refers to rewards that function in a motivating way, and the terms *positive incentive* and *negative incentive* describe outcomes an individual seeks to attain or to avoid.

An incentive, like a goal, is something one anticipates. Earlier the variable of incentive was discussed in an experiment in which some subjects were offered $100 and others were offered 10¢ for very fast performance. Money is widely used as an incentive, but many other examples exist. If one goes to a concert and hears an inspiring pianist, one may have an incentive to put more effort into one's own practicing. When the *incentive pulls* one in a certain direction and one takes energetic and effortful action directed toward that incentive, then one has *incentive motivation*.

The term incentive describes a sought-for outcome that is usually some type of concrete event that has been externally provided. Incentives can be considered as inviting or goading the individual toward an outcome. The *conditional promise of a reward* is an incentive. It is conditional, because only when certain actions are performed will the promised reward be obtained.

Persons in one's environment can provide incentives by their *modeling* behavior. If 10 year-old Jay plays in backyard baseball games and keeps missing the ball, and then goes to a major league game and sees his idol make a lot of difficult catches and hit several home runs, for the next month Jay may seek to imitate his hero who provided a "model" for him. The model gave Jay an incentive: "If I practice hard, I'll play like" the hero. When an external event, such as the promise of a reward, mobilizes action toward an anticipated reward, an external event can provide incentive motivation.

Events external to the individual, such as reward, and processes internal to the individual, like incentive motivation, are different but often closely related. Because processes that are intervening variables inside the individual, like goal and incentive motivation, are often related to those that are external to the individual, such as reward and incentive, the motivation literature has explored the relationships. Not all promises of rewards become a motivation. Some rewards serve to support behavior instigated by other motivations, yet the rewards themselves never take on motivating properties. "When I am hungry enough I'll eat spinach" would illustrate that spinach is a reward only when one is hungry.

In some cases an experimenter or a parent may believe a reward that is being offered lures the person into specific behaviors, but it turns out the offered event is not appealing to the person being lured. If an instructor tells the students that when they outline each chapter and write a chapter summary for all the assigned readings the lowest grade the student will receive is a "C," that promise may not be sufficient to motivate all the students in the class. Some students may not want to do that kind of work, and the incentive provided by the instructor fails to be motivating. Without attending to the distinction between external events and internal processes, the instructor would assume that because the incentive was provided, all the students would become motivated automatically. For some students, a "C" grade might not be sufficient incentive and they would not be motivated by that promise. All of us can think of occasions when we have been offered incentives that either had no effect or

did not have the desired effect. External events can provide motivation, but the relationship between the external and intervening (internal) variables is sometimes quite complex.

SUMMARY

Motivation can be studied in the laboratory or in the real world. In the latter case the investigation is called a *field study*.

Several ways can be used to define the construct of motivation. One involves a *stimulus definition*, which means defining the motivation in terms of conditions that induce the motivational state within the individual. An example of such a definition for hunger might involve assigning some subjects to be deprived of food for 12 hours and comparing them with those who were assigned to eat a big meal just prior to the study. The conditions define the motivation, regardless of how hungry the subjects purport to feel. A *response definition* of motivation, in contrast, relies on the way subjects react, in terms that have a bearing on the construct. Thus, a response definition of hunger might involve selecting subjects on the basis of self-ratings, and those who indicate a large amount of hunger are compared with those who gave a self-rating of a very low amount of hunger.

Motivation is an *intervening variable*. In the above examples, hunger is an intervening variable. The *independent variable* consists of the conditions used to define the variable (for example, amount of food deprivation). The *dependent variable* is some measure of performance for which one predicts the independent variable to have an effect. For example, in a study on the effect of hunger on word recognition, hunger is the intervening variable, amount of deprivation is the independent variable, and performance on a word recognition task is the dependent variable.

A *stimulus-response definition* includes aspects of both a stimulus definition and a response definition. If one used incentive motivation as the intervening variable, this kind of definition would consist of a set of stimulus conditions (like offering a lot of money for good performance to one group of subjects and a small amount of money to another group) and some kind of relevant responses (like self-ratings to indicate how much the individuals in each group believed in the promise of the money), and only those individuals within each group who believed the promises would be selected to serve as subjects in the study.

Operational definitions, like the definitions illustrated above, are used to define the intervening variable. Operational definitions need to be reliable, but they may or may not be valid. *Reliability* refers to replicability: to be able to repeat the conditions or operations. *Validity* refers to an outside criterion, usually at a conceptual or theoretical level.

Motivation differs from *emotion.* Motivation is considered action oriented and goal directed. Emotion is not considered the same way by many theorists, although some do not distinguish between emotion and motivation. By and large, the goal direction and action orientation of motivation is thought by most psychologists to be the major difference between motivation and emotion, although Adlerian psychologists consider both emotion and motivation to be goal directed and action oriented.

The *James-Lange* hypothesis, advanced independently by William James and Carl Lange, emphasizes that visceral or muscular activity leads to awareness of emotion. As James put it, we are "afraid because we tremble." This view has some support by contemporary psychologists.

Goals are internal representations that are functional at a given moment, regardless if the *anticipation* of the outcome actually occurs. *Rewards* are events that actually occur as outcomes following some action. *Incentives* are conditional promises, like money promised to be given for speedy performance. Inspiring events, other than money, can also serve as incentives. *Modeling,* when an ideal person one seeks to imitate performs in certain ways, can provide an individual with incentives. When incentives pull a person into goal-directed action, this is called *incentive motivation.*

CHAPTER 3

Arousal: The Energizing and Intensity Aspect of Motivation

Energy is necessary for all aspects of living, and the construct of "arousal" concerns the energizing characteristic of motivation. Energy mobilization and energy expenditure are important concerns for many psychologists. It has long been known that how much energy one expends in a given task or within a given hour varies, and motivation psychologists study such variation. Their research has focused on the following kinds of questions: What circumstances lead to high arousal, when in the day is arousal likely to be high and when low, what is the relationship between arousal and physiological processes, and how do different levels of arousal affect performance? A special question asks: Is performance best under high or under low arousal?

Both the energizing and directional aspects of motivation are complex. What is known today is the result of many years of study. In some periods, researchers tended to focus on the directional aspects, and in other periods they tended to focus on the energizing aspects. When behaviorism was dominant, Duffy (1932, 1934, 1951), Malmo (1957), and Hull (1951) considered motivation primarily in terms of the energizing function, and when psychology became increasingly concerned with cognitive processes, the emphasis was more on directional aspects (e.g., Bower, Gilligan, & Monteiro, 1981). Whereas direction concerns the selective way in which energy is experienced and expended, arousal concerns the quantity or intensity of that energy. The energizing aspect of motivation has been called many

names, but the term *arousal* is the one most commonly used.

Arousal has been studied in terms of sleep compared with wakefulness, and different stages of sleep show different levels of arousal (Horne, 1988). When awake individuals are drowsy or bored, their state of excitation is low (low arousal). If someone should tap us on the shoulder and say, "You have just won $10,000 in the lottery!," we would be in a state of high excitation (high arousal). We may or may not be aware of our excitation. The manner in which excitation is manifested will vary between different situations and between individuals.

THE CONSTRUCT OF AROUSAL

Arousal has been studies in terms of the *situations* that give rise to high excitation, in terms of different types of *response measures,* and in terms of *individual differences.*

Defining and Measuring Arousal

Heightened alertness, responsiveness, and an overall raised level of physiological excitation occur with high arousal. In *behavioral* terms the concept of arousal refers to greater response amplitude, vigor, and total response output. Under conditions of high arousal the individual's responses are stronger, more frequent, and more vigorous. Some researchers, like Malmo (1957), have shown that arousal leads to a greater variety of responses; yet others, like Easterbrook (1959), showed that under heightened arousal individuals may respond to a narrower range of stimuli.

In *physiological* terms the concept of arousal refers to increased physiological activity that is associated with the sympathetic nervous system. Figure 3.1 presents a schematic representation of the autonomic nervous system. From this, one can identify which organs are likely to be most responsive, and what kinds of reactions might occur under increased arousal. For example, the heart is innervated by many sympathetic nervous system pathways, and changes in heart activity, which can be measured by electrocardiogram (EKG) recordings, are often used as physiological measures of arousal. Arousal induced by various methods, such as food deprivation or presentation of fear-arousing events, has been found in many studies to increase heart rate (e.g., Watson, Gaind, & Marks, 1972); others have shown this is not always the case (Lacey, 1967; Obrist, Webb, Sutterer, & Howard, 1970). Changes in levels of arousal have also been found to lead to blood pressure changes (Anderson & Brady, 1971; Averill, 1969; Engel, 1959; Krantz & Falconer, 1995).

Effortful coping leads to cardiovascular changes, influenced by the sympathetic as well as the parasympathetic system (Light & Obrist, 1983; Obrist, 1981). Cardiovascular changes under arousal can occur due to increased activity of the sympathetic nervous system or due to decreased parasympathetic activity (Krantz & Falconer, 1995). Some evidence has shown that systolic blood pressure more than diastolic blood pressure reflects effortful coping with difficult tasks, and that systolic blood pressure may be a more sensitive measure of effortful coping than is heart rate (Wright & Gregorich, 1989; Wright, Shaw, & Jones, 1990). Depending on the task and the nature of the arousal, various kinds of physiological changes involve activity of the autonomic nervous system, which is part of the *peripheral nervous system* (PNS).

Important changes occur also in the *central nervous system* (CNS), notably in specific areas of the brain (Steriade, 1996; Steriade, McCormick, & Sejnowski, 1993).

The Reticular Activating System

Early evidence showed that when an individual experiences any of a wide array of emotions or motivating conditions, an energizing state of arousal occurs. Moruzzi and Magoun (1949), and Lindsley (1951), on the basis of their research, described how a generalized arousing state occurs in an organism. These researchers focused on the reticular activating system (RAS), whose ascending and descending pathways send signals between the reticular formation, thalamus, and cortex. Figure 3.2 presents the brain areas involved.

External stimuli were said to energize the organism by means of two routes. One was a direct pathway, which sends sensory signals to specific areas of the cortex, and the other was an indirect pathway, which nonspecifically sends sensory signals to the reticular formation and then to the thalamus and cortex. For example, in the direct route, visual stimuli reach the visual projection area of the cortex and auditory stimuli reach the auditory projection area, so that specific sense impulses are registered as being either visual or auditory. However, in the nonspecific route, the sensory signals were said to activate the cortex diffusely and, thus, via the ascending RAS to alert and energize the organism. The work of Lindsley (1951) and Moruzzi and Magoun (1949) was supported by many studies. For example, electrical stimulation of the reticular formation produced cortical desynchronization patterns (measured by the electroencephalogram, or EEG) that are typical under normal (nonexperimental) states of excitation. Compared with the work of the early researchers, more complex pathways involving the reticular formation and cortex have been identified in recent years (Carlson, 1998).

Contemporary work on brain activity under arousal uses EEG recordings as well as intracellular recording from neurons. Reticular, thalamic, and cortical intracellular recordings (Steriade, McCormick, & Sejnowski, 1993) have shown that different oscillations (rhythms) occur during sleep, waking, and states of excitation (heightened arousal). Neurotransmitters released by ascending activating systems involve the brainstem and other areas of the brain, and these neurotransmitters have

FIGURE 3.1
Schematic representation of the autonomic nervous system.

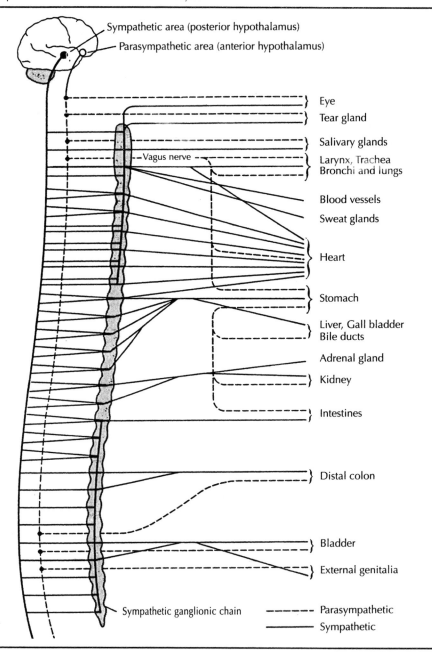

Source: From Ferguson (1982).

FIGURE 3.2
Schematic diagram of structures involved in the reticular activating system (RAS) and arousal.

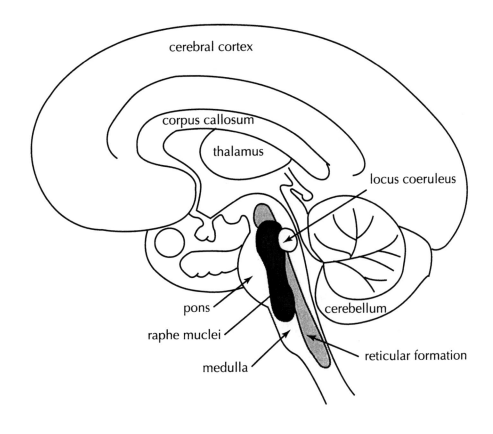

Source: Courtesy of B.E.F. Wee.

a wide influence on forebrain functions. Low-frequency oscillations are replaced by high-frequency rhythms under heightened arousal, and specific neurochemical changes (involving norepinephrine, serotonin, and acetylcholine) have been identified that mediate this process. The ascending modulatory neurotransmitter systems apparently tune the excitability of the brain, thereby aiding the individual in sensory and cognitive processes and in various types of performance.

Different systems of neurons involving various neurotransmitters have been identified as important in arousal. For example, norepinephrine-containing neurons are likely to fire according to the direction of attention to external stimuli. Neurons of the locus coeruleus send widely branching axons that release norepinephrine. Researchers (Aston-Jones, Rajkowski, Kubiak, & Alexinsky, 1994), who in monkeys recorded the electrical activity of norepinephrine neurons of the locus coeruleus, found that activity of these neurons and their neurotransmitter release was related to the monkeys' vigilance and to improved performance on a discrimination task. Serotonergic neurons found in the raphe nuclei also tend to vary their firing rate according to the individual's state of arousal. Other brain regions contain acetylcholinergic neurons, and when these have been stimulated, they have produced cortical desynchronization (Steriade, 1996) and arousal of behavior. When humans have engaged in tasks requiring alertness, measures of increased regional blood flow revealed that neuronal activity occurs in the midbrain reticular formation and specific thalamic nuclei (Steriade, 1996). In animals, stimulation of the midbrain reticular formation has increased the activation of various responses. When humans show behavioral arousal, neuronal activity is found that supports the hypothesized RAS arousal brain systems, and when the hypothesized RAS brain areas are electrically stimulated in experimental animals, these subjects show the predicted behavioral arousal. In these ways, contemporary research supports and extends the findings reported by Moruzzi and Magoun (1949) and Lindsley (1951).

Physiological Measurements

When persons or nonhuman animals are in circumstances that increase arousal, sympathetic nervous system activity increases and various neuroendocrine changes occur. One change involves the release of epinephrine and norepinephrine from the adrenal medulla. When arousal occurs due to threat and stress of the individual, corticosteroids are also produced and secreted by the adrenal cortex, as part of the arousal of the hypothalamic-pituitary-adrenocortical (HPA) system (Baum & Grunberg, 1995). The pituitary gland, stimulated via action of the hypothalamus, produces adrenocorticotropic hormone (ACTH) and this stimulates corticosteroid release from the adrenal cortex. Glucocorticoids are also released, and they provide energy (pulled from stored reserves) for action. Thus, measures of arousal and sympathetic nervous system activation may involve blood or urine samples for measuring neuroendocrine changes.

Other types of measures, which do not involve neuroendocrine measurements, are often used to measure arousal. One measure is the galvanic skin response (GSR), also known as psychogalvanic response (PGR). It records changes in skin resistance. The GSR in many studies was found to change as a function of arousing circumstances (Ferguson, 1982). The lie detector commonly used in law enforcement makes use of the GSR and other peripheral measures for diagnosing emotional activity, but controversy exists regarding such use (Kleinmuntz & Scucko, 1984; Lykken, 1980, 1984). Various measures can be used for changes in skin responses, such as a measure of conductance (umhos) that is the inverse of resistance (e.g., Levenson, Ekman, & Friesen, 1990, p. 369). Other physiological measures of arousal are EMG (electromyographic) recordings of muscle action, EKG (electrocardiogram) recordings already mentioned for identifying cardiovascular activity, and a wide array of less frequently used measures (for instance, measures of respiration rate, blood volume, and digestive motility). Heart rate can also be measured in beats per minutes (BPM). The EMG can be used to measure tension in all sorts of muscle groups, but typically the arm and forehead muscles have been investigated (see chapter 4 in Ferguson, 1982, for a fuller description of the various measures). The procedures for such measures are nonintrusive. With EMG, EKG, EEG, and PGR, surface electrodes are placed on the skin and the subject typically feels no discomfort during the experiment.

When high arousal was induced (by various procedures and for diverse conditions, such as pain, anxiety, hunger, light flashing, loud sounds, and so forth), increased physiological reactivity was found. In addition to the covariation of the different physiological measures, behavioral changes also positively correlated with the physiological changes. Summaries of early findings (Baumeister, Hawkins, & Cromwell, 1964; Ferguson, 1982; Malmo, 1975) showed that when arousal was due to external circumstances (e.g., Eason & Dudley, 1970) or was induced by direct stimulation of the reticular formation (Fuster, 1958), faster or improved performance of simple responses occurred. Malmo (1957, 1966) showed parallel results for real-life stresses, such as experienced by psychiatric patients. Additionally, when individuals are aroused, under some conditions they tend to be more vigilant in taking note of signals in their environment (Buckner & McGrath, 1963).

AROUSAL HAS MANY ASPECTS

Contemporary research has shown that in addition to generalized arousal, which varies between sleep and awake excitation, there are other aspects of arousal. For example, Beatrice and John Lacey (Lacey, Kagan, Lacey, & Moss, 1963) found that when subjects in an experiment take in information from the environment, their physiological reactions are different from when the subjects respond to and act on the environment. The Laceys found evidence that cardiac responses are controlled by cortical activity and, in turn, the heart rate signals the cortex and alters cortical activity. Thus, in arousing situations, cardiac acceleration is likely to occur if the individual seeks to decrease external stimulation, but cardiac deceleration is likely to occur if the individual seeks to increase information intake.

Situational Specificity and Response Stereotypy

Tasks and situations vary in what is demanded from an individual, and physiological arousal reactions thus also will differ. Situations may require quiet attention or robust responding, and physiological reactions will relate differently to one another and to overt behavior, according to such situational demands. Lacey (1967) described such physiological dissociations by the term *directional fractionation*. Recent studies have shown that certain brain systems and neurotransmitters are involved in attentional processing, and others are involved in behavioral activation (Robbins, 1997). Moreover, the kinds of overt responses that are required will lead to different brain and neurotransmitter activity (Carlson, 1998).

Variation in physiological and overt responses as a function of arousal has been noted in many studies. A study with infant girls (Turkewitz, Moreau, Birch, and Davis, 1971) illustrates such variation. When the neonates were 36 to 66 hours old, they were presented with varying loudness levels of white noise. The auditory stimuli were presented at the position of the ear at intensities from medium loud to an uncomfortably loud level (70, 78, 82, 90,

94, and 98 decibels). The measurements were heart rate, lateral conjugate eye movement, and finger movement. All the measures showed a significant linear increase with stimulus intensity, which would be expected as a result of increased arousal. However, the infants showed different thresholds for the different response measures. Cardiac acceleration in infants as a function of arousal was also reported in a large review of heart-rate changes by Graham and Clifton (1966). Arousal can be measured by cardiovascular and other responses, but unique patterns of reactivity are also evident. The term *response stereotypy* (Lacey & Lacey, 1958) describes the fact that over a wide range of stimulating or arousing situations each individual has stable patterns of physiological and behavioral responding that are unique to the individual. In terms of physiological indicators, one person will respond primarily with cardiovascular reactions, another person with muscular reactions, another primarily with dermatological reactions, and so on. At a behavioral level, one person will respond to arousing events with withdrawal, another with attack, another with feigned nonchalance. Unique reactivity is low under minimally exciting situations and is heightened when circumstances change to induce an increase in arousal. Thus, one person may have an increase primarily in muscular activity and another in cardiovascular activity when both see another car swerving into their lane, but whichever is the main mode of response, both persons will reveal increased reactivity as a function of the apparent danger.

A study by McNulty and Noseworthy (1966) is illustrative. The researchers identified each individual's single most active physiological function in order to assess the effect of shock threat on task performance. All subjects were measured for heart rate, blood pressure, muscle tension, and GSR. Half of the 50 male college students were told merely to do their best on a task of verbal learning and two tasks of perceptual-motor coordination, and half were told they would receive a shock if performance dropped below a set norm. The results showed that performance was not altered on the verbal learning task as a function of the shock instructions, but pursuit-rotor tracking was. Significantly better performance, in terms of mean time on target, was obtained under the shock than no-shock instructions. Moreover, when the individual subject's dominant physiological measure was considered, the highest tracking performance in the shock-threat condition was shown by the subjects who had dominant cardiovascular responsiveness (heart rate or blood pressure being the most reactive). Response stereotypy was evident, since McNulty and Noseworthy (1966) found that when the subject's dominant physiological measure was used, the rank order of individuals, in terms of physiological reactivity, remained highly consistent across the three performance tasks.

Self-report measures can yield reliable and valid data regarding internal states of arousal. However, occasionally the physiological and self-report data may be at variance with each other. For example, Lazarus and Opton (1966) presented tension-inducing films and had subjects rate their arousal. Measures were also taken of the subjects' physiological reactivity while viewing the films. Across the film viewings the subjects' rank order in autonomic reactivity was highly consistent, but their rank order was not consistent for measures of self-reported arousal and description of mood. This was true for all subjects, regardless of whether they were high or low on a personality characteristic called "defensive denial."

State Versus Trait: Arousal Compared With Arousability

Many methods of studying arousal in humans are possible. Some approaches involve self-rating scales. These may measure momentary arousal, or arousal *states,* or they may measure arousal in terms of a *trait.* This refers to the likelihood that a person is easily aroused.

One measure, developed by Coren (1988), is called the Arousal Predisposition Scale (APS). It consists of 12 items that subjects check as true for them in terms of five alternatives: never, seldom, occasionally, frequently, or always. The items contain words like mood, excitation, and emotion. An example is: "My mood is quickly influenced by entering new places." Coren considered that this scale taps cognitive arousal, in contrast to somatic

arousal. The APS was developed to measure individual differences in arousability, so that one could predict the degree to which an individual would be aroused in a stressful situation.

A significant finding in the original study was that subjects who scored high on the scale also had more night awakenings, indicative of sleep disturbance (Coren, 1988). In another study (Coren & Aks, 1991), 2 weeks before the day of the experiment subjects were pretested with the APS scale under neutral conditions. On the day of the actual study, the experimental group was given a search task to perform under conditions of visual and auditory distractions. The control group did not receive the distraction task and for 11 minutes just relaxed in an unstructured manner. At the start and end of the session both groups received a different arousal scale, described below, that was used to provide the dependent variable. The researchers found that the experimental group indeed showed an increase in their arousal scores, but more importantly, the subjects scoring high on the APS scale in the neutral pretesting showed a significantly greater increase in arousal than did those subjects who scored low on the APS in the neutral pretesting. In contrast, in the control group neither the high- nor the low-APS-scoring subjects increased their scores in arousal. Thus, the individual differences found under neutral pretesting conditions predicted who would be likely to be most aroused under subsequent arousal-inducing circumstances.

In an earlier chapter we considered the role of trait versus state definitions of motivation. The study by Coren and Aks (1991) serves to illustrate this point. The APS scale that Coren developed was designed to be a *trait* measure, which would predict who among a large group of subjects would become aroused in terms of a *state.* The measure of arousal as a state that Coren and Aks used was that developed by Thayer (1978). A state scale reveals different aspects of arousal than does a trait scale. For example, two individuals may differ significantly in their *trait,* their disposition to become aroused, but their *state* of arousal would not differ when both of them are in a calm situation. This was evident in the Coren and Aks (1991) study for the control group. Moreover, two individuals may be alike in their trait, their disposition to become aroused, but because one faces a stressful situation and the other a calm situation (let us say, in their work place), their state scores of arousal would be very different. This also was evident in the Coren and Aks data, since high-APS-scoring subjects under the experimental condition had much higher state-arousal scores than did those in the control condition. Thus, trait and state scales of arousal can be complementary, each serving a different function.

One problem with trait self-report scales is whether the obtained individual differences reflect the presumed intervening variable or whether they reflect some other characteristic, such as, say, subjects' willingness to reveal personal characteristics. For example, Coren (1990) provided normative data of 786 subjects and found significantly higher mean APS scores for women than men. One needs to ask, then, whether women are more easily aroused than men; whether they are just more willing to say they are aroused, as a difference in their verbal response bias; or whether some combination of these two factors is involved. Gender differences on a trait scale may mean that men and women differ in their response bias (as related to wanting to please the investigator, being more willing to reveal personal characteristics, being less cautious and defensive, etc.) rather than that they differ on the trait that is presumably being measured.

Tense Compared With Energetic Arousal

In a book called *The Biopsychology of Mood and Arousal,* Thayer (1989) reviewed many studies of arousal. Like Coren, Thayer assumed arousal to involve two factors. Unlike Coren's distinction between cognitive and somatic arousal, Thayer (1978, 1985) distinguished between "energetic arousal" and "tense arousal." He developed a scale to measure both types. People vary in states of arousal over time, and Thayer's work was devoted to identifying the situations in which individuals become more, and less, aroused. In his work, Thayer (1989) examined what the characteristics are of arousal, what situations heighten or lower arousal, and what physiological measures correlate with the behavioral measures.

Individuals are energized or excited by a wide range of events, some pleasurable and some aversive. A person would be in a marked state of excitement if told that a dear friend had just been killed in an accident. Also, one would be very excited if told one had just won a large fortune in the lottery. These two states of excitation are qualitatively very different. In the first case one would be "downbeat" and upset and in pain; in the other, one would be "uplifted" and jubilant. These qualitative differences Thayer (1996) described by the terms *tense* and *energetic* arousal.

Energetic arousal is related to upbeat feelings (positive mood and emotional state) while tense arousal is related to anxiety. Tense arousal occurs under threat or pain or anxiety. Thayer found that at moderate levels the two types of arousal were positively correlated, but at high levels they tended to be negatively correlated. That is, under high tension a person is not likely to feel energetic, but at medium levels of tension the feeling of being energetic is likely to be medium or high. Each type of arousal represents a dimension, calm energy versus calm tiredness, and tense energy versus tense tiredness.

The Activation-Deactivation Adjective Check List, or AD ACL, is used to measure these dimensions. A long and a short form have been developed, and both contain self-descriptive items that describe the feeling state of the individual at a given moment. The short form takes less than 40 seconds to complete and yields scores on four subscales: General Activation (energy), General Deactivation (calmness), High Activation (tension) and Deactivation Sleep (tiredness). The short form has five adjectives per subscale, each adjective being rated on a 4-point continuum. If the focus of one's investigation is high arousal, the Energy and Tension subscale scores alone can be used; if the focus is on low arousal, the Calmness and Tiredness scales alone can be used. The 4-point continuum requires subjects to indicate if the adjective describes the way they feel at the moment: vv (definitely feel that way), v (slightly feel that way), ? (cannot decide), and no (definitely do not feel that way). Examples of energetic arousal are "vigorous, lively," and of tense arousal are "jittery, tense." Thus, in a simple way the AD ACL taps two types of arousal states, and the data show the test to be both reliable and valid.

In his early work, Thayer (Thayer & Cox, 1968) tested subjects' arousal in the context of a single arousal dimension, as was the dominant view of that time. Gradually it became apparent that the data could be described best by a dual-arousal conceptualization. After developing such a conceptualization, Thayer (1989) reviewed a number of dual-arousal processes, including a metabolic one in which anaerobic (without oxygen) is contrasted with aerobic metabolism. The former can be used to produce a large amount of energy quickly, such as in emergency situations, but the latter is more efficient in using a wider supply of body stores of energy (carbohydrate, fats, proteins) and, as practitioners of aerobic exercises will testify, can lead to the subjective feeling of "health and energy."

Thayer considered a question that is important for a motivation psychologist. Can individuals increase energy without also increasing tension? Thayer (1987) explored this question by having subjects either eat a candy bar or walk briskly for 10 minutes. The experiment used a within-subject design. A fixed 2-hour period was chosen by each subject. Eighteen volunteers made self-ratings each day for 12 days in the context of their normal daily activities. For at least 1 hour before the 2-hour sessions the subjects did not engage in exercise and did not eat anything. At the start of each experimental period, subjects completed the AD ACL test and then either ate about 1.5 ounces of a candy bar of their choice or walked rapidly for 10 minutes, breathing deeply and swinging their arms freely. Thirty minutes after the start of the experimental session the subjects completed a second AD ACL form, and 1 hour later a third, with the fourth test at the end of the 2-hour period. Each subject had a snack for six experimental sessions and took a brisk walk for six sessions. The results showed that 30, 60, and 120 minutes following the onset of the session, subjects had a significantly greater increase in self-reported energy after the walking than after the snacking. A significantly greater decrease in tiredness and tension occurred after the walking than after the snacking. Of interest is the fact that, compared with pretest levels, the reported tension decreased after the walking but after the snacking it

increased! These changes from pretest levels were significant, and they were clearly opposite for the walking compared with the snacking condition. These results have important implications for a theory of arousal and they provide a practical application for the routine of one's day. In terms of a theory of arousal, it is clear that energetic arousal has different characteristics than does tense arousal, since taking a walk compared with eating a candy bar increased energetic arousal and decreased tense arousal. A single arousal dimension is thus not conceptually tenable. At a practical level, all of us can benefit from these results, by noting that when we have a choice of a sugar snack or a brisk walk, we would help ourselves feel more energetic and less tense if we took a brisk walk. Figure 3.3 shows the changes Thayer (1987) found in tense arousal as a result of snacking and walking.

When persons are depressed, they often appear to be lethargic or slow, manifesting slow movement, slow speaking, soft voice, and general diminished outward energy. Viewed from a single energy or arousal point of view, the depressed person appears to display very little energy. However, negative thoughts of many kinds are also characteristic of depression, and this may be accompanied by considerable anxiety and a great deal of mental activity. Thus, although depression appears on the surface to represent a low state of arousal, the experience subjectively is very different. It certainly differs in subjective feeling from the state of drowsiness one feels upon awakening or the calm tiredness one feels after many hours of skiing or bicycle riding.

Thayer's research addressed this issue. In one study women volunteers rated both their feelings of depression and their energy and tension over many occasions. Patterns of tiredness, low energy, and also tension, were found when the subjects were most depressed. Feeling both tense and tired, with high tense arousal but low energetic arousal, was characteristic also of subjects in a later study (cited in Thayer, 1989, pp. 151—152). Any one who has ever felt "low" because of frustration, self-blame, or other negative conditions can envision that outward energy expenditure may be low but internal tension can be very high. The work of Averill (1969) supports this observation, for when subjects saw a sad

FIGURE 3.3
Tense arousal as a function of snacking and walking.

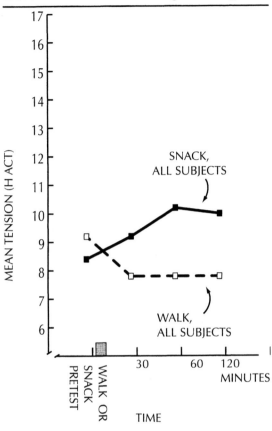

Source: From Thayer, 1987, Fig. 1.

film, they revealed cardiovascular changes characteristic of sympathetic activation. Sadness and depression may be good examples of how outward energy expenditure can be low, with self-judgments of energy also low, yet concomitantly inner tension, manifested physiologically, is high.

AROUSAL—PERFORMANCE RELATIONSHIPS

Subsequent chapters will describe how various motivations and emotions affect specific behaviors, but some general principles are considered in this chapter. These general principles concern hypotheses and findings that show how the energizing (arousal) aspect of motivation alters performance.

Motor Activity and Arousal

The discussion so far has been concerned largely with physiological reactivity and verbal self-report measures, but an important question concerns the way arousal affects various kinds of overt activities. It is useful to know not only whether *covertly* we react differently under high than low arousal, but *overtly,* in observable ways, are we more mobile, do we move faster, are we more persistent? Research before the 1980s showed that when animals and humans are aroused (or excited) they move faster, have faster latency in their responses, and traverse further, especially when the dependent measure is gross motor activity (see chapter 5 in Ferguson, 1982). Rats, chickens, humans, and a host of other species have been observed to increase speed, persistence, and effort when arousal is high, even though phenomena such as "freezing," or immobility, have also been observed. The latter typically occurs only in highly aversive situations that involve fear and "defensive reactions" (Bolles, 1970). Immobility is an exception to the more typical behavior, of heightened arousal producing increased movement and response output.

An activity wheel has been used to measure gross motor activity in rodents. The animal runs on the wheel, and with each wheel rotation a counter registers the movement. (See Figure 3.4 for an example of such a wheel.) Laboratory animals as well as pet rats, mice, and gerbils characteristically run and turn the wheel for an extended period of time if given access to an activity wheel. Running activity in such a wheel as well as in a simple runway has been found to increase significantly under various conditions of arousal. A broad review of the literature by Baumeister, Hawkins, and Cromwell (1964) showed that deprivation or need in general leads to increased activity in a variety of apparatus and test situations. However, many studies have found that wheel running is the most clearly affected by food deprivation, with other activity measures *not* showing a consistent effect (Ferguson 1982).

It is important to assess whether hunger as an arousing state leads to increased running, or whether the running increases because animals find reinforcement after running. That is, does arousal activate the behavior, or do animals learn to run because the acts of running get reinforced?

FIGURE 3.4
An activity wheel. As the drum turns, a counter records the revolutions. The resting cage is mounted to the side of the drum.

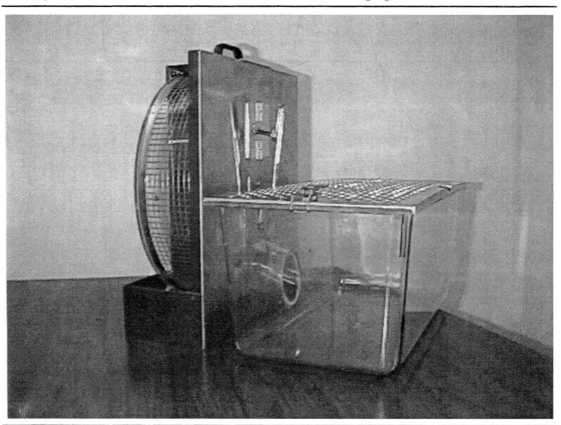

Source: Courtesy Lafayette Instrument Co.

Species differ, and this occurs in part as a function of the habitat in which the species evolved (Glickman & Schiff, 1967). If one thinks of an animal in the wild, the one that is actively pursuing food is more likely to find it than the animal that is quiescent. Thus, increased activity is likely to be reinforced by food for the hungry animal. In the laboratory, also, a legitimate question is whether increased activity occurs as a by-product of arousal or as a consequence of repeated reinforcements after the running responses.

Finger, Reid, and Weasner (1960) investigated the relative impact of both hunger-induced arousal and reinforcement on the amount of running rats did in an activity wheel. In the first part of the study,

rats that were minimally deprived (less than 3 hours of food deprivation) were tested in the activity wheel for 1 hour for 30 days. Half the animals (the experimental group) received food immediately on being returned to their home cage, and the other half (the control group) were retained in another cage for 1 hour before being returned to the home cage that contained food. After this initial phase, the experimental group given the immediate food as reinforcement showed significantly more wheel running than the control subjects that received food only after a 1-hour delay. Although this indicated the significant effect of reinforcement, it did not answer the question of whether hunger also, independently of reinforcement, would increase the running behavior. In the second phase of the study, all subjects were tested after 27, 51, and 75 hours of food deprivation and all subjects were tested under the control subjects' "delay" condition, of not receiving food immediately after removal from the activity wheel. If hunger-inducing arousal had a significant effect on running, then regardless if the animals' running had been previously reinforced (i.e., the experimental group) or not reinforced (i.e., the control group), the more the animals were deprived the more running they should do in the testing condition. That was what the investigators found for mean number of revolutions for both the experimental and the control subjects.

The control group, following 27, 51, and 75 hours of food deprivation, showed a significant increase in running as a function of increased arousal (food deprivation), although the animals had not previously received immediate reinforcement after the activity wheel running. The experimental subjects, likewise, showed increased running as a function of arousal, and they also showed more running than did the control subjects. The data clearly showed that each variable, hunger-inducing arousal and prior training with immediate food reinforcement, increased the animals' activity during the test condition. The Finger, Reid, and Weasner (1960) data can be taken generally to represent the arousal-activity relationship. Regardless of whether the various types of arousal-inducing conditions lead to identical amounts or slightly different amounts of activity, it is generally true that many types of arousing conditions lead to increased activity.

The individual who is more (rather than less) hungry, thirsty, or anxious is likely to be more persistent and vigorous and to expend more effort and action. This point was made in a review on the intensity dimension of motivation by Brehm and Self (1989, p. 111): "The greater the potential motivation, the greater is the amount of energy that a person will be willing to mobilize." These authors distinguish between potential and actual motivation, and they identify motivational arousal as a characteristic of the actual motivation. They link arousal with overt behavior by nothing that (p. 111) "The direct function of motivational arousal is . . . the production of instrumental behavior." From their

point of view, those measures of arousal that most closely reflect intensity of motivation involve (p. 112) "the sympathetic nervous system which prepares the organism for activity." Their own research focused on cardiovascular changes, such as already discussed in this chapter.

Other studies besides the one by Finger, Reid, and Weasner (1960) showed the effect of prior learning on activity. Finger et al. (1960) showed that previous experience can *increase* activity, and an area of research called "learned helplessness" (Overmier & Seligman, 1967; Seligman & Groves, 1970; Seligman & Maier, 1967) has shown that previous experiences can *decrease* activity. The latter research showed that when animals were given intense inescapable shock, which the animal could not control by any action, the animal later showed *inactivity* and nonescape behavior even after escape became possible. Such learning can occur in other aversive situations. When human subjects are given aversive conditions, they may reveal lower energy mobilization if they believe instrumental activity cannot prevent aversive consequences. Wright, Brehm, Crutcher, Evans and Jones (1990) found support for such reduced energy mobilization when subjects were given to believe that no action was possible to prevent receiving a noxious noise.

Additional variables are also important with regard to the arousal-activity relationship. Nocturnal animals are more active at night than in the day, and diurnal humans are more active in the day than at night. It is also true that, independent of activity, humans in self-report reveal being more aroused in the day than at night, and at some periods of the day more than at others (Thayer, Takahashi, & Pauli, 1988). This point is considered more fully in later chapters dealing with biological rhythms. Age-related changes also occur in the way that arousal affects the type and amount of activity. For example, one study compared young and adult cats in a special type of task that usually has arousing properties due to its novelty. It is called the "open field" because it consists of an open area in which animals display a wide range of activity. Using this task, Candland and Nagy (1969) found both the amount and type of activity to differ as a function of age: the 23-day-old kittens were more active than the $2\frac{1}{2}$- to

3-year-old adult cats; and the kittens paced back and forth, whereas the adult cats showed more exploring of the open field.

Some writers are skeptical about linking activity or effort to the intensity of motivation or to arousal because they reject the validity or usefulness of the construct of arousal. Neiss (1988, 1990), for example, pointed out that often there are low intercorrelations between measures presumed to reflect arousal, and thus to link behavior to arousal may be misleading. He argued (Neiss, 1990, p. 102) that "arousal lumps together grossly disparate states" which result "in a breadth that explains nothing."

Others disagree and point out that arousal is important in explaining various aspects of behavior. For example, at one time it was thought that the lateral hypothalamus (LH) controlled hunger and eating (Darley, Glucksberg, & Kinchla, 1986). Lesions of LH led to cessation of eating. It is now known that the LH can alter activity levels (Kalat, 1992), so a valid question is whether the LH alters *eating* or only the *activity* that enables eating. When food was put directly into the mouths of animals with LH lesions, they ate normally (Berridge, Venier, & Robinson, 1989). Thus, LH lesions decreased the animals' activity of getting food, not eating per se. Dopamine-containing axons pass though the LH, and it was found that destruction of the LH destroyed these axons. Dopamine is known to contribute to arousal (Panksnepp, 1986), especially in appetitive situations. This example illustrates that reduced eating of animals with LH lesions was interpreted mistakenly and was not interpreted more correctly in terms of the loss of arousal.

Individuals, human or nonhuman, are motivated in complex ways in their encounter with many circumstances. In adaptation and goal orientation, variable states of energy are required. Arousal involves behavioral as well as neurophysiological processes, and many studies have examined how various states of excitation affect the individual. Human and nonhuman animals' behaviors are complexly influenced by a vast variety of experiences and by biological makeup. To the extent that the arousal-activity relationship is preprogrammed in terms of the autonomic sympathetic nervous system, to that extent can we predict arousal to lead to motor activity according to certain biological and species-specific characteristics. Moreover, many kinds of learning experiences, beyond any inherent biological factors, affect the arousal-activity relationship.

Inverted-U Function and the "Yerkes-Dodson Law"

The studies reviewed thus far reveal how physiological processes relate to arousal and how simple motor activity relates to arousal. The data suggest that as arousal increases, so do physiological reactivity and motor activity. This can be stated another way: A linear, monotonic increasing, relationship exists between arousal and physiological or motor responses. Does such a linear relationship also describe the way arousal affects various forms of learning and complex task performance? Some arousal theorists have distinguished on the one hand between *physiological reactivity,* which was hypothesized to be linearly related to arousal, and *performance on a task,* which was hypothesized to be curvilinearly related to arousal by means of an inverted-U function (Malmo, 1966). Additionally the *"Yerkes-Dodson law"* was presumed to be valid, with task difficulty affecting the shape of the inverted-U arousal-performance relationship.

The inverted-U hypothesis and Yerkes-Dodson law are concerned with performance effectiveness in the way arousal presumably improves or impairs performance. "Improved performance" is a qualitative judgment based on a performance criterion, and that criterion is a function of externally imposed requirements. The requirements can be set according to the type of task one is engaged in or they can be set by the demands of some outside person, like the experimenter, a teacher, a parent, or a boss in the work place.

Controversy and inconsistent findings exist regarding the way arousal affects the success or effectiveness (i.e., the quality) of performance. In considering motor output, the issue is performance *quantity.* However, the inverted-U hypothesis and the Yerkes-Dodson law are more concerned with *quality* of performance. Quality judgments are much harder to operationalize and validate than are quantity measures, and in many circumstances psychologists as yet do not know what the task characteristics or task demands are that lead to successful performance. For this reason, it is much easier to predict the effect of arousal on physiological reactivity and motor output than it is to predict the effect on complex performance that is made up of many component processes.

When the concept of arousal first gained prominence in the literature, many investigators postulated that performance is related to an *optimum* level of arousal or excitation (Duffy, 1957; Hebb, 1955; Malmo, 1959). The hypothesis was that performance would improve with increased arousal if the optimum level had not yet been reached, whereas an arousal increase beyond that optimum level would impair performance. This was known as the *inverted-U function*. Hebb (1955) suggested that the degree of arousal a person experiences shapes the "cue" or directional aspect of behavior according to an inverted-U function: Low arousal leads to behavior of low efficiency; a medium level of arousal leads to optimum behavior of high quality and effectiveness; and beyond that optimum point, performance gets worse with increased arousal.

Hebb's hypothesized inverted-U function referred to an arousal dimension that extends from deep sleep through wakefulness and heightened alertness to extreme tension indicative of extreme stress and culminating in death. In the typical laboratory study of motivated behavior, low and high motivation states would occur in the middle two-thirds of Hebb's arousal continuum, since ordinarily researchers did not test subjects in a very sleepy state nor in conditions of extreme arousal such as terminal starvation or thirst, with the subject close to death. Thus, laboratory studies often had a hard time verifying at which slope of the inverted-U curve their motivational manipulations fell, whether just short of the optimum or just after the optimum. If short of optimum, the inverted-U hypothesis would predict that increased motivation should improve performance, but if the motivational manipulation placed the high arousal just beyond the optimum level, then increased motivation should lead to impaired performance. The concept of optimum arousal is difficult to test, especially when factors like attention and performance strategy can change

the quality of performance. That is, if arousal involves anxiety and self-preoccupation rather than a focus on task demands, the effects of heightened arousal would be different than if arousal involves alert attention to complex task requirements.

An alternative to the inverted-U formulation was proposed in the 1950s and 1960s by "drive theorists." They postulated that performance will improve with increased arousal, as long as the response is very simple and there are no competing responses (Spence, 1964). An example of such simple and noncompetitional responding is the case of classical conditioning. Spence (1964) based his formulations largely on the writings of Clark Hull (1951), with "drive" akin to arousal, in referring to the energizing aspect of motivation. In tasks with none or only few competing responses, such as in classical conditioning, the energizing aspect of motivation was predicted to improve performance. Drive theorists proposed that impaired performance would occur only because of competing responses in the task, not because some optimum arousal level had been exceeded. According to drive theorists, there was no optimum arousal. They proposed instead that impairment or improvement in performance due to drive or arousal depended on the strength of the correct response and the strength of competing responses. The Hullian assumption was that drive energized all existing habits, and if the energized habits did not interfere with task performance, increased drive or arousal would facilitate and not impair performance. Spence (1958) summarized a number of studies of classical conditioning of eyeblink, with a puff of air as the unconditioned stimulus (US) and a visual stimulus as the to-be-conditioned stimulus. The data showed that increased arousal (defined either by strength of the US or by anxiety scores of the subjects) produced a greater number of conditioned responses and did so earlier in the training.

An interesting verbal learning study gave support to the formulation of a linear arousal-performance relationship by showing the *impairing* effect of *reduced* arousal (Frith, Dowdy, Ferrier, & Crow, 1985). The investigators gave volunteer subjects an intravenous infusion of a centrally acting drug that was expected to reduce arousal by reducing noradrenaline release. Compared with injections of a neutral saline solution, the drug injections led to reduced subjective estimates of arousal and to impaired paired-associate verbal learning. Thus, a drug that lowered subjective arousal was also found to lead to lowered performance in a verbal learning task. Although some studies showed support for a linear arousal-performance relationship, others showed the inverted-U relationship with arousal. Complexities of tasks often prevented adequate tests of the linear versus the inverted-U arousal-performance relationship. Because task difficulty and not only competing responses were known to affect performance, some researchers focused on the formulation of the Yerkes-Dodson law. This is called a "law" but more properly should be labeled a hypothesis, since the formulation lacks the type of empirical support ordinarily required of a scientific law.

The formulation was first proposed by Yerkes and Dodson early in the twentieth century, long before the concept of arousal gained prominence. In the original studies (Dodson, 1915; Yerkes & Dodson, 1908), animals received various levels of shock. Discrimination learning was found to be a function of an optimum level of shock (arousal), and the optimum differed according to how difficult the discrimination was. Translated into modern terms, the law states, first, that for every level of task difficulty there is an optimum level of tension or motivation (quality of performance improves as the tension is increased up to the optimum level, and performance quality decreases when tension is increased beyond the optimum level). Secondly, task difficulty and strength of motivation interact: The optimum level of arousal is high for easy tasks, and as task difficulty increases, the optimum arousal level decreases. To attain a maximum level of performance on tasks of medium difficulty requires a medium arousal intensity, and a low arousal intensity is optimal for difficult tasks. The Yerkes-Dodson law adds the variable of task difficulty to the inverted-U function postulated by Hebb (1955).

The Yerkes-Dodson law sometimes has been used illegitimately, after the fact, to account for data that did not corroborate predictions of the investigator. That is, the "law" was used as a tool for "proving" whatever the researcher wanted to demonstrate. For a legitimate test of the law, before data are collected one must specify the difficulty of the task and what the optimum level of arousal is. Otherwise the proposition simply serves to plug loopholes in data that are embarrassing to the investigator's predictions.

A convincing support for the law came from a study by Broadhurst (1957). He used a between-subjects design in which motivational arousal was induced by air deprivation caused by underwater submersion. Task difficulty was defined in terms of brightness difference between the two branches of the underwater Y-maze. The brighter was the correct branch, permitting the animal to emerge from the water, and if the animal took the darker wrong branch, it had to retrace the path until it could exit through the correct branch. In this way, task difficulty was similarly defined as in the original studies by Yerkes and Dodson (1908) with mice and by Dodson (1915) with kittens. That is, the most difficult task involved the smallest brightness difference between the correct and incorrect paths. Broadhurst (1957) tested 120 rats for a total of 100 trials, detaining the subjects 0, 2, 4, or 8 seconds under water in a submersible cage before they could swim the maze and make the discrimination which permitted escape from the underwater maze. The larger the brightness difference, the easier was the task. Ratios of 1:300, 1:60, and 1:15 represented the easy, moderate, and difficult discriminations. If optimum arousal varied with task difficulty in line with the Yerkes-Dodson law, a higher optimum in motivational arousal (manipulated length of water submersion) would be evident for the easy than for the medium or the difficult discrimination. The data, in terms of mean number of correct trials out of a total of 100 trials, supported the prediction.

Many studies failed to support "drive theory" predictions, and many studies failed to support the Yerkes-Dodson law (e.g., Fantino, Kasdon, & Stringer, 1970). In part the difficulty related to the fact that tense and energetic arousal were not distinguished in these studies. Heightened energetic arousal may yield linear performance increases, whereas heightened tense arousal may decrease the quality of performance. Moreover, when task difficulty increases, this in itself may increase arousal.

In this way the two variables of task difficulty and strength of arousal may not be independent of one another. The strongest evidence in favor of the Yerkes-Dodson law comes from studies in which task difficulty was defined by brightness discrimination, as in the study of Broadhurst (1957) and in the early work of Yerkes and Dodson (1908) and Dodson (1915). Thus, if difficulty is defined by, and relies on, attention and information intake, the effect of arousal may be very different from when difficulty relies on motor skills, memory, or problem solving. More recent investigations have examined the effects of arousal according to specific task requirements, and increasingly researchers have examined performance in terms of attention and information processing. Whereas the majority of studies before the 1980s assessed how arousal alters physiological responding, motor output, instrumental behavior, and learning, later investigations tended to assess how arousal alters perception, attention, and higher mental processes. A few theorists built a model of motivation and of personality in which arousal serves as a key construct (K.J. Anderson, 1990; Revelle & Anderson, 1992; Revelle, Anderson, & Humphreys, 1987). Much of that research focused on perception, attention, and memory rather than on motor output and simple learning. This will be considered in a later chapter in more detail. Also, later chapters concerned with hunger, fear, and anxiety will address additional issues that bear on the relationship between arousal and performance.

SUMMARY

Arousal, which varies from sleep to wide-awake excitation, refers to the intensity of excitation and of energy mobilization. The autonomic nervous system plays a key role in arousal.

Arousal is manifested *physiologically* and *behaviorally*. Physiological manifestations are recorded by peripheral measures, such as GSR, EMG, EKG, heart rate, and blood pressure. They are also recorded by central measures of brain activity, such as EEG and intracellular measurements.

The reticular formation, thalamus, and cortex make up the reticular activating system (RAS). Additional brain systems have been found to be active under states of arousal, and several neurotransmitters have been found to play important roles in the way the brain systems affect arousal.

Some researchers have found *response stereotypy* and *situational specificity* to affect physiological responses and motor activity.

Behaviorally, various states of excitation have been shown to increase gross motor activity such as running in an activity wheel. In tasks involving simple responses, like eyeblink conditioning, heightened arousal also has been found to lead to improved performance. However, for more complex behavior, arousal has not been found to improve performance consistently.

The *inverted-U hypothesis* was suggested to describe the relationship between arousal and performance, with an optimum arousal level leading to best performance. A lesser or greater amount of arousal than the optimum level is hypothesized to lead to poorer quality of performance. The "Yerkes-Dodson law" extends the inverted-U hypothesis, by indicating that for easy tasks the optimum arousal level is high whereas for difficult tasks the optimum arousal level is low.

Contrary to the inverted-U hypothesis, other investigators propose a *linear relationship* between arousal and performance. If performance is impaired by an increase in arousal, this is explained as a result of arousal leading to an increase in competing responses.

Arousal has been studied largely as a *state,* but some research has found that the disposition to be aroused may be a *trait.* Distinct types of arousal have been suggested. Thayer separated *energetic* from *tense arousal,* and these are physiologically and behaviorally distinguishable.

CHAPTER 4

Biological Rhythms and Sleep

BETH EVA FERGUSON WEE

RELATIONSHIP OF BIOLOGICAL RHYTHMS TO MOTIVATION

So far we have considered variables that are either directly a part of motivation, such as arousal, or that have a close relationship to motivation, such as emotion and mood. Now we are going to examine a variable that modulates both motivation and behavior. It does so in ways that at times are unpredictable but in all cases are important.

All of us know that as we awake in the morning we are inclined to be drowsy and less energetic than later in the day. Some of us are slow to become alert in the morning and others of us are peppy and lively within a few moments of awakening. However, all of us follow a rhythm in which our physiological reactions and our mental alertness are likely to be higher in the day (say, around noon) than at night (say, around 2:30 a.m.). We have this type of rhythm because we are *diurnal* creatures. In contrast, rats are lively at night and not very energetic in the daytime, because they are *nocturnal* animals. Thus, the effect of motivating conditions are quite different for the human, and for the rat, in the daytime compared with the night. For example, for the human to be food deprived in the night does not lead to high activity or arousal, and for the rat to be food deprived during the day does not lead to high activity or arousal, compared with the reverse period of the 24-hour day. Musty (1976/1982, p. 199) illustrated this effect by redrawing data obtained

from Bare (1959). When rats were deprived of food for 18 hours and tested at 1:00 p.m. (during their low period of activity) they ate about the same number of pellets as nondeprived rats who were tested at 9:00 p.m. (during their active period). Thus, food deprivation used to increase motivation will have very different effects on eating, as well as on general activity, depending on whether the effects are measured in the day or in the night and whether the subject is nocturnal or diurnal.

Because many psychology students are not familiar with the literature on biological rhythms and some of the methodology and terms, the present chapter describes details of methods and definitions used to investigate biological rhythms. The next chapter will examine how such rhythms affect performance and how motivational variables interact with biological rhythms.

BIOLOGICAL RHYTHMS

Introduction

A *biological rhythm* is any process in a living organism that recurs at a constant time interval, or *period*. For example, the neural activity one can measure in a nerve cell occurs with a period on the order of milliseconds, the heart beats at intervals under a second, most adult humans go to sleep once every day, the human menstrual cycle has a period of about 28 days, and the cicada or locust emerges and sings approximately once every 17 years. When a biological rhythm has a period of about 24 hours (*circa diem,* or "about one day") it is called a *circadian rhythm.* A circadian rhythm may refer to either a single event or a pattern of events that repeats about every 24 hours. Circadian rhythms exist in organisms in all phylogenetic levels, from protozoans to humans. Many of these rhythms are not readily measured in the laboratory, but examples of rhythms that can be so measured include the circadian rhythms of feeding, drinking, body temperature, locomotor activity, hormonal secretions, and the sleep/wake cycle. Biological rhythms that have periods significantly shorter than 24 hours, usually on the order of 1 to 12 hours, are called *ultradian rhythms;* and those whose periods are longer than 24 hours, but less than one year, are called *infradian rhythms* (Halberg, Engeli, Hamburger, & Hillman, 1965). The repetition of rapid eye movements (REM) approximately every 90 minutes during sleep in humans and the repetition of short episodes of hormone secretion within the endocrine system are examples of ultradian rhythms. The human menstrual cycle and the estrous cycle of many mammalian species are examples of infradian rhythms. Rhythms such as migration or hibernation are called *circannual rhythms,* because they have a period of about one year.

In nature, circadian rhythms are synchronized, or *entrained,* to external cues that serve as *Zeitgebers* ("time givers"). Using the sun as their Zeitgeber, animals synchronize their circadian rhythms to the light-dark cycle, so that specific behaviors occur at the appropriate time of day or night. For example, nocturnal animals show increased locomotor activity, feeding, and drinking at night, and they sleep during the day. These same trends can be observed in the laboratory by placing the animal in a room that has a light-dark cycle. Nocturnal animals are active during the dark portion of the cycle, and diurnal animals are active during the light portion. Although the light-dark cycle is the most powerful Zeitgeber for most animals, entrainment by other environmental factors is also possible. For example, a variety of studies have shown that animals can entrain to a temperature cycle, periodic meal timing, or cyclic variations in barometric pressure.

In humans, pheromones (chemicals released by one organism that cause a physiological response in another organism) can serve as entraining agents, as shown by studies of college students in dormitories whose menstrual cycles were found to be synchronized (reviewed by Aschoff, 1979b; Rosenwasser & Adler, 1986).

In humans, circadian rhythms can be synchronized to the light-dark cycle. At cognitive levels, we can set our rhythms, for example, to a wristwatch that tells us when to sleep or wake up. Social cues are powerful in humans, as, for example, when parents wake us up or the end of the evening news signals bedtime. Social cues for many human actions were once thought to have a stronger Zeitgeber effectiveness than the physical stimulus of the light-dark cycle (Wever, 1982). However, subsequent research showed that light of sufficient intensity also could entrain the circadian system of normal subjects (Czeisler, 1995; Honma et al., 1995). Nonphotic stimuli, such as the activity-rest cycle, also synchronize endogenous circadian rhythms, as shown by the fact that blind subjects could be entrained to a 24-hour day (Klerman et al., 1998).

In addition to being synchronized to external cues, circadian rhythms can be generated endogenously, that is, controlled by internal factors. These rhythms do not need an external cue in order to be expressed, for they will persist under constant external conditions. If an animal or human is placed under conditions of constant darkness or constant light, various endogenously generated circadian rhythms can be measured. Under these conditions, the animal's circadian rhythms are said to "free-run," which means that they are expressed with their own intrinsic period and are not synchronized to any external cues.

Biological Rhythms Versus Biorhythms

The scientific study of biological rhythms should not be confused with the scientifically unsubstantiated theory of *biorhythms.* One might think of the relationship between biorhythms and biological rhythms as similar to the relationship between astrology and astronomy. The theory of biorhythms, which was proposed by the German scientist Wilhelm Fliess in 1897 and became popular in the 1970s, postulates that three cycles act in a concerted fashion to guide activity: a 23-day cycle that influences physical strength, energy, endurance, and physical confidence; a 28-day cycle that influences feelings, cooperation, love, and irritability; and a 33-day intellectual cycle that influences memory, learning, and creativity (Holley, Winget, DeRoshia, et al., 1981, cited in U.S. Congress, Office of Technology Assessment, 1991). According to biorhythm theory, these cycles are thought to be linked to a person's birth date and to fluctuate in a constant fashion throughout the person's life. Thus, the high and low points of each cycle can be charted and examined to see when the curves coincide, and a person's maximal and minimal performance can be predicted. Although a theory for predicting human behavior and scheduling activities may sound appealing, the theory of biorhythms has no scientific basis, and no studies have ever been able to validate the existence of any of these three cycles. Thus, one should be careful not to confuse the scientifically proven human biological rhythms with biorhythms.

Measuring Circadian Rhythms

The circadian rhythms of several physiological and behavioral variables can be measured fairly easily in the laboratory. For example, an individual's body temperature can be recorded several times over the course of 24 hours. The data gathered from such a study would show that body temperature is not constant during the circadian cycle but has peaks and troughs. When the temperature is recorded for several cycles, the circadian rhythm of body temperature will be expressed, or shown. Similarly, blood samples could be taken from an individual at specific intervals over a few days to determine the circadian rhythms of secretion of various hormones found in the blood. Measurements of food or water intake and electroencephalogram recordings (EEGs) reveal the circadian rhythm of drinking or feeding behavior and the sleep-wake cycle, respectively.

One circadian rhythm that is studied commonly in animals is that of locomotor activity. Tradition-

ally, wheel-running activity was measured in rodents as an indicator of locomotor activity, as shown in Figure 4.1. Laboratory rodents such as the golden hamster are placed in cages equipped with a running wheel that is connected to a chart recorder or computer. The animal is free to run in the wheel at any time during its circadian cycle, and the locomotor activity can be monitored for several days without disturbing the animal. Other recording devices are used that measure all of the animal's movements, not just the wheel-running activity. Either running-wheel activity or general activity (moving around in the cage) can be measured to determine the circadian rhythm of locomotor activity. Similarly, studies with birds often use "perch hopping" behavior as an indicator of the circadian rhythm of locomotor activity. The functional properties of this rhythm can be determined by manipulating the light-dark cycle to which the animal is exposed, as illustrated by results from the idealized experiment shown in Figure 4.2. Activity has been recorded continuously (black bars), and the records of successive days are plotted/pasted beneath each other. To make the rhythm easier to read, the original 24-hour record is double-plotted. In all situations, the animal has free access to food and water.

The first portion of the record in Figure 4.2 illustrates the activity pattern under conditions of constant darkness and constant temperature, when the animal's rhythm is said to free run. In this situation of no variation in the external environment, the animal's own endogenous period is expressed. The period of the free-running rhythm, called and described by the Greek letter tau, τ, depends on both intrinsic factors, such as the physiological status of the animal (e.g., hormone concentrations, age) and the animal's genetic background (e.g., the genetic strain of the animal, and whether it is a diurnal or nocturnal species), as well as extrinsic factors such as the specific environmental conditions used (e.g., temperature, light intensity) and the animal's photoperiodic history (e.g., previous experiments, breeding conditions) (reviewed in Aschoff 1979b; Pittendrigh & Daan, 1976). With the exception of light intensity, these factors have only small effects on tau, and the internal mechanisms that regulate the rhythms are remarkably stable. However,

FIGURE 4.1

Illustration of methods used to measure wheel-running activity of a hamster. The animal is placed in a cage equipped with a running wheel connected to a chart recorder or computer. The animal is free to run in the wheel at any time during its circadian cycle, and the locomotor activity can be monitored for several days without disturbing the animal. The traditional manner uses a chart recorder, in which each wheel rotation activates a sideways movement of a pen on a moving sheet of paper. When the 24-hour strips of paper are arranged one under the other, one can observe the daily rhythmic behavioral patterns. The 24-hour strips often are double-plotted for better visualization of the continuity of the rhythm (lower left). On the first line, day 1 and day 2 are plotted; on the second line, day 2 is replotted before day 3, and so on. For more objective analyses, a computer can be used, and the amount of activity can be plotted against time (lower right). Digital recordings may be necessary to distinguish between different amounts of activity during the active portion of the rhythm.

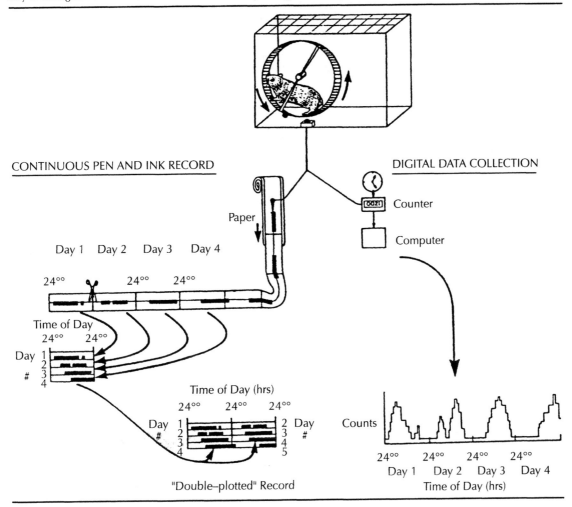

Source: Reprinted with permission from Moore-Ede, Sulzman, & Fuller, 1982.

when the intensity of the light is manipulated, one sees changes in the free-running period. For example, tau changes as the lighting conditions are changed from constant darkness to constant light (second portion of Figure 4.2), and from one intensity of constant light to a higher intensity. The way the activity rhythm is altered by a change in light intensity depends on the species of animal (Aschoff,

FIGURE 4.2

Idealized data from a hypothetical experiment illustrating the functional properties of the circadian rhythm of locomotor activity in response to manipulations of the light-dark cycle. Activity has been recorded continuously (black bars), and the records of successive days are plotted/pasted beneath each other. The data have been double-plotted as described in Figure 1. When the black bars are exactly vertical, the rhythm has a period of exactly 24 hours. Thus, the time from activity onset on one day is exactly 24 hours after the activity onset of the preceeding day. A diagonal sequence of these bars indicates that the period is longer (diagonal toward right) or shorter (diagonal toward left) than 24 hours. For example, in the first portion of the record, the activity rhythm under conditions of constant darkness and constant temperature has a period of 24.5 hours. Thus, activity onset on one day occurs approximately 24.5 hours after activity onset of the preceeding day. When the animal is transferred to conditions of constant light (LL, second portion of record), the period of the free-running rhythm increases to 25.0 hours. A change in the free-running period also would be observed by changing the hormonal status of the animal. The third portion ("ENTRAINMENT TO A ZEITGEBER") shows that when the animal is transferred from constant conditions to a 24-hour light-dark cycle, the animal's rhythm no longer free runs but becomes entrained, or synchronized, to the 24-hour Zeitgeber period. In response to displacement along the time axis (i.e., phase shift) of the light-dark cycle (fourth portion, "PHASE SHIFT OF ZEITGEBER"), the animal's rhythm also phase shifts, and the animal's rhythm again becomes entrained to the new light-dark cycle. Entrainment persists even when the Zeitgeber period is less than 24 hours (fifth portion, "ENTRAINMENT TO A ZEITGEBER T=23.25 hr"). Evidence of entrainment is shown by removing the light-dark cycle and observing that the subsequent free-running rhythm always starts at the same phase relative to that seen during entrainment (sixth portion, "POSTENTRAINMENT FREE RUN"). One technique that is used to examine how light or other stimuli such as drugs, neurotransmitters, or hormones affect the circadian clock is illustrated in the last two portions. The animal is allowed to free run in constant conditions, and at various times in the circadian cycle (indicated by the asterisk) the animal is exposed to a single administration of a stimulus. The first stimulus caused a phase advance, and the second stimulus caused a phase delay of the activity rhythm.

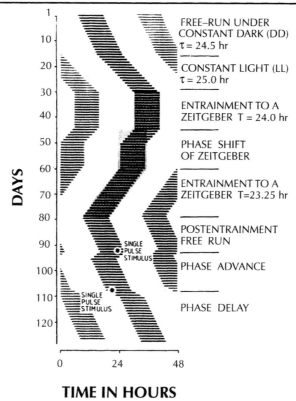

FREE–RUN UNDER
CONSTANT DARK (DD)
$\tau = 24.5$ hr

CONSTANT LIGHT (LL)
$\tau = 25.0$ hr

ENTRAINMENT TO A
ZEITGEBER T = 24.0 hr

PHASE SHIFT
OF ZEITGEBER

ENTRAINMENT TO A
ZEITGEBER T=23.25 hr

POSTENTRAINMENT
FREE RUN

PHASE ADVANCE

PHASE DELAY

SINGLE
PULSE
STIMULUS

SINGLE
PULSE
STIMULUS

DAYS

TIME IN HOURS

Source: Reprinted with permission from Wollnik, 1989.

1979a, 1979b). In general, under conditions of constant darkness the free-running period of diurnal animals is greater than 24 hours, and tau for nocturnal animals is less than 24 hours (Aschoff, 1979a).

The third portion of Figure 4.2 ("Entrainment to a Zeitgeber $T = 24.0$ hr") shows that when the animal is transferred from constant conditions to a 24-hour light-dark cycle (indicated by the shaded region), the animal's rhythm no longer free runs but takes on a period of 24 hours. The rhythm is said to be synchronized or *entrained* to the light-dark cycle. Under conditions of *entrainment,* the period of the rhythm (tau) and the period of the Zeitgeber are the same. Thus, if the light-dark cycle has a period other than 24 hours, for example 23.25 hours, tau also will be 23.25 hours during entrainment (see fifth portion of Figure 4.2). Entrainment should be confirmed in two ways. First, the light-dark cycle is displaced, or phase-shifted, along the time axis (notice how the shaded region representing the light-dark cycle has changed between the third and fourth portions of Figure 4.2), and one determines if the animal's rhythm also phase shifts. This demonstrates that the constant phase relationship between the rhythm and the Zeitgeber is stable, as one expects with true entrainment (Enright, 1981). The second step in demonstrating entrainment is to remove the light-dark cycle and determine that the subsequent free-running rhythm always starts at the same phase relative to that seen during entrainment (sixth portion of Figure 4.2 called "Postentrainment free-run").

One important point is that a circadian rhythm cannot be entrained to just any Zeitgeber period. In other words, there is a "range of entrainment" (Klotter, 1960), a specific range of Zeitgeber period under which the rhythm can be entrained. Beyond that range, entrainment usually does not occur, and the rhythm free runs with a period close to that measured in constant conditions (Aschoff, 1981). In mammals, the range of entrainment is 7 hours, from 21 to 28 hours (Aschoff & Pohl, 1978). The size of this range depends on the strength of the Zeitgeber and on properties of the circadian system of the organism.

The fifth portion of Figure 4.2 ("Entrainment to a Zeitgeber, $T = 23.25$ hr"), illustrates that the animal's rhythm can entrain to a Zeitgeber with a period of less than 24 hours. The method shown here, of changing the Zeitgeber period (compare the fourth and fifth portions of Figure 4.2), would be useful to show that an animal's rhythm really can entrain to a Zeitgeber. For example, if one wanted to test the effects of a drug on an animal's circadian system, one might determine the extent to which injections of the drug could entrain the animal's circadian rhythm (e.g., see Van Reeth & Turek, 1989a). It is possible that an animal's free-running rhythm just happens to be the same as the Zeitgeber period, even if the animal's rhythm is not really entrained to that period. By changing to a new Zeitgeber period, one can show that the stimulus (drug injections, light/dark cycle, etc.) really is acting as a Zeitgeber if the animal's rhythm is the same as the new Zeitgeber period. In the examples of entrainment illustrated in Figure 4.2, the Zeitgeber period changes from 24 to 23.25 hours, and the animal's activity rhythm also changes and becomes the same as the new Zeitgeber period.

Biological rhythms oscillate similarly to physical oscillations, such as a pendulum or a spring. A biological rhythm oscillates in the sense that once it starts, it continues indefinitely and recurs on a regular basis. Due to the similarity to physical oscillations, many of the terms used to describe biological rhythms are taken from physics. Therefore, one can talk about several characteristics of a rhythm: the period, phase, and amplitude (Figure 4.3a). One can plot the variable being studied (e.g., temperature, activity, hormone secretion) according to the intensity or level rising and falling over time. Thus, the rhythm can be represented by a sinusoidal wave that has a peak and a trough, with intensity varying above and below a mean level over the duration of the cycle. As described already, the *period* of a rhythm is the length of a cycle or the time interval over which the rhythm occurs, for example, the time from the beginning of one cycle to the beginning of the next cycle or from the peak of one cycle to the peak of the next cycle. *Amplitude* is the difference between the maximum (or minimum) and mean value in a sinusoidal oscillation (Aschoff, 1981); it is a measure of the strength of the rhythm. For example, the number of wheel revolutions

FIGURE 4.3

Schematic diagram illustrating characteristics of a biological rhythm. A biological rhythm can be visualized as a sine wave, having peaks and troughs that correspond to those times when the variable being measured is highest and lowest, respectively. (a) The period of the rhythm is the length of 1 cycle, and can be measured from the peak of one cycle to the peak of the next cycle. The amplitude of the rhythm, A, is the difference between the maximum (or minimum) and the mean value. Phase, ø, refers to the state of the rhythm at a particular point in the cycle; it is a time point within a complete cycle at which a particular event occurs. (b) A phase advance of the rhythm. The phase indicated by 2 (on the thicker curve) has been advanced (occurs earlier) with respect to the phase indicated by 1 (on the thinner curve). (c) A phase delay of the rhythm. The phase indicated by 2 (on the thicker curve) has been delayed (occurs later) with respect to the phase indicated by 1 (on the thinner curve).

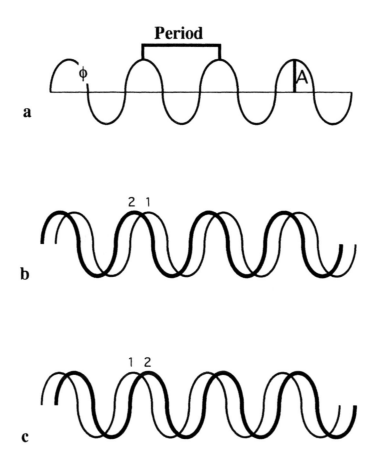

Source: Drawn by Beth Wee and Valerie Ngo-Muller.

could be measured to determine the amplitude of the circadian rhythm of locomotor activity, and the concentrations of a given hormone could be measured to determine the amplitude of the circadian rhythm of hormone release. *Phase* refers to the state of the rhythm at a particular point in the cycle; it is a time point within a complete cycle at which a particular event occurs. As a way to measure phase, one often chooses a *phase reference point,* which is a point in the rhythm upon which all comparisons will be made. When measuring the circadian rhythm of locomotor activity, the onset of activity often is used as the phase reference point because it is so precise, although one also could choose activity offset or even the middle of activity. This phase reference point can be used to describe the rhythm before and after various manipulations.

Light or other stimuli such as drugs, neurotransmitters, or hormones, or environmental manipulations such as cage changing, social interactions, and access to a novel running wheel, also can produce phase shifts, as illustrated in the last two portions of Figure 4.2. If the animal is allowed to free run in constant conditions, the stimulus will cause a shift in the phase of the animal's activity rhythm such that the onset of the activity rhythm will be shifted permanently (unless some other event occurs that again shifts the phase). A stimulus may advance the rhythm permanently, causing it to occur earlier than predicted from the previous free run. This is called a *phase advance* of the rhythm (Figure 4.3b). The rhythm also may occur later than expected, resulting in a *phase delay* of the rhythm (Figure 4.3c). The direction (advance, delay, or no change) and magnitude of the phase shift will depend on both the time during the circadian cycle that the stimulus is given and the type of stimulus that is used.

Phase shifts occur in humans when they travel rapidly across time zones or change shift work schedules. The circadian system may not respond immediately to an associated change in the light-dark cycle, but instead may require one to many cycles before the individual has re-entrained to the new light-dark cycle (see fourth portion of Figure 4.2). Indeed, several studies have shown that at least a week is required for the human circadian system to switch from a diurnal to a nocturnal ori-

entation (see review by Monk, 1986). It is easy to guess the debilitating psychological consequences of too rapid a shift in working hours if an employee is assigned to a new work schedule that reverses day and night every two to three days.

Circadian rhythms that one measures are generated by an underlying *pacemaker,* or *clock.* One way to understand the mechanisms of the clock and how it generates circadian rhythms is to manipulate the rhythm and try to infer how these manipulations have affected the underlying pacemaker. To determine if the manipulation has altered the clock, one must measure a property of the rhythm that also is a property of the clock. Only two properties of the rhythm are reliable indicators of the pacemaker system itself, which means that when the clock is changed these two rhythmic properties also are changed. These "clock properties" are the period length under free-running conditions and the steady-state (or stable) phase (Daan & Pittendrigh, 1976, see also Pittendrigh, 1981a, 1981b). Changes in the phase or period of the measured rhythm indicate that the underlying pacemaker has been changed, which implies that other rhythms controlled by the pacemaker also have been changed.

The daily rhythms expressed by different tissues and organs in an organism usually maintain distinct *phase relationships* to each other as well as to the Zeitgeber that entrains them. Together they represent a high degree of temporal order (Aschoff, 1979b). For example, if one measured the circadian rhythms of ten different hormones and a person's body temperature, one would find that there is a temporal organization of all these measures, even if all the peaks and troughs occurred at different times. That is, each rhythm has its own phase relationship to another rhythm. Thus, at any given circadian phase, the individual is in a specific physical and psychological state. It is not surprising that one's responsiveness varies according to the phase at which a stimulus is applied. For example, in responding to auditory and visual signals, the reaction time of human subjects is longest early in the morning and gets markedly shorter from noon on (Aschoff, 1979b). Other measures such as toxicity due to a variety of drugs or X-irradiation are dependent on the circadian phase at which the toxic agent is given to the organism (reviewed in Aschoff, 1979b). In addition, differences in drug effectiveness often are phase dependent. For example, the duration of anesthesia and the threshold for pain reaction, measured in a tooth after the application of a cold or electric stimulus, respectively, vary across the circadian cycle, so that medical or dental treatments are most effective in the afternoon (reviewed in Aschoff & Wever, 1981). Natural substances also produce different effects when presented at different times of the day. For example, allergic reactions of the skin to house dust or histamine are greater after exposure in the evening than in the morning (reviewed in Aschoff, 1979b).

Seasonal Rhythms

For many species, the breeding season and thus the time of birth are confined to the time of year when the probability of survival is maximal for both the adults and the offspring. Other biological activities and physiological functions such as migration, hibernation, locomotor activity, and changes in body weight and/or coat color also exhibit seasonal fluctuations. Environmental factors such as temperature, day length (*photoperiod*), food availability, rainfall, and presence or absence of competitors and/or predators can contribute to the timing of these events, and the relative importance of each environmental factor will vary from species to species. For example, hamsters, which have a short gestation period, breed during the long days of spring and summer, and their offspring are born a few weeks later, when conditions are optimal for survival. In contrast, ruminant animals, such as sheep, goats, and deer, with gestation periods of 4 to 6 months, are short-day breeders, breeding during the short days of fall and winter, and their offspring are born in the spring. Thus, seasonal breeders are able to use the environmental cues to regulate the timing of their behavior and physiology.

The human circadian pacemaker has the capacity to detect seasonal changes in day length and to make corresponding adjustments in such rhythms as hormone release and body temperature (reviewed in Wehr, 1996). However, most modern humans rarely are exposed to a purely natural photoperiod. They use artificial light to extend the day into the evening hours, and, if they remain indoors during the day, they decrease their exposure to natural daylight. Thus, reports of human seasonal changes come from studies in which humans are exposed to artificial photoperiods, and the effects of these photoperiods on circadian rhythms are assessed (Wehr, 1996). Although humans have the *capacity* to respond to natural changes in day length, such responses normally do not occur, due to the use of artificial lighting.

Nonphotic Factors that Influence the Circadian System

In addition to photic stimuli, a wide variety of nonphotic stimuli have been shown to reset the circadian clock. For example, the clock can be altered in rodents by exposing them to a novel running wheel or to social stimuli or a pulse of darkness on a background of constant light (reviewed by Mrosovsky, 1996; Turek & Van Reeth, 1996). These manipulations produce an acute increase in activity, which may be responsible for the subsequent phase shifts in the clock. Similar increases in activity and subsequent phase shifts are produced by injections of benzodiazepines, a group of drugs used to lower anxiety. Wee and Turek (1989) showed that midazolam, a short-acting benzodiazepine, induced acute increases in activity and phase shifts in the circadian rhythm of running-wheel activity in hamsters (Fig. 4.4 upper record). When the animals were pretreated with a drug that blocks benzodiazepine receptors, both the phase shifts and the acute increase in running-wheel activity induced by midazolam were blocked (Fig. 4.4 lower record).

Further support for the idea that acute increases in activity are responsible for phase shifts comes from experiments in which a hamster is confined to a small nest box or restraining tube for a period of time after the stimulus is presented. Such restraint blocks phase shifts induced by either dark pulses or benzodiazepines (Reebs, Lavery, & Mrosovsky, 1989; Van Reeth & Turek, 1989b). Providing a running wheel to an animal that does not normally have

FIGURE 4.4

Single-plotted activity records of hamsters free running in constant light (data from Wee & Turek, 1989). The hamsters were given two intraperitoneal injections indicated by the double asterisks. The injections were given 15 minutes apart, with the second injection timed to occur 6 hours prior to predicted activity onset. In the top record, the hamster was given an injection of the vehicle (V), dimethyl sulfoxide, followed by midazolam (M), a fast-acting benzodiazepine. Note the large phase advance of the circadian rhythm of running-wheel activity as well as an increase in running-wheel activity just after the midazolam injection. In the bottom record, the hamster was given the benzodiazepine receptor antagonist, RO 15-1788 (RO), followed by an injection of midazolam (M). Note that the antagonist blocked both the phase shift and the burst of activity induced by midazolam. Neither the vehicle nor the antagonist produced phase shifts or increased activity when given alone.

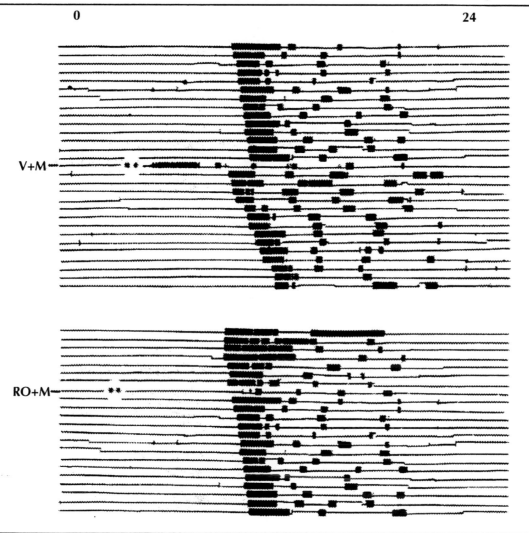

Source: Wee & Turek, 1989.

such a wheel also induces an increase in activity and a subsequent phase shift (reviewed in Mrosovsky, 1996). Phase shifts induced by the presentation of a novel running wheel as well as those produced by other nonphotic (pharmacological and nonpharmacological) stimuli are produced at times during the circadian cycle when rodents normally are not active and when light pulses are ineffective in inducing phase shifts. Another difference between light pulse-induced and nonphotic-induced phase shifts is that light pulse-induced shifts are not accompanied by acute increases in activity. These differences imply that photic and nonphotic stimuli may act on the circadian system in different ways, and that the pacemaker can be reset differently, depending on the nature and timing of the stimulus.

Although light is a very strong Zeitgeber for many animals, nonphotic stimuli may provide a potential way of adjusting clocks for humans when light is inadequate for the demands of modern existence, or in those who are blind (Mrosovsky, 1996). On the basis of findings of activity-induced phase shifts in rodents, researchers are asking questions about how exercise affects circadian rhythms in humans (Redlin & Mrosovsky, 1997). For example, exercise has been shown to cause phase shifts in circadian rhythms in humans involved in shift work (Eastman, Hoese, Youngstedt, & Liu, 1995). Although only a small number of human studies have been completed, and they have the limitations of small numbers of subjects, small effects, and ambiguities in interpretation, these studies suggest that exercise, or correlated variables, do produce phase shifts in human circadian rhythms (Redlin & Mrosovsky, 1997). Any study involving humans may be confounded by effects of light and social factors on the circadian system. However, exercise, alone, or in combination with other Zeitgebers such as light, might be preferable to pharmacological treatment of disorders of the circadian system.

CONTROL OF BIOLOGICAL RHYTHMS

The Mammalian Biological Clock

Broadly defined, the physiological system responsible for circadian rhythms must contain at least three major components: (1) a pacemaker that generates the rhythm; (2) an input pathway that allows the pacemaker to become entrained with the daily environmental cycle; and (3) an output pathway for the expression of the overt rhythm that can be measured (Takahashi & Menaker, 1984). A schematic diagram of this system illustrating these three major components is presented in Figure 4.5. In mammals, the *suprachiasmatic nucleus* (*SCN*) of the anterior hypothalamus (Figure 4.6) has been shown to be the primary biological clock responsible for the generation and entrainment of most circadian rhythms (see reviews by Klein, Moore, & Reppert, 1991; Meijer & Rietveld, 1989; Rusak & Zucker, 1979; Turek & Van Reeth, 1996). This bilaterally paired neural structure is located at the base of the third ventricle, just *above* (supra) the optic *chiasm*. Its morphology, anatomical connections, and physiology have been studied extensively and its role as an endogenous pacemaker is well established (see reviews by Meijer & Rietveld, 1989; Moore, 1997; Rusak & Zucker, 1979; Turek & Van Reeth, 1996; also Klein et al., 1991). The SCN is the target of direct and indirect retinal projections that are required for circadian rhythms to be entrained to environmental light-dark cycles (Moore, 1978, 1997). Direct retinal projections reach the SCN via the *retinohypothalamic tract* (Hendrickson, Wagoner, & Cowan, 1972; Moore & Lenn, 1972). An indirect projection from the retina reaches the SCN via the *intergeniculate leaflet* (*IGL*) of the lateral geniculate nucleus and portions of the ventral lateral geniculate nucleus of the thalamus (Card & Moore, 1989; Harrington, Nance, & Rusak, 1987; Hickey & Spear, 1976; Pickard, 1982; Swanson, Cowan, & Jones, 1974). The *geniculohypothalamic tract,* with projections from the IGL to the SCN, is not necessary for entrainment of circadian rhythms to the light-dark cycle, but it may modulate the effects of light on the circadian clock (Harrington & Rusak, 1986, 1988; Johnson, Moore, & Morin, 1989; Pickard, Ralph, & Menaker, 1987). The IGL appears to be a necessary component of the neural pathways that mediate activity- and benzodiazepine-induced nonphotic entrainment (Maywood, Smith, Hall, & Hastings, 1997). The SCN also receives afferent input from a variety of other brain regions, the most prominent projection coming from the *raphe nuclei* (Meyer-Bernstein &

FIGURE 4.5

Schematic diagram of a physiological system responsible for the generation of circadian rhythms. The system is composed of photoreceptors that can measure input concerning the light/dark cycle, a circadian pacemaker, and the associated output pathway that conveys information necessary for the overt rhythm to be expressed.

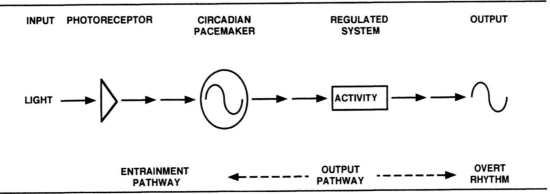

Source: Redrawn from Eskin, 1979 by Beth Wee and Valerie Ngo-Muller.

Morin, 1996; Pickard, 1982; see Meijer & Rietveld, 1989; Moore, 1995, for review). Neurons from the dorsal raphe nucleus also project to the IGL (Meyer-Bernstein & Morin, 1996). Most of the efferent projections from the SCN terminate in other hypothalamic nuclei, but some project to the thalamus and midbrain (Berk & Finkelstein, 1981; Stephan, Berkley, & Moss, 1981; Swanson & Cowan, 1975; Watts, Swanson, & Sanchez-Watts, 1987).

Recently, the human circadian clock was reported to respond to light working via photoreceptors outside the eye (Campbell & Murphy, 1998). However, the mechanism of extraocular phototransduction in humans, if this phenomenon truly does exist, is unknown. Numerous studies with rodents have led to the conclusion that photoentrainment in rodents is mediated only by ocular photoreceptors (Foster, 1998). Although the SCN is the primary pacemaker controlling biological rhythms, there is evidence that additional neural sites are involved in the control of some rhythms (see next section).

Multiple Oscillators Within the Circadian System

The various circadian rhythms such as body temperature, locomotor activity, and hormone secretion do not all show peaks (or troughs) at the same time, but they do maintain distinct phase relationships

with each other. A possible explanation for this is that the circadian system is composed of multiple circadian oscillators, or pacemakers (see reviews by Pittendrigh, 1993; Rosenwasser & Adler, 1986; Turek & Van Reeth, 1996). Under normal circumstances, the oscillators work together to ensure that the endogenously generated rhythms are synchronized to occur at the appropriate times of the day or night and at times that are appropriate relative to all of the other rhythms. However, under certain conditions the internal coordination of the circadian system becomes disrupted and the multioscillatory nature of the system is revealed most clearly. For example, if a hamster is exposed to bright constant light for an extended period of time, the circadian rhythm of wheel-running activity may split into two distinct components (Figure 4.7), each of which may be controlled by separate oscillators (Pittendrigh, 1981a). The exact nature of a given oscillator is unknown; that nature may depend on the organism in question. The oscillator may be a single neuron (Welsh, Logothetis, Meister, & Reppert, 1995) or a group of neurons such as those that make up the suprachiasmatic nucleus. In addition to the SCN, the retina of the mammalian eye also contains a pacemaker (Tosini & Menaker, 1996). The retinal oscillator is responsible for controlling the circadian rhythm of melatonin synthesis that occurs in the retina. Additional support for the idea of multiple os-

FIGURE 4.6

Schematic diagram showing the neural pathways from the retina of the eye to the pineal gland. In rodents, these pathways have been shown to mediate the responses of the reproductive system to changes in photoperiod. The direct pathway from the eye to the SCN is the retinohypothalamic tract. SCN = suprachiasmatic nuclei, PVN = paraventricular nuclei, IMLN = intermediolateral nucleus, SCG = superior cervical ganglia.

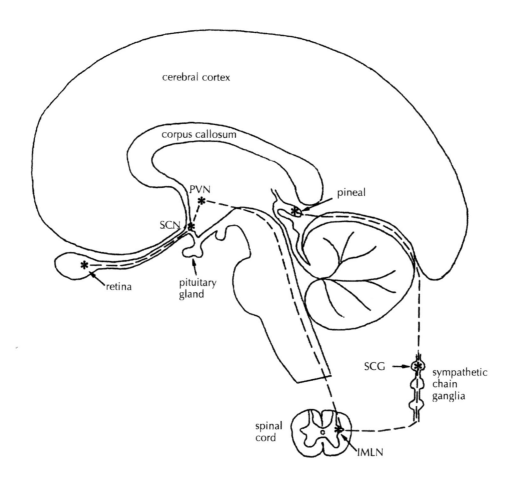

Source: Redrawn from Tamarkin, Baird, & Almeida, 1985 by Beth Wee and Tracy Muller.

cillators is that although most circadian rhythms are abolished or disrupted by lesions of the suprachiasmatic nucleus (see reviews by Moore, 1978; Rosenwasser & Adler, 1986; Rusak & Zucker, 1979), some circadian rhythms persist after SCN lesions (see review by Rosenwasser & Adler, 1986).

Melatonin

Mammals that express seasonal rhythms in reproduction use components of their circadian system (e.g., the eyes, retinohypothalamic tract, and SCN) to assess day length (photoperiod) and then to pass

FIGURE 4.7

Double-plotted activity record from a hamster free running in constant light. Note that the activity rhythm "split" into two component parts (four parts in this double-plotted figure) that are approximately 180° out of phase with each other.

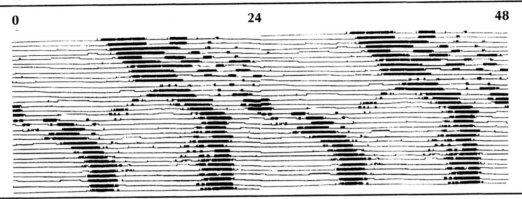

Source: Unpublished data from Beth Wee.

this information, via a multisynaptic pathway, to the *pineal gland* (Fig. 4.6). Upon receiving the appropriate neural signal, the pineal gland releases its hormone, *melatonin.* The pineal's secretion of melatonin conveys the organism's assessment of day length to the reproductive system (i.e., the hypothalamic-pituitary-gonadal axis).

Two features of melatonin secretion in mammals are worth noting: (1) melatonin secretion exhibits a pronounced circadian rhythm, and (2) in a variety of vertebrates, including humans, pineal gland production of melatonin occurs primarily during the dark portion of the daily light-dark cycle, regardless of whether the species is nocturnal or diurnal (Arendt, 1995). Due to its secretion during the night or dark phase of the light-dark cycle, melatonin has been referred to as a "darkness hormone" (Arendt, 1995). The circadian rhythm of melatonin synthesis and release is dependent upon the circadian rhythms of the enzymes that synthesize melatonin from serotonin. These rhythms are controlled by the SCN, and they are abolished by destruction of the SCN (Klein & Moore, 1979). Light acts to inhibit the melatonin-synthesizing enzymes (and therefore inhibits the release of melatonin), and also serves to synchronize the melatonin rhythm with the environment. These effects of light, inhibition, and entrainment determine when melatonin is synthesized

(the phase of the melatonin rhythm) and the length of time (duration) that melatonin will be synthesized and released (Tamarkin, Baird, & Almeida, 1985).

The important characteristic of melatonin release that conveys information about the external light-dark cycle to the reproductive system of seasonal breeders is its *duration.* During the short nights of summer, the duration of melatonin release is shorter than during the winter, when the nights are longer. This seasonal variation in melatonin duration tells the animal to breed at the correct time of year. The way this melatonin-duration signal is transduced into a change in neuroendocrine-gonadal activity is not fully known, nor are the mechanisms by which melatonin actually alters hypothalamic-pituitary function. Receptors for melatonin have been found in specific parts of the brain and pituitary in a variety of animals, including humans (Weaver, Rivkees, Carlson, & Reppert, 1991), and these melatonin receptors have been cloned and characterized (Reppert & Weaver, 1995). Melatonin has been shown to alter neuronal activity within the SCN (Liu et al., 1997; also reviewed in Gillette & McArthur, 1996), and neural actions such as these may play a role in melatonin's photoperiodic effects. Another possibility is that melatonin acts to alter feedback by gonadal steroid hormones onto the hypothalamic-pituitary axis, a possibility supported by the finding that melatonin alters the levels of estrogen receptors in the medial preoptic area (Lawson et al., 1992).

In humans, the circadian rhythm of melatonin production and secretion is closely associated with the sleep-wake cycle, with the rise in nocturnal melatonin preceding the conventional time for sleep, the peak of melatonin occurring during sleep, and its decline coinciding with awakening (Lavie, 1997). Several studies have examined the possibility that exogenous melatonin possesses sleep-inducing effects and that endogenous melatonin is involved in sleep regulation. Although these studies differed in such variables as dose, route of administration, subjects (normal versus insomniac), and time of administration, the one variable that appears to be the crucial factor with respect to melatonin's sleep-inducing effects is time of administration (Lavie, 1997). Because endogenous melatonin is released exclusively at night, the administration of exogenous melatonin at night results in different levels of circulating melatonin compared with levels produced by daytime melatonin administration. Further, any sleep-inducing effects of melatonin given during the night are confounded by the endogenous increase in nocturnal sleepiness. Lavie (1997) concluded that sleep-inducing effects of nighttime administration of melatonin occur only with high pharmacological doses. In contrast, daytime administration of melatonin consistently produced increased sleepiness (as measured by increased scores on sleepiness questionnaires, shortened latency to sleep onset, increased sleep duration, and decreased performance levels) even at relatively low doses. On the basis of these findings and the close temporal relationship between the endogenous rhythm of melatonin secretion and the sleep-wake cycle, Lavie (1997) suggests that melatonin participates in the regulation of the sleep-wake cycle by inhibiting wakefulness-generating mechanisms of the central nervous system.

In addition to its photoperiodic and sleep-inducing or hypnotic effects, melatonin has specific physiological and neurobiological effects such as phase shifting and entrainment of mammalian circadian rhythms, regulation of core body temperature, regulatory functions in the vertebrate retina, and acute neuronal inhibition (see reviews by Arendt, 1995, 1997; Cagnacci, Krauchi, Wirz-Justice, & Volpe, 1997; Liu et al., 1997; Reppert & Weaver, 1995). These effects probably are mediated through the specific melatonin receptors mentioned above. Melatonin has received much publicity from the media and the health food industry for its reported ability to reverse aging, improve one's sex life, and treat everything from high blood pressure to cancer to sleep disorders. Many of these claims have not been substantiated scientifically, so caution needs to be used before assuming that melatonin is the proclaimed cure-all. Although only minimal side effects have been reported for acute melatonin treatment, long-term studies (use of melatonin for more than six months) examining its safety and/or levels of toxicity are lacking (Arendt, 1997; Weaver, 1997).

ADVANTAGES OF BIOLOGICAL TIMEKEEPING

An advantage of having a biological clock that tells an animal when to breed is the animal's increased probability of finding a mate and having the young born when environmental conditions are optimal for survival. A biological clock that measures seasonal information also will be useful to the animal that needs to hibernate or migrate. Preparation for these *seasonal* events may include altering the diet to add body fat, storing up food, and/or preparing a place to hibernate, as well as undergoing a variety of physiological changes.

Physical features in the environment such as light, temperature, and humidity fluctuate on a *circadian* basis. Therefore, individuals whose behavior and/or physiology are influenced by these features must restrict their functions (feeding, activity, sleep, etc.) to the appropriate times of the day or night. Some animals need sufficient light to be able to see to catch prey or gather food and/or to escape from predators. Thus, maximal adaptiveness for these animals occurs when they are diurnal. Alternatively, an animal that has developed sufficient night vision might be active at night, thus avoiding predators as well as decreasing the competition for food with diurnal animals. Animals that are susceptible to water loss are more likely to be active during times when humidity is high. Animals that cannot regulate their body temperature will be active during times when temperature is optimal, depending on the environment (temperate, arctic, desert, etc.) in which they live. An animal's survival is dependent not only on the ability to behave or respond physiologically in a certain way, but also on the animal's ability to do these functions at the proper time.

In humans, many physiological functions such as activities of the nervous and cardiovascular systems slow down at night and increase during the day. During the slowing down, the body has a chance to rest. Without this daily chance to rest, the body would have to maintain its daytime work load throughout the night. For organs such as the heart, this prolonged high level of activity could be detrimental. Indeed, more heart attacks occur between the hours of 6 a.m. and noon, when a variety of physiological variables such as heart rate are increasing (Muller et al., 1985). Thus, physiological fluctuations throughout the 24-hour day, which provide the body with a chance to rest, appear to be necessary for good health. Another example of a circadian rhythm that is necessary for healthy functioning is the alternation between sleep and wakefulness (see below). Any college student is aware of the need for sleep after staying up all night, either for studying or socializing. Although the biological clock does not cause sleep to occur, it is responsible for the timing of sleep, so that sleep is synchronized to the 24-hour day as well as to the body's other circadian rhythms. One advantage of having several rhythms (e.g., hormones, urinary constituents, body temperature) synchronized to the sleep-wake cycle, particularly so that they start to increase just before wakefulness (for review, see Aschoff, 1979b), is that preparations for the stresses of the day have already started before the individual awakens. The importance of this temporal synchronization will be discussed further in the next section.

EFFECTS OF DISRUPTING BIOLOGICAL RHYTHMS

The circadian system provides temporal organization between an organism and its environment and also maintains a high degree of temporal organization within the individual. Such temporal order is necessary for the maintenance of normal health. If this temporal organization is disrupted, the normal health of the individual also will be disrupted. Three categories of circadian rhythm disorders are recognized. These pertain to the major effects observed when the subject is studied under standard 24-hour conditions: *phase disorders,* in which the person is not able to sleep at the appropriate times of day or night; *period disorders,* in which a person fails to entrain to the normal 24-hour cues in the environment; and *amplitude disorders,* which involve reduction of the amplitude of the rhythm, or, in extreme cases, loss of rhythmicity altogether. Although further discussion of these types of disorders is beyond the scope of this book, it is worth mentioning that some of these disorders are associated with mental disorders such as depression.

Seasonal Affective Disorder and Phototherapy

In addition to disturbances of the circadian system, one can talk about rhythmicity of psychiatric illnesses themselves. That is, certain psychiatric illnesses occur at certain times and not at others. Much attention has been given to a syndrome of cyclic depression, known as *seasonal affective disorder,* or *SAD,* that recurs annually during the winter and undergoes spontaneous remission in the spring (Rosenthal et al., 1984). Symptoms include marked changes in energy level, appetite (often cravings for carbohydrates), sleep, weight, and mood (Skwerer et al., 1988). In addition, in patients with SAD circadian rest-activity rhythms are significantly phase delayed and poorly entrained to the 24-hour day (Teicher et al., 1997). The great interest in SAD is due, in part, to the fact that it presents a rare instance of a major psychiatric illness that is readily susceptible to treatment with light, or *phototherapy.* Both clinicians and patients are attracted to phototherapy, because unlike many other treatments for mental illness, phototherapy is noninvasive and not drug based. Unlike drug treatments that may take weeks for the effect to be seen and have the potential of side effects, phototherapy produces its clinical effects rapidly, within hours or days, and does not produce side effects. Treatment usually involves exposing patients to bright light (usually 2,500 lux or more; normal room light is 500 lux or less) for a couple of hours each day, and the improvement is measured as a reduction in the patient's scores on various depression rating scales. Several factors appear to influence the efficacy of phototherapy, including the intensity, duration, and timing of light (Rosenthal, Sack, Skwerer, Jacobsen, & Wehr, 1988). Bright-light treatment mimics sunlight, and it is believed that the reduction in sunlight during the winter is the main trigger for SAD in vulnerable individuals (Eastman, 1990). The wintertime reduction in light exposure at temperate latitudes is due to shorter photoperiod (day length), reduction in the maximum intensity of sunlight, and lower temperatures that limit the time most people spend outdoors (Eastman, 1990).

The treatment of SAD with phototherapy was influenced by the finding that exposure of humans to bright light, but not ordinary room light, can depress the production of nighttime melatonin (Lewy, Wehr, Goodwin, Newsome, & Markey, 1980), the hormone believed to convey information about day length. This finding, coupled with the finding that the antidepressive effects of light occur only after exposure to bright light, but not to ordinary room light, led to the theory that bright-light treatment exerts its antidepressant effects by modifying the pattern of melatonin secretion (see review by Skwerer et al., 1988). However, experimental evidence has not provided strong support for this "melatonin hypothesis." Another hypothesis was that bright-light supplements satisfy a general "need" for light, which is intensified during the dark winter months (reviewed in Terman et al., 1989). If that were the case, light therapy should be effective at any time of day, although its effectiveness would be modulated by diurnal variation in the eye's sensitivity (Terman et al., 1989). The antidepressive effectiveness of phototherapy has been shown to depend on the time during the circadian cycle when the bright light is given. The question of effective time of light treatment has important theoretical implications for understanding the specific action of light that underlies the therapeutic effect (Terman et al., 1989).

Other researchers explain the success of pho-

totherapy by the "phase-shifting hypothesis" which predicts that an abnormality of circadian rhythms is the basis for the seasonal changes in mood and behavior found in SAD patients, and light therapy exerts its antidepressant effects by correcting these abnormal rhythms by causing appropriate phase shifts of the rhythms (Skwerer et al., 1988). The timing of bright-light exposure has been shown by several groups of researchers to be critical for its antidepressant effects, with treatment during the early morning being more effective than evening light treatment (see review by Lewy & Sack, 1996; Rosenthal et al., 1988). However, individuals differ in their sensitivity to the timing of phototherapy, with some patients showing a therapeutic response to phototherapy at times other than the early morning. The variation among subjects in terms of the optimal time of phototherapy may be due to variability among subjects' circadian systems or to some other factors. For example, new subjects appeared to be much more responsive to bright-light treatment during the evening than did subjects with substantial prior experience (Terman et al., 1989). Conclusions about optimal time of phototherapy also must consider how the timing of bright-light exposure relates to the timing of sleep. So far, no definitive conclusions have been made as to how phototherapy works, and there are problems with all of the hypotheses proposed so far. In addition, individual phototherapy studies have differed with respect to the severity of the subjects' depression; the duration of light treatment, both in terms of how long the subjects were exposed to the bright light each session and the number of days the subject received treatment; and the control procedures used. Consequently, the optimal variables such as the duration and timing of treatment are not agreed upon by all researchers and clinicians who administer light therapy. The wide range of the subjects' severity of depression makes it unlikely that any single treatment regimen will be optimal for every SAD patient (Terman et al., 1989). For example, longer light exposures (either per session or by adding more sessions) might be required for therapeutic effects in more severe cases. Alternatively, increasing the intensity of the light (e.g., from 2,500 lux to 10,000 lux), over a shorter duration might be more effective for other individuals (Terman et al., 1989). Finally, light treatment is not a viable option for treating circadian rhythm disorders in people who are totally blind (Lewy & Sack, 1996). For these patients, melatonin may be the preferred treatment. Nonetheless, results from studies with bright-light treatment (e.g., Czeisler, 1995; Czeisler et al., 1989), indicate that the sensitivity of the human circadian pacemaker to light is far greater than previously recognized. Phototherapy also has been useful for the treatment of other disruptions of the circadian system such as those associated with shift work and jet lag (reviewed in Lewy & Sack, 1996).

"Jet Lag"

The biological clock of most healthy individuals is synchronized to the daily light-dark cycle and to social cues. When people travel rapidly across time zones, however, their biological clock must adjust to the new time zone. Many travelers experience a condition known as "jet lag," whose symptoms may include sleep disturbance and daytime fatigue, loss of appetite, decreased vigilance and attention span, headaches, tired muscles, poor psychomotor coordination, irritability, dizziness, gastrointestinal disturbances, and a general feeling of malaise (Graeber, 1994; Moore-Ede, Sulzman, & Fuller, 1982). Deterioration in performance is frequently a consequence of crossing several time zones (Moore-Ede et al., 1982). This has profound implications for diplomats, business people, and many others who must make difficult decisions shortly after their arrival in the new time zone.

Jet lag should not be confused with the fatigue and stress and/or sleep loss that is a direct consequence of travel and independent of the timing conflict. For example, flying from north to south does not involve crossing of any time zone, but the stress of the flight itself may influence a traveler's performance. The symptoms of jet lag result from the circadian system's inability to adjust rapidly to a sudden shift in the timing of such external Zeitgebers as the light-dark cycle, meal timing, electromagnetic influences, social cues, work-rest schedules, and knowledge of clock time (Graeber, 1982). The severity of jet lag is related to both the direction of

flight and the number of time zones crossed. The direction of flight determines the direction of the phase shift in the light-dark cycle and, thus, the shift that the passenger's circadian system will have to make to adjust to the new time zone. Westward flights lengthen the day, and the circadian system must undergo a phase delay, or a slowing down to stretch the endogenous rhythms out over the extended time period of the new Zeitgeber. Eastward travel shortens day length, and the system must undergo a phase advance, or a speeding up of the endogenous rhythms. The extent of the delay or advance depends upon the number of time zones crossed. When 12 or more zones are crossed, various rhythms may undergo either an advance or a delay to achieve resynchronization with the new environment. For example, crossing 13 time zones going west is the same as crossing eleven time zones going east. The traveler's circadian system can either undergo a delay associated with a 13-hour shift, or an advance associated with an 11-hour shift. Because our endogenous rhythms have a period greater than 24 hours, humans adjust more easily to a phase delay (i.e., having to stay up later) than to a phase advance (i.e., having to fall asleep earlier than normal). Thus, jet lag is not as severe when traveling westward compared with traveling eastward.

Jet lag has three major components: external desynchronization, internal desynchronization, and sleep loss (Graeber, 1994). *External desynchronization* refers to the disparity between external and internal body time. The internal clock is either too far ahead or too far behind the external Zeitgeber. This discrepancy causes the traveler to feel tired at inappropriate times of the day, have difficulty sleeping through the night, feel hungry at mealtimes, and exhibit an irregular daily pattern of urination and bowel movements (Graeber, 1982). Performance also is likely to suffer. For example, if five time zones have been crossed going eastward, the traveler will have difficulty operating with maximal efficiency at a 9 a.m. meeting, when his or her internal clock says that it is only 4 a.m., a time when the individual normally is asleep. Under normal circumstances an individual's many circadian rhythms maintain fixed temporal relationships to each other (*internal synchronization*), but this synchrony does not persist after transmeridian flights (those that cross the east-west axis), resulting in *internal desynchronization,* in which different endogenous rhythms adjust to the new time zone at different rates. Thus, the circadian rhythm of the urinary secretion of one metabolite may adjust its phase more rapidly than that of another metabolite, which in turn may adjust more rapidly than the circadian rhythm of body temperature. Performance rhythms also have been reported to adjust at different rates, depending on the task (Klein, Wegmann, & Hunt, 1972).

The third component of jet lag is the sleep loss that results from the combined impact of both types of circadian desynchrony (Graeber, 1994). One of the most common complaints of jet lag is fatigue. This symptom may be caused by (1) loss of sleep during the usual sleep span while aboard the airplane, (2) wakefulness during local daytime while the sleep-wake cycle still is externally desynchronized and at a point more appropriate for sleep, or (3) loss of sleep due to awakenings at night resulting from an unadjusted sleep-wake cycle or the need to void (Graeber, 1982). Although some travelers try to eliminate these factors by resorting to mild sedatives, hypnotics, or alcohol, such agents often are unsuccessful in inducing sleep. Also, they typically lead to undesirable side effects that compound the desynchronization problem. For example, if the pharmaceutical agents are taken at an inappropriate time in the circadian cycle, they could cause the circadian rhythms to be shifted in directions opposite to the way the person is traveling (e.g., cause rhythms to be phase delayed when the light-dark cycle has been phase advanced).

The best advice for the traveler who wants to adjust rapidly to a new time zone is to be active during the new daytime, go to bed during the new night, eat meals at local times, and spend the day in well-lit environments with maximum social contact (Moore-Ede et al., 1982). Although a number of pharmacological agents have been found to phase shift circadian rhythms in a variety of organisms, most of these are not effective in treating jet lag. However, considerable attention has been given to melatonin, which has been used successfully to treat jet lag and some circadian-based sleep disor-

ders (Arendt, 1995; Arendt, Skene, Middleton, Lockley, & Deacon, 1997). The improvement is greater when larger numbers of time zones are crossed and when the traveler is flying in an eastward direction (melatonin causing a phase advance) compared with westward travel (melatonin causing a phase delay). Following melatonin treatment to phase advance over eight time zones, subjects reported improved latency and quality of sleep, greater daytime alertness, and more rapid re-entrainment of endogenous cortisol and melatonin rhythms (Arendt, 1995). Travelers should use caution when taking melatonin to treat jet lag, because effective results are obtained only when melatonin is given at the *appropriate doses and times in the circadian cycle.* A nonpharmacological method of treating jet lag is to expose the traveler to bright lights at appropriate times in the circadian cycle (phototherapy). In principle, scheduled exposure to bright light should alleviate symptoms of jet lag by accelerating circadian re-entrainment to the new time zones. However, both laboratory and field studies have given mixed results, and their applicability to the general public remains uncertain due to limited sample sizes (Boulos et al., 1995).

SLEEP

Sleep for most lay persons is considered to be the opposite of arousal. Early postulations by psychologists, as well, considered sleep to be a state of very low arousal (Hebb, 1955). However, research on sleep has shown that distinct stages exist and that in some stages the sleeper is in a relatively excited state. Thus, sleep is not merely calm quiescence.

Stages of Sleep

The state of sleep is measured by recording the electrical activity of the brain. Electrodes are attached to the scalp to pick up the electrical potential changes emanating from the cortex. These changes then are magnified to produce an electroencephalogram (EEG) recording. The EEG represents an average of the waveforms of many small zones of the cortex that underlie a given electrode. EEG recordings have revealed four distinct stages of sleep (Fig. 4.8).

FIGURE 4.8

Electroencephalographic (EEG) recordings of human sleep stages. Wakefulness shows alpha activity (subject relaxed) and beta activity (subject alert). Theta activity is seen in stage 1 sleep. Spindles and K complexes are characteristic of stage 2 sleep. The large slow waves, called delta activity, are seen in stage 4 sleep, and to a lesser extent in stage 3 sleep. Stages 3 and 4 together are called "slow wave sleep" (SWS). The EEG of REM sleep resembles that of stage 1, and contains a mixture of beta and theta activities. However, eye movements and chin muscle tonus are different between stage 1 and REM sleep.

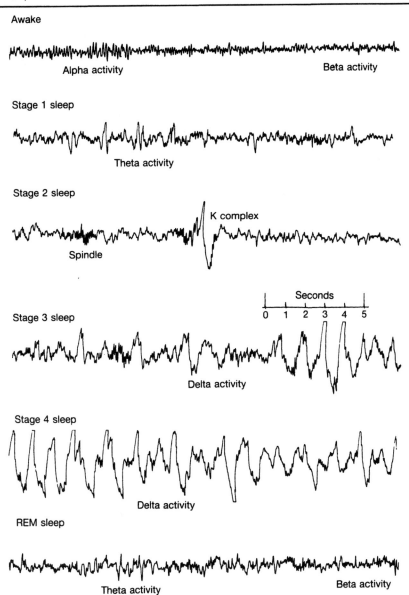

Source: Reprinted with permission from Horne, 1988.

A regular waveform occurs if the cortical activity over an area of several square centimeters is synchronous, meaning that several neurons are producing the same type of neural message. The waves are slow (low frequency) and of relatively high peak (amplitude). When the activity is not synchronous (desynchronous), the recorded waves are of high frequency with low amplitude. In measures of EEG, amplitude usually refers to the voltage between the peak (maximum) and the trough (minimum) of a wave (Horne, 1988, p. 8), measured in millionths of a volt, or microvolts (μV). This definition contrasts with that of amplitude for oscillations that measure biological rhythms, in which amplitude is defined as the difference between the peak or trough and the midpoint (mean value) of a wave (Aschoff, 1981). There are different ways of defining amplitude, but in all cases the term refers to the height of a wave. In measures of EEG, frequency refers to the number of complete waves or cycles occurring in one second, and it is expressed in hertz (Hz), cycles per second (Horne, 1988, p. 8).

Beta waves of around 15 Hz and of low amplitude occur when a person is alert and attentive to events in the environment. *Alpha waves,* in the range of 8 to 11 Hz, with higher amplitude, are characteristic of relaxed wakefulness. Amplitude rises with increased "deepness" of sleep. *Theta waves,* in the range of 3.5 to 7.5 Hz, reflect drowsiness or light sleep, and *delta waves,* less than 3.5 Hz, are characteristic of deep sleep. These different waveforms help to define the different stages of sleep. Stage 1 sleep, marked by the presence of theta activity, is actually a transition between wakefulness and sleep. Stage 2 has periods of theta activity plus irregularly occurring *sleep spindles* (12–14 Hz) and high voltage *K complexes.* Stage 3 sleep has 20 to 50 percent of the large and slow delta waves. When delta activity is more than 50 percent, the deepest sleep of stage 4 has been reached (Horne, 1988). *Slow wave sleep* (SWS) is the collective term for stage 3 and stage 4 sleep. Figure 4.9 shows the various sleep stages during the course of a night's sleep. Soon after sleep onset, stage 4 sleep occurs. *REM* (rapid eye movement) sleep occurs on a periodic basis (on a 90-minute cycle). During the first half of the night, SWS predominates, but REM and stage 2 sleep predominate during the second half of the night. The large amount of beta activity during REM sleep indicates that the brain is highly active during this type of sleep, and, thus, quiescence is not characteristic of all sleep. Due to the presence in REM sleep of beta activity that normally is characteristic of wakefulness, REM sleep also has been called "paradoxical sleep."

FIGURE 4.9
A simplified "hypnogram" of sleep stage changes over the night in young human adults.

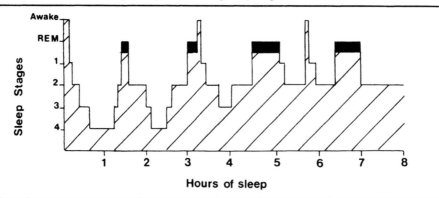

Source: Reprinted with permission from Horne, 1988.

Why Do We Sleep?

Researchers have not found a definitive answer to the question of why we sleep. However, two major suggestions have been made. One idea is that sleep is an *adaptive* or *evolutionary process* (Webb, 1974). Because all animals are known to have some type of sleep, or at least a period of quiescence, sleep must serve an adaptive function. The adaptive theory of sleep is based on the postulate that survival requires periods of minimal behavioral interaction with the environment. When an animal sleeps, it conserves energy and avoids exposure to predators. The duration of sleep characteristic of each species is related to factors such as the length of time necessary to acquire food, an animal's rank in the predator-prey hierarchy, how long energy is stored after food is eaten, and so on. A second explanation of why we sleep is that sleep serves a *repair and restorative function*, enabling the body, especially the brain, to repair itself following the exertions carried out during the prior period of wakefulness. Most likely, the true function of sleep is a combination of both of these ideas.

Evidence in support of the repair and restoration idea comes from results from *sleep deprivation studies*. Earlier sleep deprivation studies were somewhat inconclusive, because they lacked good controls (reviewed in Horne, 1988). However, Rechtschaffen and his colleagues designed sleep deprivation experiments that controlled for the effects of the forced exercise that was required to keep the experimental animals awake (Rechtschaffen, Bergmann, Everson, Kushida, & Gilliland, 1989). An experimental rat was paired with a control rat by housing each animal on either side of a divided horizontal disk suspended over water. Both rats had their EEG recorded continuously. Whenever the experimental rat started to sleep, the disk was automatically rotated, which awakened the experimental rat and forced both rats to walk opposite to the direction of disk rotation to avoid falling into the water. (Rats dislike water, so they do their best to avoid falling in!) Thus, both rats received the same physical stimulation, but the stimulation was timed to awaken the experimental rat. Although the control rat was awakened if it was asleep when the

disk rotated in response to the experimental rat's attempt to sleep, the control rat could sleep ad lib when the experimental rat was awake. In different experiments, this technique was used to deprive the experimental rat of all sleep or of just paradoxical (REM) sleep, or to disrupt and/or deprive from non-REM sleep.

All types of sleep deprivation caused a progressive debilitated scrawny appearance, weight loss (despite increased food intake), skin lesions, increased energy expenditure, decreased body temperature during the late stages of deprivation, increased plasma norepinephrine level, decreased plasma thyroxine level, and finally death (Rechtschaffen et al., 1989). These changes developed more slowly in the rats that were deprived only of paradoxical sleep compared with the totally sleep deprived rats. For example, survival ranged from 11 to 32 days for rats that were totally sleep deprived and 16 to 54 days for rats that were deprived only of paradoxical sleep. Thus, both total sleep and paradoxical sleep serve vital functions. The authors of the study concluded that sleep may be necessary for effective thermoregulation. When a subgroup of rats was allowed to sleep ad lib after they had shown major effects of sleep deprivation, most of the rats showed complete or almost complete reversal of the deprivation-induced changes. Interestingly, recovery sleep featured huge, immediate rebounds in paradoxical sleep and inconsistent or relatively small rebounds of other sleep stages.

In contrast to rats, results from sleep deprivation studies with humans suggest that sleep is less important for the rest of the body than it is for the brain (Horne, 1988). Although a decrease in body temperature is a common outcome of sleep deprivation in humans, it is unclear whether this indicates a problem with thermoregulation as in the rat. There is little evidence that sleep is an essential tissue repair process for most of the human body or that sleep deprivation causes impairments to organs other than the brain. Rather, adverse effects of sleep loss in humans are confined to the cerebrum and behavior, with such effects as hallucinations or visual illusions and confusion. One major difference between animal and human sleep deprivation studies is that human subjects are less stressed, simply because they know that they can end the experiment at any time. In addition, human sleep deprivation studies have ended much earlier than the nonhuman animal studies, so the debilitating effects on the human body have not been seen. Obviously prolonged sleep deprivation studies with humans, which would cause the results seen in rats, would be unethical.

Horne (1988) separated sleep into two components. *Core sleep* is essential for repairing the effects of waking wear and tear on the cerebrum and is evident in studies in which subjects are given a chance for recovery after sleep deprivation. During recovery sleep, much greater percentages of stage 4 sleep and REM sleep are made up than stage 1 and stage 2 sleep. The other component of sleep is motivational, which Horne called *optional sleep*. The motivational component refers to the fact that people and nonhuman animals want to sleep after they have been sleep deprived, and, when given the opportunity, they will sleep, even if only for small naps. One role for optional sleep in nonhuman mammals may be as a time filler when the mammal is constrained by darkness and cannot carry out its other activities.

Relationship of Sleep to Circadian Rhythms

Normally, the circadian rhythm of sleep and waking is tightly coupled to other circadian rhythms, such as the circadian rhythm of body temperature. Sleep onset occurs as body temperature is decreasing. The constant association that normally exists among rhythms is biologically adaptive, so in the evening, body temperature and plasma adrenaline concentration fall, we feel tired, and it is easy to have unbroken sleep (Waterhouse, 1993). By contrast, even if a subject has been awake all night, unbroken sleep is difficult if it starts at 0800 hours because the rhythms of body temperature, adrenaline, and general alertness will all be in their rising phases. Although the circadian rhythms of body temperature and other psychological and physiological functions are influenced by the alteration of sleep and wakefulness, they are not caused by it, as shown by the fact that the body temperature rhythm persists during prolonged sleep deprivation (Aschoff & Wever, 1981). Plasma cortisol and adrenocortico-

trophic hormone (ACTH) also show a characteristic pattern of release that persists under several constant conditions, indicating that its release is controlled primarily by a circadian pacemaker (Van Cauter, 1990; Van Cauter, Plat, Leproult, & Copinschi, 1998). In contrast to these variables whose rhythm appears to be independent of sleep, there are other variables, such as growth hormone, whose secretion is largely "triggered" by sleep and thus shows no rhythm during the first 24 hours of sleep deprivation (Aschoff & Wever, 1981).

One might believe that the length and quality of sleep are determined by the length of the prior period of wakefulness. However, even after extended periods of sleep deprivation, "recovery" sleep rarely exceeds 11 to 16 hours. Several studies have shown that the length of prior wakefulness affects only some aspects of sleep, and that other characteristics of sleep are dependent upon circadian factors. In other words, the timing of sleep and wakefulness and sleep structure result from an interaction between a circadian component and a sleep-dependent, or homeostatic, component or process (Borbely, 1982; Daan, Beersma, & Borbely, 1984). In his "two process model," Borbely refers to the sleep-independent circadian component as process C and the sleep-dependent component as process S. The consistent finding among sleep studies using a variety of protocols is that sleep propensity and REM sleep peak at or shortly after the trough of the endogenous component of the core body temperature rhythm (Dijk & Czeisler, 1995). In contrast, non-REM sleep, particularly SWS, appears to be controlled primarily by a *recovery process* that is dependent upon prior wakefulness and is largely independent of endogenous circadian phase. This process S reflects a homeostatically regulated process of sleep intensity, in which non-REM sleep intensity declines during sleep but rises during wakefulness (Achermann & Borbely, 1990). Sleep onset is possible when the homeostatic S factor is at a high level, and spontaneous awakening from sleep occurs when it is at a low level. When sleep follows an extended period of wakefulness, the initial level of SWS is increased. Naps taken later in the day contain more SWS than naps taken earlier in the day (Borbely, 1994). In contrast to the homeostatic component, the sleep-wake independent component of sleep regulation, process C, is generated by a circadian pacemaker. (Horne [1988, p. 149] notes that his "core sleep" and "optional sleep" are subdivisions of Borbely's process S and that Borbely's process C is the circadian temperature rise that normally determines the end of optional sleep.)

Dijk and Czeisler (1995) used a forced desynchrony protocol in which the circadian and sleep-dependent components of sleep regulation could be separated from each other. Male subjects lived in the sleep laboratory for 33 to 36 days, and were scheduled to a 28 hour rest-activity cycle so that sleep episodes (9.33 hr each) occurred at all phases of the endogenous circadian cycle, as indicated by the core body temperature rhythm, and variations in wakefulness preceding sleep were minimized. Core body temperature was recorded throughout the study period, and EEG and other variables associated with sleep were recorded during all sleep episodes. The results showed that although sleep could be initiated rapidly at all circadian phases, sleep latencies (interval between time of lights out and first occurrence of any sleep stage) varied significantly with circadian phase. The shortest sleep latencies were observed at the minimum of the endogenous component of the temperature rhythm, and sleep latencies increased gradually, reaching a peak (i.e., longest latency to onset of sleep) during the plateau of the body temperature rhythm, which, in the entrained state, would correspond to the interval between 0600 and 2200 hours. In other words, the subjects were taking longer to fall asleep during times when they otherwise (i.e., during nonexperimental situations) would be awake. Total sleep time also varied significantly with circadian phase. REM and non-REM sleep were affected in different ways by both circadian and sleep-dependent factors. Thus, Dijk and Czeisler conclude that their data confirm the pivotal role of the endogenous circadian pacemaker in the regulation of sleep in humans and show that sleep propensity and sleep structure result from (sometimes nonadditive) interactions of circadian and sleep-wake-dependent oscillatory processes. The probability of waking from sleep also results from an interaction between these two processes.

The probable circadian pacemaker is the suprachiasmatic nucleus (SCN), which is involved in the *timing* of sleep and wakefulness. Lesions in the SCN (or an area homologous to the SCN in humans) severely disrupt sleep-wake rhythms in rats (Mistlberger, Bergmann, Waldenar, & Rechtschaffen, 1983), squirrel monkeys (diurnal primates) (Edgar, Dement, & Fuller, 1993) and humans (Cohen & Albers, 1991). SCN-lesioned monkeys continue to sleep and wake, but the *timing* of sleep and wakefulness is altered, such that the rhythm of sleep and wakefulness is lost (Edgar et al., 1993). In fact, total sleep time was actually higher in SCN-lesioned monkeys. SCN-lesioned rats exhibit recovery sleep after sleep deprivation (Mistlberger et al., 1983). This suggests that a homeostatic sleep-promoting process can function independent of the circadian effects on sleep (Edgar et al., 1993).

On the bases of the finding that SCN-lesioned squirrel monkeys had increased total sleep times, but decreased wake bout lengths during the day, Edgar, Dement, and Fuller (1993) suggested a variation on the "two-process model" proposed by Borbely (1982, Daan et al., 1984). They consider sleep-wake regulation in probabilistic terms such that the circadian pacemaker promotes wakefulness and thus *opposes* the homeostatic process of sleep. According to their "opponent process" model, physiological sleep tendency (or its converse, alertness) is determined by the sum of these two opponent processes. This model implies that the circadian rhythm of sleep is caused indirectly by SCN-dependent mechanisms that impose prolonged intervals of waking (sleep loss) each circadian day. The role of the SCN in promoting wakefulness fits with their finding that wakefulness is decreased (and total sleep time is increased) in SCN-lesioned monkeys. The authors add that if the circadian timing system were not responsible for promoting wakefulness, it would be difficult to understand why shift work and jet lag result in waking at inappropriate times, even when subjects have experienced considerable sleep loss.

Regardless of the terms used to describe the various factors that regulate sleep, a major purpose of the human circadian system is to prepare the body and mind for restful sleep at certain times of the 24-

hour cycle and active wakefulness at other times. Thus, the internal physiological milieu is prepared for the state the person is about to enter (Monk, 1991). In a normal healthy person, as night approaches the circadian system will "shut down" any processes that oppose sleep (e.g., hunger, cortisol excretion, renal function) so the person can have seven or eight hours of restful sleep. Toward the end of the night, processes that promote wakefulness (e.g., suppression of melatonin, cortisol excretion, rising body temperature) will increase, so productive wakefulness can occur as soon as possible after the individual awakens in the morning.

EFFECTS OF AGING ON BIOLOGICAL RHYTHMS AND SLEEP

The elderly face many problems (e.g., failing health, retirement, financial restrictions, loss of family and friends, social isolation, poorly appreciated sexual problems, increased use of medications, lack of physical exercise, increased bed rest, and postmenopausal hormonal changes). People vary in how well their chronological age compares with their biological age. Some people are "old" at 50, and others are relatively vigorous and youthful at 80. Numerous surveys have been conducted on various populations of elderly (arbitrarily defined as persons over the age of 65 years) which show that the elderly often wake up earlier, go to bed earlier, nap more during the daytime, and have increased time in bed. They also have increased use of sleeping pills, and marked increase in "wake after sleep onset" (WASO) (Lieberman, Wurtman, & Teicher, 1989; Miles & Dement, 1980; Minors, Rabbitt, Worthington, & Waterhouse, 1989). Reports have suggested that the EEG of awake elderly people tends to be interrupted by brief episodes of sleep-like EEG recordings, and the incidence of these "microsleeps" (bursts of sleep lasting 1–10 s while the person is in an eyes-closed resting state) increases with the age of the subject (Liberson, 1945). Characteristics of delta wave activity (0.5–3.0 Hz) also change (e.g., reduced amplitude, slowing of delta frequencies) with increasing age (Smith, Karacan, & Yang, 1977).

Increasing age has different effects on the time spent in the different stages of sleep (Williams, Karacan, & Hursch, 1970). In general, absolute amounts of REM sleep fall slightly, but relative amounts of REM are well maintained until extreme old age, when they do show some decline (Miles & Dement, 1980). At that age, individuals tend to be awake in the latter part of the night, when REM is most prevalent. This may explain the reduction in the percentage of REM sleep. A decline in their REM sleep is accompanied by a decrease in the physiological changes associated with REM, such as rapid irregular respiration and heart rate, penile tumescence, muscular twitches, and increased cerebral blood flow.

The biphasic pattern of sleep and wakefulness, seen in young and middle-aged adults, seems to break down with age, with a return to the polyphasic sleep-wake pattern seen in babies and young children. However, the amplitude of the cycles (measured by the amounts of SWS and REM) is decreased in the elderly (Miles & Dement, 1980). Sleep in the elderly tends to be more fragmented, which may be due, in part, to sleep apnea. However, regardless of respiratory status, daytime sleepiness in one study of elderly subjects was greater than in children or in young adults, recorded in identical circumstances (Miles & Dement, 1980). A substantial number of elderly people may be pathologically sleepy, even when they do not complain of hypersomnia (excessive sleeping). Aging leads to a paradox in that the elderly may be plagued by an inability to sleep during the night, with excessive sleepiness, often leading to increased napping, during the day. Some of this nocturnal insomnia and daytime hypersomnia may be explained by a weakening in the circadian rhythm of alertness reported for the elderly, especially in men (Monk, Buysse, Reynolds, Kupfer, & Houck, 1996).

The effects of age on various circadian rhythms are evident in other age groups besides the elderly, although the effects may be more pronounced in individuals over 60, who have been studied most extensively. In individuals between the ages of 20 and 59 the effects of age were studied with respect to characteristics of sleep and to morningness/eveningness (Carrier, Monk, Buysse, & Kupfer, 1997). Increasing age was related to increased morningness (e.g., earlier wake time, earlier bed-time, less time in bed, better mood and alertness at wake time). When polysomnographic sleep characteristics were recorded in the laboratory, increasing age was associated with less time asleep, decreased sleep efficiency, increased number of awakenings, lower percentage of SWS and REM sleep, higher percentages of stage 1 and 2 sleep, reduced REM activity and density, and shorter REM latency. The authors concluded that both age and degree of morningness are important predictors of habitual sleep patterns and polysomnographic sleep characteristics of this young and middle-aged group.

A variety of human circadian rhythms, such as body temperature, motor activity, and cortisol, melatonin, and growth hormone rhythms, are altered with age (Lieberman et al., 1989; Richardson, Carskadon, Orav, & Dement, 1982; Sharma et al., 1989; Van Cauter et al., 1998; Weitzman, Moline, Czeisler, & Zimmerman, 1982). In some cases, aging affects one rhythm more than another in the same individuals. The circadian rhythm of subjective alertness was weakened with advancing age, even in those subjects with intact temperature rhythms (Monk et al., 1996). In that study, older men fared the worst, showing the lowest amplitude and most phase-advanced alertness rhythms compared with older women and younger men and women. Compared with younger people, older people have more severe and longer lasting symptoms of jet lag, show decreased tolerance to shift work, and show a shift toward morningness (that is, a phase advance of their circadian rhythms and a reduction in amplitude) (reviewed in Reilly, Waterhouse, & Atkinson, 1997). The combination of decreased circulating levels of melatonin associated with advanced age (Sharma et al., 1989) and melatonin's reported effects on sleep (Lavie, 1997) have led some researchers to suggest that sleep disruptions (e.g., insomnia) observed in the elderly may be a consequence of low melatonin production (Hughes, Sack, & Lewy, 1998). However, melatonin replacement may not be as effective for treating age-related insomnia as currently available hypnotics or bright-light treatment (Hughes et al., 1998).

Many aging studies have been limited to the effects of age on the *amplitude* of circadian rhythms (reviewed in Myers & Badia, 1995; Turek & Van Reeth, 1996). However, such alterations do not necessarily imply a change that is intrinsic to the circadian pacemaker. One could explain such age-related changes as resulting from changes either upstream (input) or downstream (output) from the clock. The suggestion that the circadian clock itself (and not just the rhythm being measured), is altered by age is supported by the observations that the *period* of the circadian rhythm of locomotor activity is decreased in old hamsters (Morin, 1988; Pittendrigh & Daan, 1974). As mentioned earlier, the only two clock properties that are reliable indicators of the pacemaker system itself are phase and free-running period length (Daan & Pittendrigh, 1976; also see Pittendrigh, 1981a, 1981b). Thus, changes in period that occur with increasing age reflect changes in the circadian system itself. Many of the effects of aging on the circadian system of hamsters can be simulated in young animals by depleting brain monoamine levels, suggesting that aging alters monoaminergic inputs to the clock (Turek et al., 1995).

Because circadian rhythms in older subjects are influenced by both endogenous (clock-driven) and exogenous (lifestyle-driven) factors, rhythm changes observed in the elderly could arise from either or both types of factors (Minors, Atkinson, Bent, Rabbitt, & Waterhouse, 1998). Retirement from a full-time job provides the opportunity for daytime naps and more flexible schedules, and older people vary in the extent to which they are physically active during the daytime. Another possibility is that the biological clock does not entrain as well under less structured lifestyles, and the decline in its output with increasing age reflects a more general neurological decline (Minors et al., 1998). For example, age-related changes in the circadian system may be due to changes in sensory capacities or altered sensitivity to subtle environmental changes (Van Gool & Mirmiran, 1986). However, alleged visual impairments cannot be the sole explanation for age-related changes in observed biological rhythms, because a decrease in period length was observed in older animals housed in constant darkness (Pittendrigh & Daan, 1974) as well as in blinded older animals (Morin, 1988).

Other possible explanations include age-related reductions in neurotransmitter content or release, or structural and functional changes in the hypothalamus or pineal gland (see review by Myers & Badia, 1995; Van Gool & Mirmiran, 1986). For example, aging alters the circadian rhythm of glucose utilization in the SCN, which is related to the timing of the luteinizing hormone (LH) surge of females (Wise, Cohen, Weiland, & London, 1988). Changes in the integrity of the SCN or in the ability of the SCN to entrain other neurochemical events may underlie some of the reproductive changes observed in older individuals.

A significant decrease in the volume and the number of neurons in the SCN was observed in both men and women ranging in age from 80 to 100 years compared with subjects in a 0- to 20-year-old group (Swaab, Fliers, & Partiman, 1985). The reduction in SCN cell number was especially pronounced in patients with senile dementia of the Alzheimer type (SDAT). Some Alzheimer's patients also show degeneration of the retina and optic nerve (reviewed in Swaab, Van Someren, Zhou, & Hofman, 1996), which are part of the visual input to the SCN. These results suggest that the presence of a structural defect in the SCN and/or input of the visual system to the SCN may underlie the general disturbance of biological rhythms in senescence and SDAT (Swaab et al., 1985; Swaab et al., 1996). Understanding the effects of aging on the expression and control of biological rhythms and sleep will become increasingly more important, especially as the average age of the human population increases.

SUMMARY

This chapter describes details of the methods and definitions used to investigate biological rhythms. The distinction was made among the different types of biological rhythms, which differ in their period, or time interval. Many different kinds of circadian rhythms can be measured in both human and non-human animals, and often these rhythms are entrained, or synchronized, to a *Zeitgeber*, such as the light (sun), social cues, or other "time givers." A variety of photic and nonphotic stimuli can produce phase shifts of circadian rhythms, such that they occur earlier (phase advance) or later (phase delay) than they ordinarily would without exposure to the stimulus.

In addition to circadian rhythms, many animals exhibit seasonal rhythms, in which various aspects of their physiology and/or behavior vary in response to changes in day length, or photoperiod. Such seasonal rhythms as migration, hibernation, and breeding enable the animal to survive and reproduce during optimal conditions related to climate, food and mate availability and avoidance of prey. Although modern humans have the *capacity* to respond to natural changes in day length, such responses normally do not occur, due to our use of artificial lighting.

Rhythms that persist and "free run" under constant environmental conditions are thought to be generated endogenously by an underlying pacemaker, or biological clock. In mammals, the biological clock is the suprachiasmatic nucleus of the hypothalamus, but the circadian system may be composed of additional pacemakers. The hormone melatonin which is produced at night by the pineal gland is involved in the control of seasonal rhythms. When administered exogenously, melatonin also has such varied effects as being able to entrain circadian rhythms, regulate core body temperature, and induce sleep.

Biological timekeeping is important for a number of reasons. Within the organism, the various rhythms of hormone release, body temperature, and system (e.g., cardiovascular) functioning are synchronized to each other. In addition, the organism's behaviors need to be synchronized to the outside world. Thus, sleep, motor activity, feeding, drinking, and breeding need to occur during the day and year when conditions are most appropriate. The internal rhythms are directly associated with these behaviors in a normal, healthy individual. However, if environmental conditions change dramatically, for example during rapid travel across time zones, the body needs to adjust to these changes. Until the adjustments are made, the individual will experience assorted symptoms of discomfort. In addition, psychiatric illnesses such as seasonal affective disorder (SAD) vary throughout the year in their severity. Administration of melatonin and other pharmacological agents and/or bright-light exposure are used to treat disorders of circadian timekeeping. Proper functioning of the circadian system is essential for the good health and well-being of the individual.

An important function that exhibits a circadian rhythm is the sleep-wake cycle. Electroencephalographic (EEG) recordings reveal distinct stages of sleep that differ in the type and proportion of brain waves found in each stage. Although the exact function of sleep is unknown, we know that sleep is adaptive and that all animals sleep. Results from sleep deprivation studies support the idea that sleep is a biological necessity, perhaps because it enables the brain to repair itself after the wear and tear of the prior period of wakefulness. Sleep also may have a thermoregulatory function in nonhuman animals. The sleep-wake cycle is tightly coupled to other circadian rhythms. Some circadian rhythms, such as the rhythms of body temperature and cortisol and ACTH secretion, are independent of sleep, while other variables, such as the secretion of growth hormone, are sleep dependent. Various models have been proposed to explain the regulation of sleep. The general agreement is that the timing of sleep and wakefulness results from both sleep-independent circadian factors, and homeostatic sleep-dependent processes.

The biological clock and its overt rhythms and various parameters related to sleep undergo changes as the individual ages. Increasing age affects the amount of time spent in different stages of sleep, the timing of when sleep occurs, and the quality of sleep that the individual gets. Although the biological clock is stable in many respects, it also is subject to changes in neural structure and/or integrity with advanced age.

CHAPTER 5

Time of Day, Alertness, and Performance

In unusual circumstances, such as jet lag and shift work, circadian rhythms affect human functioning in dramatic ways. The internal biological clock also affects functioning during normal routine. Many external and internal changes occur during the course of a person's day. These in turn affect all kinds of behaviors as well as cognitive and affective processes. *Motivation and alertness change in the course of a day,* and many other functions also change. Motivational processes have peaks and lows during the day, including hunger, thirst, and sexual motivation.

Circadian rhythms influence when one wants to eat or drink. People are hungry and thirsty during their waking and active hours and not during those times in the 24-hour day when they would normally be asleep. This is true also for nonhuman animals, like rats (Rosenwasser, Boulos, & Terman, 1981) and rabbits (Gieselman, Martin, Vanderweele, & Novin, 1980). The feeding and drinking behavior of animals as well as humans has identifiable patterns, with peaks and troughs over the 24-hour day (de Castro, 1987, 1991; Siegel & Stuckey, 1947; Spiteri, 1982; Stricker, 1991; Young & Richey, 1952). Moreover, when certain neurotransmitters, like norepinephrine, that alter feeding behavior (in terms of appetite-enhancing or appetite-reducing effects), are injected into specific sites in the hypothalamus of research animals, the effects are greatest at certain times in the 24-hour day (Rowland, Li, & Morien, 1996).

Researchers have assessed if taste preference varies according to time of day and not just according to hunger. Warwick, Costanzo, Gill, and Schiffman (1989) studied the sweetness preferences of women college students. The researchers gave subjects a rating scale to determine if they were restraining from eating in an effort to control food intake (high restraint) or if they ate in an unrestrained fashion (low restraint). They were given six concentrations of sucrose dissolved in water. Over several days, the subjects were given samples of the various sweet solutions and they gave what the researchers called "hedonic ratings" for each solution. The results showed that in the morning, the preference was significantly higher for the high-restraint women than for the low-restraint, and the preference difference between the two groups increased the more the solution was concentrated with sucrose. For subjects tested in the morning, low-restraint persons decreased their hedonic ratings the more the solution became sweet; high-restraint persons either increased or maintained their liking for the solution except when it reached the most concentrated sweetness level. In the evening the pattern was reversed. The high-restraint women showed a dislike of the concentrated solutions, and the low-restraint women had an overall greater preference than the high-restraint persons for the sweet solutions. Judgments and preference of sweetness thus interacted between amount of restraint (and thus possibly amount of hunger) and time of day of testing.

From the point of view of planning one's eating

patterns, these data have practical consequences. If people know their preferences across the time of day for certain foods, and they wish either to increase or decrease their overall daily food intake, such information can guide them in which foods to eat at what time of the day. Various explanations have been given for the change in sweetness judgments and preferences from morning to evening, but regardless of the explanation, practical applications are possible from such findings.

Alertness, mood, and performance vary during the 24-hour day in ways that can affect people's everyday lives. In daily life one can observe loss of concentration, increased errors in task performance, drowsiness, and a host of other changes as a result of difference in time of day. Subjective changes also occur, such as how peppy or sleepy one feels, how eager one is to do challenging work, and how one's mood changes. The present chapter considers both observable behavior and subjective assessment of internal states as a function of time of day. Arousal and energy mobilization clearly change across the span of a day, and for this reason time of day is an important factor in understanding motivation and action.

VARIABLES OF IMPORTANCE IN ADDITION TO TIME OF DAY

Time Since Sleeping

All of us have noticed that if we do not have a full night of sleep, the next day we can be groggy and drowsy. Studying all night for an upcoming exam can lead to unusual energy levels the next day. Equally, if we have more rest than usual, the following day we may feel more peppy than usual. In addition to considering *how much sleep* we had the night before, to assess our performance at a given time of day it is necessary to consider *how long ago that sleep occurred*. Reactions at 9:00 a.m. will be different if we have just awakened from a night's sleep or if we have been awake for 3 hours. How a person reacts at different times of the day may thus be a function of both the duration of sleep the previous night and the length of the preceding waking time (Koulack, 1997). Because sleep has a strong

impact on waking performance, some researchers have examined whether the sleep-wake cycle is more important than, for example, the temperature cycle in affecting specific reactions (Folkard, Wever, & Wildgruber, 1983).

Prior Activity

How a person reacts at different times of the day may be due to the types of prior activity engaged in by the person. The prior activity is likely to affect both the quality of performance and the degree of arousal that is present at a certain moment. Prior activity can alter performance independent of what time of day it happens. This has been found in studies of learning and cognition. Before one can conclude that performance is changed due to time-of-day effects, one needs to know the nature of the individual's prior activity. Studies of learning and cognition have shown that such activity can alter performance due to (1) *interference,* caused by negative transfer or fatigue, or (2) *facilitation,* resulting from warm-up, learning-how-to-learn, positive transfer or priming.

Interference. This effect occurs when prior activities have a negative impact on actions of the moment. One type of interference is called "negative transfer," which means that doing one activity intrudes into the effective performance of the subsequent activity. For example, if a student is studying for an exam in 19th century European history and then tries to write an essay on women's efforts to obtain the right to vote in the United States early in the 20th century, interfering ideas from the first task may slow down performance on the second task.

A second type of interference relates to fatigue. If one has performed many tasks, a temporary inhibitory process can set in, which interferes with performing additional tasks. This can occur at any time of day. If performance on cognitive tasks is compared at 4:00 p.m. with such performance at 10:00 a.m., by 4:00 p.m. many cognitive events will have occurred that leave an inhibitory effect, compared with 10:00 a.m. when one is relatively "fresh." If a researcher tests subjects at different times and wants to assess "time-of-day" effects, the researcher needs to control the amount of activities subjects engage in prior to testing.

Facilitation. Prior activity also can facilitate performance. For example, athletes, musicians, and a host of other individuals know that peak performance is not attained without previous warming-up activity. Pitchers do not throw their first ball in a game without prior throwing activity, runners do not run a race without first doing limbering-up and stretching exercises, and pianists as well as other musicians would not perform a concert without considerable prior exercising of the appropriate actions. Research has shown the effect of warm-up in verbal tasks. If someone learns two or three lists of words and each list has no specific transfer effects (not specifically interfering with or facilitating the learning of the subsequent list), the more the person practices learning the word lists, the more will learning improve in a nonspecific way. Some nonspecific effects are due to "learning-to-learn" (Postman & Schwartz, 1964), but some are due to warm-up (Thune, 1951). The effect of warm-up is short term, lasting up to about 1 hour, whereas learning-to-learn can lead to facilitation up to a much longer time (24 hr). When considering the effects of circadian rhythms on performance, it is important to note that a later time in the day could permit more facilitation than an earlier time simply because no warm-up activity preceded the earlier observation.

In addition to the nonspecific types of transfer like warm-up and learning-how-to-learn, specific transfer can facilitate performance. It is called "positive transfer" (Dallett, 1962). For example, if one learns to drive a stick-shift Honda, one does not need to learn all over again to drive a stick-shift Toyota, since learning to do the first task easily transfers to the second task. In verbal learning, similar facilitating effects from a prior activity occur in learning or performing a subsequent task.

Performance also can be facilitated by priming, which affects a number of cognitive processes. For example, if the person has just seen the word "nurse" and the word "doctor" is quickly flashed on a screen, the second word will be recognized sooner

than if the first word had been "purse" or "horse." A great deal of research has shown that semantic relatedness and simple associations can speed up processing of relevant information (e.g., Ratcliff & McKoon, 1981). In the laboratory, facilitation due to priming has been shown in experiments on lexical decisions (Meyer, Schvaneveldt, & Ruddy, 1974), in which subjects have to indicate whether visual stimuli are words or nonwords. Priming also has been shown in anagram studies, in which subjects have to make words out of scrambled letters (Dominowski & Ekstrand, 1967). If items are the same on two or more tasks, or if they are associated or semantically related, faster and more accurate performance will be evident. This type of priming can be found in many kinds of tasks. For this reason many clerical jobs, and work that involves processing of related concepts, will likely show improved performance after enough preceding related activity has occurred. For one to conclude that variables involved in time of day (and possibly circadian rhythms) are responsible for performance peaks, we need to be sure that priming is not the reason for certain work being performed better late, rather than early, in the day.

Stimulation and Goals

An important variable that can affect performance and motivation, and that can mask the effects of time of day, is the *amount of stimulation* that is present in one's environment at a given moment. If at 9:00 a.m. the room is very quiet and the input for action and thought comes primarily from internal factors, the way an individual reacts will be different than if much stimulation occurs in the surroundings. Thus, at 9:00 a.m. on a weekend morning, with little external stimulation, one is likely to react very differently than at the same time on a Tuesday morning, when one is at a busy office in a work environment or in a student cafeteria with bustle and noise. External stimulation as well as amount of sleep, time since sleeping, and type of intervening activity may all play a role as "masking" factors, which is a term used by Folkard, Marks, Minors, and Waterhouse (1985). Such factors have an impact on behavior and can mask what would otherwise be assumed to be time-of-day effects due to endogenous circadian rhythms.

Studies of normal subjects going about their routine activities at various times in the day may involve different stimulation, like social and family interactions (Folkard, Minors, & Waterhouse, 1985), and these experiences can limit conclusions about time-of-day effects. To overcome these problems, controlled laboratory experiments provide the most convincing data about behavioral and physiological rhythms. Under controlled conditions subjects are isolated from their normal routines and are provided with prepared schedules of stimulation, tasks, and amount of allowed sleep. When all subjects receive controlled stimulation and activities, more valid conclusions can be drawn about circadian rhythms as well as their possible interaction with individual differences. In normal daily routine, both the surrounding stimulation and the individual's goal for activity at a given time in the day will affect how the person reacts. If at 9:00 a.m. one is busy studying for an examination that will take place in 2 hours, focus of attention, arousal, and directed motivation will all be different than if at 9:00 a.m. one faces a long day of boring work or chores. If one is under time pressure and directing one's energies toward specific accomplishments, the effect of time of day may be relatively negligible in comparison with other variables.

Many factors can diminish or heighten the outward manifestation of the working of an internal clock. This is important to consider when one examines the results of studies on effects of time of day. Many studies reveal that some individuals perform better on certain tasks in the morning and other persons perform better on the task later in the day, and caution is required in interpreting such data. Until one can determine that volitional sleep patterns (when the individuals go to sleep and when they awaken), contextual stimulation, prior activity patterns, stimulation exposure, and individual goals are comparable for these persons, differences in their reactions at a given time of day may not be due to effects of the internal clock as much as a function of other important but nontiming variables.

ARE THERE SEVERAL RHYTHMS?

Sleep Compared with Temperature Rhythms

The sleep-wake cycle relates to various other circadian rhythms, and the cycle is altered by changed conditions, such as shift work. Controlled laboratory studies and observation of night workers have shown that daytime sleep differs from night sleep. One difference is that from 1 to 4 fewer hours of sleep occur in the day than at night (Folkard, Minors, & Waterhouse, 1985). This would help explain why night workers tend to fall asleep at work more than do day workers, why they sleep more during their off-work days, and why they have more naps during nonworking time. In other words, sleeping in the daytime rather than at night creates a sleep deficit, which is made up at other times. Day sleep also differs from night sleep in the distribution of sleep stages throughout sleep. Whereas during normal night sleep the slow-wave stages (3 and 4) occur toward the beginning, daytime sleep does not show this dominance early in sleep. Moreover, stage 2 and REM sleep rather than the slow-wave stages tend to get lost with the briefer day sleep, and instead of REM sleep lasting longer as sleep continues, it may even become shorter at the later end of sleep. One possible explanation for these differences between day and night sleep is that the body temperature rhythm does not coincide with the sleep-wake cycle when the latter is altered. It is difficult to fall asleep when body temperature is high, and sleep duration is shortened if the temperature does not fall just before starting sleep (Folkard, Minors, & Waterhouse, 1985). Temperature rhythms and sleep-wake cycles are important in their interrelationship as well as in their joint effects on performance.

Laboratory studies have assessed these two variables in controlled environments. Two types of environments have been used to study the relationship between sleep and temperature rhythms. One is an isolated environment in which the light-dark schedule is maintained at the normal 24 hours but all other external stimuli are artificially controlled. In the second environment a "fractional desynchronization technique" is employed that progressively shortens or lengthens subjects' days by use of artificial zeitgebers, as used in one study by Folkard, Wever, and Wildgruber (1983). In this study the subjects were isolated for close to 28 days. They received artificial light and dark zeitgebers, and some were on a schedule that was progressively shortened by 5 minutes per cycle, shortening the day from 24 to 22 hours. Other subjects had a schedule in which the zeitgebers progressively lengthened by 10 minutes per cycle, lengthening the day to be up to 26 to 29 hours. Rectal temperature was taken regularly, and sleep onset and sleep offset were recorded by the subjects' pushing buttons when they retired and awakened. The sleep-wake cycle was found to follow the zeitgeber period during the study. After a number of days, the temperature rhythm separated from the sleep-wake cycle and showed a free-running period between 24 and 25 hours. This separation has been found to occur in many other studies, including one that employed the same fractional desynchronization technique but recorded sleep by means of polygraph recordings (Folkard, Hume, Minors, Waterhouse, & Watson, 1985) rather than relying merely on subjects' button pressing to signal start and stop of sleep.

Because the sleep-wake cycle appeared to be influenced by external stimuli more than the temperature rhythm, researchers concluded that temperature was the more endogenous rhythm, set by the biological clock. Because the temperature rhythm seemed to be the more endogenous, some researchers initially thought that time-of-day effects on performance were influenced by the temperature rhythm. However, additional findings suggest that performance may relate to an independent alertness-sleepiness variable that is separate from both the sleep-wake cycle and the temperature rhythm (Folkard, Marks, et al., 1985).

Alertness-Sleepiness

The usual assumption by lay people is that "feeling sleepy" as a subjective experience is highly correlated with "being sleepy" as an objective condition. However, as noted by Horne (1988), the need for sleep has two components, one being a biological necessity and the other an optional, nonbiological,

state that is a motivation. Coming from different perspectives, other researchers have also pointed out that objective sleepiness is different from subjective sleepiness (Monk, 1987).

Several ways of measuring subjective sleepiness exist. Thayer (1989), for example, had a "tiredness" component in his AD ACL (Activation-Deactivation Adjective Check List) multidimensional activation test, which measures the strength of deactivation-sleep with items like sleepy, tired, drowsy, and sluggish. Subjects give self-ratings on a 4-point scale, according to the extent that the item word describes their feelings at the moment: vv (definitely feel that way at the moment), v (slightly feel that way at the moment), ? (the word does not apply at the moment), no (definitely do not feel that way at the moment). This method of measurement permits direct ratings of tiredness or sleepiness, separate from direct ratings of activation or alertness. There are advantages to such measurements in which each type of item receives its own score. Other researchers prefer a different approach (Folkard, Hume, et al., 1985; Monk, 1987), in which subjects place a mark on a line that goes from "very sleepy" at one end to "very alert" at the other end. A score is obtained by the experimenter's measuring the distance of the mark from the left end. Monk (1987), in describing this as a visual analogue scale, stated that when subjects are required to make numerous repeated indications of their sleepiness, this is a useful, sensitive, and brief procedure.

In reviewing several studies, Monk (1987) pointed out that when subjects were in a constant environment in an isolated experimental setting for 72 hours under conditions of uniform food intake and without knowledge of clock time, their sleepiness-alertness correlated significantly with body temperature. When temperature fell, so did alertness, with low temperature indicating high sleepiness. In field studies, in which measurements were taken in actual work settings and subjects lived normal lives, sleepiness again correlated with body temperature, with maximum sleepiness and lowest body temperature occurring around 6:00 a.m. Of greatest interest, however, in terms of comparing objective sleepiness with subjective sleepiness, is the fact that objectively people tend to be sleepy in the early afternoon, which is just the time people report high subjective alertness (low subjective sleepiness). Figure 5.1 illustrates data from a study by Monk and Embrey (1981), with highest subjective alertness evident at noon although body temperature peaks at 8:00 p.m.

To identify the separate roles of the temperature and the sleep-wake cycles, researchers in a different study (Monk, 1987) used the desynchronization technique already described. Four subjects in an isolated environment were given sleep-wake cycles different from 24 hours, and although "day length" defined in this way varied from 23 to 26 hours, the temperature cycle remained between 24.3 and 24.8 hours. In that study subjects were asked to rate only sleepiness, not also alertness, on the visual analog scale. Subjects marked on a line how sleepy they felt, from "very little" at the left end to "very much" at the right end. Recordings were made about six times each day. Bedtime and wake time were prescribed and not voluntary. The least sleepiness occurred about 6 hours after subjects awoke, which

confirmed the overall finding of other studies done in the laboratory and in normal life environments, with the lowest subjective sleepiness occurring at what would be around 1:00 p.m. in the normal sleep-waking day. As in other studies, the four subjects experienced the least sleepiness at the time of their peak temperature. The overall conclusion from that study is that both temperature and time since awakening affect how sleepy (and by implicating the reverse, how alert) subjects feel themselves to be. Moreover, subjective sleepiness and objective sleepiness (measured by physiological and other behavioral measures) appear to differ markedly. Especially in isolated environments, when subjects do not know what the time is nor when other normal external zeitgebers are present, objective sleepiness is high at the very time of day when subjective sleepiness is low. Other studies, with different subjects, have provided data that support this conclusion (Monk, Moline, Fookson, & Peetz, 1989).

Monk (1991) suggested that subjective sleepi-

FIGURE 5.1

The circadian rhythms of oral temperature (●—●) and self-rated alertness (O- - -O). Two cycles of the 12 points defining each rhythm have been plotted.

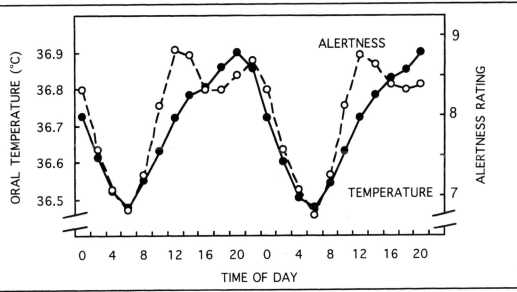

Source: From Monk & Embrey, 1981, p. 475.

ness functions like a "circadian messenger" and that it is adaptive and beneficial for subjective sleepiness to be linked to the temperature rhythm. Following a temperature peak at about 8:00 p.m. both temperature and alertness drop in parallel fashion. Since under normal circumstances subjective sleepiness leads to the decision to go to sleep, it is adaptive for subjective sleepiness to increase (and thus trigger the decision to go to sleep) in the later evening. Additionally, for cultures in which people do not take naps after lunch, it is adaptive that subjective and objective sleepiness peak at different times. Subjective sleepiness is low around 1:00 p.m. even though at that time objective sleepiness is high, which means that in nonnapping societies it is easy for people to refrain from going to bed in the early afternoon.

The complex relationship between alertness, temperature, and objective sleepiness also suggests that *arousal* is not manifested as a single dimension. Not only are alertness ratings high near midday when temperature is high and objective sleepiness is high, but subjective alertness peaks earlier than does temperature. A divergence between temperature and alertness occurs between 4:00 p.m. and 8:00 p.m. The data show that subjective and objective sleepiness peak at different times in the day and that subjective sleepiness is partly determined by the temperature rhythm and partly by the sleep-wake cycle (Monk, 1991; Monk & Moline, 1989). These data do not fit a simple arousal pattern.

PERFORMANCE VARIES WITH ALERTNESS AND TIME OF DAY

Many studies have investigated how performance and mood vary with time of day, but only a few have held the most relevant variables constant. Fortunately, enough studies used important controls, which permits valid conclusions to be drawn that are relevant to the field of motivation.

Performance and Alertness

An ingenious study controlled for the sleep-wake time and the types of intervening activities (Folkard, Marks, & Froberg, 1986). It compared the effect of

time of day on several physiological measures, on alertness, and on different types of performance. Subjects were placed on a constant routine for 75 hours after they had had a normal night's sleep. Starting at 8:00 a.m., the room temperature, light, and noise levels were held constant, and subjects had no knowledge of clock time. Following a short time for relaxation, subjects performed the same group of tests every 3 hours over the 75-hour session. During each 3 hours they recorded temperature and pulse and made affective ratings. Factor analysis of these ratings revealed two factors, one of alertness and one of fatigue. Food and water intake were of controlled amounts and given at prescribed times. Urine samples were taken, from which data on adrenalin and noradrenalin were obtained. All subjects had a preset routine, so that any differences in performance on the various tasks could be explained by time-of-day effects and not by any effect due to a difference in prior activities.

Several tasks were investigated in this study. Subjects were given performance tests that involved different kinds of abilities, such as sustained attention in the vigilance task, short-term memory (STM) in the digit span task, a complex mix of STM and longer-term memory in a coding task, and complex information processing in a syllogistic reasoning task. Subjective alertness was related to performance in different ways, depending on the nature of the task: for some tasks an increase in alertness related with improvement in performance, for other tasks it related with impairment in performance. An important question for the motivation psychologist is whether the correlation observed between such endogenously generated subjective alertness and performance is also obtained when alertness is induced exogenously. That is, in a time-of-day study like that of Folkard and colleagues (1986), the alertness-performance relationships are correlational in nature. It is not possible to identify whether the endogenously generated alertness alters the performance, or whether both are altered by some common influence.

In digit span, subjects recall a series of digits. Peak and trough levels of performance on this task showed a shorter period (21.66 hours) than on other tasks. Poorest STM digit recall occurred in the hours from late morning to early afternoon (depending on when in the 21-hour period the digit span task was performed). The poor STM performance occurred when body temperature and self-rated alertness were high. This inverse relationship between subjective alertness (and body temperature) and performance on a short-term memory task appears to be a general finding. It contrasts with performance on a vigilance task, in which the subjects have to give sustained attention to a simple, unchallenging, series of events or signals. Vigilance typically covaries with subjective alertness and body temperature, and under the present controlled and constant conditions, the study confirmed this relationship.

Alertness (based on self-ratings) had a mean period of 25.65 hours, which was longer than the periods of most of the other variables. (The alertness period was similar to the 25.48 hours found in another study by Folkard, Hume, et al. (1985), in which the body temperature rhythm was dissociated from that of the alertness rhythm.) The subjects' temperature, adrenalin level, amount of fatigue, and most of the performance measures, however, revealed periods that were approximately 24 hours. Noradrenalin secretion and pulse rate tended *not* to have endogenous periods, which corroborates findings of other studies that suggest these two variables are largely under external influences. Only when rhythms are largely under endogenous influence do they tend to show clear periods under constant routine conditions such as were used in the present study. Thus, several *performance* measures showed clear periods, whereas some physiological variables (noradrenalin secretion and pulse rate) did not.

Subjective fatigue had a slightly different rhythm than did subjective alertness. Although a number of performance measures covaried with subjective fatigue, the performance covariation was less than with subjective alertness. That fatigue (extracted from factor analysis of affective ratings) is not quite the inverse of alertness suggests that measuring these two factors with separate scales, as done by Thayer (1987), is justified.

A different study, done by Horowitz, Wolfe, and Czeisler (1998), duplicated as well as extended the findings of Folkard and colleagues (1986). Under very tightly controlled conditions, which permitted analysis of circadian rhythms independent from extraneous variables, reaction time (RT) was found to be far faster later in the day, when temperature and alertness were highest. Errors in a search task (whether or not a target was present among distractor stimuli) were greater when temperature and subjective alertness were low. Allocation of attentional resources, measured by a complex cognitive search task, did not mirror the circadian pattern for simple RT: Although subjects slow down at certain times of low alertness, their search efficiency is not necessarily worse for large compared with small sets of stimuli.

Different Tasks Show Different Effects

Monk (1990) showed that various types of tasks have different effects on performance, depending on when the task is done. Tasks emphasizing perceptual search have a different peak than those involving reasoning and abstract cognitions, and these in turn have different peaks for memory tasks. When Folkard, Wever, and Wildgruber (1983) studied subjects in isolation for approximately 28 days, the verbal reasoning task showed peak performance (maximum speed on the task) around the middle of the waking day. Letter cancellation and verbal reasoning performance differed in their sensitivity to external versus endogenous factors. The researchers suggested that performance on these two tasks may be controlled by different circadian oscillators: performance that does not rely primarily on memory is controlled by an oscillator responsible for body temperature, whereas a 21-hour oscillator controls more memory-demanding performance, such as is required in a reasoning task.

Because the Folkard et al. (1986) study showed that performance on a pure memory task (digit recall) is related inversely to an endogenous rhythm like subjective alertness, the question remains whether different oscillators control different types of performance (as Folkard et al. [1983] suggested). Considerable evidence shows that different kinds of memory are affected differently by time of day. Monk (1990) indicated that when memory is tested shortly after the material is presented, the performance is best fairly early in the morning and is poor later in the afternoon or evening. A study by Oakhill (1988) supports this hypothesis. Oakhill gave university students text material to read, and the exact wording was to be recalled 2 minutes after subjects read the paragraph. The task involved relatively short-term memory. Oakhill found better recall of the text paragraph in the morning between 9:00 and 10:00 a.m. compared with late afternoon between 5:00 and 6:00 p.m.

The superiority of morning for immediate recall contrasts with performance on a memory task that involves a day or a week delay. According to Monk (1990), long-term memory is best in the later part of the waking day. This was found with schoolchildren and also with night nurses. The latter were shown a training film either at 4:00 a.m. or at 8:30 p.m. Regardless of when the recall test was given, the material presented early in the morning was remembered best for *immediate recall* and the material presented late in the day was remembered best for *delayed recall*. For schoolchildren as well as night nurses, the time of day when the recall test was given proved to have no significant effect. The time-of-day effect can be said to influence encoding and, probably even more importantly, the *storage* stage of learning, but not to influence the *retrieval* stage during recall.

Studies on mood and memory, to be further discussed in a later chapter, show that mood tends to affect learning but has a weaker effect on retrieval (Bower, 1981). The variables of mood and of time of day thus in part are similar, since retrieval conditions appear not to be crucial for either time of day or mood. These variables also are different, however, since time of day seems to affect primarily storage and mood affects primarily encoding. The data cited by Monk (1990) suggest that subjects store information differently in the morning versus the late afternoon or evening. This is only a tentative conclusion. More clear-cut data are required to verify that these variables differ in terms of encoding versus storage effects.

Monk (1990) pointed out that search tasks with high memory loads (e.g., six letters to search) produce peaks and troughs in performance similar to those produced by immediate memory tasks involving other kinds of remembering, such as recall of prose. That is, when search tasks involve a fairly high memory load, performance is best in the early morning and tends to be poorest in the late afternoon or early evening. Figure 5.2 illustrates some of these findings.

An answer to the question of how time of day affects digit span or any other type of STM performance will depend on when the peak occurs for a person's subjective alertness and body temperature. If sleep deprivation is induced, the peak performance and the time when the best performance occurs are likely to change further. For example, Monk and his colleagues (Monk, Buysse, Reynolds, Jarrett, & Kupfer, 1992) found that although temperature rose after a trough that appeared about 20 hours following the start of a 36-hour study, in which subjects were isolated and sleep deprived, many performance scores continued to drop, probably due to the sleep deprivation. The drop in performance was found for young (mean age of 25.6 years) as well as old (mean age of 82.0 years) men, but it was more marked for the older subjects.

It is clear that for tasks relying on *simple perceptual and attentional* processes, the *endogenous rhythms* of the individual are likely to affect peak performance, whereas on tasks of problem solving, reasoning, and more demanding cognitions, these rhythms are less likely to be influential. However, the correlation between body temperature and performance on certain tasks may simply be due to independent circadian rhythms that are "in phase" with each other (reviewed in Wilkinson, 1982). Monk, Buysse, et al. (1992), in line with others, suggested that cortical rather than lower-level circadian processes may influence various psychological functions. The data of studies reviewed above have relevance for the demands of a complex society in a modern world. In that society humans are increasingly required to engage in problem-solving and reasoning tasks, so that a relative "freedom" from endogenous noncortical rhythms for this type of performance would be highly adaptive.

Performance on a wide range of tasks (both mental and physical) varies considerably at different times of the day. Many human performance

FIGURE 5.2

The time-of-day function for low- (two-letter), medium- (four-letter), and high- (six-letter) memory load versions of a serial search task (●—●) plotted together with rectal temperature (O—O).

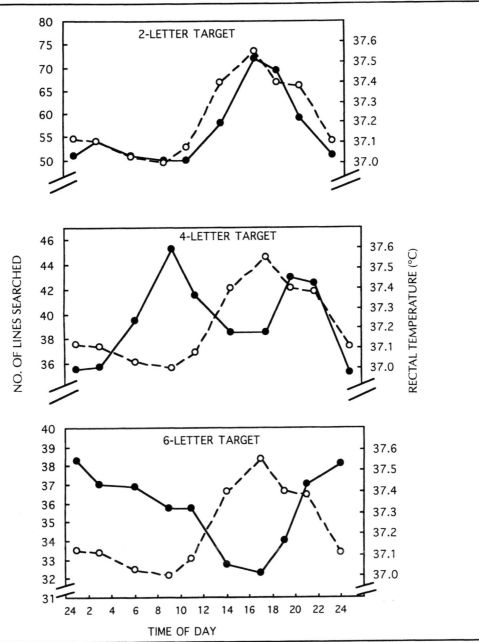

Source: From Monk, 1990.

measures follow a pattern of high performance in the late afternoon/evening, reaching a nadir (low point) in the early morning hours (Reilly, Waterhouse, & Atkinson, 1997). A number of factors can affect the phase, amplitude, and detailed shape of these circadian variations. The existence of a circadian rhythm of performance suggests that it might be affected by alterations in external timing cues, such as those associated with shift work.

TIME OF DAY, SHIFT WORK, AND MOOD

Two major variables have important effects on all performance measures: *body temperature* and the *sleep-wake cycle*. Time since awakening and amount of sleep or extent of sleep deprivation also are very important.

Monk, Buysse, et al. (1992) reviewed the model proposed by Borbely (1982). A rhythmic process, like temperature, acts like a "self-sustaining oscillator with a momentum of its own" (Monk, Buysse, et al., 1992, p. 221). A homeostatic process, which is involved in the sleep-wake cycle, "acts like a capacitor, building up during wakefulness and discharging during sleep" (Monk, Buysse et al., 1992, p. 221). This homeostatic process relates to the wear and tear experienced during the time that the individual is awake.

Shift Work

Most people can tolerate an occasional adjustment to a new time without too much discomfort, but repeated shifts in rest-activity schedules, such as those associated with rotating shift work schedules, present much greater stress. Although definitions of shift work vary, 15% to 25% of the working population in industrialized countries are shift workers (Moore-Ede, Sulzman, & Fuller, 1982). Shift work has developed because of the demand for 24-hour service in hospitals, transportation, and emergency services; because of the economic demands for expensive equipment to be used around the clock; and because of the need for continuous attention to technological processes in the steel, energy and chemical industries. Shift work schedules vary in the length of work per schedule (e.g., 6–12 hours in length), rotation interval of the schedule (workers may rotate every few days or every month or simply shift to a permanent schedule), and the direction of the rotation (some workers may rotate by successive delays and others may rotate by successive advances). Some workers always work the night shift, but they may be subject to shifting environmental schedules if they are active during the daytime on weekends and vacations. The ability of shift workers to phase shift to a different schedule is highly variable and is dependent upon a number of factors. These include both intrinsic factors, such as sex, age, and circadian propensity ("morningness" or "eveningness"), and extrinsic factors, such as shift work schedule, intensity of social interactions, and amount and timing of light exposure (Sack & Lewy, 1997).

The health consequences of night work and shift work include increased risk of cardiovascular illness, gastrointestinal disorders including ulcers, infertility, and sleep disorders such as chronic fatigue and insomnia (Moore-Ede et al., 1982; see review by Czeisler et al., 1990). Studies have shown that even after several years, workers on permanent or rotating night shifts do not show a complete physiological adaptation of endogenous circadian rhythms to such an inversion of the daily routine (see review by Czeisler, et al., 1990). Physiological maladaptation to an inverted schedule results in diminished performance and alertness during nighttime work, with the number of fatigue-related accidents increased during nighttime and early morning hours (Czeisler et al., 1990; Moore-Ede et al., 1982). The neural processes controlling alertness and sleep produce an increased sleep tendency and diminished capacity to function during certain early morning hours (circa 2–7 a.m.) and, to a lesser degree, during a period in the midafternoon (circa 2–5 p.m.) whether or not the person has slept (Mitler et al., 1988). The incidence of work errors, including the number of errors in reading meters or in answering warning signals, or the delay before answering the telephone, all increase in the early morning hours (see review by Moore-Ede et al., 1982). These findings are in agreement with results from laboratory tests of human performance that show that psychomotor ability and the capability for mental arithmetic fall to a minimum between 3 and 5 a.m. Unfortunately, this pattern is reflected in mistakes made in a whole range of tasks as well as catastrophic events that implicate human error at night. Many of the major accidents at nuclear power plants have occurred when workers were on the night shift. For example, the 1979 accident at the Three Mile Island nuclear power plant occurred at 4 a.m., the middle of the night shift (11 p.m.–7 a.m.) with a crew that had been on night duty for only a few days and had been rotating shifts around the clock on a weekly basis for the previous 6 weeks (Moore-Ede et al., 1982). Another example is the Chernobyl nuclear power plant catastrophe, which occurred at 1:23 a.m. as a result of human error (Milter et al., 1988). The operator in a control room at a nuclear power plant works with a wide array of instruments and instrument panels. In this monotonous environment, the operator must demonstrate a high degree of vigilance and performance on psychomotor tasks such as responding to emergency calls and reading meters. Unfortunately, these actions often are impaired during the night shift when the workers are forced to perform mental and/or physical tasks at an inappropriate time relative to the internal clock.

Superimposed on the normal two peaks of sleep vulnerability are the cumulative effects of sleep deprivation, which might occur during accommodation to an unusual work schedule, and sleep disruption, which could occur as a result of a sleep disorder (Mitler et al., 1988). The effects of such sleep loss are cumulative, and continued sleep loss, or "sleep debt," increases the chance of error due to sudden overwhelming sleepiness. Although most individuals cope with sleep debt by physical activity and dietary stimulants, coping mechanisms can temporarily make an individual completely unaware of a dangerous accumulated sleep loss (Mitler et al., 1988). Even a brief episode of sleep, such as the "microsleeps" described by Liberson (1945), could result in serious error.

Disruptions of mealtimes and rest periods are the obvious causes of gastrointestinal and sleep disorders experienced by shift workers (Moore-Ede et al., 1982). For example, food is provided at times that may not be compatible with the endogenous circadian rhythms of gastrointestinal function. Similarly, if workers are not able to sleep at the normal phase of the circadian cycle, they may try to sleep at the maximum of their endogenous rhythm of alertness, resulting in failure to obtain the needed rest. Shift work schedules also cause stress in family and social life because workers are out of synchrony with their family and friends. Thus, environmental cycles, such as light-dark, social cues, and food availability, that normally synchronize the circadian system are disrupted and may even provide conflicting phase information. With continuous shifting, the body is constantly in a state of transient internal desynchronization, in which the internal rhythms are not synchronized to each other.

The simplest treatment for shift workers with medical problems resulting from their work schedule is to avoid shift work altogether and to work during regular daytime hours (Moore-Ede et al., 1982). If shift work must be done, there are some treatments to choose from. Melatonin, when given at the optimal circadian time, has been shown to facilitate phase shifting of shift workers (Sack & Lewy, 1997). The effect may be caused by melatonin's phase-shifting effects or its sleep-promoting actions, or both. Physical exercise has been suggested as an aid to adjust to a new light-dark cycle. In a laboratory study, a single episode of nocturnal intense exercise induced, within one day, 1- to 2-hour phase delays in endocrine markers in young volunteers (Van Reeth et al., 1994). Field studies also have shown the beneficial effects of physical exercise in adjusting to a new shift schedule, as well as improved sleep quality and performance (e.g., Eastman, Hoese, Youngstedt, & Liu, 1995; Harma, Ilmarinen, Knauth, Rutenfranz, & Hanninen, 1988a, 1988b).

Scheduled exposure of shift workers to bright light at night and darkness during the day effectively treated the maladaptation of the circadian system to night work (Czeisler et al., 1990). Night workers in the control group did desk work under ordinary lighting conditions (approximately 150 lux), then went home to sleep in their usual bedrooms. In contrast, night workers in the experimental group worked under bright artificial light

(7,000–12,000 lux), then returned home to bedrooms that had been modified so that incoming sunlight was blocked. On the sixth night of this rigorous schedule of exposure to bright light and darkness, workers in the experimental group exhibited a successful circadian adaptation to daytime sleep and nighttime work. In addition to shifts in the circadian rhythm of body temperature, patterns of 24-hour plasma cortisol concentration, and urinary excretion rate, workers in the experimental group showed appropriate shifts in subjective assessment of alertness and cognitive performance. These shifts resulted in a significant improvement in both cognitive performance and alertness. The control workers did not adapt to the nighttime work schedule. Czeisler and colleagues (1990) attributed their results to the synchronizing effects of bright light on the human circadian system. However, exposure to darkness during the period of daytime sleep also may have facilitated the adaptation to the work schedule, directly or indirectly (Van Cauter & Turek, 1990). In animals housed in constant light, exposure to darkness can cause phase shifts in the circadian activity rhythm; these phase-shifting effects of dark pulses may be mediated by behavioral events such as the associated increase in locomotor activity (Van Reeth & Turek, 1989). Thus, in the Czeisler and colleagues (1990) study the differences between control and experimental subjects in their rate of adaptation to the night work schedule may be due to a combination of behavioral differences (e.g., the experimental subjects slept an average of 2 hours longer during the dark portion and were more alert during the light portion than the control subjects) and differences in the light-dark cycle. The very intense light used in the initial study may not even be necessary, because ordinary room light has been shown to reset human circadian rhythms of melatonin and cortisol concentrations (Boivin & Czeisler, 1998).

When scheduling shift workers, managers must look at the entire situation, including the job type and social and domestic issues, before deciding on the speed of the rotation (Monk, 1986). In addition, whether an individual will or will not cope with shift work is affected by the individual's age (increasing age is associated with decreased tolerance

of shift work) and his or her circadian type (individuals of the "morning type" seem to have a lower tolerance of shift work than do "evening types") (Reilly, Waterhouse, & Atkinson, 1997). Some workers prefer to be assigned permanently to a given shift so that they have ample time to adjust to their work schedule. However, the disadvantage of this schedule is a gradual buildup of sleep loss. Other workers prefer fast-rotating schedules with 1 or 2 days on each shift, which does not allow enough time to resynchronize to any new schedule, but results in less accumulation of sleep deficit. Both of these rotation speeds are well represented in the scheduling practices of thousands of companies involving millions of employees (Monk, 1986). Because the period of the endogenous rhythm is longer than 24 hours, the human circadian system adjusts more rapidly to phase delays than to phase advances of the sleep-wake cycle (Czeisler, Moore-Ede, & Coleman, 1982). In other words, it is easier to stay up later on a subsequent work shift than to go to sleep earlier. Thus, shift workers adjust better to clockwise rotating schedules (morning shift to afternoon shift to night shift) than to a counterclockwise rotating schedule (night to afternoon to morning shifts). The most unsatisfying schedules seem to be those that change once a week, because the individual is always in a state of readjustment to a new schedule and yet has enough time to accumulate a sleep debt (Moore-Ede et al., 1982). An educated decision about the speed of the shift rotation should lead to optimal employee morale, productivity, health, and safety.

Mood Changes

Monk, Buysse, and colleagues (1992) did a sleep deprivation study in which young (20–30 years) and old (80 years and over) men went without sleep for 36 hours. Throughout that time, subjects rated their mood according to a method developed by Monk (1989). In a visual analog scale rating along 10-cm lines, subjects made a checkmark to indicate how much "effort is it to do anything?" as well as how alert, tense, sleepy, and so on they felt. The lines were anchored with end points that extended from "very little" to "very much." Two measures resulted from these ratings: global vigor (representing felt alertness and weariness), and global affect (representing happiness and calm).

When each subject's ratings were compared with his own mean, global vigor decreased steadily for the older subjects and generally decreased for the younger subjects, with a trough for the younger men after 24 hours of sleep deprivation and confinement, from which vigor rose somewhat. Global affect for the younger men had an even more severe trough followed by a rise after 24 hours. As can be seen in Figure 5.3, the manual dexterity measure and the visual search speed tend to covary with the global affect trough and rise for the younger men, but the pattern is different for the older men. The temperature trough (not shown) occurred at about the same time as the global affect trough for the younger men, but neither their global affect nor their performance rose to the height of the temperature rebound. The loss of vigor and positive affect appear to be a function of the time of confinement and sleep deprivation as well as of the temperature drop.

Performance more closely resembled the vigor and affect loss than the temperature curve, especially as the duration of the deprivation continued. This loss appears to be a good indicator of the homeostatic process, related to the "wear and tear" of sleep deprivation. Thus, when subjects are in a confined and relatively constant environment, mood is complexly related to both rhythmic and homeostatic processes. One can expect that in a varying rather than constant environment, even more complexity exists regarding the factors that influence mood.

Social processes also have been studied in regard to 24-hour patterns. The "Social Rhythm Metric" measures the extent to which the events in an individual's daily life are social rather than solitary (Monk, Flaherty, Frank, Hoskinson, & Kupfer, 1990). Typical daily activities were marked by subjects in terms of the persons involved, such as "have breakfast" or "start work" with, for example, spouse, or friend, or alone. This social measurement has been studied with younger and older subjects (Monk, Reynolds, Machen, & Kupfer, 1992). It is well established that sleep disturbances are characteristic of older age. Early indications with

FIGURE 5.3

Ratings of global affect (A), speed of manual dexterity (B), and speed of visual search (C), expressed as a percentage of each subject's own 36-hour mean, averaged over nine young men (broken line) and nine older men (solid line), plotted as a function of time of day.

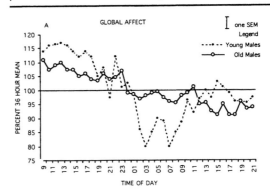

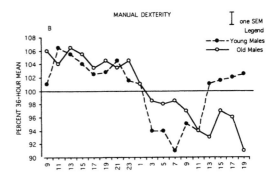

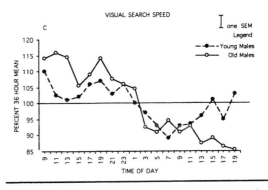

Source: From Monk, Buysse, Reynolds, Jarrett & Kupfer, 1992.

research using the Social Rhythm Metric shows that the sleep disturbances in older people are not attributable to disturbances in their "social rhythm," that is, in the social patterns that occur during a 24-hour day. For young as well as older people, complex factors shape the way mood and performance covary and the way mood and performance change over a 24-hour day. Aging affects the mood-performance relationship, and it is important to understand how mood and performance covary in older compared with young persons.

Mood relates to the 24-hour day differently in real-life settings than in isolation laboratories. In the above research by Monk and colleagues, mood was measured by nine visual analog scales, which yielded global measures of vigor and affect. Because the isolation laboratory provides standardized measures, with individuals rising and sleeping and performing tasks on a standardized schedule, comparisons over the 24-hour day yield meaningful data that are not comparable in studies of "everyday life," in which people have various experiences and at different times of day.

Using mood tests different from those used by Monk, Buysse et al. (1992), Clark, Watson, and Leeka (1989) had college students use a form for affective ratings (which the researchers called mood ratings). The form included items such as "interested," "excited," "determined," and "attentive" for positive affect and "distressed," "guilty," "hostile," "afraid" for negative affect. Subjects marked each affect description from 1 (not at all) to 5 (very much) according to how much that affect was felt at the moment of rating. In contrast to the method of Monk and colleagues, who measured global vigor and global affect, Clark and co-workers examined how time of day affects mood, which they defined in terms of positive and negative affect. In the week-long study, over 100 subjects made daily ratings at rising and retiring and at 3-hour intervals after awakening. Subjects followed their regular routines, which varied greatly. For example, some people rose at 6:00 a.m. and some at noon. The data were averaged for the approximately seven ratings per day for one week, and the investigators found that positive affects rose markedly from early morning until noon. Positive affect rose in a clear-cut pattern from morning to 9:00 p.m. but negative affect did not show clear-cut changes over the time subjects were awake. The greatest rise in positive affect, from 9:00 a.m. to 3:00 p.m., was in the "attentive" items, but all subcategories of positive affect on the average rose from 9:00 a.m. to 9:00 p.m. Very low ratings for positive affect were given at 3:00 a.m. and 6:00 a.m. by those subjects who were awake at these hours. Interestingly, the generally unchanged negative affect was not markedly higher at these hours, even though positive affect dropped noticeably. Figure 5.4 reveals the overall pattern for positive and negative affect in two studies by Clark, Watson, and Leeka (1989). Although the averages across each data point were not standardized in the manner of Monk and colleagues, and although different measures of mood were used, it is important to note that the two kinds of studies found some comparability in peaks for mood across the 24-hour day.

To date it is not clear what processes lead to the effects of time of day on mood, defined either as Monk (1989) and colleagues did or as Clark et al. (1989) did. It is evident that the sleep-wake cycle is related to subjective ratings of alertness and sleepiness, and the daily effects on ratings of *mood* mirror the data on ratings of *alertness* and *sleepiness*. In the studies just cited, self-rated vigor, strength, and alertness were found to increase as a function of time since waking, and heightened arousal covaried with both performance effectiveness and positive mood.

Thayer (1987) had college students (six women and two men) fill out the short form of the Activation-Deactivation Adjective Check List (AD ACL) for measuring energetic and tense arousal. The items on the *energy* and *tension* subscales were quite similar to items described in the studies of Monk (1989) and Clark et al. (1989): for *energy,* they were energetic, lively, active, vigorous, full of pep; for *tension,* they were tense, clutched-up, fearful, jittery, intense. The subjects agreed to make ratings five times a day for 10 days over a period of 3 to 4 weeks. Ratings were made immediately after awakening, in late morning (about 11:00 a.m.), in late afternoon (about 4:00 p.m.), just before night sleep, and at one other self-set time that occurred 1.5 hours from the

FIGURE 5.4
Diurnal pattern of positive affect (PA) and negative affect (NA) in studies I and II.

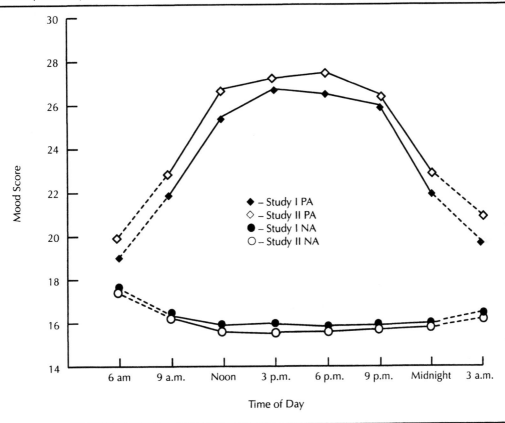

Source: From Clark, Watson, & Leeka, 1989.

other ratings and immediately followed a brisk walk of 10 minutes. The 10-day ratings were to be made on days that were comparable in terms of schedules for awakening, night sleep, and general daily activities, and the brisk walk was to occur at a prescheduled time on all the rating days. In this way a log was kept that yielded time-of-day effects for tense arousal and energetic arousal, which are the two variables that in Thayer's conceptualization represent the fundamental dimensions underlying mood, affect, and motivation.

These same subjects also made ratings regarding personal problems. On one scale they rated how se-

rious the problem appeared to be at the time of the rating, with 20 representing "extremely serious" and 1 "not serious at all." On a second scale they rated how difficult the solution for the problem appeared to be, with 20 representing "extremely difficult" and 1 "not difficult at all." On the third scale they rated how likely it was that the problem would be solved, with 1 representing "very likely" and 20 "not likely at all." All volunteer subjects had indicated prior to participating in the study that they had bothersome and continuing personal problems. All AD ACL ratings preceded each occasion of rating the personal problems. Although some subjects kept the ratings for less than the prescribed 10 days, the main time-of-day effects still were significant.

In line with many other studies that have been reviewed already, late morning showed the highest self-rated *energetic arousal,* whereas late afternoon showed the highest self-rated *tense arousal.* Both energetic and tense arousal ratings were lowest after subjects' awakening and before sleeping. In line with the ratings of tension, the most negative perception of problems occurred in late afternoon and before subjects went to sleep. When problem perception of individual subjects was analyzed, it also was found to be less negative when subjects' energy was highest and tension was lowest. In addition, problem perception was most severe when subjects' tension was highest and energy was lowest. Thus, perception of personal problems is associated with self-rated levels of energy and tension, and late afternoon seems to be when problems appear more serious and least likely to be solved.

Other studies reveal how mood or other assessments of internal states are influenced by the interaction between a given experience and the time of day in which it occurs. For example, in one study (Babkoff, Casy, & Mikulincer, 1991) the effect of a specific set of task experiences led to an alteration in subjects' assessment of their internal state only at certain times of the day. In a sleep deprivation laboratory, subjects were given a battery of tasks that included reaction time, reasoning, and recall and recognition. After sleeping about 8 hours, subjects received their first testing at 8:00 a.m. and the same task experiences were given every 2 hours thereafter until the end of the 3 days of sleep deprivation. Before and after each testing session the subjects gave subjective sleepiness ratings on scales that utilized descriptions of how the subjects felt at the time. These ratings were similar to those employed by Thayer (1987) and Monk (1989), such as feeling "alert, wide awake, functioning with no problems" to "extremely drowsy, very tired, almost asleep."

Babkoff and co-workers (1991) found that, as expected, self-reported sleepiness increased significantly across the 3 days of sleep deprivation. Sleepiness ratings did not increase uniformly after the test taking, however. Compared with ratings before the testing, ratings after the testing showed in-

creased sleepiness only at those times when normal sleepiness was at its peak. That is, the effect of cognitive testing on sleepiness ratings depended on the time of day. Between 8:00 and 10:00 a.m. and between 6:00 and 8:00 p.m., which were the hours when overall sleepiness was minimal, testing gave a minimal increase in sleepiness ratings. Testing gave maximum increase in sleepiness ratings between 2:00 and 6:00 a.m., when subjects overall felt the most sleepy. In spite of the fact that subjects were feeling overall more sleepy over the 3 days of sleep deprivation, a change in self-assessed sleepiness due to the task experience was not significantly altered by the sleep deprivation.

The relationship between sleep-wakefulness and effective functioning is not found exclusively in humans. A careful study was done with cats by Livingstone and Hubel (1981). They assessed if effectiveness in visual responding relates to sleep-wakefulness and to arousal, and they tested cats under different stages of sleep as well as under wakefulness. Single cell recordings were made at different locations in the visual pathway. Cats were presented with visual stimuli and aroused by noise or pinching (tactile stimulation). The investigators found that neural cell firing was different when the cats were aroused compared with nonaroused. When the animals were in slow-wave sleep and then aroused, for example, visual evoked activity was depressed, especially in the deeper layers of the visual cortex. Overall, in terms of neural activity in cells in the visual pathway (lateral geniculate body and primary as well as deeper visual cortex), arousal enhanced evoked responses to visual stimuli and increased the signal-to-noise ratio (gave finer or sharper perception). The fact that single cell activity reveals sharpened perception with wakefulness and with externally induced arousal in an animal may have a bearing on the mood data obtained with humans. That is, if humans also have a circadian rhythm of neural and brain activity, then human functioning can be expected to differ across the circadian cycle, that is, at different times of the day. Because individuals probably are aware that they function more effectively at different times of the day, this is a possible reason why they might rate themselves as feeling greater strength, vigor, and alertness from morning to evening. The rise in positive affect from early morning to evening could be a direct result of circadian physiological changes.

People differ in how time of day affects stress-related chemical excretions. This was observed in studies of young children, in which urine samples were taken frequently throughout the day for many days (Restoin, et al., 1981). The children differed in who was dominant, appeasing, or aggressive in behavior, and these differences were reflected in the time-of-day patterns in their stress-related chemical excretions. The children with high interpersonal effectiveness showed different chemical excretion patterns across time of day than did children who were less effective in their interpersonal relationships. Studies with adults found similar results when their urinary excretions were analyzed. Adrenaline excretion is assumed to reflect emotional and motivational processes, and variation in time-of-day patterns in adrenaline excretion was found to follow affectively laden experiences (Vokac, Gundersen, Magnus, Jebens, & Bakka, 1981). Thus, physiological time-of-day changes may follow affective reactions, and affective reactions can follow physiological time-of-day effects.

In normal living, when many variables are operating, mood or other self-assessments of internal states may not vary as strongly with time of day. Thayer, Takahashi, and Pauli (1988) noted the need for naturalistic observations, and many clinical studies of patients with mood disturbances have shown that factors in daily living play a large role in whether and how time of day affects mood.

PERSONALITY CHARACTERISTICS AND "MORNINGNESS" VERSUS "EVENINGNESS"

It is well known that the brain generates complex patterns of neural activity spontaneously (Steriade, McCormick, & Sejnowski, 1993), and different patterns occur for the sleeping compared with the aroused brain. This could bear on whether sensory, motor, cognitive, and motivational processes are differentially effective at different times within an individual's sleep-arousal cycle. However, in humans, sensation, cognition, motivation, and behavior are complexly determined. Many variables have effects, either alone or in interaction with endogenous rhythms.

Morningness-Eveningness

Some people have their best performance and vigor in the morning, and others in the evening. In laypersons' language, using an analogy from bird species, these individuals have been referred to as the "fowls" and the "owls." To measure the differences a "morningness-eveningness" questionnaire (Horne & Ostberg, 1976) was developed, which can be abbreviated as MEQ. A large body of literature has examined how the two types of individuals differ.

The questionnaire in English was adapted from an earlier one in the Swedish language, which had proven useful in predicting adaptability to shift work. The questionnaire asked subjects about times of day in which they function best. For example, one item asked, "At what time would you get up if you were entirely free to plan your day?," and another asked about when subjects would go to bed. Other questions asked how easy it was to get up in the morning, and how alert subjects feel after first awakening. The 19 questions provided a composite score, and the scores fit into five categories: definite morning type, moderate morning type, intermediate type, moderate evening type, and definite evening type. Men and women students between ages 18 and 32 were selected. They consisted of three groups (definite morning, definite evening, and intermediate) and they took oral temperatures daily, for 3 weeks. Temperatures were taken upon awakening and at approximately half hour intervals until bedtime. Subjects also kept a log of sleep length, bedtime, and time of awakening. Horne and Ostberg (1976) found that morning types had higher temperatures than intermediate and evening types up to 6:00 p.m., and after 9:00 p.m. the evening types had higher temperatures than the intermediate and morning types. The average peak temperature time for morning subjects was 7:32 p.m.; for evening subjects it was 8:40 p.m. The intermediate subjects had an average peak temperature at 8:25 p.m.

In this naturalistic study the subjects led normal lives except for their data collecting, which means they selected their own schedules of activities and times for waking and sleeping. The evening subjects went to bed nearly 100 minutes later than did the morning subjects; intermediate subjects were close to the morning subjects on this variable. Because this was a student population, their rising times and bedtimes were later than would be expected of other persons, with morning subjects going to bed at about 11:30 p.m. and evening subjects only retiring after 1:00 a.m. Equally, morning subjects arose on the average at 7:24 a.m., while evening subjects arose on the average at 9:18 a.m. Although sleep length did not differ significantly for the three groups, rising time was significantly different. The morning subjects awakened 114 minutes before the evening subjects, with intermediate subjects arising roughly midway between the other two groups. Scores on the MEQ were significantly correlated with peak temperature times, rising times, and bedtimes. The data show clearly that for people having choices of when to do normal daily activities, some follow a "fowl" pattern and others an "owl" pattern, and their temperature peaks reflect this difference. Later studies (reviewed by Monk, 1991) show that temperature and the sleep-wake cycle are complexly intertwined.

The above findings have interesting implications, since answers on a simple questionnaire were found to be related to physiological and behavioral measures. Subjects who were identified by a questionnaire as being morning types were found to have on the average earlier peak temperatures than did those subjects who were identified as evening types, and morning subjects were found to rise and retire earlier than evening subjects. These findings reveal, first, that people can reliably assess their own daily rhythm, noting when they perform best and at what times they engage in their sleep and waking activities. Second, individual differences in circadian rhythms of temperature and sleep-wake cycle are evident. Third, individual differences in sleep-wake patterns appear to be stable across a long time period. This suggests that activity rhythms may be related in some way to stable personality differences.

Individual differences of the sort measured by the MEQ have been thought to relate to phasic differences in motivation and performance, and to sta-

ble differences such as subjects' personality. In line with the latter, some psychologists have examined time-of-day effects in conjunction with personality traits.

Extraversion, Impulsiveness, and Morningness-Eveningness

According to the formulation of Eysenck (1967), extraversion and neuroticism constitute two independent personality dimensions, with extraversion related to cortical arousal and neuroticism related to arousal associated with limbic and autonomic nervous system activity. That is, introverts are presumed to be more cortically aroused than extraverts, and persons with high neuroticism are presumed to be more autonomically aroused than normal or low neuroticism individuals. Thayer, Takahashi, and Pauli (1988) interpret Eysenck's conceptualization of cortical arousal to be closely related to Thayer's "energetic arousal" and Eysenck's conceptualization of autonomic arousal to be closely related to Thayer's "tense arousal."

In their study, Thayer and co-workers (1988) had subjects fill out the short form of the AD ACL for energetic and tense arousal items. This took less than 30 seconds and could be completed many times during the day. Subjects also filled out items from Eysenck personality inventory forms for measures of extraversion and neuroticism, and they completed the Horne and Ostberg (1976) MEQ. The AD ACL items were completed for 6 days: upon awakening, every hour thereafter, and just before bedtime. Individual interviews with subjects assessed best and worst hours for doing various tasks, including intellectual and physical tasks and getting along well with other people. This sample of subjects had a tendency toward "morningness" rather than "eveningness," and in line with this the subjects also had a rather early average waking time (6:19 am).

Thayer et al. (1988) also found that introverts had higher levels of energetic arousal than did extraverts, but not to a significant extent. However, neuroticism scores correlated significantly with tense arousal scores, and a significant interaction was found between extraversion-introversion and time of day, the introverts being more tense in the first two-thirds of the day and extraverts more tense in the last third. Additionally, morningness was related to greater energetic arousal in the early part of the day and eveningness was related to greater energetic arousal in late afternoon and evening, although the relationship fell short of being significant. Morningness scores did predict significantly which hours were reported in the interview as the best and worst times for the various task performances and other functions. The hours reported in the interviews as best and worst were corroborated by differences in energetic arousal scores for these hours. Thus, stable personality characteristics, as measured by tests of extraversion and neuroticism, appear to lead to different arousal levels, and they also interact with what time of day subjects experience energetic and tense arousal. A large number of studies have found Eysenck's personality dimension of introversion-extraversion to interact with time of day. Although many researchers investigating this personality dimension *assume* arousal to differ for extraverts and introverts, they do not usually report measured arousal scores, as did Thayer and colleagues (1988).

Some researchers (Humphreys & Revelle, 1984; Revelle, Humphreys, Simon, & Gilliland, 1980) tested the role of arousal in the way personality and time of day interact by giving subjects caffeine. Caffeine is a known stimulant that increases excitation or arousal. If subjects' performance on tasks improved after use of caffeine, this would suggest the subjects were underaroused before caffeine ingestion. Studies have shown that introverts' best performance occurs in the morning or early afternoon, while extraverts perform best in the late afternoon and evening. Revelle and colleagues found a third variable, impulsivity, to play an important role (Humphreys & Revelle, 1984; Revelle et al., 1980). These researchers found that the critical dimension that altered the performance of introverts and extraverts according to time of day was impulsivity. The Eysenck test of extraversion was found to be made up of two components, sociability and impulsivity. Revelle and colleagues (1980) found that sociability did not show the interactive time-of-day effects, whereas impulsivity was significant.

Caffeine use improved performance of highly impulsive persons (extraverts) but lowered performance of subjects low in impulsivity (introverted)

in the morning, and the reverse occurred in the evening. The researchers presumed that subjects with low impulsivity were highly aroused in the morning but not in the evening. The researchers reasoned that low impulsive subjects improved their performance with caffeine in the evening because they had lower arousal in the evening compared with the morning; the added stimulant in the evening provided what was needed to improve their performance in the evening. In contrast, the researchers reasoned that caffeine improved the performance of extraverts in the morning because these highly impulsive people were less aroused in the morning than in the evening. The caffeine by extraversion-introversion by time-of-day effects illustrate a triple interaction, three variables interacting to affect performance.

Humphreys and Revelle (1984) added another postulate, that whether performance was better in the morning or in the evening was a function of the nature of the task and not merely of an interaction among arousal, impulsivity, and time of day. They postulated that high arousal is not advantageous for tasks involving STM but improves performance on simple perceptual tasks. Studies already discussed in an earlier section of this chapter showed that performance on simple tasks, which did not require much memory, is likely to improve with increased arousal. In his review, Monk (1990) stated that simple perceptual motor tasks are improved by increased alertness, excitation, or arousal. Thus, the Humphreys-Revelle hypotheses received some support. The discussion of how alertness and performance vary according to time of day is in line with their assertion. Based on the hypotheses concerning the complex interplay of task, arousal level, time of day, and impulsivity (which underlies the important dimension of extraversion-introversion), the Humphreys-Revelle hypotheses predict that low impulsive subjects should perform better on simple perceptual tasks in the morning and high impulsive subjects should perform better on such tasks in the late afternoon or evening. The hypotheses reverse the prediction for tasks involving memory.

In this regard one can consider the studies by Folkard et al. (1986). They showed that good performance on short-term memory tasks was better in the late afternoon and evening, and as already described, various studies have shown that alertness tends to peak in the late afternoon. From the perspective of defining arousal according to time of day, high arousal or alertness leading to improved performance on STM tasks is contrary to the Humphreys-Revelle postulation. However, the formulations of Humphreys and Revelle (1984) add a useful perspective. By their considering a personality variable, their prediction concerning STM performance may be supported even in the Folkard et al. (1986) studies, because those studies reported many individual differences. From the perspective of Humphreys and Revelle (1984), a possible source of these differences may be the personality factor of impulsivity. Because highly impulsive subjects are presumed to have low arousal in the morning, and low impulsive subjects are presumed to have low arousal in the evening, Humphreys and Revelle (1984) would predict for STM performance that the low impulsive subjects should do worse in the morning and high impulsive subjects should do worse in the evening. Findings from several studies reviewed by Revelle (1989) support these predictions.

Alternative explanations besides an interaction involving arousal and task demands, as well as time of day and impulsivity, may explain the findings. For example, extraverts may have many more items they attend to at night due to their liveliness at night, and this could interfere with their performance on STM tasks. Nevertheless, the hypotheses put forth by Humphreys and Revelle (1984) provide structure for ongoing research involving time-of-day effects. Research is only slowly emerging to reveal how personality factors, time of day, and task demands interact. Whether personality factors can be equated with arousal, in the manner proposed by Humphreys and Revelle (1984), remains an open question.

Although they did not directly test the hypotheses of Humphreys and Revelle, Folkard and colleagues (Vidacek, Kaliterna, Radosevic-Vidacek, & Folkard, 1988) investigated the interaction between personality factors and time of day. The study used a factorial design to assess how physiological and performance measures are affected by time of day, extraversion-introversion, and morningness eveningness. Translations of Eysenck's personality inventory and the MEQ were given to university students in the country that at the time was Yugoslavia. No impulsivity scores were obtained, but introversion-extraversion and morningness-eveningness scores were obtained. Extreme-scoring subjects on both dimensions were selected so that four groups were established: morning extraverts, morning introverts, evening extraverts, and evening introverts. Prior to the experiment, subjects came to the laboratory to practice the tasks and gain familiarity with the recording techniques. On the test day they arrived for the study at 6:30 a.m. and stayed for about 24 hours. Subjects were tested individually. Every 4 hours following the first testing at 7:45 a.m. they received the experimental procedures. Between these procedures they could engage in activities of their own choice within the laboratory.

The results showed that all the measures varied significantly with time of day, but unlike findings reported in other studies already discussed, physiological and performance measures did not vary according to either alertness or temperature. The main interactions between morningness-eveningness and time-of-day effects occurred for alertness and oral temperature measures. Peak alertness for morningness subjects occurred about 2:00 p.m. and for eveningness subjects about 8:00 p.m. Temperature peak times also differed for these two main groups, and the peak was higher and the trough was lower for morningness than eveningness subjects. Physiological and task performance measures did *not* interact significantly with time-of-day effects for morning versus evening types of subjects. For extraversion-introversion, the main difference as a function of time of day was obtained for subjective alertness ratings. Performance measures were not different for the interaction of time of day with either morningness-eveningness or extraversion-introversion.

Because alertness was significantly different as a function of time of day in interaction with each of these other two variables, if the Humphreys-Revelle hypotheses were supported, simple RT and vigilance detection also should have varied in line with the alertness ratings. This did not happen. However, partial support for the Humphreys-Revelle hypotheses was found in the significant triple interaction of time of day, extraversion, and morningness for the choice-RT performance task. The evening-extraverts peaked (with faster RT) later than the other three groups. Their peak was between 4:00 and 8:00 p.m. The study by Folkard and colleagues provided important data, in that a factorial design separated the variables of morningness-eveningness from extraversion-introversion. Of interest is the fact that more significant effects were found for morningness-eveningness than for extraversion-introversion.

The above study reveals how complex the time-of-day effects are. At present, one can safely conclude: that different tasks are more effectively performed at different times of the day; that arousal (defined in a variety of ways) influences both the time-of-day and task effects on performance; and that morningness-eveningness in many cases will interact with the time-of-day variable and with task demands. The nature of these interactions is presently not clearly understood. Also not clear is the extent to which the individual differences in morningness-eveningness are inborn or learned. They could result from patterns of early childhood rearing, or to some extent they could be inborn (due to prenatal factors and not necessarily genetically determined). It is known that aging alters the pattern toward morningness (see Monk, Reynolds, et al., 1992). If aging can change that pattern, possibly other variables can do so as well.

Whether extraversion-introversion or impulsiveness are learned or inborn, and whether they change with aging, is still not clearly established. How arousal interacts with morningness-eveningness and with extraversion-introversion is also still an open question. For now, interesting hypotheses, such as those by Humphreys and Revelle (1984), are offered. These in turn have generated additional studies to answer in what way time of day interacts with task characteristics, personality characteristics, and arousal.

SUMMARY

The sleep-wake cycle has an important effect on performance and learning. How long the period is between the end of sleep and performing a task is very important. The kinds of activities that precede performance also affect the quality of performance, independently of the time of day in which a task is performed. Prior activities can facilitate or impair performance on a given task. Thus, when assessing the role of time of day, it is important to control for the types of activities engaged in previous to the task under investigation.

The amount of stimulation present, and the goal of one's performance, affect how well one does on a task. Day sleep differs from night sleep. The sleep-wake cycle is influenced by external stimuli more than is the temperature rhythm.

An alertness-sleepiness rhythm has been identified as being independent of the sleep-wake cycle. Subjective and objective sleepiness often do not coincide. For example, objectively people tend to be sleepy in the early afternoon, but for many people that is the time they report low subjective sleepiness and high subjective alertness. After 8:00 p.m., body temperature and alertness level both drop, but at other times of the day their rise and fall may not coincide. Temperature tends to be high near the middle of the day, and between 4:00 and 8:00 p.m. temperature and alertness differ. Subjective sleepiness (alertness) is partly determined by the temperature rhythm and partly by the sleep-wake cycle.

How performance varies with time of day depends on the type of task. Digit span has a period shorter than 24 hours. Digits are least well recalled in the middle of the day. Short-term memory (STM) is poor when body temperature and subjective alertness are high. Vigilance, sustained attention to a simple series of events, varies with subjective alertness and body temperature. Whereas digit span has a period less than 24 hours, subjective alertness has a period greater than 24 hours. When rhythms are endogenously rather than externally influenced, they show clear periods, but not all physiological variables show periods. Although alertness can be induced by external factors, as in incentive motivation, alertness is also induced endogenously in terms of the subjective alertness-sleepiness cycle.

Shift workers and their performance are affected by many variables. Verbal reasoning performance of shift workers adjusts well to altered external zeit-gebers, whereas letter cancellation performance seems to be more related to the endogenous temperature rhythm.

On memory tasks, time of day influences encoding and storage of information more than the retrieval of learned material. Material presented in the early morning is best remembered with immediate recall, and material presented late in the day is best remembered with delayed recall, with time of day of learning rather than time of day of testing playing the major role. Tasks with a high memory load are performed best in the early morning and poorest in the early evening.

When subjects in a study are confined in a relatively constant environment, mood is complexly related to rhythmic and homeostatic processes. Positive affect (pleasantness of emotional reactions) rises from early morning to noon, and continues to rise until near bedtime in the evening. Negative affect ratings do not show clear patterns of change during the waking hours.

People differ according to their "morningness" or "eveningness," the time of day when they have most energy and vigor. Persons who are the morning type have earlier peak temperatures than per-sons identified as the evening types. Temperature rhythms and sleep-wake cycles differ between the two types.

Various researchers sought to relate Eysenck's personality dimension of introversion-extraversion with time-of-day effects. Introverts' best performance seems to occur in the morning or early afternoon, while extraverts perform best in the later afternoon and in the evening. Impulsivity appears to play a role in these time-of-day effects. Extraverts tend to be more impulsive than introverts, and Humphreys and Revelle found with caffeine studies that impulsivity had a significant effect on performance for extraverts versus introverts in the morning compared with the evening.

Depending on how one measures it, arousal has complex effects at different times of day. On the one hand, arousal varies with time of day, and on the other hand, arousal (endogenous and externally caused) affects performance differently at various times of day. For this reason as well as other reasons, the way motivation affects performance is not comparable throughout the day. Knowledge of time-of-day effects is very important in understanding the relationships among motivation, mood, and performance.

CHAPTER **6**

Emotion and Mood: I. Problems of Definition and Measurement

Emotion is closely related to the construct of motivation. Following the lead of Duffy (1934, 1951), many psychologists in the 1950s and 1960s considered emotion and motivation as being the same. Increased research by psychologists has provided new insights, as well as brought forth new controversies, regarding the relationship between emotion and motivation. This chapter considers how researchers have conceptualized, defined, and measured emotion in general. Later chapters focus on specific emotions, like fear and anger.

HOW ARE MOTIVATION AND EMOTION DIFFERENT?

Excellent reviews of emotion exist (e.g., Fiedler & Forgas, 1987; Lazarus, 1991b; Leventhal & Tomarken, 1986). Some theories of emotion have not related emotion to motivation, and some textbooks on motivation have not included emotion as an important topic. This chapter selectively considers issues in the study of emotion that have a meaningful relationship to the topic of motivation.

The view taken in the present book is that motivation sets the guideline within which emotion takes shape. That is, motivation provides the broad direction, and different emotions can be experienced for any given motivation. For example, when one is hungry and sits down to a meal, a wide range of emotions may occur, such as joy, eagerness, or anger, depending on whether the food tastes good, the food is ready to be served and is attractively displayed, or there is a delay before the food will be served. Psychologists have distinguished between emotion and motivation in various ways, and the present perspective encompasses many of these ways.

Emotion and Motivation: Duration and Congruence

Although emotion and motivation sometimes have been distinguished according to their duration, on the whole this is not a reliable way to differentiate these two constructs. Both emotions and motivations may be relatively brief, and some emotions and some motivational states can last for an extended period. Eating very salty food leads to thirst, and as soon as one drinks a lot of fluid the motivation of thirst is gone. Stubbing one's toe on a rock may lead to an emotion of anger, but this emotion diminishes as soon as one continues to walk. Contrasting to such brief durations are the enduring emotion of sadness by a widow or widower and the ongoing motivational state reported by some parents of teenagers, "That kid is always hungry!" Consideration of duration also is relevant to the distinction between *state* and *trait*. The point was made in chapter 3 that arousability, as the tendency to become energized or aroused, can be studied as a trait, even though arousal, as heightened excitation, is a state. Emotionality, the tendency to have strong emotional reactions, also has been studied as a trait, even though the more usual way of discussing emotion is as a state.

Human motivation often entails long-term processes due to the long-term nature of human goals.
Some goals from childhood may last a lifetime, and
the associated motivation traits may endure also for
a lifetime. Moreover, brief motivational states tend
to be congruent with the motivations that are oriented toward long-term goals. An example is the
motivation to get a college degree. For the sopho-
more in high school, "seeking to obtain a college
degree" describes a long-term goal and a long-term
motivation. The motivation directs and energizes
specific behaviors of the high school student. The
student is likely to select specific courses in high
school that may be useful for gaining entrance to
college, or they may be useful for successful completion of college work. Curriculum choices at one
age may reflect long-term motivation that is directed toward goal attainment at a much later age.

Just as short-term motivations are congruent
with long-term ones, so emotions are congruent
with motivations. That is the meaning of the earlier
statement, that "motivation sets the guideline
within which emotion takes shape." For instance, if
a class is full, but the student wishes to take it and it
fits the student's career planning, the emotion of
anger may occur. If then the student sets a new sub-
goal of winning the instructor's favor and gaining
special permission to enter the class, the student
forms a new short-term motivation and new emotions are likely to be experienced. Brehm and Self
(1989) pointed to motivational arousal as the momentary state that leads to a given instrumental behavior. To this one can add that momentary motivations also engender momentary emotions. Emotion
and motivation can change rapidly, and emotion is
congruent with the motivation, that is, the emotion
occurs within the guideline of the motivation.

Debate exists regarding "how long emotion
lasts," with some theorists considering emotion to
last for seconds and others saying it can last for
hours. In spite of theorists differing on the duration
of emotion, most agree on two points: that *mood* is
like emotion, and that mood is of far longer duration. Duration separates out *mood and emotion,*
even though duration is not generally useful for distinguishing between motivation and emotion.

Situational Variables and Goals

Motivation has both biological and social aspects.
For human beings the vast majority of adaptive
challenges are social, since the demands for effective living come largely from the person's culture
and society (Cacciopo & Berntson, 1992). Nonhuman animals as well as humans relate adaptively
and dynamically to their inner and outer worlds,
that is, to stimulus conditions occurring both within
the individual and external to the individual. Goals
direct the individual with respect to the stimulus
conditions, and motivation mobilizes actions. Emotion is congruent both with the motivation and with
the changing stimulus array.

Lability of emotion and of motivation in part depends on the situation. Both motivation and emotion can change when the situation changes. An example is a child who "wants the toy truck" (her
motivation) and who is happy (her emotion) on seeing the truck. When a playmate reaches the truck
first and prevents the child from obtaining it, the
child experiences the emotion of anger. The motivation did not change (the child still wants the
truck), but the altered stimulus array (the playmate
now has the truck) changes the emotion from happiness to anger. This illustrates how emotion is congruent with motivation and with the total stimulus
situation.

DEFINITIONS AND CLASSIFICATIONS OF EMOTION

The role of emotions has been emphasized in many
psychological theories, from those of William
James (1884) and Freud (1901/1960) to current theories. Many concepts continue from older to contemporary theories, like the emphasis on hedonic
pleasure seeking and pain avoidance. That was a
major part of Freud's theory, and some contemporary researchers also emphasize pleasantness-unpleasantness as an important aspect of emotion.

Emotion has been studied in terms of: the stimulus events that lead to specific emotional reactions
and to various intensities of reaction; the neurological and neuroendocrine systems that are active in

states of emotion; the motor patterns that are most likely to occur when individuals are experiencing emotions; the cognitions that modulate (heighten or dampen) emotions; the self-report verbalizations that accompany emotions and that provide the verbal cues indicative of specific emotional stress; and the social and biological value of emotions.

Historical Considerations

Within the history of psychology the construct of emotion was important for some early writers. Wundt (1902) had emphases that are still prominent. One was his concern with the importance of the intensity of arousal, and the other was his belief that emotions can be described best in terms of dimensions.

Wundt's Approach.   Early psychologists measured emotion by introspective methods. Wundt (1902, p. 196) distinguished emotion from feeling and emphasized "the arousing effect which comes from a special combination of particular affective contents." He considered feelings as discrete, and he called "a succession of feelings an *emotion*" (Wundt, 1902, p. 186, emphasis in original). Wundt believed that (p. 187) "a large number of single affective processes are grouped because of certain common characteristics." He also linked emotion and cognition (p. 187): "Emotions such as joy, hope, anxiety, care, and anger, are accompanied in every case by new ideational contents."

Wundt noted that physiological changes accompany emotional experiences and that emotions lead to expressive movements. He wrote that qualitatively different emotions may have common underlying physiological substrates (p. 193): "It may sometimes happen that emotions with very different, even opposite kinds of affective contents, may belong to the same class so far as the accompanying physical phenomena are concerned," and he cited joy and anger as examples. This question, of how specific or how general the physiological reactions are that accompany specific emotions, has been a concern for researchers long after Wundt's writings. In chapter 2 the James-Lange theory of emotion was considered in relation to the statement "we

are afraid because we run." Wundt considered that physiological and expressive movements are not unique to a given emotion, and he rejected James' and Lange's theory of emotion (Wundt, 1902, p. 193): "when they describe the emotions as psychical processes which can be aroused only through expressive movements, we must reject their paradoxical view."

Wundt classified emotions into three affective *dimensions* in terms of their primary characteristics, but secondary characteristics provided further qualitative variations. According to their primary characteristics, emotions may be pleasurable or unpleasurable, exciting or depressing, and straining or relaxing. Wundt cited joy as primarily a pleasurable emotion which is also exciting, and sorrow as unpleasurable and depressing. However, when sorrow becomes intense, he posited (p. 196) "it may become exciting." The observations of Wundt relate to contemporary controversies concerning the intensity and dimensionality of emotions.

Watson's Approach.   Contrary to Wundt's emphasis on dimensions, the early Behaviorist named John B. Watson (1925) proposed that there are some basic emotions, and he also focused on the conditionability of emotions. He considered fear, rage, and love to be innate, in the sense that at birth the human infant shows these three emotions as specific responses to specific stimuli. He thought that these basic emotions were limited to only a very few stimuli, and he proposed that the large range of emotions in adults are learned reactions. Many of these could be learned during infancy by means of classical conditioning. Psychologists tested these formulations, and their studies showed that many of the stimuli that elicit emotional reactions in humans and nonhumans do so as a result of learning, and that such learning is highly resistant to extinction.

In a famous study, a young boy named Albert learned to fear a white rat by means of *classical conditioning,* in which the white rat was the conditioned stimulus (CS) and a loud sound was the unconditioned stimulus (US). According to Watson and Rayner (1920, p. 12), Albert "was of an extremely phlegmatic type." He was selected as a subject for that reason. When he was between 8 and 9 months old, he was shown various stimuli (a white rat, a rabbit, a dog, cotton wool, etc.), which he tried to touch and none of which he feared. After that, he was tested for a fear response to a sudden loud sound. Initially, he halted his breathing, then he puckered his lips and trembled, and the third time he heard the sound he (Watson & Rayner, p. 2) "broke into a sudden crying fit. This is the first time an emotional situation in the laboratory has produced any fear or even crying in Albert." When Albert was 11 months and 3 days old, he received the pairing of the white rat and the loud sound. Just as his hand touched the animal, the bar was struck behind his head to produce the loud sound. Two such pairings occurred. When Albert was tested a week later, he withdrew his hand after starting to reach for the animal's head. In contrast to that reaction, Albert played actively with blocks that were subsequently presented to him. Further conditioning and testing were done within the next month, and the fear to the rat became generalized to other furry white stimuli. In summary, this study showed that on pretesting, Albert willingly approached the rat and other furry animals. However, after the researchers repeatedly presented a loud noise at the same time as they showed the rat to the child, Albert gradually withdrew from the animal and eventually whimpered when the rat was presented on its own, without the accompanying noise. The withdrawal behavior was identified as a function of learned fear to the animal. That fear was found to generalize to other white and furry objects and it persisted for some time.

Later researchers studied emotion within the context of classical conditioning, and they defined emotion as a *conditioned response* (CR). It was conceptualized to be an internal response, mediated by the autonomic nervous system, and its training and extinction were said to follow the laws of conditioning. That definition for emotion was used in psychology for many years. For some researchers it is still a valid way of defining and conceptualizing emotion.

Issues Raised by Early Theorists. J. B. Watson, Wundt, and James focused on entirely different aspects of emotion. Some of their disagreements remain as debates in contemporary writing and research.

1. Many contemporary psychologists follow the work begun by Watson, and they emphasize the *learned* aspects of emotions (by studying the effects of training, imitation, and the influence of culture). However, other psychologists, like Ekman (1992a, 1992b), emphasize the innate rather than the learned aspects of emotions in line with the theorizing of Darwin (1872/1965). Although acknowledging that individual learning experiences influence emotions in the adult, the evolutionary researchers emphasize that emotions are a product of evolution. This question will be considered again in the discussion concerning basic emotions.

2. Modern psychologists recognize that *physiological processes* play a major mediating role in emotion. Wundt had emphasized excitation and physiological arousal. This was congruent with points discussed in chapter 3 on arousal, and it also bears on the emphasis placed on the autonomic nervous system by certain contemporary psychologists (e.g., Levenson, 1992; Levenson, Ekman, Heider, & Friesen, 1992).

3. Many modern psychologists take a strong stand on whether emotions should be conceptualized, as Wundt did, in terms of common underlying *dimensions*. Some contemporary researchers actively investigate emotion in terms of its pleasantness-unpleasantness, and others argue that emotion should not be defined in terms of dimensions but rather in terms of *categories*. Contemporary theorists of emotion like Lazarus (1991b) have given serious attention to this question.

4. James and Wundt were concerned with *expressive movements* in relationship to emotion. Today expressive movements are given major emphasis by a number of theorists. The role of expressive movements in emotion is a topic of controversy and debate in contemporary research on emotions.

5. Wundt pointed out the importance of *cognitions* with respect to emotions, although this term was

not used in his time and instead he spoke of "ideational content." Modern researchers tend to approach the study of emotion from a cognitive point of view and attempt to assess the nature of the cognition-emotion relationship. In that regard, contemporary researchers are closer to the introspective era of James and Wundt than to that of Watson. The question of the relationship between emotion and cognition is discussed later in more detail.

Categories, Classification of Basic Emotions, and Face Muscle Movement

Theories of emotion differ according to several important issues. One relates to the question of whether emotion is best studied in terms of categories and in terms of basic (primary) emotions.

Basic Emotions. Some psychologists sought to classify emotions by having large groups of subjects provide ratings of words considered by the general public as being emotional terms, with the raters relying on subjective evaluations of what, for example, joy represents. Such judgments integrate memory and classification of many previous experiences which the rater judges to have involved joy. In one such approach to classification, Shaver, Schwartz, Kirson, and O'Connor (1987) had college students rate 213 emotion terms for "emotionness." From these data, the researchers obtained clusters that represented emotion categories. Other ways to classify emotions have been used. Using facial expression as the basis for classification, Ekman, Friesen, and Ellsworth (1972, p. 64) proposed "happiness, surprise, fear, anger, sadness, disgust/contempt, and interest." These are similar but not identical to the terms that Shaver et al. (1987) obtained- love, joy, anger, sadness, surprise, and fear clusters.

For some researchers the classification of emotions is important to allow separating basic or primary emotions from secondary emotions, with basic emotions postulated to be innate and universal in all humans. Ekman and his colleagues conceptualized emotion as being highly specific and very brief reactions that last no more than about 5 seconds. Ekman and his colleagues found the same

short duration patterns of facial and autonomic responses in people at different ages (Levenson, Carstensen, Friesen, & Ekman, 1991) and of many different cultures, including the matrilineal and agrarian Minangkabou of West Sumatra (Levenson et al., 1992). Further support for this was found when experimental subjects had no knowledge of the emotion experienced by the person being observed. In one study (Gottman & Levenson, 1985), experimental subjects observed social interactions on videotape, and they gave empathic responses that duplicated the same autonomic patterns of emotions as those given by the target person the subjects viewed in the videotape. Psychologists like Ekman take an evolutionary perspective, which postulates that certain emotions and emotional expressions follow characteristics of the species rather than the dynamics of an individual's unique life experiences. Ekman (1984) also did not think of startle as an emotion, because it is a reflex. It is the reflexive nature of startle, not its short duration, that led him and others (Lazarus, 1991b) to reject startle as an emotion.

Researchers focusing on expressive movements tend to argue that emotions are examples of biological, species-wide preprogramming, and that these movements provide an answer to the question, "What is an emotion?" Ekman, Friesen, and Ellsworth (1972) concluded from studies of facial expression that there are certain basic emotions such as fear and anger (see Figure 6.1). After more than 20 years, Ekman and his colleagues continued to demonstrate that not only are facial expressions specific for given emotions but that these specific expressions have a universal nature (found in many cultures), which is why these emotions are called *basic* (Ekman, 1994).

Classification of emotions by Ekman and colleagues is dependent on which specific facial muscles the person uses. For example, Ekman and Friesen (1982) distinguished between smiles that represent enjoyment from other types of smiles. There are "false smiles" that fake enjoyment, and "masking smiles" that conceal the experience of negative emotion. In many cultures, pretending to feel certain emotions is considered polite, and Ekman and colleagues pointed out that the "true" spontaneous emotion has different muscular con-

FIGURE 6.1
Basic emotions. Muscles in the face differ for six categories.

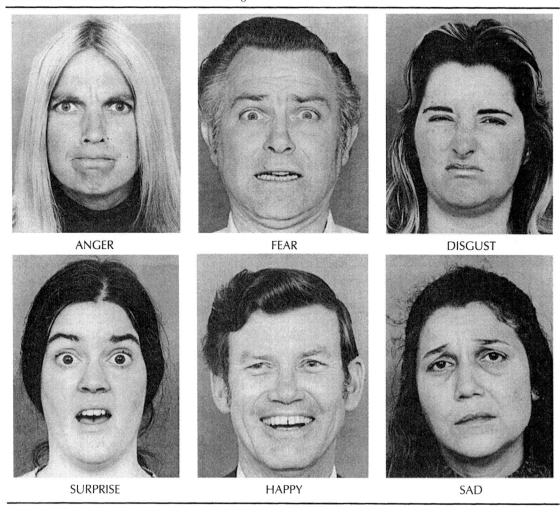

ANGER FEAR DISGUST

SURPRISE HAPPY SAD

Source: From Paul Ekman, *Unmasking the Face;* copyright 1975 by Paul Ekman.

figurations than does the "pretend" emotion. Ekman, Davidson, and Friesen (1990) described the "Duchenne smile," which is named after the scientist who first described it, as an illustration of a smile that does not reflect the emotional experience of joy normally associated with smiling. For Ekman and colleagues, specific facial muscle activity is used as a response definition of emotion. Their point is that one need not know the stimuli or events to which the person responds; one need only look at

the specific muscles the person uses in order to identify which emotion the person is experiencing.

Ekman (1992c) and others have had actors and other persons move specific muscles, and such induced muscle activity has led to the experience of emotion. Although they emphasize facial muscles, Ekman (1992c) and colleagues do not explain emotion in terms of a "peripheralist" view. They note that induced muscle activity can create the pertinent emotion, but they theorize that the effect is through a command action of the brain. According to their theorizing, when a person is deliberately told by the researchers to move specific muscles that correlate with a specific emotion, the motor cortex and other brain areas activate a hardwired network that leads to the various facial and other physiological responses that are specific to each basic emotion. These researchers postulate that it is not merely feedback from the muscles that sets off an emotion experience, but instead, when a person hears the verbal commands the person, via the motor cortex and other brain regions, activates the emotion network. This involves subjective experience, autonomic reactions, and facial muscle activity (Levenson, Ekman, & Friesen, 1990). Results of many studies support this view. Ekman and colleagues found that when subjects are told muscle by muscle to make specific face movements, these subjects then state that they experience the correlated emotion, and their autonomic nervous system responses also match the emotion.

Highly specific motor and autonomic reactions were found to occur when subjects relived a previous emotional experience (Ekman, Levenson, & Friesen, 1983), and cerebral as well as facial responses were specific when subjects viewed emotion-arousing stimuli, such as a videotape that graphically depicted a surgical procedure (Davidson, Ekman, Saron, Senulis, & Friesen, 1990). The measures of heart rate, skin conductance, and finger temperature were found to differentiate significantly between the six basic emotions of anger, fear, sadness, disgust, happiness, and surprise. Figure 6.2 shows data from one research report, based on 10-second recording periods (Levenson, Ekman, & Friesen, 1990). It illustrates change in autonomic responses (panels 1, 2, and 3) and overall body motion (panel 4) between the "directed" face configuration, in which each subject was coached muscle by muscle for the six emotions, and the neutral "control" face condition.

Face Muscles and Emotions. Zajonc, Murphy, and Inglehart (1989, p. 395) made the strongest case of all contemporary writers in arguing that "facial muscular movements alone are capable of altering subjective feeling states," and they posited

unequivocally that facial muscular movement of the kind that is normally involved in emotional expression (Zajonc et al., 1989, p. 405) "is a sufficient condition for the induction of affective reactions." They cited as support the results of studies in which experimental subjects were asked to read aloud stories that induced facial muscle action involved in making certain vowel sounds (such as the German *ü*). Following that procedure, subjects rated their own emotion and their liking of the material they read, and affective ratings were in line with the face-muscle condition.

Several researchers believe that movement of the facial muscles leads to the elicitation and modulation of emotion (Izard, 1990; Tomkins, 1982; Zajonc, 1985; Zajonc et al., 1989), and some believe that the peripheral nervous system and not cognitive processes or control by the brain (which is part of the central nervous system) leads to emotions. Zajonc et al. (1989) proposed that muscle action leads to a change in temperature and blood flow to the brain, and this leads to positive or negative emotion. A feedback hypothesis was proposed by Izard (1990) as the basis for emotion in infancy. He posited that in early infancy, the baby gives emotional expressions as automatic reactions to evoking stimuli. Then, by means of feedback mechanisms from the facial muscles, the emotion experience takes place without any modulation. Izard hypothesized that only with learning and maturation does this reflex-like process change.

In reviewing the literature on how emotion is affected by inducing specific muscles to move in special ways, Izard (1990) distinguished between two kinds of circumstances: those when muscle activity is imposed arbitrarily by some external agent (such as an experimenter in a research project), and those when muscle activity is induced by oneself. Izard was not convinced the way Zajonc was that arbitrary and external methods were effective in inducing changes in emotion. Rather, Izard (1990) concluded that facial muscle changes could alter emotions if the facial movements were self-induced, because then they were congruent with the individual's goals for change, whereas externally and arbitrarily induced facial muscle activity was not likely to yield major changes in emotion. Mat-

FIGURE 6.2

Heart rate (panel 1), finger temperature (panel 2), skin conductance (panel 3), and muscle activity (panel 4) changes and standard errors during six emotional configurations. AN = anger, FE = fear, SA = sadness, DI = disgust, HA = happiness, SU = suprise.

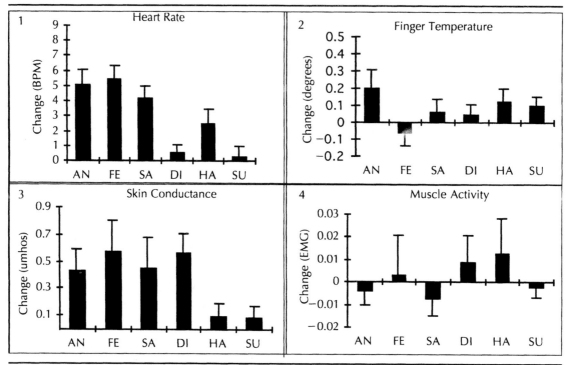

Source: From Levenson, Ekman, & Friesen, 1990, p. 369.

sumoto (1987) stated a similar skeptical conclusion regarding emotion change as a function of externally and arbitrarily induced facial muscle change.

An explanation of emotion in terms of a "response-produced state" is in line with the James-Lange formulation, that first the response occurs and then the emotion follows. The idea that facial expression leads to the experience of emotion is a controversial viewpoint. Most theorists consider that the facial expression that accompanies emotion is merely a consequence or readout of the emotional experience (Buck, 1985), and whatever its function, the facial expression is not the cause or antecedent of the emotional experience (Lazarus, 1991a, 1991b).

Emphasizing a peripheral muscle system as the basis for emotion is contrary to the current focus on

central processes. Most contemporary researchers emphasize a "top-down" approach, which posits that thought or attention or motivation directs the kind of emotional response a person or animal makes to external stimuli. For many psychologists, the role of facial muscle activity is secondary, such activity being a consequence, not a precursor, to emotion, and is only a part of an individual's total pattern of emotional reactions.

Autonomic Nervous System and Emotions.   The relationship between the autonomic nervous system and emotions has been of interest to psychologists since the early part of the 20th century. In contemporary research, data concerning the role of the autonomic nervous system in emotions have come from two areas of research, studies concerned with *basic emotions* and expressive movements of the face, and studies concerned with *arousal.* Data that revealed highly specific autonomic nervous system (ANS) responses supported theorists like Ekman, who argued for the selective specificity of emotional reactions, and data that revealed more generalized ANS activity supported arousal-based theories of emotion.

Gottman and Levenson (1985) studied married couple volunteers and compared lived emotions versus relived emotions. Instead of the usual rating scales, a joystick was used for the self-rating procedure. In the laboratory, subjects' baseline data were obtained during 5 minutes of silence, and then the couple discussed the day's events in the way they would at home at the end of the day. Subsequently, they discussed a problem area of conflict in their marriage. Several days later they returned, separately, to view the videotape recording of the session. During the interactive first session, heart rate, pulse transmission time to the finger, skin conductance level, and general body movement level were taken as physiological and somatic measures. In the second session, the physiological measures were again taken, and additionally, each subject observed the session on videotape and made continuous emotion ratings with a joystick that could be moved to settings over an arc of 180°. Very negative was at 0°, neutral at 90°, and very positive at 180°. The rating task required subjects to move the rating dial according to how they felt during the actual interaction, not how they felt at the time of viewing the videotape. This type of rating involves reliving of emotions, but with the aid of graphic visual cues.

Not only did the spouses observe their own interactions, but separate from the subjects, independent outside observers also viewed the videotapes. These observers made emotion ratings of the spouses on the basis of a highly detailed coding system that took into account verbal content, voice tone, facial expression, gestures, and so forth. For all the data sets the response measures were divided into 10-second units. This permitted comparisons between all the obtained measures. Interesting results were found. In viewing their interactions, the spouses, as predicted, gave considerably more negative ratings to themselves during the high conflict than during the low-conflict discussion. Also, prior attitudes affected the ratings. The more the couples had expressed dissatisfaction with their marriage in a pretesting questionnaire, the more negative were their dial ratings for the interaction that involved the high-conflict discussion segment. The correlation was not significant but in the same direction for ratings made on the low-conflict segment. On both the high-conflict and the low-conflict segments, emotion ratings were similar for the two spouses, and the observers' ratings of emotion were consistent with the spouses' ratings.

The physiological and somatic measures in the *initial sessions* were significantly similar to these same measures in the *relived session,* when the subjects viewed the videotapes. This gives support for the hypothesis that in this type of reliving situation the subjects validly replicate their initial emotional experience. Because in the present study extensive visual cues existed to help the subjects remember their initial emotions, one cannot be sure that under other circumstances the relived emotions would as fully duplicate the original emotional experience. The situations that subjects recalled in the Gottman and Levenson (1985) study were highly specific, and research on memory has shown that encapsulated, specific episodes are easier to remember than are other types of events (Kintsch, 1977). Thus, it is safe to say that some emotional episodes are easier to relive than others.

Of interest were the physiological data. Only the physiological reactions, and not the emotion self-report dial ratings, were duplicated between the initial and relived session.

The above study showed that highly specific physiological reactions relate to specific emotions. Other studies (Ekman, Levenson & Friesen, 1983; Levenson, 1988, 1992) also have shown that specific emotions involve specific physiological responses. The overall results show: highly specific facial muscle activity occurs for different emotion-inducing stimuli (Ekman et al., 1990; Ekman, Friesen, & Ancoli, 1980); when subjects are trained to move those same muscles without any evoking stimulus they give verbal self-report of the relevant specific emotion; and specific autonomic nervous system activity occurs with the specific emotions

(Ekman, Levenson, & Friesen, 1983; Levenson, 1992). Repeated findings that emotions involve autonomic specificity support what Ekman and colleagues had proposed, that there are only a small, limited number of *basic* emotions (Levenson, Ekman, & Friesen, 1990).

Intensity and Arousal of Emotions

Arousal-based and intensity theories of emotion differ from the study of basic emotions in several ways. Contemporary researchers who focused on classifying emotions, either according to categories (Lazarus, 1991b; Levenson, et al., 1992) or according to their associative characteristics (Bower, 1981), focused on classification of *qualitative* rather than *intensity* characteristics of emotion. Other theorists have focused on the intensity of emotions (Diener, Larsen, Levine, & Emmons, 1985) as important for understanding "what is emotion?" As already described, Wundt had proposed that an intensity change in emotions can lead to qualitative differences. Moreover, his example that sorrow could be either depression or excitation, depending on its intensity, raises questions that still require further investigation.

The Schachter and Singer Hypothesis. Another approach to the study of intensity is the cognitive-arousal formulation of emotion by Schachter (1967). Latané and Schachter (1962) proposed that general patterns of physiological reactions in emotion are mediated by the secretion of adrenaline. Early researchers (Cantril & Hunt, 1932; Landis & Hunt, 1932) sought to discover if injection of adrenaline would produce emotion. They found that the majority of subjects who had received an injection of adrenaline merely showed autonomic arousal and its observable effects (blanching of skin, muscle tremor, palpitation). These individuals either reported "as if" they were emotionally aroused, or they merely reported the physiological symptoms. However, some subjects did report feeling emotionally upset, even though no characteristic environmental events normally associated with emotion were present. They reported experiencing an emo-

tion merely because of the autonomic activity, not because any event had precipitated the emotion. Because the majority of subjects had *not* reported feeling any emotion merely because of the adrenaline, psychologists concluded that emotional experiences require more than physiological arousal.

Schachter (1967) expanded the concept of adrenaline-induced arousal and added that environmental cues were necessary for inducing emotion. Schachter (1971, p. 2) formulated his "cognitive-physiological formulation of emotion," proposing that emotions are determined by cognitions about the external environment and by the way a person interprets the internal cues of physiological arousal. That is, physiological arousal is necessary for emotion and so are the environmental cues and antecedent events that provide contextual meaning for interpreting the arousal.

In their classic experiment, Schachter and Singer (1962) showed that there were no emotion-arousal effects when control subjects were given a placebo of a saline solution (and thus had no symptoms of physiological arousal) and when they were in the presence of a confederate of the experimenter who (unbeknownst to the subjects) had been instructed by the researchers to provide either "happy-" or "angry-" producing cues. That is, environmental cues alone, without physiological arousal, did not produce emotional arousal. Adrenaline-injected subjects, who were given correct information about what physiological effects to expect subsequent to the injection, also had no emotional experience congruent with the happy or angry cued behavior of the confederate. In other words, physiological arousal interpreted correctly as due to the injection was not sufficient to lead to the cued emotion. However, subjects given no information about their subsequent physiological symptoms, and subjects given the wrong information, did show either euphoria or anger in line with the actions of the experimental confederate. Schachter's conceptualization about the basis for emotion was accepted for many years: that emotion was a function of the joint action of both physiological arousal and cognitive factors concerning the external environment and the internal cues.

An Experimental Test of the Schachter and Singer Hypothesis. Maslach (1979) tested the Schachter and Singer (1962) hypothesis. Her study illustrates how data from questionnaires and self-report ratings can be compared with both physiological indicators of arousal and behavioral data. Schachter and Singer had induced arousal by epinephrine (adrenaline) injection. Instead of using adrenaline injections, Maslach used hypnotically induced instructions to create physiological symptoms of arousal for the experimental subjects. These subjects were told they would experience moist hands and increased heart beat and breathing rate upon the presentation of a target word, but that they would not remember being so instructed. This "amnesia" was crucial for testing the Schachter and Singer hypothesis, which predicted that external environmental cues would be salient for emotion only if subjects had no other basis for judging the source of their physiological arousal. Three groups were in the experiment and received words for serial learning. The experimental-hypnotized subjects received the target word as the last one in the word series. Hypnotized subjects who were controls for the arousal condition were given a neutral last word instead of the arousal-inducing target word. An unhypnotized control group had no arousing instructions associated with the target word and they received the target word as the last in the word series. (It should be noted that *all* the subjects were thoroughly debriefed and all hypnotic suggestions were removed at the end of the experimental session.)

Physiological measures (heart rate and skin resistance) and responses on the Nowlis (1965) Mood Adjective Check List showed that the experimental-hypnotized and the control-unhypnotized subjects differed significantly in their reactions to the arousal target word. The physiological reactions of the hypnotized experimental subjects were in the expected direction (higher heart rate and higher galvanic skin response) and their mood was less positive and less passive. Thus, physiological arousal was demonstrated. Duplicating the design of the Schachter and Singer study, the subjects in Maslach's study were then exposed to a confederate whose behavior for half the subjects was "happy"

and for the other half was "angry." All subjects' verbal and nonverbal behavior was observed in the experimental sessions, and the subjects made ratings on bipolar scales that asked about emotions such as happy-sad, angry-peaceful, and confident-apprehensive.

Maslach (1979) found that the "angry" or "happy" confederate conditions did not produce significantly different self-reported emotion ratings, and rather than showing happy or angry observed behavior, the experimental as well as the two groups of control subjects showed more *sociable* behavior in the presence of the "happy" compared with the "angry" confederate. Of interest was the finding that the self-report measure of the experimental subjects revealed an overall angry emotion regardless of the confederate conditions, whereas the two sets of control subjects showed an overall happy self-report emotion regardless of the confederate conditions. Table 6.1 shows the behavioral and self-report data for the three groups as a function of the confederate conditions, with the "Unaroused" group being the hypnotized subjects who did not receive the target-arousing word.

Maslach interpreted the anger of the experimental-hypnotized subjects as being due to distress created by their not knowing (i.e., their "amnesia") why they had such physiological responses, whereas the other two groups were prepared to be comfortable and content in the experimental situation. This study demonstrates that self-report of emotion (happy versus angry) can differ from overt behavior. Moreover, physiological arousal need not interact with cognitive processes according to the way predicted by Schachter and Singer (1962). Maslach's results were not due to the hypnotic procedure for inducing arousal, since, Marshall and Zimbardo (1979) obtained similar results even though they induced arousal by means of epinephrine injections, the method used by Schachter and Singer.

EMOTION AND EVERYDAY LIFE

Joy or anxiety or anger have meaning and intensity for each individual in terms of uniquely personal

TABLE 6.1
Expressed and experienced emotion: A Test of the Schachter–Singer hypothesis

Condition[a]	Mean no. of observed sociable behaviors				Self-reported emotion (happy minus angry)[b]	
	Verbal		Nonverbal			
	Confederate		Confederate		Confederate	
	Happy	Angry	Happy	Angry	Happy	Angry
Hypnotized-Aroused	4.4	0.7	10.5	0.8	−1.0	−1.2
Hypnotized-Unaroused	4.3	0.4	8.2	0.4	+1.8	+2.5
Unhypnotized	2.5	0.9	6.0	1.6	+0.8	+0.4

[a]$n = 12$ for each condition (6 per cell).
[b]Mean scores are based on the Schachter and Singer (1962) index, which ranges from +4 (most happy) to –4 (most angry).
Data from Maslach, 1979, p. 961.

and complex experiences, thoughts, and goals. In daily life people are not concerned with the question of whether emotion is characteristic of the human species or whether emotion is basic or a blend. Pleasantness or unpleasantness as dimensions are often more readily identified in everyday life than are emotion categories, even though research with humans (Hupka, Zaleski, Otto, Reidl, & Tarabrina, 1997) and experiments with animals (Jitsumori & Yoshihara, 1997) have found strong support for characteristics of categories in emotions. Although in everyday life people normally do not concern themselves with whether emotion has reflexive or hard-wired components, categories, or dimensions, research from the laboratory, from field studies, and from case studies help psychologists answer the question, "What is an emotion?," and how emotion can be altered.

Dimensions of Emotions

Maslach's subjects reported emotions during a relatively brief experimental session. Ekman and Levenson (Levenson et al., 1990) investigated emotions that lasted around 5 seconds. Other researchers have had subjects use rating scales to report emotions in their daily life over a considerable course of time. Thayer (1989) used that approach in a number of his studies on arousal, with subjects rating their states of arousal over the course of days. Studies not concerned with basic emotions or with arousal have in-

vestigated *dimensions* of emotions in terms of intensity, duration, and frequency, and they use ratings made during the subjects' normal routines.

Studies by Diener and Colleagues. Diener et al. (1985) focused on affect in terms of pleasant-unpleasant, and noted (p. 1253) that in the past "most researchers had conceptualized affect as a single hedonic dimension in which positive and negative affect were defined and measured as bipolar opposites." They suggested, instead, that two independent dimensions exist. That is, positive and negative are each experienced in its own right and, at times, independently of the other. One can experience both a positive and a negative emotion at a given moment. These researchers investigated emotion in terms of the two dimensions.

Diener and colleagues (1985) asked subjects to complete a rating form (which the authors, on p. 1256, called a "mood form" although they state that it was used for subjects "describing their emotions for that day"). In one study, the subjects were to complete the form for 10 weeks. On each evening before retiring, they were to describe their emotions for that day. The subject volunteers were given 23 monopolar scales. Each item was rated from 0 to 6, with 0 indicating that the subject did not at all feel that way during the course of the day and 6 indicating that the subject felt extremely much in the way described by the item. Examples of "positive affect" items were *happy, pleased,* and *joyful,* and examples of "negative affect" items were *unhappy, frustrated, angry/hostile.* Such monopolar scales differ from the bipolar scale used by Maslach, which had polar opposite descriptions and subjects had to rate their emotions by checking some point between the two extremes.

Diener et al. (1985) added the scores across positive items independent of scores for negative items. That yielded a daily "positive affect" and "negative affect" score. A person's total positive score could range from 0 to 24, and a total negative score could range from 0 to 30. By averaging methods to equate the scales, the researchers obtained daily scores that described the frequency and intensity of positive and negative affect for each subject on a daily basis for a total of 10 weeks. Intensity was measured by taking the mean positive score for happy days (on those days when positive exceeded negative affective scores) and the same for negative scores on unhappy days. The rationale for measuring intensity in this way was that it measured how strongly the emotion was experienced regardless of how frequently subjects reported feeling the emotion.

By pooling descriptors for many specific emotions into hedonic dimensions of positive and negative, Diener et al. (1985) did not refer to specific emotions in the way that Ekman and Levenson had done. Moreover, although intensity might be related to specific emotions, such a relationship could not be ascertained from the kind of measurements Diener and colleagues (1985) used. For example, if on happy days some very intensely angry moments occurred, they would not be evident by this method of reporting. In part to correct this problem, and to assess momentary emotions when they actually occurred, the investigators asked subjects in a second study to rate emotions at bedtime (as was done in the first study) and at two random moments each day, as well as at a time when they felt a very strong emotion. A third study used this procedure with persons who were older than college students, to permit broader generalization of the results.

The researchers found a nonsignificant relationship between mean positive and negative emotions. Correlations were sometimes plus and sometimes minus. The statistical analyses suggested that positive and negative emotions were independent and not related, and the researchers hypothesized that

intensity might play an important role. When the researchers removed intensity as a contributing factor from the correlations they found negative correlations (inverse relationships) between positive and negative emotions. The researchers concluded, in line with results found by Diener and Emmons (1984), that although positive and negative emotions may be independent, overall they are not likely to be experienced at the same time.

Diener et al. (1985) considered intensity rather than frequency of emotions to be the important variable. The second study found close to zero correlations between frequency and intensity, and in all three studies intensity of the two types of emotions was highly and positively (directly) correlated. That is, subjects who scored high on intensity for positive emotions also scored high on intensity for negative emotions, and the same was true for the low intensity scores. The researchers concluded that emotional intensity is a personality variable and reflects stable individual differences.

Later research (Diener, Smith, and Fujita, 1995) focused on positive versus negative affectivity instead of intensity as a personality variable. Subjects made both retrospective ratings and ongoing self-ratings for 52 days. They rated positive emotions of love and joy and negative emotions of shame, anger, fear, and sadness. The data showed high intercorrelation between love and joy and between the unpleasant emotions. The experience of love and joy were both likely to occur in a given person, and likewise, if a person had negative emotions, various ones were likely to be experienced. Diener et al. (1995) concluded, in line with Watson and Clark (1992), that negative affectivity occurs as part of personality, with people tending to experience not just one but various unpleasant emotions. Diener, et al. (1995) further concluded that pleasant and unpleasant emotions are separable but not independent. That is, one person is likely to experience pleasant emotions and another to experience negative emotions, but clear-cut (statistical) independence does not occur. For example, those people who tended to experience love frequently also tended to experience fear or anxiety frequently.

Ratings and Memory of Positive and Negative Emotions. Some self-report measures describe immediately ongoing emotions and some describe past events from memory. For example, one study described by Frijda, Mesquita, Sonnemans, and Van Goozen (1991) measured how long emotions last. The subjects reported an emotion they experienced in the previous week, and they indicated the duration on a 5-category scale. The data showed that durations lasted from 5 seconds to over 1 hour, and in some cases, for over 1 week. The researchers noted that the measures of duration of an emotion is dependent on how one defines an emotion, and from their perspective, emotions may, indeed, last far longer than an hour and may have several peaks over a number of days.

Self-rated emotions reported *retrospectively* may differ in important ways from those that occur *at a given moment.* Memory can bias reporting of prior emotions. Diener et al. (1985) attempted to control for this by having subjects give both retrospective and momentary ratings of emotion. Their work differed from that of Frijda et al. (1991) in a number of ways, and the two types of studies reveal different information about emotions. In both cases, however, the problem of comparing remembered emotions with ongoing experiences of emotion remains an important one.

Larson (1987) addressed the problem of relying on remembered versus immediately experienced emotion in his studies. He asked adolescents (under age 18) as well as adults (aged 19 to 64) to carry electronic pagers for a week. In response to a signal received on the pager, each subject was to fill out a self-report rating of emotion at that moment. To ensure that prior emotions did not mask the immediate momentary emotion, and given that emotions may last considerably longer than 2 hours, Larson used data points spaced at least 2 hours apart. Ratings were along 7-point bipolar scales. They included not only happy-sad but friendly-angry and active-passive types of items. Thus, the emotions subjects rated were a mixture of specific categories and dimensions (anger being categorical, active and passive being dimensional).

Larson used the same type of frequency measure that Diener et al. (1985) employed. That is, frequency referred to whether or not a given emotion rating was absent or present within a given momen-

tary time sampling, not how often an emotion occurred. An emotion that was brief and repeated within the time sampling would be counted as a frequency of only one occurrence. As discussed earlier, Diener et al. (1985) found subjects to be stable in terms of the *intensity* of their emotions. In contrast, Larson found that subjects were quite stable in the *frequency* of their emotions. That is, over the course of the week subjects reliably experienced either few or many positive emotions and few or many negative emotions. He found that the frequency of positive and negative emotions was relatively independent: some subjects could experience many emotions of both kinds or very few of both kinds, and some subjects had asymmetry in the frequency of their positive and negative emotions.

Larson used a bipolar scale in contrast to the unipolar scale used by Diener et al. (1985). With a bipolar scale the subjects could place a rating on the positive end at some point in the day and on the opposite end at other times in the day, but they could not rate themselves as experiencing the two opposite emotions concurrently. Larson found that the majority of emotions lasted at most a few hours and he found support for independence between positive and negative emotions. For any single moment a negative correlation between positive and negative emotions would be present, the two emotions not occurring together, but over the course of the day a near-zero correlation was evident. The subjects could and did experience opposite types of emotion over the period of a day. This suggests two dimensions rather than one for pleasantness versus unpleasantness of emotions.

Since the data Larson obtained with immediately occurring emotions showed long durations for emotions, as was also reported by Frijda et al. (1991) with remembered emotions, memory may not be severely biasing for durations of emotions. However, it is not clear to what extent memory is biasing for frequency of emotions or for the independence of positive versus negative emotions. The research in which Diener et al. (1995) found separability rather than independence of positive versus negative emotions used measures of both retrospective and immediately occurring emotions. From their writing it is not clear to what extent memory biases the subjects' reporting toward one or two dimensions of pleasantness versus unpleasantness of emotions. However, it is clear that when units of time are longer term than short bursts of emotions, pleasantness versus unpleasantness of emotions does *not* represent a single dimension. Over the course of a day or even an hour, a person can have both pleasant and unpleasant emotions.

Person-Environment Relationships

Several theories of emotion and motivation were derived from observation of how people function in their daily lives. Several theorists have emphasized person-environment relationships. They consider that human emotion and motivation can be understood only in terms of the way an individual relates to the environment.

Lazarus and the Person-Environment Relationship. Lazarus (1991b) emphasized the role of cognition in the study of emotion, and he conceptualized that emotion is steered by motivation. The position taken in the present book is congruent with his viewpoint. Lazarus (1991b, p. 6) defined emotion in the following way: "Emotions are complex, patterned, organismic reactions to how we think we are doing in our lifelong efforts to survive and flourish and to achieve what we wish for ourselves." He conceptualized emotion as a "psychosociobiological construct" and that emotions (p. 6) "combine motivational, cognitive, adaptational, and physiological processes into a single complex state that involves several levels of analysis." Emotions occur when a person or a nonhuman animal appraises the situation as one involving gain or loss in relation to goals and well-being, with motivation delineating the goals. For Lazarus (1991a, p. 352), motivation is crucial for emotion: "Without some version of a motivational principle, emotion makes little sense, inasmuch as what is important or unimportant to us determines what we define as harmful or beneficial, hence emotional." Because in his theory motivation defines what is important for the individual at any given time, motivation plays a major role in defining emotions. Emotions and motivation have biological as well as social functions.

Lazarus (1991c, p. 819) viewed emotion as *relational,* stating that emotion is "always about person-environment relationships" that involve harms or benefits. Because his focus is on human emotion, the word *person* is used, but since his formulations also pertain to nonhuman animals, the word should be interpreted broadly as "the individual" and not given exclusively human attributes. He conceptualized the process of appraisal as one in which the individual gives meaning to the "adaptational encounter" (Lazarus, 1991a, p. 355), and "meaning" refers to the personal significance of the event in terms of harm or benefit. Appraisal can be nonverbal and out of awareness. Thus, infants and nonhuman animals can have emotions, as long as they apprehend the relational characteristic between the environment and the individual.

To clarify what he meant by cognition, Lazarus stated that both knowledge and appraisal are cognitions and represent thought. *Appraisal* involves evaluation of the significance of a transaction with the environment, whereas *knowledge* (Lazarus, 1991a, p. 354) "consists of what a person believes about the way the world works in general and in a specific context." Because knowledge need not involve a personal relevance in terms of harm or benefit to the self, knowledge alone need not lead to emotion. For Lazarus (1991a, p. 354), knowledge is "necessary but not sufficient" to lead to emotion, "whereas appraisal is both necessary and sufficient." Motivation provides the personal relevance and the meaning of whether the outcome of the transaction with the environment has personal stakes, so that emotion occurs within the framework set by motivation.

Lazarus related both motivation and cognition to emotion. Motivation defines what is important or unimportant and therefore of emotional relevance, and cognition, by means of appraisal, defines whether harm or benefit is occurring at a given moment and thus whether emotion is or is not aroused. Since startle, which occurs as a rapid response to a sudden stimulus like a loud sound, does not rely on appraisal nor is it modified by characteristics of the environment-person relationship, Lazarus (1991b) rejected startle as an emotion.

Lazarus considered a broad range of emotions,

ı included basic emotions (in the sense used by Ekman, 1994) and blends of basic emotions. He focused on the *individual* and on *phenomenal* (derived from "phenomenon," of how things appear to us) subjective experience. His concern was with individual appraisal more than with expressive movements, and thus he had a different emphasis than did others who linked species characteristics to emotions (Eibl-Eibesfeldt, 1972; Ekman, 1972; Izard, 1971, 1990; Tomkins, 1982; Zajonc et al., 1989). Others who studied basic emotions differed from Lazarus, in that they focused on phylogenetic ("phylogenetic" coming from the term *phyla* in zoology) and species characteristics regarding emotion. They sought to identify what aspects of emotion are true for the whole human species, and to link these characteristics to evolution. In the nineteenth century, Darwin (1872/1965) formulated an evolutionary perspective with his descriptions of emotions for various animal groups. Many contemporary psychologists and ethologists (animal-behavior zoologists) take this evolutionary perspective rather than focus on appraisal of the person-environment relationship.

Adaptation and Coping With the Environment. Various viewpoints exist whether emotion aids in the way individuals adapt to and cope with the environment. Evolutionary psychologists consider that at a species level emotion is adaptive, in that emotions help organisms deal with disruptions in the environment. The question remains whether emotion is adaptive at the individual level. Some writers emphasize the protective "fight or flight" response as a reaction to danger (Selye, 1976), and many psychologists conceptualize emotion as having a protective survival quality for the individual, not merely for the species. Some (Levenson, 1988) suggest that emotion has evolved in a phylogenetic way as a shorthand and rapid way for the individual animal or human to take in information that is potentially harmful. Thus, many theorists agree that in terms of the species, emotion is very adaptive, and in circumstances of danger, emotion is also adaptive for the individual. Not all theorists consider adaptiveness to rely on appraisal, however. Zajonc (1989) emphasizes the adaptive nature of facial expressions and emotion in terms of the relationship between facial muscles, brain blood flow, and temperature. This differs radically from the views of Lazarus and others who consider adaptiveness in terms of the way the organism appraises the environment.

Although Lazarus considers that emotion may be adaptive, his research on stress and illness has shown many cases of maladaptive appraisals and emotions (Folkman & Lazarus, 1988). It is also well known from the field of psychopathology that individuals have a wide range of inappropriate and damaging emotions. Dramatic illustrations are hatred that kills innocent people, mania or depression that prevents the person from adequately meeting real-life demands, and flattened emotional responses that represent withdrawal from the life situations of the individual. Other illustrations of maladaptive emotions appear in connection with stress and illness. Psychological variables play an important role in many types of disease. Lazarus (1966; Folkman & Lazarus, 1988) has written extensively on the relationship between emotion, coping, stress, and disease. Lazarus considered that a major part of emotion is learned and social, not biologically preprogrammed. In contrast, Levenson (1988) focused on preprogramming for facial muscle and autonomic responses, and he focused more on harms than benefits, whereas Lazarus also considered positive emotions, like joy. When the person appraises a situation as *beneficial* or *harmful*, Lazarus considers emotion as adaptive if the appraisal is appropriate.

Some theorists consider appraisal not to be necessary for the occurrence of emotion (Levenson, 1988) and some like Izard (1990) and Levenson (1988) emphasize harm in their discussion of emotion and do not include the appraisal of benefit as an important aspect of emotion. Levenson (1988, p. 18) posited that "the essential function of emotion is organization." That is, humans and nonhuman animals need "an efficient mechanism" that "can mobilize and organize disparate response systems to deal with environmental events that pose a threat to survival."

Levenson (1988) pointed out that people encounter situations in which responses must be quickly organized, without time for deliberation or planning. Fine coordination is required in face muscles and visceral organs, and behaviors that are not ordinarily displayed need to become dominant. The specific emotions guide which responses will be made within the major response systems. For example, emotions guide which facial muscles to move or whether in one's body movement one needs to fight or flee or freeze. The specific emotions also guide how the heart, stomach, and other organs should respond. Because the parasympathetic branch of the autonomic system has specific patterns of control over internal organs, Levenson postulated that in moderately intense emotions quite specific processes take place. Normal emotional intensities differ from extremely intense emotion. In intense emotion the adrenal medulla releases its hormones into the bloodstream and thereby generates a strongly diffuse sympathetic nervous system activation, but with normal emotional intensities, Levenson rejects the idea that a generalized arousal state occurs.

Mandler (1975, 1984), like Levenson, considered the adaptive nature of emotion, but unlike Levenson, Mandler linked emotion with arousal and motivation. In his earlier writings Mandler (1975) focused on the negative aspect of emotion, that is, on fear or anxiety. For Mandler (1975, p. 165), interruption to completion of tasks was basic for emotion: "Whenever an organized sequence is interrupted we expect the occurrence of some emotional responses." His point was that the emotional response itself need not be disorganized or disruptive, just because the disruption of ongoing behavior leads to emotion. He pointed out (Mandler, 1975, p. 167) that a "fine rage is as well organized and may even be as productive of desired consequences as the most banal and unemotional organized sequence."

Mandler said fear and happiness are easily identified as involving different evaluations, but to separate out the two emotions of "nervous and afraid" one "must rely on an intensity factor" (Mandler, 1992, p. 123). He considered variations in arousal as adaptive (Mandler, 1992, p. 117): "for primates accustomed to gathering fruits and seeds in the daytime while looking out for predators, conserving

energy by sleeping at night is a very useful adaptation to lowered visual acuity and associated higher risk of predation at night." Referring to the work of Thayer on arousal, Mandler (1992, p. 124) stated that, "Energetic arousal and positive affect covary strongly as do tense arousal and negative affect. . . . The negative affect experienced while watching a horror movie is accompanied by an increase in tense arousal. The positive affect associated with a lively party is also associated with an increase in energetic arousal." The adaptive nature of emotion was said by Mandler to derive from two aspects. One is the adaptive aspect of conserving or using energy, and the other is the "desired consequence" (Mandler, 1975) of responses that are triggered by the experience of emotion. Thus, one way emotions may be adaptive is in their being goal directed toward an outcome.

Alfred Adler and the Goal Directedness of Emotions. Whereas the majority of theorists writing on emotion focused on *antecedent events* that triggered emotion because of harm or benefit, Alfred Adler (1928, 1929/1969, 1933/1964) put primary emphasis on the goal directedness of emotions. When Mandler considered a well-organized rage, he described the rage as leading to a consequence. The theory of Adler includes as an integral part of emotion the *appraisal of consequences,* and it emphasizes consequences more than did any of the theories discussed so far. Whereas Mandler and Lazarus gave credit to the concept of consequences, Adler made it essential in his formulation of emotion. That is, Lazarus (1991b, p. 145) did consider consequences with his concept of "secondary appraisal" (which "is an evaluation of the person's options and resources for coping with the situation"), but the term *secondary* gives lesser value to this type of appraisal. In contrast, Adler focused primarily on consequences.

Adler was a younger colleague in Freud's circle, and he broke with Freud over the latter's emphasis on sexual motivation. Adler also rejected Freud's emphasis on internal conflicts. Adler stressed the unity of the person, which led to his theory being called *individual psychology* (A. Adler, 1927/1971). His use of the term *individual* did not mean opposition to social, for his theory was based on a social psychological view of motivation. Instead, the term was used to focus on the whole individual rather than on a divided self. He rejected Freud's concept of a divided self (with id, ego, and super-ego) and developed a holistic theory of psychology that emphasized (a) social motivation, (b) goal direction, and (c) motivation oriented toward the outer environment rather than toward internal intrapsychic conflicts.

To quote directly from Adler (1928, p. 316): "We do not believe that anxiety arises from suppression of sexuality nor as the result of birth." Physiology and bodily reactions are important but do not explain emotion. Rather "what we see in mind and psyche is the use of this material toward a certain goal." Adler gave the example of (1928, p. 316) "a child who is accustomed to be accompanied by the mother uses anxiety . . . to arrive at his goal of superiority to control the mother. In this we are not concerned with a description of anger, but we are experienced enough to see that anger is a means to overcome a person or a situation."

Because Adler based his theory on a fundamentally social motivation (Ferguson, 1989, 1995), that placed emphasis on human striving to belong and to feel of value in a human group, his theory considered "social" an aspect of "evolutionary." Humans as a species are social, and this phylogenetic characteristic makes human actions understandable only in social terms. Furthermore, his is a cognitive theory. All goals are based on beliefs. For Adler, emotion always is directed to fulfill the individual's goal, and in that sense it is adaptive. Emotion helps move the person toward his or her goals. If there are maladaptive aspects, it is not the emotion but the *goals* that are maladaptive. To change pathological emotions, one needs to change maladaptive goals.

Adler was perhaps the first cognitive psychotherapist. He emphasized a person's goals and related beliefs as important in psychopathology. The goal need not be conscious. When emotions occurring in cases of illness and disease are maladaptive, the cause of the maladaptiveness lies in the goal and in the underlying cognitions on which the goal is based. A goal may be constructive or it may be destructive from the perspective of society or from the point of view of the person's own welfare. The goal fits the person's beliefs, and some of these beliefs are "private logic," which means they are idiosyncratic and may deviate markedly from more realistic or consensual beliefs (Dreikurs, 1950/1992).

The theory of Adler has not received as much attention as has that of Freud, yet Adler's theory in many ways is more akin to contemporary psychology. Adler emphasized holism and goal direction, and cognitive and social factors. That contrasted with Freud's emphasis on hedonic and sexual characteristics (Freud, 1901/1960). These two men's theories differed fundamentally in their conceptualization of emotion and motivation (see Ferguson, 1995, for a fuller description of Adler's theory). From the point of view developed by Adler and others (e.g., K. A. Adler, 1961; Dreikurs, 1967b), emotion may be, but ordinarily is not, a fleeting experience. Emotion may be brief or it may last some time, depending on the consequences being sought.

That emotion is goal directed means that in one situation an antecedent event may lead to anger, in another it may lead to joy, and in another it may lead to fear. The difference is a function of one's *appraisal of consequences* that one seeks to attain. Under ordinary circumstances, seeing a car come crashing toward oneself will engender a highly intense reaction of fear, in line with the formulations of Lazarus, Levenson, Selye, and many others. However, the fear reflects the goal of the person, of seeking a long life. For a person with a goal of suicide, the same event is likely to engender other emotions, possibly even of joy. To the lover who wants to break up a relationship, an ardent love letter by the partner may engender rage; to the lover who seeks close bonding with the partner, the letter would engender great joy. In this way, from the standpoint of Adler's theory, appraisal of "harm" or "benefit" as leading to emotion are defined by the person's goal. The emotion fits, not to the event as such but to its consequences.

The theory of Adler was developed as a broadly therapeutic and rehabilitative model. It arose from the perspective of clinical psychology and was part of the pioneering work in modern psychiatry. By the late 1930s it was applied to real-life problems in marriage, parenting, classrooms and schools, and in work relationships. Empirical support for the theory came from case studies rather than from laboratory experiments.

One can imagine a scene involving two friends going to the movies to illustrate how goals direct emotions. One person arrives early because of eagerness to see the friend, and the emotion is some variant of joy or positive anticipation. The other person arrives later but at the prearranged time and experiences distress (such as anxiety or mild anger) because of wishing to see the whole movie and wanting not to miss any part of it. The emotion (of anger or anxiety) is oriented toward the consequence (goal), to facilitate the activity of hurrying both of the friends through the process of buying the tickets and racing to get seated in the theater. The first-arriver could react to this whirlwind with various emotions. However, if the first-arriver has the goal of visiting with the friend at the moment of their encounter, she or he will respond with anger, directed toward the consequence of slowing down the later-arriver in order that some time can be spent visiting, rather than merely racing into the theater.

The above illustrates that the emotion selectively facilitates those actions that bring about goal attainment. The emotion may directly alter one's own actions or the actions of others. The emotion may facilitate succinct signaling of one's intention(s) to other persons. Thus, according to Adlerian theory, emotion helps move the individual in one or another direction. *Appraisal* occurs both in the sense of appraising the immediately antecedent events and in appraising the outcome of actions or events that are anticipated to follow the emotion.

Usually a person is not aware of how emotions fit outcomes. According to Adlerian theory, goals may be conscious but they need not be. Adler's theory has no counterpart to Freud's postulate of "the Unconscious." Adler's theory did not distinguish between conscious and unconscious in the way Freud's theory did, and appraisal of outcomes may or may not be conscious. People often wonder why their emotions occurred as they did and why at

times emotions may shift rapidly. Adler's theory postulated that people typically are not cognizant of their goals and they ordinarily do not realize that their emotions fit a goal. Many case studies illustrate the Adlerian postulation regarding emotions and their goal directedness (A. Adler, 1929/1969, 1939; Dreikurs, 1946/1990, 1948/1990, 1971/1992; Dreikurs, Grunwald, & Pepper, 1998; Ferguson, 1989; Mosak, 1977; Shulman & Mosak, 1967).

How Can Emotions Be Changed?

Adlerians recommend that the way to change emotions is to help alter an individual's specific goal(s). Adlerians have devised special and effective techniques for helping to change goals (e.g., Dreikurs, 1947, 1972), and they report consistent success with their methods. Other theorists may emphasize conditioning principles, and still others focus on cognitive processes and their modification (Barlow, 1993). Since the time when Watson and Rayner (1920) demonstrated the classical conditioning of an emotion (fear toward a white rat), many additional studies of classical and operant conditioning have demonstrated that emotions are learned reactions that also can be altered by counterconditioning or extinction (Lang, 1964, 1968; Lang, Melamed, & Hart, 1970; Wolpe, 1958, 1997). Likewise, cognitive therapists have provided many methods for modifying emotions (Beck and Young, 1985; Beck & Greenberg, 1996; Burns, 1989; Ellis & Dryden, 1997; Freeman & Davison, 1997; Kopp, 1995; Werner, 1982).

Some psychologists (e.g., Izard, 1990) link emotion to evolutionary determinants as well as to learning experiences. Levenson, Ekman, and Friesen (1990) posit that at birth, (p. 381) a "central connection would be hard-wired," but beyond early childhood, individual learning experiences then modulate and regulate these processes. Theories of change will be different for researchers in artificial intelligence (Levine & Leven, 1992) than for researchers who emphasize the intensity or arousal aspect of emotion (Duffy, 1941), and different from clinicians (A. Adler, 1928; Lazarus, 1991b) who are concerned with the welfare and mental health of the individual as well as of society. If one considers the emotion maladaptive, efforts will be spent on re-training the emotion; if one considers the cognitions and the goals set by the individual as maladaptive, the reorientation will be focused on changing the cognitions and goals.

Even though some laboratory studies appear to be far removed from everyday experiences, several such studies have provided application to real-world phenomena. For example, Gottman and Levenson (1985) studied married couples who were willing to discuss both high-conflict and low-conflict problems in a laboratory setting. Gottman and Levenson suggested that extensions of their work could help predict or improve marital relationships. Other applications of laboratory studies to real-life emotions extended research on various types of conditioning to the treatment of excess fears and phobias (Wolpe, 1997), panic disorders (Craske & Barlow, 1993), and anxiety disorders (Brown, O'Leary, & Barlow, 1993).

EMOTION, MOOD, AND AFFECT

A broad range of studies from a variety of theoretical perspectives have assessed what effects emotion and mood have on behavior. A large literature exists, but inconsistent use of terms made it hard to separate out whether the studies concerned emotion, mood, or "affect."

Are Emotion, Mood, and Affect Different?

Many terms, like feelings, affect, emotion, and mood, have been used, often interchangeably. For example, Gilligan and Bower (1985, p. 547) discussed the assumption that "perceptions, thoughts, and actions are strongly biased by our emotional feelings" and they added that they have "examined how emotional mood states might influence such cognitive processes as learning, memory, perception, and judgments." This illustrates that "feelings," "emotion," and "mood" have been used interchangeably. In recognition of this difficulty, in later writings Bower (1992, p. 3) explained he "used only an informal, layman's view of emotions. I advanced no particular conceptualization of what

an emotion is." In seeking a more careful analysis, he noted (p. 11):

> An emotion has many of the properties of a reaction: It often has an identifiable cause or stimulus; it is usually a brief, spasmodic, intense experience of short duration; and the person is typically much aware of it. Emotional states typically have bodily concomitants the person is well aware of. A mood tends to be more subtle, longer lasting, less intense, more in the background, a frame of mind, casting a positive or negative light over experiences.

Not all writers distinguish between emotion and mood, but the above distinction captures characteristics described by other writers (e.g., Ekman, 1984, 1992a; Lazarus, 1991c). Some writers distinguished emotion from mood not only in terms of duration but on the basis that emotion but not mood has some kind of a target "object." Frijda, et al. (1991) as well as Lazarus (1991b) postulated that moods, contrary to emotions, refer to one's relationship to life or to the world in *general,* and not to a specific object. Frijda and colleagues (1991, p. 220) pointed out that "moods can be described as appraisals of the world as a whole" and as "feeling states that do not bear upon a particular object." Lazarus (1991b, p. 48) stated that "moods refer to the larger, pervasive, existential issues of one's life," whereas emotions refer to immediate adaptational encounters with some specific aspects of the environment.

Mood is considered a diffuse reaction that deals with relatively abstract and long-lasting life contexts, compared with the acute reactions of emotions. One way to describe mood is that it primes certain emotional reactions, that is, mood biases the individual for "readiness to react" in certain ways. Mood provides a guiding set within which some emotions are more likely to occur than others. Mood can be thought of as an emotional "tone." Analogous to muscle tone, mood provides a certain kind of emotional response readiness in the same way that a certain kind of muscle response readiness occurs in muscle tone. Both types of tone can change as a result of new experiences, but a change in tone usually takes longer than does the occurrence of a specific emotional or muscular response.

Various instruments for measuring specific emotions and general mood have been developed, like the scales for measuring anger (Spielberger, Jacobs, Russell, & Crane, 1983), anxiety (Spielberger, Gorsuch, & Lushene, 1970), depression (Beck, Ward, Mendelsohn, Mock, & Erbaujh, 1961; Lubin, 1965), empathy (Mehrabian & Epstein, 1972), and general mood (Nowlis, 1965).

In contrast to the way mood and emotions are identified, some writers (e.g., Frijda et al., 1991) identify a hedonic meaning for the term *affect*. (The *noun* "affect" and the *verb* "affect" need to be kept separate in this discussion.) Frijda et al. (1991, p. 195) described the noun "affect" as the "basic aspect of emotional feeling, the experience of pleasure or pain." Other writers (e.g., Lazarus, 1991b) disavow that pleasure and pain should describe "affect," because pleasure and pain are experiences without reference to specific kinds of person-environment transactions.

Many meanings have been used when affect, emotion, and mood are linked to the construct of personality. John (1990, p. 66) noted problems of definitions in his review of measurement scales used to study personality: "scales with the same name often measure concepts that are not the same, and scales with quite different names overlap considerably in their item content." John pointed out that personality and mood have been linked in studies of individual differences, and measures of "positive" and "negative" emotionality appear to relate to mood and personality but are measured by scales with the label of "affect" (e.g., a scale by Watson, Clark, & Tellegen, 1988). Interchangeability between "affect" and "mood" was evident when Emmons and King (1989, p. 478) stated that they examined "affective reactivity (intensity and variability of mood)" within a personal striving framework. Labeling a scale for mood as one of affect (Watson et al., 1988) and identifying affective reactivity in terms of characteristics of mood (Emmons & King, 1989) illustrate difficulties encountered in terminology. Whereas the term *affect* tends to refer to the positive or negative hedonic quality of a specific emotional experience, often the term *mood* also refers to positive or negative hedonic qualities, but unlike affect, lacks a specific situational target and refers to a long-lasting orientation.

Pleasantness-Unpleasantness: Dimensions Are Different from Categories

A controversy exists between theorists conceptualizing emotion in terms of categories versus dimensions. Ekman et al. (1972) and Levenson (1988) noted that research in the field of emotion differs according to whether the emphasis is on discrete emotions, which differ in *categories,* or on *dimensions* of emotion. Although in his later writings Ekman argued that emotions fit categories rather than dimensions, early in his work, when reviewing studies of facial expression in photographs, Ekman et al. (1972, p. 71) concluded that "the only consistent finding across experiments is a dimension of Pleasantness/Unpleasantness," and several early researchers in the field of facial expression emphasized emotion dimensions like pleasant-unpleasant and active-passive as fundamental to emotional experience. This agreed with Wundt (1902), who had concluded that various categories of emotion like anger or sadness were not fundamentally distinct but, instead, that the underlying dimensions were crucial.

The dimension of pleasant versus unpleasant refers to hedonic tone. From the time of the earliest philosophers, writers have emphasized pleasure seeking (i.e., hedonism) and pain avoidance as fundamental motivational characteristics. A psychology of hedonism played a major role in the theory of Freud (1920/1975). Many considered pleasant-unpleasant to provide a dimension on which a simple scale could be devised and easily applied for data collecting. Untrained observers can recognize fairly easily if a person is feeling "good" or "bad," and expert judges can respond to photos fairly reliably in terms of whether a given face displays a pleasant or an unpleasant emotion. Pleasant versus unpleasant became a key aspect in some research on emotion, and this led to one use of the term *affect.*

Controversy about whether pleasant-unpleasant is important for the study of emotion in part pertains to how much one seeks to relate emotion to motivation and action. For example, in an opening address in an early international symposium on the topic of emotion, Jastrow (1928, p. 24) noted that emotion and motivation are very closely linked:

"The common root of several energetic words, *m-o-t*, . . . leads to our moving in that we are moved to response. Motive, emotion, and motion are of one psychological as well as philological family." This statement links *movement, motivation,* and *emotion.* From this perspective, motivation and emotion are dynamic processes involved in the adaptive movement of the individual, and hedonic characteristics of emotion, like pleasantness-unpleasantness, would be less important than are other characteristics of emotion.

EMOTION AND OPPONENT PROCESSES

Opponent Process Theory

A very different approach than that taken by Schachter and Singer (1962), Lazarus (1991b), Ekman et al. (1983), and Diener et al. (1985) is the approach of Solomon and Corbit (1974; Solomon, 1980, 1991). That approach was developed from the perspective and background of conditioning experiments, in contrast to the work discussed so far which derived largely from social, personality, or clinical psychology.

The work of Solomon (1980, 1991) had its origin in the field of motivation, and emotion was conceptualized within the motivational perspective. The work of earlier conditioning theorists provides the background of "opponent process theory." Early conditioning researchers posited opposing excitatory and inhibitory processes. A well-known example is the work of Pavlov (1927), the famous Russian physiologist who demonstrated the power of conditioning and who had great influence on the development of American psychology. Pavlov (1927) used the concept of internal inhibition to account for data in his conditioning studies, and he postulated that every time a response occurs it reflects both excitatory and inhibitory processes that are opponents of one another. Solomon and Corbit (1974) used this concept of opponent processes for hedonic characteristics, which differed from the work of Pavlov. Solomon and Corbit postulated that hedonically positive and negative reactions are crucial in motivation and emotion.

Their theory goes as follows. If the subject experiences an event that leads to a positive or pleasurable reaction, after a short lag of time an opponent process of displeasure will occur. This displeasure reaction will decay after the pleasurable reaction ceases, so that the hedonic state that remains is the opponent reaction. At first, this opponent afterreaction is weaker than the initial reaction. This means that on first encountering the positive event an initial pleasure is stronger than the opponent remaining displeasure. However, after many such experiences with an initial positive reaction, the negative afterreaction becomes the stronger. The strength of the initial reaction weakens and the strength of the afterreaction increases with repeated experiences, so that the cost of pleasure becomes greater with time. This formulation fits equally to pleasurable and painful states. Thus, if the subject has a painful event that initiates a hedonically negative state, after a short lag a pleasurable opponent process begins and it remains after the negative state has stopped. After many repetitions it becomes the stronger and will be the remaining hedonic state.

By means of this formulation, Solomon explained the phenomenon of addiction: what initially is a pleasurable experience becomes with repetition less and less pleasurable due to the displeasurable afterreaction, since the displeasure remains and becomes increasingly stronger with repetition of the addictive behavior. Studies with nonhuman animals as well as with humans have lent support to this formulation. The processes that are assumed to occur in this sequence are not cognitive. Rather, they are assumed to occur in the same type of noncognitive way that many writers assume takes place in simple conditioning.

Test of the Opponent Process Theory

Mauro (1988) tested the opponent process formulation by means of hypnotically induced hedonic states. His dependent variables were physiological reactions and self-report measures of emotion. The dimensional emotion ratings were obtained with a bipolar scale, in which 1 was very unpleasant and 9 was very pleasant. At an early stage of the experimental session, bipolar ratings provided a global assessment of how pleasant or unpleasant the subject felt. Categories of emotion were measured with unipolar scales, in which 1 was "not at all" and 9 was "extremely," for ratings of happy, sad, angry, afraid, and disgusted.

Muscle action recordings were obtained from above the eyebrows (corrugator activity) and from the cheek area (zygomat activity). Heart rate was also recorded. Mauro (1988) hypothesized that if opponent process theory is correct, subjects should show similar muscle activity and self-rating of emotion when the emotion is an opponent reaction (e.g., a happy reaction as an afterreaction to an unpleasant stimulus) as when it is an initial reaction (e.g., a happy reaction as an initial reaction to a pleasant stimulus). For the hypnotic induction, Mauro had subjects experience reliving of real-life emotions from the past, with subjects being urged to recall a very happy (or sad) previous time. When the relived emotion was created, the subject was also instructed that a light (blue, green, yellow, or red, assigned randomly to emotions for different subjects) will be associated with that emotion, and the more intense the light, the stronger that emotion.

The lights were presented against a blank screen. After the subjects saw the lights that had just been associated as the happy and sad lights, their initial emotions were rated. Compared with baseline measures, self-ratings showed that the light associated with the *happy* emotion gave significantly more pleasant ratings and the light associated with the *sad* emotion gave significantly less pleasant self-ratings. Heart rate was not significantly different, but significantly more zygomatic activity was found when subjects initially saw the happy light and corrugator activity was significantly higher when subjects saw the sad light.

Opponent process theory would predict that when the happy and sad lights were terminated, the reverse reactions should occur. To a large extent the data confirmed this. Subjects reported feeling significantly more unpleasant, less happy, and more sad (compared with baseline) after the happy light was terminated. Moreover, the face muscle activity was in the predicted direction: the zygomatic activity decreased after the happy light went off, compared with the high activity during the happy light; the corrugator activity increased after the happy light went off, compared with the low activity while the happy light was on.

The study by Mauro (1988) had additional conditions that, in their complexity, won't be described here. However, one interesting finding worth noting is the asymmetry of the opponent process effect. The data for the happy and after-happy light were in line with the Solomon predictions, but data for the after-sad condition were not. Following the sad light termination, the opponent process should have led to positive emotion. Instead, the self-report of emotion was significantly less pleasant, less happy, more disgusted, and sadder compared with baseline. In other words, when the sad light stopped, instead of experiencing happy or positive emotions, subjects continued to experience negative and sad emotions. The face muscle activity duplicated this effect, with the direction of activity continuing toward negative and sad emotion rather than revealing the opponent process. Although with the "happy-sad" conditions the asymmetry occurred, Mauro suggested that the asymmetry might not occur with other negative emotions. For example, it is not known whether the predicted effect of opponent processes, rather than the asymmetry effect, would occur with an emotion such as fear. One cannot conclude at this time if the asymmetry data obtained by Mauro is due to an overall difference between positive and negative emotional states or if it is limited to the negative emotion of sadness. Mauro suggested that until negative emotions other than sadness are investigated, it is premature to conclude that positive emotions lead to the opponent process whereas negative emotions do not.

SUMMARY

Emotion and motivation have similarities, but usually emotion is more specific and more influenced by the immediate situation. Motivation sets the broad direction or guidelines within which emotion occurs. Emotions may change as situations change. In a given situation, emotion is determined by the motivation and goals of the individual at that time. Emotion is usually briefer than mood, whereas emotion and motivation are not distinguishable in terms of duration.

In the early years of the 20th century William James, W. Wundt, and J. B. Watson had different approaches to the definition and study of emotion, and those early controversies remain as unresolved issues in the writings of contemporary researchers. Early theorists raised issues that are still controversial today: the role of expressive movements; the kind of physiological changes that accompany emotion; the role of emotional intensity versus qualitative differences in emotion; and whether emotion is best described in terms of categories, like basic emotions, or in terms of dimensions, like pleasantness-unpleasantness.

In the history of psychology, various theorists defined emotion in different ways. Wundt considered three dimensions for emotion and emphasized that intensity of emotion is important. Wundt rejected the James-Lange theory, with its emphasis on expressive movement for defining emotion. Watson considered three emotions innate and basic (fear, rage, and love), but he emphasized that most emotions are learned. He demonstrated with a young boy and a white rat that emotions can be conditioned. He also assumed that just as emotions can be learned by conditioning, so they can be eliminated by procedures of extinction.

When Ekman and colleagues directed persons, for example actors, to move specific face muscles, these persons experienced the associated specific emotion and they experienced the associated autonomic nervous system activity. Several other researchers also believe that emotions occur as a result of face muscle movement, and this lends support for the James-Lange view of emotion. Although data show such response-produced emotions can occur, most researchers believe that face muscle activity in general is a consequence, not a precursor, to an individual's emotion.

The Schachter and Singer hypothesis proposed that emotion is a function of physiological arousal and a person's cognitions concerning the external environment and internal bodily cues. Tests made by others of the Schachter and Singer hypothesis did not support the hypothesis. They failed to replicate earlier findings of happy or angry self-reported emotions as a function of environmental cues (provided by a happy or angry confederate.) Also,

overt behavior was not congruent with self-reported emotions.

Emotions rated over days in one's daily life show that although pleasant and unpleasant emotions can be experienced separately, they are not fully independent. People who experience love more frequently than others also tend to experience fear or anxiety more frequently. Both positive and negative emotions can be experienced at generally the same time if the time frame is long enough, but if the time frame is very brief, then a person would experience only a pleasant or only an unpleasant emotion.

Lazarus considers emotion to reflect an appraised relationship between the person and the environment. Appraisal occurs in terms of benefit or harm, that is, in what way the person believes the environment benefits or harms himself or herself. Such appraisal is necessary for the person to experience emotion. Motivation defines the personal significance of the person's transaction with the environment.

Emotion serves an adaptive function at the species level. It allows fast organizing of overt behavior and activity of internal organs in the face of threat (Levenson), and emotions can be intense or calm according to what the energy demands are on the individual (Mandler). Emotions are adaptive in that they bring about consequences. At the individual level the adaptiveness or maladaptiveness of an emotion depends on the appropriateness of the person's person-environment appraisal (Lazarus) or on the degree of realism and social interest of the individual's goal (Adler).

Adlerian psychology is holistic, social, and cognitive, and postulates that the fundamental motivation of humans is to feel belonging and contribute to others. Emotions are directed to goals, and to change emotions one needs to change the goals and their underlying beliefs. This contrasts with Behavioral approaches, which seek to change emotion in terms of conditioning theory or behavior modification techniques.

Most theorists consider emotion a directional internal state that differs from motivation. All theorists consider emotion to differ from mood. Mood is less specific than emotion in its antecedent and target—

mood is more global. Mood can be considered to involve emotional tone in a way that is analogous to muscle tone. Mood is not targeted to specific events the way emotion is, and mood has longer duration than emotion. Affect is thought by some (Frijda) to refer to specific pleasure or pain experiences. "Affect" tends to be considered as the hedonic quality of emotional experiences, but there is no general agreement on the meaning of the term *affect.*

Some researchers consider categories and others consider dimensions as the most useful way to study emotion. Dimensions of emotion in terms of pleasantness or unpleasantness have been found useful to describe everyday emotions and, depending on whether the emotion is brief or long, pleasantness can be considered as a different dimension from unpleasantness.

Various measures have been used to answer if pleasantness-unpleasantness refers to one or two dimensions. Subjective ratings have been used to measure emotions in everyday life and in laboratory studies. These ratings may, but need not, agree with behavioral observation of emotion.

Emotions and motivations can be conceptualized to involve opponent processes. Solomon applied the concepts of excitation and inhibition from research on conditioning to the study of motivation, and he proposed that hedonically opponent processes occur to produce afterreactions. The strength of the initial reaction weakens and the afterreaction increases in strength with repeated experience. Mauro found support for this formulation for the afterreaction of sadness following a happy emotion but he did not obtain the afterreaction of happiness following a sad emotion. Thus, opponent process theory may explain some, but not all, emotional shifts.

Although memory can distort aspects of an emotional experience, remembered emotions can be congruent with presently experienced emotions. Contrasting theories provide different ways for conceptualizing the relationship between emotion and motivation. The present book focuses on emotion as a dynamic process that occurs when the individual is in transaction with the environment, and motivation provides the goal toward which emotion is directed.

CHAPTER 7

Emotion and Mood: II. Cognition and Information Processing

Cognition was discussed in the previous chapter in various ways, as in the description of appraisal by Lazarus (1991b) and in the arousal-cognition formulation by Schachter and Singer (1962) that was tested by Maslach (1979). The present chapter relates emotion and mood to cognition and information processing from additional perspectives. For example, questions considered here are: How do cognitions of the individual alter emotion and mood, and how do emotion and mood alter cognition? How does the emotional content of stimuli, such as found in emotional words, alter the way we encode, store, and retrieve that information? Does the brain process emotional stimuli differently than it does nonemotional stimuli? Furthermore, do different parts of the brain process different kinds of emotions? Firm answers to these questions are not as yet fully available, but psychologists have begun to give tentative answers and to form hypotheses to help guide further research regarding these questions.

COMPLEXITY OF EMOTION AND COGNITION

In the previous chapter we noted that emotions can last for as brief a time as a few seconds and for as long as several hours. From an evolutionary viewpoint (Ekman, 1992a, 1992b, 1992c), basic and inborn emotions are theorized to be very brief, and what appear to the observer to be long emotional experiences are explained to be sequences of brief

bursts of basic emotions and blends. More cognitive perspectives provide other explanations for long durations of emotions. Emotions can be brought about not only by specific momentary stimuli but also by thoughts and memories (cognitions). The next section will consider alternative explanations for why research with self-report measures shows emotions to last from a few minutes to several hours or even days. Experiences in daily life often involve complex emotions that consist of possible contradictions, various nuances, and different durations.

Multiple Targets at a Given Moment

Many times, people experience two or more very different emotions at apparently the same time. One way this can happen is that several concurrent targets can each involve different emotions. An illustration would be the following scene: Jane is berating the boss to her partner while the puppy is licking her hands. Jane is angry at her boss, has a strong emotion of love to her partner, and experiences happiness as the puppy licks her hand. Here there are three targets for emotions, the boss, the partner, and the puppy. Each of these emotions can be assumed to have associated with them quite different cognitions.

Theorists like Levenson (1988, 1992), who argue for very brief bursts of emotion, would say that being angry at a boss, love filled toward a partner, and happy with a puppy's affectionate behavior at apparently the same time is an illusory effect.

That is, different momentary bursts of emotions are occurring, singly rather than concurrently, over a span of time that covers many minutes. From that point of view, the acute emotion of anger, which lasts a few seconds, is interspersed with acute emotional experiences of love as the partner nods sympathetically to the story, and it is interspersed with the acute happiness that occurs when the puppy's warm tongue soothes Jane's clammy hand. Each of these emotions is accompanied by different cognitions. Careful analysis in the above example might well show that during some of the 5- to 10-second periods the emotions were brief bursts in succession. However, subjectively a person is not likely to experience the emotions as short bursts in succession, but rather as occurring simultaneously during a single "moment" that might last many minutes.

The size of the subjective moment is likely to vary according to the immediate stimuli (such as the puppy licking the hand) as well as the flow of ideas and memories (cognitions) the individual is generating. The vivid recall and image of the boss's actions during the prior week will give rise to the stream of anger within the time period, during which the partner nods sympathetically and the puppy licks Jane's hand. Emotions are generated by one's thoughts and memories and by specific stimuli present within a given period. Thus, the complexity of emotional experiences is in part due to the complexity of cognitions interacting with stimuli that occur in the immediate environment.

Developmental Factors and the Question of Blends Versus Pure Emotions

The last chapter described the fact that some writers (e.g., Lazarus, 1991b) have sought to distinguish pure emotions from blends. Other writers, like Ekman and colleagues (Ekman, Friesen, & Ellsworth, 1972), have contrasted basic emotions, like anger, with love, which they do not consider a basic emotion (Ekman, Levenson, & Friesen 1983). Theorists differ in the specific way they distinguish between pure and blended emotions, and the important question is to what extent any distinction between pure and blended is fruitful.

In nonhuman animals and in human neonates a few simple emotions exist, and many theorists identify these as basic emotions. As humans develop with age, their emotions become increasingly complex and so do the accompanying cognitions. The fact that emotions become increasingly complex as individuals develop and as their cognitions become more subtle requires a developmental perspective that differs from a concern with distinguishing pure (or basic) from blended emotions.

Certain characteristic changes occur in the way children's emotions gain complexity, and these changes are intricately related to cognitive development. Fischer, Shaver, and Carnochan (1990) reviewed a number of studies that reveal increasing complexity in the way children can conceptualize and behaviorally express emotions. These authors considered that emotions fit into groupings ("families") within which specific emotions share resemblances but not universal features. They state it this way (Fischer et al., 1990, p. 85): "In the terms of cognitive theory, emotions fit the prototype model of categories, in which all category members can be related to a best instance (prototype) defining the category but few members have all characteristics of that prototype." Instead of calling "contentment" a blend, for example, these authors suggested it is part of a subordinate category that contains similar emotions (like pride and bliss) and is related to a developmentally more elementary emotion of joy. Emotions such as contentment and bliss, according to the scheme of these authors, are developmentally more complex and are experienced at a later age than simpler, basic emotions.

Developmentally, increasing complexity in emotions occurs in relationship with increased cognitive complexity. This dual development permits adult emotions to have many nuances. The developmental characteristic of emotions may be more important for understanding emotion than is a concern with pure versus blends of emotion. Data from several studies (Fischer et al., 1990) showed that in the first 4 months only partial expressions of anger and joy are apparent, but by the age of 2 years, children can display anger even in pretense, such as making a doll act angry. By the age of 10 or 12 years, children experience complex emotions that reflect their increasingly abstract thinking.

Beyond the age of 3 or 4 years, children's understanding of their own and others' emotions becomes more sophisticated. Already at ages 2 and 3, children understand their own and others' emotional and motivational states, and they seem to understand these better than they do internal beliefs. For example, Hadwin and Perner (1991) showed that the young child can understand that another person's desire may not be fulfilled before the child can understand that another's beliefs may be false. Astington and Gopnik (1990) found that 3-year-olds can remember their own past unfulfilled desires. Unlike 4-year-olds, they cannot readily report the content of their past desires that were fulfilled, as found in a study by Gopnik and Slaughter (1991). These investigators gave children sets of two sequential conditions that involved changes (in perception, desire for objects or events, intention about actions, and belief about objects or events). At age 3 children could easily report their past perceptions, they could report their past desires and intentions somewhat less easily, and they had great difficulty reporting their past beliefs. By age 4, children had no difficulty in recalling any of these. Thus, understanding desires and intentions, one's own as well as others', seems to fall developmentally midway between understanding what one perceives and what one believes.

Fischer et al. (1990) point out another and later shift in the child's representation of emotion. These investigators suggest that under age 10 children's emotions have a strongly concrete quality, but in later years more abstract processes shape the emotions. From the expanding literature on the development of emotions, it appears that in infancy quite undifferentiated and limited emotional experiences occur, and with age and experience the child has increasingly complex emotions. Some writers (Fischer et al., 1990; Watson & Rayner, 1920) argue for the full or partial appearance of a limited set of basic emotions in the newborn and young infant, whereas others (Werner, 1940/1961) point out that only undifferentiated excitation is evident, and this state gradually becomes differentiated into distress, excitement, and delight. According to Werner (1940/1961), these three emotions differentiate only at a considerably later age into fear, anger, distress, excitement, delight, joy, and affection. With increasing age and cognitive complexity these emotions differentiate further. Thus, controversy exists whether basic emotions occur at birth or within the first year, and which emotions in fact are basic, although there is general agreement that developmental changes in emotion occur.

Fischer et al. (1990) separate basic emotions from subcategories of emotions in their emphasis on prototype. The search for prototypes permits the scientist to posit conditions that lead to idealized emotions. This is useful, but still does not yield full understanding of the way complex and multifaceted emotions occur in the practical course of human transactions, especially in adults. In daily life, a wide range of cognitions and motivations are involved in the generation of any given emotion. The search for prototypes or for pure and blended emotions may aid in understanding the emotions of young children, but the normal emotional experiences of individuals beyond early childhood also need to be understood within the context of people's transaction with their complex environments.

An Ecological Perspective

Emotions can be considered ecologically in terms of environmental contexts and in terms of the direction of a person's actions within an environmental field. In adulthood, a given stimulus might lead to the type of appraisals Lazarus (1991b) described for adult anger, in which self-esteem is appraised as being assaulted or threatened, but ordinarily a wide range of additional reactions are generated in response to an emotion-arousing stimulus. For example, one might have anger directed toward a rude person who appears to be insulting, and this might be accompanied by the emotion of fear of greater insults about to happen, with an additional emotion of disgust at the boorishness of the other person's actions.

An example of how the complexity of emotions relates to cognitive processes can be seen for a driver hurrying to make a tight deadline, who is angry at the stoplight that just turned red. He may have a private logic thought of "how dare the light do this to me," by considering the light to have assaulted his self-esteem, but accompanying dreads, such as worry about getting to his destination, or concern that his late arrival will have negative consequences, are likely to create a mix of emotional reactions. In general, nuances and complexities of emotions are the rule. Ecological concern with a total context focuses on the function of emotions with respect to goals and the flow of actions in the person's normal life events.

This viewpoint was expressed some years ago by ecologically oriented psychologists. Werner (1957) argued for permitting the study of psychological processes in their normal flow. In the field of perception, Bachmann (1991) has described how arbitrary introduction of perceptual experiences can distort the ongoing perceptual process. The study of isolated emotions outside of normal life experiences may likewise artificially truncate (abbreviate) what is observed, so that the recorded emotion may be distorted and may not fully represent a normal self-generated and adaptive emotional process. Although the study of pure and basic emotions has increased understanding of emotion, efforts to isolate emotions from the flow of self-generated emotions within normal motivational and cognitive complexities can create distortions analogous to those reported by Bachmann (1991) in perception studies.

Long-term Versus Short-term Targets

Not only can a person have two or more different emotions with different targets at a given time, but a person can have emotions of different durations directed at apparently the same target. Different cognitions would accompany the different emotions. Although researchers who tied emotion to physiological reactivity (e.g., Levenson, 1992) considered emotions as being of short duration, from a cognitive and ecological perspective, emotions directed at a given target have long-term as well as short-term characteristics.

Emotions like love may be part of complex states that are a mixture of cognition, emotion, and motivation. In the previous example, cognitions about the partner are likely to affect the specific emotion of love at the given moment, such as the knowledge that one's partner will be supportive while one is speaking. One's belief regarding one's own and the partner's commitment to the relationship is also important. The long-term motivational process of commitment to a given relationship enters into the nuances of the emotion of love in the example. Long-term beliefs shape emotions, and emotions can be long-term and broadly directed to a target. Because they have a specific target, long-term emotions differ from moods. Schwarz and Clore (1988, p. 58) used the term *global* to refer to moods, which they distinguished from specific emotions, and what is here described as long-term emotions are not the same as moods.

Anger has been identified by many researchers as a more clear-cut emotion than love. For older children and adults, cognitions play a role in anger. In the hypothetical example concerning anger with the boss, the intensity and nuances of the anger might be influenced by knowledge of the boss's untrustworthy actions taken in the past. Thus, even with emotions like anger, which many writers presume to be pure or basic, knowledge of the past and belief in future happenings shape emotions that humans experience from the time of early childhood.

From a dynamic and adaptive point of view, one can note that feuding neighbors, estranged spouses, and warring populations can have long-term hates or rages that are very different from moods. The long-term emotion is not a *trait*, which refers to a *disposition* to experience the emotion or motivation. Rather, it is an ongoing and long-term *state*, directed specifically to a limited set of circumstances or individuals. If the feuding neighbors or estranged spouses only rarely get angry in other relationships, there is no evidence that the person has a trait (general disposition) of anger. The distinction made in an earlier chapter, between tonic and phasic, is appropriate here. The concept of tonic versus phasic emotions distinguishes between emotions that last hours versus seconds, and also applies to longer-term emotions.

In the previous chapter we noted that Lazarus (1991b) and Frijda, Mesquita, Sonnemans, and Van Goozen (1991) suggested that, in contrast to emotions, moods lack specific objects or targets. One can have long-term hates and long-term loves, and at a tonic level these can be identified as emotions, not moods. In the hypothetical example of Jane, the target for the love is the partner. Many theorists do not consider the tonic characteristic as emotion, and they consider emotion only in terms of phasic characteristics. However, from an adaptive and ecological perspective, humans have long-term emotions that direct and organize actions in a way that is comparable for short-term emotions. If one says, "I am happy at the party," this refers to an event of possibly several hours, and yet a variety of short-term emotions are likely to arise in terms of specific events at the party. The last chapter described that Diener, Larsen, Levine, and Emmons (1985) and Larson (1987) argued for the independence of pleasant versus unpleasant emotions. Their view was that although a person cannot have both sets of emotions at the same time, within some hours or on a given day one can have both sorts of emotions. In the same way, one can experience both love and anger toward the same person in a given hour or day. Two kinds of emotions, love (which is presumably pleasant) and hate (which is presumably unpleasant), can be experienced in a way that appears to be concurrent. From a cognitive perspective, varied and even contrary emotions can occur together if one separates short-term from long-term reactions.

The distinction between long-term and short-term helps clarify how what seem to be two contrary emotions may occur concurrently. If one's partner does some specific offensive act that engenders anger, one is likely to think, "I feel anger toward this person." Strictly speaking, however, it is *the act* that is the target of the anger. Although the *general* target is one's partner, components of emotions toward the general target can be specific, with each component having its own associated cognitions. A fuller description might be: "I am angry that my partner broke the vase (short-term target) and I love my partner (long-term target) and I am grateful that my partner cooked dinner tonight (short-term target)." The general target is the partner, but specific targets and emotions, some short-term and some long-term, are involved. Many components shape the complexity of emotions.

This distinction helps clarify problems in social interactions and is the basis for many types of counseling and training procedures. For example, in advice given to parents and teachers by Adlerians

(Dreikurs, 1948/1990; Dreikurs & Cassel, 1990; Dreikurs & Grey, 1992; Dreikurs, Grunwald, & Pepper, 1998; Dreikurs & Soltz, 1992), the focus is on the child's *action,* not on the child. The specific action is the antecedent to the parents' or teachers' anger. Telling the child, "I am angry with you," is not as rehabilitative as saying, "I like you very much, but I do not like what you have just done." The latter statement helps the child focus on the appropriate target, that is, the action. It is much easier to change specific actions than one's whole self.

In discussing love, Lazarus (1991b) distinguished between love as a *social relationship* and love as a *momentary state.* Only the latter he called an emotion. Lazarus distinguished sentiment from emotion. He labeled love (Lazarus, 1991b, p. 274) "in the aggregate . . . as a sentiment." Thus, what the present book describes as long term emotion, Lazarus (1991b) called a *sentiment.* The present distinction between long-term and short-term emotion may be more fruitful than the distinction between "sentiment" and "emotion," however, because it permits study of the real-life complexity of human emotions, including emotions that have different targets and involve different spans of time.

EMOTION AND MOOD HAVE A RECIPROCAL RELATIONSHIP WITH COGNITION

What Kinds of Cognitions Relate to Emotion?

Cognitions are of many types. Some of the more obvious ones are expectancies, beliefs, attitudes, biases, judgments, thoughts, opinions, knowledge, and information. Strategies for organizing and categorizing of information involve cognitive processes. Many writers have indicated that cognitions range from "hot" to "cold" (e.g., Sorrentino & Higgins, 1986): the "hot" have a highly emotional loading and the "cold" have very little personal relevance. What has been called "cold" cognition refers to knowledge or belief about the outer world that has no direct personal meaning, and so one can deal with that knowledge in a detached way. Many illustrations can be given. The belief that the earth is round and is a planet that orbits the sun is a "cold" cognition for most people. However, in the 15th and 16th centuries, when religious dogma placed great emphasis on the concept that the earth is flat and that all heavenly bodies, including the sun, revolve around the earth, that belief would have had enormous emotional loading. The personal consequence of a belief in the round earth that orbits the sun could have been imprisonment and even death.

The relationship between cognition and emotion is two-way: cognitions influence emotions, and emotions influence cognitions. Cognitions influence emotions in varied and complex ways. Theories like that of Beck (1963, 1983) point out that the content of thought can increase the emotional condition of depression, and when one is depressed, the emotion in turn leads to cognitive changes (Ottaviani & Beck, 1988, p. 217): Depressed people "view themselves, their situation, and their future in a consistently negative fashion. In addition to the negative content, systematic errors in reasoning—cognitive distortions—occur which further hinder the accurate appraisal of experiences." According to this theoretical formulation, latent or dormant thoughts become activated by specific stressors. These thoughts bring an altered emotional state, and that state in turn alters appraisal of experiences and leads to a wide range of altered cognitions.

Bower's Studies of Emotion and Mood

In studies reported by Bower (1983), sad and happy subjects were found to spend different amounts of time taking in sad or happy information. As can be predicted from that finding, their judgment of self and others was also congruent with the sad or happy state. Forgas, Bower, and Krantz (1984) had normal (nonclinical) subjects interact with randomly assigned partners. Various types of interaction episodes occurred and were videotaped. The next day, subjects had either a happy or a sad emotion hypnotically induced, and they were asked to look at the videotapes and interpret the behavior of their partners and themselves. In the happy state, the subjects identified more positive acts (desirable characteristics, such as skilled acts) and fewer negative

behaviors (undesirable characteristics, such as unskilled acts) in the videotaped interactions; the reverse occurred for the sad state. As seen in Figure 7.1, the number of positive and negative behaviors subjects observed in a given state differed as a function of two variables: according to the type of emotional state the subject experienced; and according to whether the observations were of their own or their partners' behavior. In the sad state, judgments of self were far more negative than judgments of the partner, but in the happy state, positive observations were high for both the self and partner's actions.

In another study, Forgas and Bower (1987) gave subjects detailed positive and negative descriptions to read about hypothetical other persons (the target persons). Before they read these details, the subjects were given mood manipulations (by means of false feedback concerning unrelated performance on a prior task). The time spent reading each statement about the target persons was recorded. The data showed that happy subjects spent a lot more time reading about positive details and sad subjects took more time reading negative details about the target persons. Additionally, subjects in a happy state made far more positive judgments and less negative judgments about the target persons than they did in a sad state. As shown in Figure 7.2, subjects in the happy state also took a lot less time to make their judgments than they did in the sad state. The difference was especially strong for positive judgments, with happy versus sad mood showing a very large difference in the judgment latencies. A much smaller difference in judgment speed was evident for the negative impression formations. Of interest is the fact that when the slopes of the happy and sad subjects are compared in Figure 7.2, it is evident that a slight downward slope occurs for the sad subjects and a steep upward slope occurs for the happy subjects. This indicates that the happy subjects gave their positive judgments much faster than they did their negative judgments, whereas in the sad state the judgments were slightly faster for the negative than the positive judgments.

Everyday experiences are likely to reveal the same patterns reported by Forgas and Bower (1987, 1988). In line with Figure 7.1, people in daily life

FIGURE 7.1
The effects of good and bad mood on perceptions of positive and negative acts in the self and in a partner.

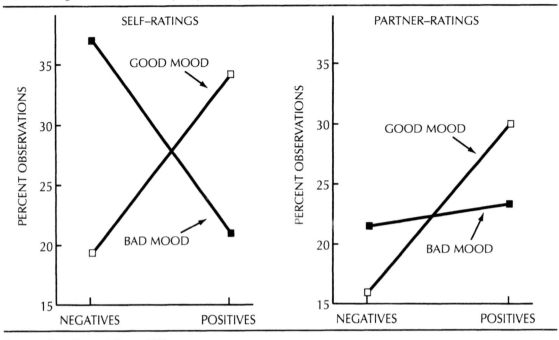

Source: From Forgas & Bower, 1988.

FIGURE 7.2
The effects of mood on the latency of positive and negative impression formation judgments.

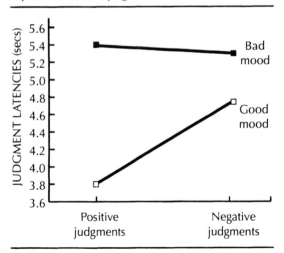

Source: From Forgas & Bower, 1988, p. 200.

are likely to notice more of the events that fit their emotional state of the moment. Regarding speed of judgments, in line with Figure 7.2, people in daily life are likely to draw conclusions slower about noncongruent events than about events that are congruent with their emotional state. Also, people are generally slowed down in processing information when they are sad or depressed.

Results from research have led a number of writers (e.g., Schwarz & Clore, 1988) to point out that emotions organize people's cognitions. Various theorists give different explanations for why or how emotions influence cognitions and why or how cognitions influence emotions. According to the goal-directed theory of Adler (Ferguson, 1995), input of information from the environment is selective and goal directed, thereby providing congruent information that maintains and supports the emotion. To maintain the emotion in its strength and direction, according to Adlerian theory, cognitions congruent with the emotion will be sought or generated, and information from the environment will be sought that supports the emotion (for example, positive events supporting and stimulating a happy state).

Other explanations follow traditional and less dynamic information-processing conceptualizations. For example, the "associative network formulation" (Bower, 1981; Anderson & Bower, 1973; Gilligan & Bower, 1984) has stimulated a large amount of research on the effects of emotion on memory, and this approach is presented next.

EMOTION AND INFORMATION PROCESSING

Are Emotion and Cognition One or Two Separate Systems?

Much of the literature reviewed so far has conceptualized emotion to be different from cognition in function and in physiology. Debate exists whether emotion represents a separate system from cognition, or whether emotion and cognition have common characteristics that fit into one type of system.

Physiological Perspectives. The previous chapter noted that some theorists (e.g., Levenson, 1988) have linked emotion to specific patterns of autonomic (sympathetic) nervous system activity. Other researchers have related emotion to precortical structures such as the limbic system (Izard, 1977). Data show that emotions have a link both with cortical functions and with structures of the brain that are older, in an evolutionary sense, than the parts of the brain used in higher mental processes. The amygdala and hypothalamus have been identified for emotional reactions. For example, Flynn (1967) showed that direct electrical stimulation of the hypothalamus in cats leads to rage reactions and to attack behavior.

The amygdala has gained increasing recognition as important for emotions. LeDoux (1989, p. 274) suggested that "the amygdala receives sensory inputs from the thalamus both directly and by way of the cortex. The thalamo-amygdala projections appear to be involved in the processing of the affective significance of relatively simple sensory cues" and these projections have a different function from those that are involved in processing of complex stimuli. For LeDoux (1989, p. 284), "affect and cognition are separate information processing (computational) functions mediated by different brain systems."

The focus on precortical and phylogenetically older parts of the brain as the source of emotions is one physiological perspective. Another is that taken by Davidson (1984, 1992, 1993, 1994) and colleagues (Davidson & Fox, 1982; Davidson & Tomarken, 1989; Ekman, Davidson, & Friesen, 1990; Fox & Davidson, 1988; Sutton & Davidson, 1997), which involves relating a person's emotional state to measures of the anterior regions of the cerebral hemispheres. This approach has used electroencephalogram (EEG) and other recordings. The researchers found increased "relative" activation of the left hemisphere anterior region to be associated with heightened positive emotion or with decreased negative emotion. Heightened negative emotion or decreased positive emotion was found to be linked to an increased "relative" right hemisphere activation. It is relative, since for many subjects the overall pattern is a higher left hemisphere activation. However, when negative emotions are experienced, the right hemisphere tends to become more active.

Davidson and colleagues postulate that the anterior portions of the brain respond differentially for *emotional experiences* and the parietal portions are more involved in the *decoding of emotional information* (Davidson & Tomarken, 1989). They also postulate that precortical and cortical activity are linked. Davidson and colleagues distinguish between emotion and cognition in terms of anterior versus posterior brain regions.

Another way of distinguishing emotion versus cognition was provided by studies seeking to demonstrate that left hemisphere activity is linked with analytical thought and rigorous cognition whereas right hemisphere activity is linked with emotional processing. The breakthrough work of Sperry (1961) and colleagues (Gazzaniga & Sperry, 1967) led to a new understanding of the functions of the right and left hemispheres, and early studies revealed different modes of processing for emotional compared with nonemotional material. Studies found that pictures of faces with emotional compared with neutral meaning were recognized faster or more accurately for stimuli presented in the left visual field such that the right hemisphere initially processed the input (e.g., Ley & Bryden, 1979; Suberi & McKeever, 1977). These studies led researchers to conclude that emotional stimuli were processed in the right hemisphere and nonemotional stimuli in the left hemisphere. Davidson (1984) indicated that emotions were processed by both left and right hemispheres, the left being biased for positive and the right for negative emotions. Data from other types of studies on hemispheric differences for processing emotions suggested two kinds of processing, one being a very rapid intake of emotional information that permits simple emotional judgments and represents a primitive appraisal, and the other being a slower process that involves more complex cognitive elaboration concerning emotional content (Raccuglia & Phaf, 1997).

Contrary to the more psychophysiological approaches, many cognitive psychologists argued for a single-system view in which emotion and cognition have common characteristics. Some cognitive psychologists considered both emotion and cognition in terms of computer models and studied emotion and cognition from a single-system perspective. Other ways to integrate emotion and cognition into a single coherent system have been suggested from the viewpoint of artificial intelligence, automata, as well as neurochemical and neuroanatomical processes that can mediate both emotion and cognition (Levine & Leven, 1992).

Computer-based Perspectives

Using the computer as an analog for human functioning has proved fruitful for clarifying processes involved in concept formation, thinking, and problem solving (e.g., Anderson, 1985; Newell & Simon, 1961; Simon, 1978). It is not yet certain how effective this strategy is for scientific understanding of motivation and emotion in nonhuman animals and humans, but the models have led to new studies and unique designs for obtaining data. Some laboratories have successfully utilized the computer-based models for studying the way emotion relates to learning, memory, and cognition, and it is their work that is considered next.

The majority of cognitive single-system points of view have relied on abstract functional models that emphasize information processing. One group of researchers formulated models based on memory networks (e.g., Anderson, 1985), and other researchers related emotion and cognition in terms of models of attention. Formulations of emotions in terms of these two approaches differed. An associative network model focused on learning and memory, whereas an information-processing model placed emphasis on attentional capacity and resources (Ellis, Ottaway, Varner, Becker, & Moore, 1997).

In daily life people do not think that emotion provides information, yet when one experiences strong emotion one is cognizant of a change in physiological activity (such as change in heart rate, blood flow, and breathing), and when one is emotionally aroused one gains information about oneself and the environment. When one is angry and not in denial, one has some self knowledge even when one is unsure about the exact cause or target of one's anger. In the next section some cognitive models of emotion will be considered, which focus on the way emotion is related to learning, memory, and attention.

Emotion as a Node in an Associative Network

Gilligan and Bower (1984, p. 571) described emotion as a node in a network of associations, and they referred to it as "a network theory of affect." The general network theory from which it was derived was first formulated to account for learning and memory in general, that is, in the way people encode, store, and retrieve information. Many persons found the theory useful for predicting and explaining a wide range of cognitive phenomena (Anderson & Bower, 1973; Collins & Quillian, 1969; Loftus & Loftus, 1976). Sometimes referred to as "semantic network theory" or as "propositional network theory," the basic terms include the following: ellipse, which represents a proposition or event; nodes, which contain propositions, concepts, or relations; and links, which connect the nodes. The links indicate associations between nodes. An example of such a network that does not involve emotion is given in Figure 7.3. The diagram is taken from Anderson (1985) and represents the sentence, "Children who are slow eat bread that is cold."

Inspection of the network leads to the prediction that after subjects learn the sentence, if asked to respond with the first word from the sentence that comes to mind, they should say "cold" to the cue of "bread." They should say "cold" rather than "slow," even though the latter occurred temporally closer to "bread" in the original sentence. Since "bread" is separated from "cold" by only three links, compared with five links for "slow," the links in the network, rather than the stated word order, are predicted to determine the free association.

The Approach of Gilligan and Bower. These authors studied emotions from the perspective of such a network. Gilligan and Bower (1984) posited that emotion is associatively connected to a wide range of responses (physiological as well as other types of responses) and to semantic processes in the same way that all types of nodes are interconnected. According to these authors, the process of thinking involves excitation of specific nodes in a network, and these nodes may be concepts, emotions, or propositions. When one node in a network is stimulated, excitation travels to interconnected nodes, with the closest nodes being the most excited. They drew an analogy to an electrical system that has interrelated wires and electric current flowing along the wire, with terminal points of connection being a node. This analogy fit data in studies of memory retrieval, and the process was coined "spreading activation" (Collins & Loftus, 1975).

Activation in the sense used by Bower and his colleagues and students is not what Duffy (1962) meant in her discussion of activation as physiological arousal. She referred to a generalized arousal or excitation, not to the analogy of electrical current flow along an associative network, and she did not postulate that nodes were excited. Because the Bower formulation emphasized memory and associative processes, Bower's term *activation* was conceptualized outside the framework of arousal and motivation processes.

The Gilligan and Bower (1984) model refers to a single system in which emotions are like cognitions or any other nodes. Whether the node that is stimulated is an emotion or a concept does not matter. Exciting a concept node can lead to activation of an emotion node, and exciting an emotion node can lead to activation of a concept node. If by prior association the nodes have become connected, than

FIGURE 7.3
A propositional network representation of the sentence, "Children who are slow eat bread that is cold."

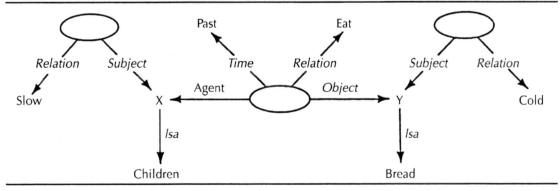

Source: From Anderson, 1985, p. 121.

FIGURE 7.4
A semantic network encoding of a proposition ("medical school admitted Carol") and an emotion it causes. Lower nodes represent preexisting concepts, and lines represent new associations. S = subject; P = predicate; R = relation; and O = object.

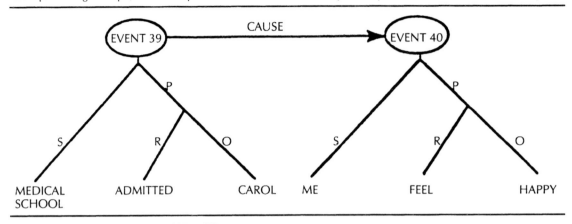

Source: From Gilligan and Bower, 1985, p. 572.

either can activate the other. Figure 7.4 shows how Gilligan and Bower (1984) illustrated a situation in which one asks a person, "How do you feel about your friend being accepted into medical school?" Excitation of the one node of information or knowledge leads to the corresponding excitations of associated nodes.

In their model, Gilligan and Bower suggested that emotional intensity is represented by the amount of activation (excitation) of an emotion node. If a low-intensity emotion occurs, only minimal spreading activation occurs to the nearby nodes, whereas a high-intensity emotion leads to a large spread, i.e., to many associated links and to distant segments of the network. In this way, a strong emotion would lead to more ideas being linked to that emotion. Researchers working with this model tend to equate the terms *emotion* and *mood,* so that in the title of many of the reports of studies testing the network theory, the term *mood* or *mood induction* can be found. This is particularly evident in studies dealing with the effect of depression on learning and memory.

Bower and his colleagues investigated a number of variables, each dealing with different questions. Other researchers assessing the effect of emotion on

learning and memory have also explored these questions.

1. The first question relates the content of the mood with the content of the material being learned or remembered. A question of this type asks if different emotions or moods selectively improve the learning or memory of congruent material. For instance, does a happy emotion or mood lead to better learning and retention of happy compared with sad material? This can be called "the mood-congruent effect."

2. A second question relates the intensity of the emotion or mood to the amount that is learned and remembered. A question of this type asks if strong emotions or moods heighten learning and memory. For instance, does a strong happy emotion lead to better learning and retention than does a mild happy emotion? This is called the "emotion intensity effect."

3. A third question relates the state under which learning takes place with the state under which remembering occurs. A question of this type asks if memory is better when the same mood, compared with a contrary mood, exists under conditions of learning and of remembering. For instance, is recall better when material is learned and remembered under a happy emotion (or learned and remembered under a sad emotion), compared with when emotion is switched between learning and recall? This is called the "state-dependent effect."

In studying the effect of emotion on learning and memory, Bower and his colleagues explored various issues. However, a major focus was the mood-congruent effect. The work of other researchers who focused on evaluating the state-dependent effect will be considered after reviewing the work of Bower and his colleagues. Because the computer-based perspective tends to avoid the energizing aspects involved in social-biological functioning, relatively less work has been done on the emotion intensity effect within the computer-oriented models. The review in this chapter of the associative network theory therefore focuses on studies of the mood-congruent effect.

What Is the Evidence Concerning a Mood-Congruent Effect? The previous chapter presented the study by Maslach (1979), in which she tested a specific arousal-cognition hypothesis. Her study used hypnosis and posthypnotic cues to induce emotion. In many of their studies, Bower and colleagues used hypnosis in a comparable way to induce what they described as "mood." To assess if a happy or sad mood alters the amount of information that subjects learn about happy or sad content, Bower, Gilligan, and Monteiro (1981) prepared a short narrative. It dealt with two people who played tennis. The happy character, Andre, was jovial and won the game, and the sad character, Jack, was morose and lost the game. Within the story, an equal number of statements occurred of happy (Andre) and sad (Jack) content. Mood was induced in subjects by means of a posthypnotic cue and, following mood induction, subjects read the narrative. They also filled out a questionnaire to indicate with which of the two characters they identified more. The next day, in a neutral mood, subjects wrote out what they recalled of the story. The recall statements by those who had been in the happy mood were 55% about Andre, and those who had been in the sad mood had

80% of their recall statements about Jack. As expected, the subjects indicated more identification with the character who had the same mood as theirs at the time of story reading. The results *showed the mood-congruency effect for learning,* in that the subjects' happy or sad mood biased their selective intake of information.

A follow-up study was done and reported by Bower (1981). To test if a story about only one person would yield the same kind of results, the subjects read a story in a hypnotically induced happy or sad mood. The story was about one person who had happy and sad memories. Twenty minutes later, in either the same or opposite type of hypnotically induced mood, they recalled the story. That is, some subjects during recall were in the same mood as they had been during learning and some subjects were in the opposite mood during recall. The results showed that recall mood did not influence the selectivity of incidents remembered. Mood congruence for *memory* was not found, in that the type of mood subjects had during recall did not relate significantly to which type of material was better remembered. Also, a state-dependent effect was not found, since recall was not different for matched versus opposite moods. The study did not show mood congruence for memory or a state-dependent effect, but it did find a mood-congruent effect for *learning.* The subjects recalled far more happy incidents when they took in the information under the happy mood, and subjects recalled far more sad incidents when their story reading had been under the sad mood. Figure 7.5, taken from Bower (1981), illustrates the results. Because the same character occurred in the happy and the sad incidents, Bower's (1981) finding, verified with further investigation, revealed that it was the mood congruence for the incidents and not for the character in the story that had the impact on learning.

Gilligan and Bower (1984) concluded that emotions such as "happy" and "sad" selectively bias the *learning* of new material but not the memory of material learned under neutral emotion. Neither retrieval under free recall nor performance on tests of recognition showed mood-congruent effects (of happy content remembered more when the person was happy, or sad content remembered more when

FIGURE 7.5
Number of happy versus sad story incidents recalled by
readers who were happy or sad. (One character in the story
described both types of personal incidents.)

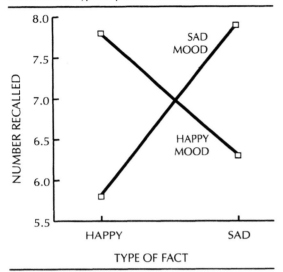

Source: From Bower, 1981, p. 144.

the person was sad). Only when state-dependent effects also were involved did emotions show effects
on memory measures, and then only when two different lists of materials for learning and recall were
used.

Although the evidence is far stronger that emotion or mood alters *learning* rather than *memory* in
a mood-congruent way, other researchers did find
mood-congruent effects in recall. That is, subjects'
mood at the time of retrieval selectively affected
what was remembered, even when the material was
originally learned in an emotionally neutral condition (Teasdale & Russell, 1983). In discussing the
role of emotion on retrieval in later years following
the work of Gilligan and Bower (1984), Bower
(1992) suggested that when emotion does affect
memory performance, it does so with *free recall*
rather than with recognition or cued recall. Moreover, the effect is more likely when the subjects
generate the material to be recalled (such as autobiographical memory).

Formulations in the field of learning and memory, unrelated to the study of emotion, provide a

plausible explanation for the mood-congruent effect for learning. Phenomena called "elaboration"
and "priming" have explained a host of learning
and memory data. Priming refers to the fact that a
given cue activates a word or concept, and this
leads to activation of associated material (in line
with what was already described for the associative
network and its nodes). Gilligan and Bower (1984)
suggested that the subjects' mood primes associations that are similar to the mood. Additionally, subjects more readily might elaborate mood-congruent
material once it was activated, by imaging events or
thinking more broadly about events that are mood
congruent. The researchers further pointed out that
when the emotion node is activated, emotion-relevant information enters into short-term memory.
(Short-term memory is a kind of working memory,
which contains all items of information the subject
is actively processing at a given moment.) Gilligan
and Bower (1984) suggested that under extreme
circumstances the emotion-relevant ideas would be
so overwhelming that unrelated external information is not processed. Under extreme emotion, the
person could be fully preoccupied with handling
only emotion-relevant information in thought,
memory, and attention.

Research with content unrelated to emotion
(Craik & Tulving, 1975) has shown that elaboration
significantly enhances learning and memory performance. Kintsch (1977, p. 233), in discussing the
role of levels of processing of material that is to be
remembered, pointed out: "It is not only the nomi-
nal level of processing that matters; the elaboration
of a code within a level is equally significant."
Thus, mood congruence may affect learning due to
selective elaboration and rehearsal of the congruent
information. Alternative explanations will be considered when studies are presented that relate to the
attention model, but for the moment the hypothesis
that differential elaboration and priming lead to
the mood-congruent effect in learning is a tenable
explanation.

Bower (1992) postulated a "causal belongingness" hypothesis to explain why in only certain instances the mood-congruent effect occurs in memory tests. Bower (1992, p. 24) stipulated that recall
will be affected by mood congruence only if sub-

jects "causally relate their emotional reaction to the occurrence of that stimulus" or situation. If subjects "form a strong association in memory between the stimulus event and the emotion it evoked," the mood-congruent effect should be evident in memory performance. Put another way, "the incident-to-emotion association, which underlies" the mood-dependent retrieval, "would have been strongly formed initially, hence to be retrieved upon later testing when subjects re-enter a similar mood." Bower (1992, p. 28) distinguished the role of motivation and emotion with regard to the cognitive system. He conceptualized motivation as mobilizing resources for action, directing attention, and guiding execution of plans. In contrast, emotions evaluate both the present situation and the plans (their execution and outcomes). Emotion thus has a prominent role in the information-processing network, and that role is different from the way motivation affects learning and memory. It is the former, emotion, to which Bower directed his research within the framework of an associative network.

Emotional States Regulate Allocation of Capacity

The work of Bower is linked with the term *associative networks,* and Henry Ellis is identified with a *resource allocation* model. Ellis and Ashbrook (1988, p. 26) posited that "emotional states can affect the amount of attentional capacity that can be allocated to a given cognitive or motor task." They discuss emotion in terms of a capacity or resource model of attention, with emotion regulating the amount of capacity or resources allocated to a task. Because they emphasized sad or depressed emotion states in their work, they considered that sadness ties up capacity. Subjects think about their sadness, and in this way sadness takes up capacity that would otherwise be available for the task. Their approach has relevance for the question of emotion intensity in that they (Ellis & Ashbrook, 1988, p. 27) pointed out: "weak or mild mood states are unlikely to have much impact on performance," and the most likely impact of mood or emotion on performance occurs "when demands on encoding are relatively high or when the mood state is relatively intense."

They translated allocation of capacity into the concept of cognitive effort. Generally, when more effort is made during encoding, the individual's retention of information is also improved, and thus one can predict that sadness or depression would lead to less learning and to less memory for new material. Whereas the studies reviewed in the previous section used hypnosis to induce "mood" and the researchers compared sad and happy mood, Ellis and colleagues tended to compare depressed mood with a neutral state and they used the "Velten mood-induction procedure" devised by Velten (1968). In this procedure the subjects read self-referent derogatory statements. The Velten method has been criticized as not leading to reliable mood-induction effects, but Ellis and colleagues found in postinduction assessments that the procedure did lead to a depressed state. Ellis, Thomas, and Rodriguez (1984) assessed if such an induced depressed state impairs learning. Following the mood induction, subjects were given words to learn under a variety of encoding demands. For the conditions that the experimenters considered to demand more encoding effort, performance of the sad subjects was found to be worse than that of the subjects in a neutral state.

In their review, Ellis and Ashbrook (1988) indicated that a depressed mood at time of retrieval impairs performance. In one study subjects learned words under neutral conditions and the depressed mood was induced only after the learning. Recall for these subjects was worse than for the subjects who were given the memory test in a neutral state. The important issue for Ellis and Ashbrook (1988) was that learning and memory impairment for depressed subjects will occur only when the encoding or retrieval demands are high. No impairment of performance would be expected if the processing resources required by the task are not severe. That is because even with loss of processing capacity due to the depressed state, the task could still be done well. Furthermore, when the depressed mood is not intense, performance should not be impaired because the loss of processing capacity is not sufficient.

The emphasis placed on capacity by Ellis and colleagues helps to relate the nature of the task with the state of the person. This is useful, but the formulation does not fully explain how emotion affects cognitive processes. For example, the formulation does not predict performance effects under happy states, although others have made such predictions and compared happy versus sad states (e.g., Isen & Gorgoglione, 1983). Reviews of such studies (Isen, 1984; Leventhal & Tomarken, 1986) have shown that happy states alter a wide range of attitudes and actions and that they improve performance on cognitive tasks. The evidence suggests that happy and sad states do not have merely opposite effects. Rather, happy states seem to bring about a whole new set of cognitive processes.

As is discussed later in this book, some motivational variables have emotional concomitants, like the need to achieve which is linked with positive emotions and expectations of positive outcomes. A large literature that includes motivation and emotion has shown that positive and negative emotional states have complex effects on performance. Positive and negative emotions influence, and are influenced by, expectations, attributions, and self-concept ascriptions.

Ellis and Ashbrook (1988) treated *attention* capacity and *processing* capacity synonymously, but the two variables are not necessarily the same. A very bright person may give very little attention to a task, yet high performance can be attained as a function of excellent processing capacity. Likewise, a person with limited intellect may be highly attentive to a task, but due to low processing capacity the person's performance may be quite low. Effective performance on difficult tasks requires both high attentional and high processing resources, but each is different.

In spite of several difficulties with the Ellis and Ashbrook (1988) formulation, that approach nevertheless made important contributions, by linking *task variables* with emotion, and by relating emotion or mood to *effort*. It is important to predict effects of emotion according to task characteristics, and because effort bears on the way motivation affects performance, Ellis and Ashbrook (1988) provided a link between emotion and motivation.

State-dependent Effects

Some studies using Bower's associative network formulation tested state-dependent effects, and

studies described by Ellis and Ashbrook (1988) also examined such effects. When subjects learned material under a neutral emotion and then for some subjects a depressed mood was induced before recall, these subjects' recall was impaired relative to the subjects whose recall was under a neutral emotion. Because the depressed state occurred only under recall, Ellis and Ashbrook (1988) interpreted the results to indicate that depression affected retrieval rather than initial encoding. However, a switch in state can impair performance, and the results reported by Ellis and Ashbrook (1988) could be due to a state-dependent effect. Subjects who learned and recalled under the same neutral state were compared with the subjects tested for recall under depression, which meant a switch of state from the encoding to the retrieval task. The mere fact of switching and not the depressed state could have accounted for the impaired performance. The *state-dependent effect,* of memory being better when the subject recalls and learns the material in the same state rather than in different states, plays an important role in the field of emotion and motivation. The underlying processes are not fully understood, but considerable research has given credence to the phenomenon. Studies have been done in which subjects learned material under the influence of alcohol (Goodwin, Powell, & Brenner, 1969) or in a sober state, with their recall later tested under the same or the altered state. A wide range of drugs, including narcotics and stimulants, have been used for this type of study and results overall showed poorer recall for the switched compared with the unswitched conditions.

Task characteristics as well as arousal conditions play a role in state-dependent memory. For example, Bower, Monteiro, and Gilligan (1978) found a robust state-dependent effect in a study that used two lists of words rather than the same list for learning and recall. The experimental subjects felt either happy or sad while learning the first list of words and had the opposite emotion induced before they learned a second list. Twenty minutes later they recalled the first list either in the emotion they had during the first list or in the emotion they had during second-list learning. State-dependent effects were evident according to whether first-list recall was under a switched or a nonswitched emotion. If subjects learned and recalled the first list in the same state, recall was over 70% correct; if learning and recall of the first list occurred in the opposite state, recall was between 40% and 50%. Whether the subjects were sad or happy at the time of learning or at the time of recall was not significant. The significant variable was whether the emotion was switched or not. Experimental groups were compared with each other and with "control" subjects. Control subjects did not experience a shift in emotion, only a shift in lists. They were given the two lists to learn without a state change, learning both lists while either happy or sad and recalling the first list in that same state. Their recall levels were between those of the two experimental groups (i.e., 50% and 60% correct). They suffered the normal performance loss that tends to occur under *retroactive inhibition* (Underwood, 1945, 1948). When a person learns one list, then another list, and subsequently tries to recall the first list, very often the second list retroactively interferes with the recall of the first list.

In the Bower et al. (1978) study, the experimental "nonswitch subjects" (whose recall of the first list occurred while they were under the same emotion they had while learning the first list) did not suffer retroactive inhibition as did the control subjects. It is as if the discontinuity of emotion between first-list and second-list learning protected the memory of the first list from the retroactive interference of the second list. In contrast, the experimental "switch subjects" (who recalled the first list under the emotion they experienced while learning the second list) had more extreme retroactive inhibition than the control subjects. Thus, state-dependent memory helped performance for one experimental group and impaired performance for the other experimental group. The phenomenon of state-dependent memory interacted with task characteristics, either facilitating or impairing performance.

Emotions can provide context and thus affect learning and recall. Although not all subsequent studies were able to show the state-dependent effect (e.g., Bower & Mayer, 1985), the overall evidence is that for many types of states the effect does occur, and in this way emotions can influence recall of previously learned material.

Are There Additional Issues?

A number of additional important issues have been investigated that relate how emotion affects cognition and in turn how cognition affects emotion. Some researchers have assessed whether it is the intensity of emotion or arousal that alters cognition (e.g., Clark, Milberg, & Ross, 1983). Others have examined the extent to which emotions have a selective effect on what details are attended to and learned (e.g., Christianson & Loftus, 1987). A large literature in motivation also has addressed these issues, as have studies assessing how cognition affects emotion.

Researchers in the field of personality and in clinical psychology have been concerned with the way self-concept affects emotions. The Velten (1968) method of mood induction uses a self-referencing procedure, and many additional self-oriented approaches have been examined in interaction with emotion. Clinical studies have demonstrated that low self-confidence, expectation of distressing outcomes, and a sense of despair or discouragement go together in a recycling pattern. Pessimistic beliefs (measured as "explanatory styles") that emanate from childhood experiences can lead to a wide range of discouraging emotions (Peterson & Bossio, 1991), and feelings of discouragement can lead to expectation of failure (Dreikurs, 1960, 1967). In turn, false expectations lead to discouragement, depression, and despair (Adler, K. A., 1961; Mosak & Dreikurs, 1973; Shulman, 1968). Autobiographical memory has been studied as it relates to emotion, with considerable evidence suggesting that thoughts and memory can shape emotions. In turn, emotions influence thoughts one has concerning the present, and they can direct what specific events of the past one remembers (see reviews by Horowitz & Reidbord, 1992; Williams, 1992).

APPROACH AND WITHDRAWAL

Emotion and Cerebral Asymmetry

The work of Davidson and colleagues was described in reference to areas of cortical activity involved in cognition and emotion. That work provided interesting data regarding positive and negative emotions, and the next section discusses the relationship of these emotions to approach and withdrawal.

The Work of Davidson and Fox. Davidson (1984) reviewed many studies with clinical subjects and concluded that in patient populations, lesions in the right hemisphere (which means decrease in control by that hemisphere) led to different emotional effects than lesions in the left hemisphere. When the left hemisphere was dominant due to a right-hemisphere lesion, patients tended to show exaggerated laughing and joking; when the right hemisphere was dominant due to a left-hemisphere lesion, patients tended to show excessive crying and other signs of depression. Such asymmetry in emotional reaction occurred when the lesions were in the frontal but not in the posterior brain area. In follow-up work, Davidson and colleagues found that normal subjects also showed differences in responding. One effect depended on whether emotional or cognitive stimuli were presented, and the second effect concerned whether positive or negative emotional stimuli were presented.

In one study of positive and negative emotional responding, Davidson, Schwartz, Saron, Bennett, and Goleman (1979) showed right-handed subjects videotaped segments of television programs. Subjects rated the degree to which they had negative or positive emotional reactions to the programs by pressing down or up on a pressure-sensitive gauge. This provided a measure of emotional self-report. Brain activity was measured by EEG recordings from the frontal and parietal areas by surface electrodes. When the 30-second epochs that each subject judged to be most positive were compared for EEG activity, the data showed more left-frontal activation. Subjects also had facial muscle recordings (electromyographic, or EMG, recordings), and the positively rated epochs showed more zygomatic (smile) muscle activity. In contrast, the negative epochs had less left-frontal activation, and the frontalis muscles (used for frowning) yielded more EMG activity than was obtained for the positive epochs.

Studying infants, Fox and Davidson (1986) found that 2-day-olds showed an increase in rela-

tive left-frontal activation immediately after being given a taste of sugar water. Recordings of their facial expressions showed the infants giving what could best be described as an "approach" response. When given distilled water to taste, the face expression was an "avoidance" or aversion response, and the EEG showed an increase in relative right-hemisphere activation. Emotions of "interest" and "disgust" seemed to be represented by these facial expressions, and the difference was reflected in the EEG asymmetry. Both frontal and parietal regions of the brain revealed the EEG asymmetry of the neonates, whereas recordings of 10-month-old infants in another study (Fox and Davidson, 1988) showed the asymmetry only in the frontal region. With age, specialization in cortical functioning is thus evident in EEG measures of emotional reactions.

To induce the two kinds of emotions in 10-month-olds, Fox and Davidson (1988) at different times had the child's mother and a stranger approach the subjects. The researchers found that when the mother approached, the infants had a significantly different type of smile than when the stranger approached, and relatively more left EEG activation occurred when the infant gave the type of smile shown when the mother approached. Right activation was evident when the infant smiled in the manner of the stranger's approach. The EEG asymmetry was found only for the frontal, not the parietal, region in these 10-month-olds.

Individual differences were evident when subjects of that age were observed in response to maternal separation for up to 1 minute (Davidson & Fox, 1989). EEG measures were taken just before the separation episodes. Those infants who cried revealed greater right-frontal and less left-frontal activation during the resting (preseparation) period, and no asymmetry was found in the parietal EEG recordings. Davidson and Tomarken (1989) interpreted this type of predisposition for a strong aversive reaction as probably due to individual differences in propensity for positive approach versus negative withdrawal emotional reactions. Not all negative emotions should show this asymmetry, because not all negative emotions represent withdrawal from the environment. Anger is not an emotion of withdrawal, whereas sadness is. As Tomarken, Davidson, Wheeler, and Doss (1992, p. 684) noted, neither should all positive emotions show such asymmetry, for "only some of these states may be characterized by strong approach motivation, which is hypothesized to be the critical component linked to relative left anterior activation. In this view, *approach* is denoted by such features as heightened incentive motivation and task engagement" (emphasis in original).

A conceptualization that positive versus negative states are linked with approach and withdrawal was advanced some years earlier in other areas of psychology that were not related to cortical measurements. For example, Atkinson (1964; Atkinson & Littwin, 1960) conceived of achievement motivation and anxiety in terms of a special type of approach/avoidance. In a different context, Lacey, Kagan, Lacey, and Moss (1963) suggested that physiological responses differ according to whether one seeks or shuts out information from the environment. Ferguson (1987) also described the difference between effects of appetitive and aversive motivations on the basis of approach versus avoidance or withdrawal with respect to attentiveness to stimuli in the environment. Likewise, the work of Thayer (1989) suggested that one type of arousal energizes a person's action directed toward the environment (being "peppy") while a different type of arousal energizes the person for withdrawing actions (being "tense" or "anxious"). Thus, what Davidson and colleagues formulated is congruent with a large literature and is compatible with the viewpoint taken in the present book, that both motivation and emotion are characterized in terms of approach toward or withdrawal from the environment.

Davidson and colleagues related emotion to motivation (Tomarken et al., 1992) in the way that the present book conceptualizes emotion to be linked with the concept of motion. Conceptualizing animal or human emotion in terms of movement toward or away from the environment, i.e., approach versus withdrawal, is dynamically a more fruitful way to consider emotion than is a focus on hedonic qualities of pleasantness for positive emotions and unpleasantness for negative emotions. Although positive and negative, or pleasant and unpleasant, are

important, the hedonic quality in itself is less important than how it affects actions. Pleasure and pain affect a wide range of psychological and physiological processes. Later chapters will address how they affect not only behavior and thought but also health. For now one can note that it is the approach and withdrawal characteristics of pleasantness and unpleasantness that provide their potency. The understanding of emotion and motivation in a multifaceted way goes beyond hedonic qualities and is concerned with the transaction between an individual and the environment. Approach and withdrawal pertain to the dynamics of motion, overtly in action and covertly in a wide range of internal processes.

Other Research on Brain-Emotion Relationships. Various researchers have sought to identify the way emotion and brain functions are related. Whereas most studies in the past have related reinforcement only to motivation, Edmund T. Rolls (1990) sought to relate reinforcers also to emotion:

> Only some of the states produced by reinforcing stimuli are emotional states. First, emotional states are normally initiated by external reinforcing stimuli, such as an (external) noise in the environment associated with pain (delivered by an external stimulus). In contrast, drive-related or motivational states, such as hunger and thirst, are normally initiated by internal stimuli, such as hypoglycemia (for hunger) or hyperosmolality (for thirst), and these states then make external stimuli, such as the taste of food or of water, become reinforcing. (p. 165).

Rolls considered that an emotional state arises if an external stimulus is associated with a reinforcer and then remembered. Rolls placed special emphasis on the amygdala in connection with emotion. Bilateral removal of the amygdala in animals has resulted in emotional deficits, such as lack of emotional responsiveness, tameness, and lack of fear for stimuli linked with shock. Animals seemed to be deficient in making associations between stimuli and reinforcers, both positive and negative. In conjunction with the amygdala, the orbitofrontal cortex also is involved in reactions involving stimuli with reinforcement value. Rolls (1990, p. 176) suggested that: "Cortical cells found in certain of the temporal lobe regions ... which project into the amygdala have properties which would enable them to provide useful inputs" to the associative activity of the amygdala. He continued (p. 176), "These cortical neurons in many cases respond differently to the faces of different individuals."

Both in monkeys and humans, emotional responding to faces was found to be a function of cortical and amygdala neuron activity. In the highly social human and monkey species, face recognition plays a powerful role in emotional responding. Fox and Davidson (1988) showed that human infants gave strong cortical reactions to their mother's approach compared with the approach of a stranger, and Rolls emphasized that the amygdala as well as specific regions of the cortex have specialized neurons that respond to the visual stimulus of a face.

In monkeys and humans, emotional facial expression has a special social function. It is crucial for communication and bonding. Rolls (1990) considered it significant that face recognition is actively mediated by specific neurons in the amygdala and cortex. Rolls added that the hypothalamus is also important for emotion, in approach to stimuli associated with positive reinforcement and avoidance or withdrawal from stimuli associated with punishment. Rolls did not refer to these brain regions in terms of left versus right hemispheric asymmetry, but it is possible that specific links between the amygdala and anterior cortical regions involve asymmetric activation for approach versus withdrawal emotions.

Other researchers related emotions to reinforcers and focused on additional brain regions. Kentridge and Aggleton (1990) noted that the temporal lobe plays a critical role in the relationship between external reinforcers and emotion. These authors, like Rolls, were concerned with the intricate relationship between learning and memory on the one hand and emotion on the other hand. Although learning need not involve emotion, reinforcers play an important role in learning, and according to Rolls (1990) and Kentridge and Aggleton (1990), reinforcers have their effect on learning because of their emotional quality. Moreover, emotion occurs only because of the association (learning) of primitive (primary) reinforcers or punishers with exter-

nal stimuli. For example, a signal can evoke an avoidance emotion only if the individual remembers that the signal had been followed by an aversive event in the past. The interplay between emotion and cognitive processes is complex, and the representations of the various processes in the brain involve multiple areas and pathways.

It is not known how hemispheric asymmetry for approach versus withdrawal emotions is developed, but one study, based on the work of Davidson and colleagues, may provide relevant information. The researchers (Dawson, Klinger, Panagiotides, Hill, and Spieker, 1992) sought to identify response patterns of infants from two types of mothers, depressed versus nondepressed. Previous data had shown that infants of depressed compared with nondepressed mothers exhibited lower levels of positive emotion while playing with their mother. On that basis, the researchers tested 11- to 17-month-old infants whose mothers either did or did not have symptoms of depression. For the sample of 31 infant-mother pairs, 15 mothers had indication of elevated depressive symptoms. During the testing, the infants sat in a high chair and their EEG recordings were taken under several conditions. One was a video skit for the infant to view, another had an interaction between mother and child in which they played peek-a-boo, another had a stranger entering the room, and in a final segment, the mother left the room. Behavioral measures were taken of the infant and its mother.

On a number of measures, infants from depressed mothers did not differ from the other group of infants, and mothers in the two groups were similar in their emotional behavior toward their infant while playing with the child. The two groups of infants did not differ in their emotional responding during the play period. However, when the mother left the room, the infants of the depressed mothers showed less behavioral distress, and in their EEG responding, the infants of the two sets of mothers differed. The frontal EEG data showed that for nondepressed mothers, when the mother left the room the infants had greater right-frontal activation (indicative of distress or withdrawal) whereas the infants of mothers with depressive symptoms had greater left-frontal activation. Congruent with this result, the infants of nondepressed mothers had greater left-frontal activation when the stranger left the room (indicative of positive or approach reactions), and the infants of depressed mothers had greater left-frontal activation when the stranger entered the room. During the peek-a-boo game, the infants of the nondepressed mothers had more left-frontal activation than the infants of the depressed mothers.

Since under baseline conditions the two groups of infants did not differ in their EEG patterns, the authors concluded that the difference in the frontal EEG patterns between the two sets of infants was not due to long-term trait-like characteristics. Rather, the researchers suggested that the two types of infants probably learned different coping modes, which would be revealed for both the playtime pleasures as well as the stressors. The contrasting frontal EEG pattern by about 1 year of age could reflect differences in how infants learned to deal with positive and aversive circumstances, especially in such situations as separation from the mother. One possible interpretation of the fact that the left-frontal brain area showed activation in infants of the depressed mothers, in circumstances that ordinarily would be distressing (and thus should lead to right-frontal activation), is that these infants had developed (Dawson et al., 1992, p. 735) "a reliance of self-directed rather than other-directed strategies for regulating negative affect."

These findings help to clarify how hemispheric asymmetry in the frontal brain regions can develop for the approach and withdrawal emotions. The EEG data gave more sensitive indications of the way the infants reacted to emotionally arousing situations than did the infants' overt behavior. Overall, the approach-withdrawal formulation regarding frontal brain activity has promising diagnostic value, as well as providing a method of research for studying a wide range of emotions.

Visual Recognition of Emotional Stimuli

Since the 1940s, researchers sought to discover whether under brief viewing, emotional stimuli are recognized sooner than are stimuli with nonemotional content. Another issue was whether positive emotional stimuli are recognized more easily than negative emotional stimuli. Bower (1983) showed that positive versus negative information is acquired differently according to whether subjects are in a happy or sad state, but the question remained, how does the content of stimuli affect cognitive processes regardless of people's happy or sad state? When a person in a neutral emotional state encounters emotional stimuli, are these stimuli processed differently than nonemotional stimuli, and are pleasant stimuli processed more readily than unpleasant stimuli?

Ley and Bryden (1979) used a tachistoscope to present pictures of faces that expressed emotional content. This type of apparatus displays visual stimuli extremely rapidly, on the order of milliseconds. (One second is made up of 1,000 milliseconds.) When stimuli of a duration under 200 milliseconds are presented left or right of a center fixation, the hemisphere opposite the presentation field initially encodes the stimulus. Ley and Bryden were able to present the pictures of faces so that they were initially encoded by either the left or the right hemisphere. Thus, stimuli presented rapidly to the left visual field were initially encoded by the right hemisphere, and stimuli presented rapidly to the right visual field were initially encoded by the left hemisphere. Ley and Bryden (1979) found overall a right hemisphere advantage for recognizing various emotional kinds of faces, and Suberi and McKeever (1977) found a right hemisphere advantage, in terms of faster reaction times, for recognizing emotional compared with nonemotional faces. Both studies found hemispheric asymmetry for positive versus negative emotional faces in line with Davidson's (1984) approach-withdrawal dichotomy. Thus, whether *emotional faces* are recognized sooner than nonemotional faces depends on which hemisphere initially encodes information, and whether pleasant or unpleasant emotional faces are processed faster also depends on which hemisphere initially encodes the stimuli.

With very fast tachistoscopic presentations of stimuli to the left or right visual field, stimuli involving spatial relationships tend to be more easily recognized by the right hemisphere, whereas verbal stimuli (that involve linguistic processing), tend to be more easily recognized by the left hemisphere. The spatial characteristics of faces thus may tend to bias their recognition in favor of the right hemisphere. A different study (Ferguson, 1989) presented *words* of emotional content to college students. Subjects said the word aloud and then gave a pleasantness rating on a scale from 1 (most unpleasant) to 7 (most pleasant). Table 7.1 presents the reaction times for word naming for the three categories, and it is evident that no visual field (and thus no hemispheric) advantage was found. The pleasant words had significantly higher ratings and they were named significantly sooner than the unpleasant words. Thus, under fast tachistoscopic presentation, pleasant words were named significantly sooner than were unpleasant words, but no evidence was found for hemispheric asymmetry for speed of emotional word naming.

In studies that did not test for hemispheric asymmetry, word recognition differed according to the pleasantness of the words. Broadbent and Gregory (1967) presented words of varied length to housewives rather than to college students. The researchers found a recognition difference as a function of affective content, with a disadvantage for the recognition of unpleasant words. In two studies by Ferguson (1983), negatively emotional words were less readily recognized than were more pleasant animal and food words. Thus, in studies (Broadbent & Gregory, 1967; Ferguson, 1983) that did not involve hemispheric asymmetry, negatively emotional words were recognized less readily than pleasant words, and in a study that presented words in the left

or right visual field (Ferguson, 1989), pleasant words were named with faster reaction time than unpleasant words. The likelihood is that subjects encoded the pleasant words sooner, and not that they held back from saying the negatively emotional words aloud. Holding back did not occur in the Suberi and McKeever (1977) study in which subjects said the negative-emotion words aloud, and faster responses were found for the sad faces when these negatively emotional stimuli were initially encoded by the right, versus the left, hemisphere.

The approach versus withdrawal model of emotion is pertinent to these findings. Hemispheric asymmetry representing approach versus withdrawal was found with pictures of faces, and independent of the question of asymmetry, faster encoding for pleasant than unpleasant words is congruent with an approach versus withdrawal perspective. When subjects encode stimuli that suggest pleasantness, an approach toward the environment is initiated and this increases subjects' information intake. When subjects encode stimuli that suggest unpleasantness, there is less approach to the environment than with encoding of pleasant stimuli.

To what extent pleasant and unpleasant stimuli lead to approach and withdrawal depends on a number of factors, a major factor being the state of the subject at the time of stimulus encoding. Complex interactions between variables are involved in individuals' processing of information. In ratings of pleasantness and unpleasantness, Davidson (1984) found a big difference between subjects' emotional rating of the *stimulus* and of their own emotional

TABLE 7.1
Mean Ratings and Mean Reaction Times (RTs) for Word Naming

	Mean ratings		Mean RTs for naming	
	LVF	RVF	LVF	RVF
Food	5.10	5.06	1,226.10	1,099.78
Animal	5.10	5.11	1,191.02	1,031.38
Neg. emot.	2.33	2.22	1,268.65	1,235.05

Note: For ratings, 7 is pleasant and 1 is unpleasant. Neg. emot. = negatively emotional words. LVF and RVF = left and right visual fields, respectively.
Source: From Ferguson, 1989, p. 309.

experience. If subjects experience a negative emotion they may well withdraw from information intake. However, they may rate a stimulus as unpleasant and yet themselves not experience a strong negative emotion. How the experience of emotions and the emotional content of stimuli interact in information processing still remains in part an open question.

SUMMARY

Emotion and cognition have a reciprocal relationship—each affects the other. Memory, thoughts, and information processing all shape emotion and, in turn, emotion shapes cognition. Various emotions, aimed at different targets, can occur concurrently. Emotions are generated by one's thoughts and memories and by specific events present at a given moment.

From birth on, emotion changes in complexity and variety and is in line with developmental changes in cognition. By the age of 10 or 12, children's complex emotions reflect their increasingly abstract thinking.

An ecological perspective seeks to understand the function of emotion and how emotion fits the context of the environment and a person's pattern of actions. A developmental and an ecological approach to emotion tends to focus more on the totality of life patterns of the individual and less on the distinction between pure (or basic) and blended emotions.

Long-term emotions can be distinguished from short-term emotions. When emotions are directed to a general target, like one's partner, one can have both long-term emotions, based on long-term characteristics of the partner, and short-term emotions, based on specific target aspects or actions.

Cognitions that have strong personal relevance have been described as "hot" and cognitions with minimal or no personal relevance have been described as "cold." The interface of cognition and emotion occurs at many levels. For example, when one is sad one is more likely to notice and to make quicker judgments of sad events than of happy ones, and the reverse occurs when one is happy.

Some theorists consider emotion and cognition to be best understood within a single system, others emphasize two distinct systems. Physiologically based theories tend to emphasize two distinct systems, whereas some computer-based theories formulate emotion and cognition as part of a single system.

Different approaches have examined the neurophysiology of emotion and cognition. Some researchers suggest that emotional experiences are due to subcortical processes, compared with cognition that is cortical, and other researchers suggest that hemispheric differences are involved in emotion compared with cognition. Davidson and colleagues suggest that the anterior portions of the brain respond to emotion experiences and posterior portions to cognitive processing.

A network theory of affect describes emotion as a node in a network of associations. Nodes in a network are linked, and nodes may be concepts, emotions, or propositions. When linked nodes are excited they become activated. In this way, Bower explains how cognitions and emotions can activate one another. A strong emotion can activate more ideas than can a weak emotion.

"Mood congruence" is more effective for learning than for memory of material. People learn happy information better in a happy state and sad information in a sad state, so the congruence between the material and the state has a significant effect on the learning of the material. Recall of the material is not as clearly affected by the emotional state of the person at time of recall. *State-dependent* effects for emotion refer to better performance when a person has the same emotional state under both recall and learning compared with when there is a switch in emotion states. State-dependent effects for emotion have been found but not in all studies.

Resource allocation models describe the fact that emotion can take up attentional and processing capacity. Ellis showed that performance is impaired in tasks requiring encoding effort when a person is in a depressed compared within a neutral emotional state. Task demands and emotion intensity affect performance. For low-demand tasks, a depressed state is not likely to impair performance.

Approach and withdrawal represent two ways

emotions can direct individuals toward or away from the environment. Using EEG recordings, Davidson found approach emotions to activate left-frontal brain regions and avoidance emotions to activate right-frontal brain regions. The approach-avoidance conceptualization for emotion integrates emotion with motivation and is congruent with the perspective of the present book.

The relationship among emotion, reinforcement, and memory has been highlighted by a number of researchers. The exact relationship among these variables and between their neuroanatomical sites is still not known.

Under some conditions of testing, pleasant stimuli, regardless of the person's emotional state, tend to be recognized sooner than unpleasant stimuli, in line with an approach to versus a withdrawal from information intake. Hemispheric asymmetry has been reported for recognition of positive versus negative emotional faces, but to date this has not been found for positive versus negative emotional words.

Emotion and cognitive processes intertwine and influence one another in many ways. Both can be studied neurophysiologically and in terms of information processing, and both are closely intertwined with motivation.

CHAPTER 8

Hunger and Thirst: Biological and Cultural Processes

The present chapter deals with two motivations that are crucial for survival of the individual, hunger and thirst. The chapter first considers the behaviors most closely related to these motivations, that is, eating and drinking.

BIOLOGICAL PROCESSES AND THE REGULATION OF ENERGY IN HUNGER

Problems of Definition: Motivational States Versus Consummatory Responses

Hunger and thirst are motivations, that is, internal states (intervening variables), and thus are different from the related overt responses of eating and drinking. Eating and drinking are known as *consummatory responses,* and these deal with the specific actions of ingestion. Consummatory responses differ from other, broader categories of behavior.

Consummatory, Appetitive, and Instrumental Responses

Grill and Kaplan (1990) distinguished between appetitive and consummatory responses in relation to hunger and thirst. Consummatory responses refer to acts of ingestion, whereas appetitive responses refer to behavior involved in seeking and procuring food or water. Appetitive responses *lead to* consummatory responses. Many researchers do not use the terms in precisely these ways, but all agree that these kinds of behaviors need to be distinguished from instrumental responses.

The term *instrumental responses* refers to a wide range of behaviors that are directed to the environment and that are not uniquely related to any specific type of motivation or to a specific kind of ingestion. The range of behaviors is extremely wide, and includes cleaning house, reading a book, washing one's hands, or running to a store. For laboratory animals, instrumental responses include acts like pressing a lever, pushing knobs, or running a maze. Instrumental responses can be made under any of a wide range of motivations. For instance, hunger, thirst, or fear can increase the rate of bar pressing in a laboratory rat. In contrast, consummatory behavior is more closely linked with specific motivational states, such as eating with hunger, drinking with thirst, and copulating with sexual arousal.

Although consummatory responses are closely linked with specific motivational states, it is not the case that one can unequivocally make an inference about the state merely from observing these responses. When researchers in earlier years investigated whether stimulation of a specific area in the brain led to hunger, they defined hunger on the basis of how much consummatory response was elicited by the brain stimulation. This led to confounding, with the investigators not knowing whether the stimulation led to the internal state of *hunger* or merely to the overt consummatory eating response. Often consummatory responses are *not* linked to the appropriate motivational state. Persons or animals can eat without being hungry and drink without being thirsty, and animals and humans can be hungry without eating, or thirsty without drinking (Ferguson, 1993). Thus, one has to distinguish between instrumental and consummatory responses and between internal states and their related consummatory responses.

Consummatory Responses and Subjective Descriptions

Nonhuman animals do not give introspective descriptions about their internal state, but percentage of body weight loss does provide a good response measure to define hunger. Animals at 80% of normal body weight are defined as being more hungry than those at 95% of normal body weight. With human subjects the researcher can make use of *subjective* measures, and the subjective report then can be compared with consummatory responses, stomach motility, and various other measures. The subjective report also can be correlated with hours of deprivation (time since last eating).

Subjective measures involve ratings or other recordings of conscious awareness. A subjective description of being *hungry* might include statements such as "my stomach growls, I feel queezy, I can't think of anything but food, there is a gnawing feeling inside of me." Different kinds of statements would be used for describing *eating,* such as "I picked at my food" or "I stuffed my mouth" or "I ate everything in sight." Research with humans often uses rating scales to indicate the extent to which the subjects feel hungry (de Castro, 1987, 1988; Ferguson, 1984, 1992b).

Subjective hunger ratings typically relate positively to both deprivation duration and consummatory responses. One study found ratings to correlate significantly with the amount of food that was eaten after subjects made the ratings (de Castro, 1988), and ratings also were found to be significantly different as a function of the deprivation duration since the subjects' last eating (Ferguson, 1984; Placentini, Schell, & Vanderweele, 1993). Although considerable individual differences are evident, subjects with longer time since last eating tend to have higher ratings. Verbal descriptions of how hungry a person feels subjectively are generally a close match with how hungry the person is in terms of objective measures. Ratings as well as descriptive categories can provide subjective measures. In one investigation (Baldeweg, Ullsperger, Pietrowsky, Feham, & Born, 1993) the subjects had to indicate whether a given statement was a true or false description of their immediate motivational state, and those who had just eaten selected different descriptors than did those who were food deprived.

Introspections are useful, but research in the field of eating disorders shows that subjective statements often do not provide a valid index of the internal state of hunger. Persons with weight and eating disorders, such as obesity, anorexia, and bulimia, have been found to report their hunger differently, and they reveal different sensitivity to hunger cues, than do persons who have normal weight and eating patterns (Halmi, Sunday, Puglisi, & Marchi, 1989; Stunkard & Koch, 1964). The relationships between internal states and their measurement, and how internal states relate to consummatory responses, have proven to be complex.

In studying hunger and thirst, researchers have asked the following: What environmental and physiological variables give rise to the intervening variable (of hunger and of thirst)? What processes lead to consummatory responses? In what ways can consummatory behavior become dissociated from the corresponding internal state?

Concepts and Terms

Hunger, food seeking, and food consuming are closely linked. Food ingestion is required for survival of the individual, yet it is not fully understood by what mechanisms or processes the internal state of hunger leads to food seeking and to food consuming. Food ingestion provides the individual with energy, and energy is required for normal life processes and for overt activity. Studies of hunger, conducted with humans as well as with many species of nonhuman animals, have focused on identifying by what means hunger leads to the initiation of food consumption and by what means satiety leads to the cessation of food consumption.

Primary Versus Secondary

At one time psychologists used the term *primary* to describe innate (biologically determined) motivations, and they used the term *secondary* to refer to learned or acquired states. Hull (1943) described hunger as a "primary drive," which contrasted with learned or acquired motivations, called "secondary drive." Fear was studied as an example of a learned or secondary drive. An animal that has had light repeatedly paired with pain will come to fear the light. Such fear is learned and not innately programmed. Food deprivation, however, leads to hunger without learning. The secondary drive of learned fear presumably can be extinguished, but the primary drive of hunger cannot. The assumption is made that primary motivations, like hunger and thirst induced by deprivation of food or water, are characteristic of a species and involve survival of the individual. Other motivations, like sexual motivation, are linked to survival of the species but are not required for survival of the individual.

The terms *primary* (innate, biologically preprogrammed) and *secondary* (learned, acquired by experience) were applied not only to motivations but also to rewards (Simon, Wickens, Brown, & Pennock, 1951). Some rewards ("primary") were considered innately satisfying, like solutions of sucrose (Young & Greene, 1953) or saccharin (Young & Richey, 1952). Other rewards ("secondary") were considered to be learned. For example, if a light is always associated with consumption of a sweet-tasting substance, in time the light takes on powerfully rewarding characteristics. Researchers working within the framework of classical conditioning consider secondary rewards to become satisfying by their frequent association with primary rewards. Because they are learned and not innately satisfying, under certain conditions they can also be extinguished and cease to be rewarding. The distinction between primary (involved with survival and biological preprogramming) and secondary (not related to a species characteristic) proved useful. It delineated powerful biological states like hunger, induced by food deprivation, from motivations that were the result of learning and could be extinguished.

In time, critics argued against this distinction. One reason was that the distinction gave too little weight to childhood experiences and culture, which shape many aspects of even the supposed primary

motivations. Moreover, most human motivations are not innate but learned. Idiosyncratic learning experiences shape many aspects of motivations, even of thirst and hunger. Learning experiences and many environmental variables shape what conditions lead to hunger and satiety and what specific behaviors result from hunger (Capaldi, 1996). At one time a distinction between inborn and learned ("primary" and "secondary") appeared reasonable, but contemporary researchers recognize that for many psychological variables that dichotomy is too all-or-none. Although food is a primary reward in the sense that it is necessary for the survival of the individual, a great many practices concerned with food are learned.

Homeostasis, Negative Feedback, and Feedforward Regulation

Until recently, the concept of homeostasis has shaped much of the direction of research on hunger and thirst. The term *homeostasis,* coined by the famous physiologist Walter B. Cannon (1929, 1932), referred to the fact that living organisms seek to keep an equilibrium or constancy in their internal environment. He wrote the following (Cannon, 1932, p. 24): "The coordinated physiological processes which maintain most of the steady states in the organism are so complex and so peculiar to living beings—involving, as they may, the brain and the nervous system, the heart, lungs, kidneys and spleen, all working cooperatively—that I have suggested a special designation for these states, *homeostasis.*" The evidence for homeostasis came from data that showed that in a changing environment, animals and humans maintain an inner constancy in basic physiological systems, such as constancy of blood sugar, water content of the blood, and body temperature. The internal environment is not kept at a fixed value, but stability exists within certain limits. An intricate set of checks and balances, or feedback mechanisms, maintains this internal stability. Cannon described a number of regulatory mechanisms, which he considered to be at a subcortical level and to operate automatically.

A disturbance in an internal system gives rise to signals, and compensating actions take place to bring the system back to its steady state. The organism is in constant interaction with an external environment, and homeostasis is facilitated by storage of needed substances and elimination of excesses or waste. Homeostasis may be modified according to the demands made on the individual by the external environment. Although physiologists and psychologists in the 1920s through the 1940s thought of homeostatic regulation as involving primarily the *peripheral nervous system* (which contains nerves leading to diverse body organs, glands, and muscles), by the 1950s a number of sites in the brain (part of the *central nervous system*) were identified as playing a crucial role in homeostatic regulation. A broad review by Musty (1982) details the way physiologists and psychologists conceptualized and studied hunger and satiety before the mid-1970s. Research on onset and offset of eating as related to hunger and satiety was initially stimulated by the work of Cannon on homeostasis and was later expanded to include the study of glucostatic receptors (Mayer, 1952, 1953) and hypothalamic centers (Epstein, 1960; Teitelbaum, 1955). These earlier approaches have been replaced by a variety of newer types of research. A review of contemporary studies on brain mechanisms, and how the action of specific hormones and neurotransmitters at brain and peripheral sites affect onset and offset of eating, is provided by Rowland, Li, and Morien (1996).

The type of homeostatic function Cannon described is called "negative feedback," in which a perturbation is sensed and behavioral adjustments (like eating) are made to reduce the disturbance and restore a state of equilibrium. This contrasts with "feedforward regulation," which emphasizes behavioral adjustments being made reliably *prior* to the actual perturbation (Ramsay, Seeley, Bolles, & Woods, 1996). Although research continues to identify the relevant negative feedback loops involved in hunger signals controlling eating behavior, an increasing focus in contemporary research is on feedforward processes. Thus, researchers seek to identify the means by which animals and humans modify their behavior in anticipation of a major perturbation. Normal eating in humans and nonhuman animals starts and stops before the occurrence

of major homeostatic imbalances, and research on feedforward regulation seeks to understand such anticipatory processes.

Short-term Versus Long-term Regulation

Food intake can be studied on a short-term or daily basis and on the basis of weight maintenance over a long time. The two types of regulation are different. How hunger relates to eating is studied typically in terms of *short-term regulation,* following a few hours of food deprivation. Humans eat several times a day, and a person's daily energy intake shows a zero correlation with daily expenditure of energy, although over a week there is a substantial positive correlation between food intake and expenditure of energy (Martin, White, & Hulsey, 1991). Frequency and size of meals (energy intake) vary across species, with some animals eating often but consuming only a small amount of food at a given meal, and other animals eating less often and consuming a larger amount of food. Nevertheless, in all species, the act of eating and ceasing to eat a meal involves different regulatory processes than occur for the maintenance of a stable body weight over a period of time. Studies of short-term regulation only partially help in understanding long-term effects of deprivation, as in starvation.

Studies of *long-term regulation* deal with weight loss and gain and how body weight is maintained stably over a long period, independently of what happens in short-term energy regulation. Studies of long-term processes have assessed how continuously restricted food intake by dieters or by persons with diagnosed pathology affects body weight loss and how humans and animals can regain their lost weight. These approaches do not answer questions pertaining to short-term hunger states. Weight maintenance over a long time period involves body energy regulation and body energy stores (Keesey & Powley, 1986). Body weight is presumed to reflect a balance between energy expenditure and energy intake. Corbett and Keesy (1982) made estimates of heat production for rats whose energy expenditure was equal to their energy intake. They estimated that approximately 75% of the ingested energy was available for bodily functions, such as resting heat production (basal metabolic needs), heat production during eating and processing of food, and activity-related heat production.

Calories. Calories refer to energy; the term refers to the amount of energy required to raise the temperature of a gram of water by 1°C. Because this refers to a very small amount of energy, in studies with human subjects the caloric content of food or of a preload (food given before a specific experimental treatment) is described in terms of kcal, or a thousand calories. For the lay person and in everyday use, descriptions such as found on cereal boxes are likely to speak of, for example, 100 calories, but in the research literature that same designation would be 100 kcal. In studies with human subjects, a small amount of energy is described as SC or "little calories" (de Castro & Elmore, 1988).

Important Terms in the Study of Eating. How much and how regularly one eats are essential questions in the study of eating. A special vocabulary involving "phagia" refers to the amount eaten: *hyperphagia* means eating a large amount; *hypophagia* means eating a small amount. Regularity of eating and time between meals is also important. Animals in their natural terrain time their meals according to species characteristics and the availability of food. Laboratory animals are either fed on some type of schedule or they have food freely available. When food is always available in the laboratory and the animal can eat freely at any time, this is called "ad libitum" feeding. The term *ad libitum* is used for animals, whereas with humans the terms *nonrestrained* and *restrained* are used to describe whether the subjects do, or do not, eat freely when they feel hungry. Restrained eating means that the person purposely restricts food intake, as a method of weight control or dieting (Stunkard & Messick, 1985); unrestrained refers to normal patterns of eating. The concept of "unrestrained" does not mean the person eats continuously, but rather that there are no systematic controls to refrain from eating.

Humans and nonhuman animals do not eat continuously. Eating is in various-sized intervals, with the term *prandial* referring to "meal." Thus, the term *preprandial interval* refers to the time between the onset of a designated meal and the start of the previous meal, whereas *postprandial interval* refers to the time elapsed between the onset of the designated meal and the start of the next following meal.

The beginning of eating is called the *preabsorptive* phase, and it also has been called the "cephalic phase of insulin release" (Le Magnen, 1985; Pinel, 1990). The period during eating is called the *absorptive phase.* The period after eating is complete, when the stomach and intestines have emptied and nutrients are no longer in the blood, is called the *post absorptive phase.* This represents fasting or deprivation between meals.

Hunger and Satiety, Onset and Cessation of Eating: The Role of the Central Nervous System

Research on hunger and satiety in nonhuman animals and humans has focused on identifying (a) what variables lead to initiation and cessation of eating at a given feeding or mealtime (short-term regulation), and (b) what variables lead to regulation of body weight over a duration covering weeks, months, and years. Although far greater knowledge is now available than at the time of Cannon's work (1929, 1932), many questions and considerable controversy remain regarding which processes govern hunger and eating, and satiation and cessation of eating. During the 1950s, researchers identified areas in the hypothalamus thought to play crucial roles in these processes. Although still considered important today, these areas are now thought to have very different functions from those once described.

The Role of the Lateral Hypothalamus

The lateral hypothalamus (LH) once was identified unequivocally as the "hunger center." Some researchers (Le Magnen, 1985) still consider the LH to be the primary area involved in hunger and eating, but the majority of researchers contradict this view. To help make clear the methods used by researchers who assessed the role of brain areas in hunger and satiety, a brief presentation is made to describe electrical stimulation and lesion studies.

Electrical Stimulation and Lesion Studies. *Electrical stimulation* of specific cells or areas in the brain can be produced with very fine electrodes and very low voltage. This type of stimulation mimics the cells' natural (neural) firing and causes the *cells to become active.* Researchers then observe what behavioral or neurochemical effects occur as a result of the activity of that brain area. In addition to this method for determining the role of a brain region for eliciting or maintaining a specific behavior, a different method involves making a *lesion* that destroys the neurons or severs the neural pathways leading to and from a given brain region. The lesion prevents the cells from receiving and sending their normal signals and thus *prevents the cells from having their normal effects.* Lesions thus tend to produce opposite effects to those of stimulation. If a researcher wants to demonstrate that a given region is responsible for certain effects, such as a region involved in hunger, stimulation of cells in that area should heighten hunger, and lesions of the region should inhibit hunger (lead to satiety).

In the 1950s and 1960s, researchers suggested that excitation or firing of neurons in the LH was solely responsible for the experience of hunger and for the onset of eating, and excitation of cells in the ventromedial hypothalamus (VMH) was thought to be solely responsible for the experience of satiety and for the cessation of eating. Studies had shown that lesions of the LH led to noneating and serious weight loss, whereas lesions of the VMH led to excess eating and obesity. Additional data that suggested that the LH was responsible for hunger and the VMH for satiety came from studies in which the animal rather than the experimenter provided stimulation. This type of study deals with *intracranial self-stimulation.*

Intracranial Self-Stimulation Studies. In this procedure electrodes are inserted into specific parts of the brain and mild electrical pulses are given immediately after the animal makes some prescribed response. A large literature on operant conditioning has shown that responses increase in frequency when a reward is given immediately after that response is made. Thus, if electrical pulses (given to a specific brain region immediately following a response) lead to a significant increase in that response, one can infer that the electrical pulse was rewarding. Figure 8.1 gives a schematic diagram of the electrical self-stimulation procedure. In self-stimulation studies, the animal can move about freely. When the designated response is made, mild electrical stimulation is given to the specified brain region according to an operant conditioning approach: the animal presses a lever and this is followed by small bursts of intracranial stimulation. It is called self-stimulation because the animal's action of lever pressing, not the experimenter's action, determines the number of bursts of stimulation. If the animal makes more lever presses, this results in more stimulation, and less lever pressing results in less stimulation.

From self-stimulation and lesion studies researchers found that the LH initiates the activity of eating, and most researchers assumed therefore that the LH is responsive to hunger as an intervening state. However, it was not clear unequivocally whether the *motivation* (internal state), or the consummatory *response,* or both were involved in the activity of the LH.

According to Le Magnen (1985), stimulation of the LH involves both hunger and the consummatory response of eating. He cited self-stimulation studies that showed hunger, and not merely eating, was involved in the activity of the LH, with hunger defined according to the amount of weight lost due to food deprivation. When food had just been presented, the hungrier the animal the more lever presses for LH self-stimulation occurred. Le Magnen (1985) indicated that the LH self-stimulation did not substitute for eating, because the animals ate normally when food was presented. This was important, because in some types of self-stimulation studies (in which electrodes were not in the LH but placed in a presumed "pleasure center") animals pressed a lever for brain stimulation as a "reward" and they refrained from eating even though food was readily available. Le Magnen (1985) concluded that (1) animals given an LH self-stimulation procedure eat normally when food is presented, and (2) the hungrier the animal, the more eating occurs. Hunger altered the amount of self-stimulation only when the implanted electrodes were in the LH

FIGURE 8.1
Self-stimulation.

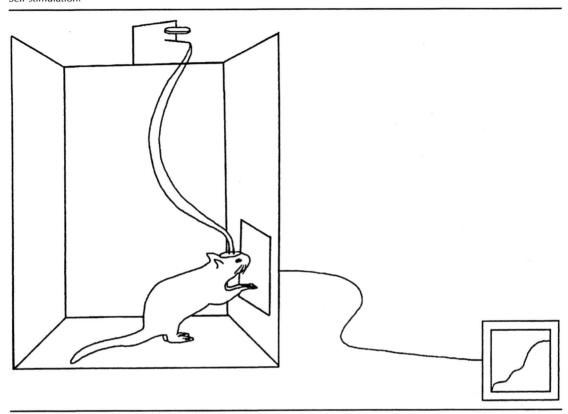

Source: Courtesy of B. E. F. Wee.

and when the animals had just been presented with palatable food.

Recording of Single Cell Activity. Electrodes can be used not only to provide stimulation but, under different testing procedures, to provide recordings of activity of cells in specific areas of the brain. Implanted electrodes can record neural pulses when the cells "fire." In this type of study, Le Magnen (1985) showed that LH cell firing is altered by hunger induced by food deprivation. Moreover, individual neurons in the LH responded actively to food-related stimuli, but only when the animal was hungry. Le Magnen proposed that the LH is responsible for initiating eating because the LH is sensitive to a de-

crease in blood glucose. He distinguished between glucose *sensitivity* of the LH and *control* of blood glucose levels. He proposed that the LH neurons are glucose sensitive and thus bring about eating when glucose levels are low, but the LH neurons do not directly control the blood glucose levels.

Le Magnen (1985) also pointed out that stimulation of the LH activates a number of neuronal systems and does not lead merely to a single type of response like eating. Depending on what response the animal made just before the stimulation, and depending on what stimuli are present in the environment, animals may drink, eat, or engage in sexual activity in response to electrical stimulation of the LH.

Controversy Regarding the Role of the LH. Other researchers do not give as much importance to the role of glucose or to the LH as did Le Magnen, and considerable controversy remains regarding the role of the LH in hunger and eating. In support of the importance of the LH, the LH cell firing (Le Magnen, 1985) is altered by hunger (induced by food deprivation), and hunger affects animals' intracranial self-stimulation. Also, some researchers consider the LH to be important for energy regulation and for weight regulation (Keesey & Powley, 1986), and studies have shown that lesion of the LH lowers food intake as well as body weight (Harris, 1990). Blood-glucose levels were found to play a significant role in modulating food intake (Martin, White, & Hulsey, 1991), and neurons in the LH have been identified as a major site for glucose chemoreception (Le Magnen (1985). Thus, in spite of criticism regarding the importance of the LH, many studies show it plays a significant role in hunger and eating. On the other hand, various researchers propose that peripheral organs and specific peptides are more important in hunger and satiety than is the LH or any other specific brain region. Other researchers accept the importance of brain regions but question the importance of the LH in hunger. The LH is known to affect motor activity, so presumably the LH is involved in the motor activity of eating.

Recently a new perspective has been offered on the role of the LH. Winn (1995) considered that the LH functions to assess internal signals and external sensory qualities. The LH makes computations about the relationship between the internal state of the organism and the sensory qualities of stimuli. If the individual is hungry and desirable food is present, the LH neurons are activated and signals are sent to the frontal cortex, which then generates behavior. He proposed that the paraventricular system regulates the internal environment and the LH functions as an interface between this system and the frontal cortex. Winn (1995) proposed that a number of brain regions function together to coordinate activity in hunger and eating.

In addition to the LH, the paraventricular hypothalamus and the perifornical hypothalamus (Stanley & Gillard, 1994) play crucial roles, especially in the way neuropetide Y (NPY) initiates and maintains eating. The paraventricular nucleus is also thought to help maintain nutrient balance (Martin et al., 1991). The LH thus plays an important role in conjunction with other hypothalamic regions with respect to hunger and initiation of eating. Figures 8.2 and 8.3 illustrate a number of the relevant hypothalamic areas.

The Role of the Ventromedial Hypothalamus

Before the 1970s the role of the VMH was given major importance, in that researchers assumed that the VMH was a satiety center that controlled cessation of hunger and eating. Neurons in the VMH are still considered important, but the VMH is no longer assumed to be a satiety center. Early studies had found that rats with VMH lesions became obese and ate more per meal than did normal rats (Teitelbaum & Campbell, 1958). The lesion was thought to prevent the normal function of this presumed satiety area, but questions about the weight gain and eating arose. For example, these animals were found to be "picky eaters" in the sense that good-tasting food was eaten but less tasty food was not. Later research found that the VMH lesions had damaged other neural pathways, which in turn led to the altered eating pattern and obesity. Today it is thought that neurons in the VMH play a role in cessation of eating, but the VMH is clearly not a satiety center.

The Role of the Caudal Brainstem

The hypothalamus and the caudal brainstem carry out regulatory and integrative functions (Grill & Kaplan, 1990). The caudal brainstem, located at the base of the brain near the spinal cord, has been identified as playing an important role in onset and offset of eating. Research has shown that sensory input and motor output associated with eating are integrated by neurons in this area. Grill and Kaplan (1990) report studies of decerebrate rats in which hypothalamic pathways have been surgically separated from the caudal brainstem, and these animals show normal discriminative consummatory responses to taste. That is, they reject bitter tastes like quinine, and they consume sweet-tasting substances like sucrose solutions. In order to survive, decerebrate animals need to have nutrients placed directly in their mouths. Because they do not show

FIGURE 8.2

Hypothalamus from the lateral aspect: *A,* ventromedial nucleus; *B,* neural pathway from hypothalamus to the vagus nucleus and nerve; *C,* lateral hypothalamus; *D,* anterior hypothalamus; *E,* paraventricular hypothalamus; *F,* supraoptic hypothalamus; *G,* posterior pituitary gland or hypophysis; *H,* anterior pituitary gland or hypophysis; *I,* vagus nucleus; *J,* vagus nerve; *K,* pre-optic hypothalamus.

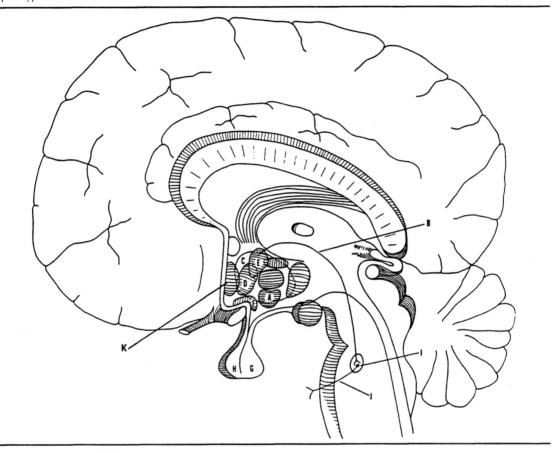

Source: From Musty, 1982.

food seeking or other active appetitive and avoidance behaviors, no evidence is available to show that their taste experiences lead to behavior modification, such as is found in normal animals. From this fact, Grill and Kaplan (1990) concluded that (a) the hypothalamus integrates hunger and satiety signals in a more fine-tuned way than does the caudal brainstem, and (b) motor activity that leads to procuring food is due to hypothalamic rather than brainstem neurons.

Chapter 3 described how the reticular formation (located in the brainstem) is important for excita-tion and arousal of the individual. Grill and Kaplan (1990) suggest that caudal brainstem neurons respond in a general way to reduction of metabolic fuels. When decerebrate animals are food deprived they show an increase in *general activity* level even though they do not manifest food-seeking behavior. Grill and Kaplan (1990) note that although specific control of eating onset and offset is a function of areas in the hypothalamus and that brainstem neurons do not involve such specific areas, brainstem neurons have an effect on behavior by increasing the general activity of hungry animals.

FIGURE 8.3

Schematic details of hypothalamic areas important for eating and drinking. lpoa = lateral preoptic area; mpoa = medial preoptic area; son = supraoptic nucleus; scn = suprachiasmatic nucleus; arc = arcuate nucleus; ah = anterior hypothalamus; pvn = paraventricular nucleus of the hypothalamus; pfh = perifornical hypothalamus; dh = dorsal hypothalamus; dmh = dorsomedial hypothalamus; vmh = ventromedial hypothalamus; ph = posterior hypothalamus; lh = lateral hypothalamus; mb = mammillary body.

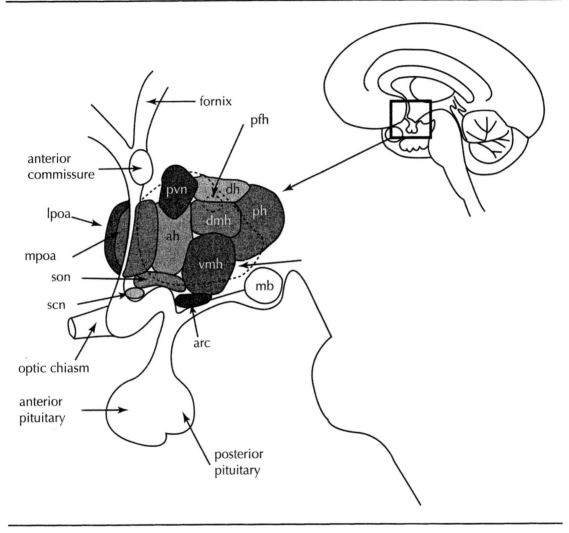

Source: Courtesy of B. E. F. Wee.

Hunger and Satiety, Onset and Cessation of Eating: The Role of Peripheral Sites

The Autonomic Nervous System

The previous discussion concerned the role of the brain (in the central nervous system). The question remains, how much of a role is played by the periphery for providing "eating" and "stop eating" signals? The autonomic nervous system has two subsystems (sympathetic and parasympathetic) and is part of the *peripheral nervous system*. The autonomic nervous system increasingly has been found to be important in the control of both eating and weight stabilization.

In regard to hunger and eating, the brain and autonomic nervous system communicate by means of the hypothalamus. For example, descending *parasympathetic pathways from the LH* involve the gastrointestinal tract and the pancreas, and descending *sympathetic pathways from the medial hypothalamus* involve the liver as well as specialized cells of the pancreas (Le Magnen, 1985). Sympathetic and parasympathetic activity affect a variety of neurochemical processes that play a crucial role in onset and offset of eating. Thus, hypothalamic areas have input to, as well as from, various autonomic nerves, and these in turn involve various organs and neurochemicals. The vagus nerve (part of the parasympathetic nervous system) has been specifically identified as playing an important role in modulating the influences of hypothalamic areas and in influencing the action of a wide range of neurochemicals.

Researchers have focused increasingly on the role played by peripheral receptors, such as in the stomach. Campfield and Smith (1990) provided evidence that peripheral receptors, which depend on neural signals mediated by the vagus nerve, determine onset and offset of eating. The stomach and liver have been shown to play important roles in providing signals for the initiation and cessation of eating. Considerable data obtained in recent years (Deutsch, 1990) indicate that satiety signals emanate from the stomach and that these stomach signals affect consummatory responses. The distention of the stomach involves stretch receptors that provide important signals. Thus, whereas earlier research on hunger and satiety focused mainly on brain regions, increasing emphasis is now given to various peripheral sites.

Cholecystokinin (CCK)

Some of the controversy about mechanisms and processes involved in short-term and long-term energy regulation concerns questions of regions of control (where are the important ones, and how do they function). Researchers continue to discover what kinds of neurochemical signals are crucial for short-term and long-term energy regulation. Recent emphasis has been given to the peptide cholecystokinin (CCK), which was found to reduce food intake. CCK is a brain-gut peptide that may function as a neurotransmitter/neuromodulator or a hormone/paracrine substance (De Giorgio, Stanghellini, Maccarini, et al., 1994). The functions served by this peptide are mediated by a type A receptor, present largely in peripheral sites like the stomach, and a type B receptor, present largely in the central nervous system. Debate is ongoing whether CCK plays a major role in gastric motility. However, it is known that CCK receptors are located in the esophagus, stomach, small intestine, and colon (Belinger, 1994), as well as in the brain. By the 1980s over a thousand studies had investigated the role of CCK (Ervin, 1994). Smith and Gibbs (1994) postulated that endogenous CCK released by nutrients in the gut during a meal helped lead to satiation as a short-term mechanism for control of meal size and to the termination of eating. They concluded that this is proven in rodents but not yet firmly established in humans.

Because CCK receptors are in the periphery as well as in the central nervous system, the debate has become somewhat moot whether peripheral *or* central sites control hunger and eating versus satiety and cessation of eating. The answer is that *both* do. Brain receptors (in the hypothalamus) process information concerning CCK. The lateral hypothalamus, specifically, is sensitive to the satiating action of centrally acting CCK (Schick, Schusdziarra, Yaksh, & Go, 1994). CCK released from hypothalamic neurons during eating plays a role in cessation of eating and in satiety. Ritter, Brenner, and Tamura (1994) confirmed that the types of nutrients being ingested affect CCK-mediated satiation signals. They suggested that CCK functions in multiple ways, possibly altering eating in response to intestinal, metabolic, or environmental signals. In conditioning studies, Balleine and colleagues (Balleine, Davies, & Dickinson, 1995; Balleine, & Dickinson, 1994) found that CCK decreased instrumental conditioning in rats by diminishing their incentive learning due to satiety.

The Role of Glucose, Insulin, and Lipids in Onset and Offset of Eating

Glucose

Some of the controversy regarding which sites play the dominant role in onset and offset of eating (brain versus periphery) relates to the importance of glucose sensitivity in eating onset. Researchers who emphasize glucose receptors tend to place emphasis on brain areas, and those who emphasize peripheral sites tend to minimize the importance of glucose receptors. For example, the stomach not only provides signals from stretch receptors but also provides signals regarding caloric content, and that is not the same as information about glucose (Deutsch, 1990).

Chapter 3 discussed sugar as providing energy in reference to a study on arousal by Thayer (1987). That study sought to assess which provides more vitality and a heightened sense of energetic arousal, a sugar snack or a brisk walk. The brisk walk was found to lead to more alertness and to be subjectively more energizing. Sugar has a variety of effects, and the effect of sugar on alertness is likely to be different from its effect on hunger and satiety. Increasing evidence suggests that sucrose and glucose serve different functions. Glucose has received major attention with respect to hunger and satiety, in part because glucose is the major nutrient for most cells. For brain cells it is thought to be the sole nutrient. Normal brain functioning is not possible without glucose, and short-term maintenance of energy balance also relies on glucose. This provides the basis for the *glucostatic hypothesis,* which posits that glucose and glucose receptors determine onset and offset of eating.

Immediately before the start of a meal, a small decrease in serum glucose occurs (Martin et al., 1991). Studies with humans and with many species of nonhuman animals have shown that the blood glucose level determines whether eating onset is initiated or retarded. If the level is low, eating will begin. After eating, when nutrients enter the blood and blood glucose level is high, eating will stop. At that stage the glucose receptors in the LH become less active, and glucose receptors in the VMH increase their firing (Harris, 1990). If blood glucose levels are high, eating will not begin. For example, Le Magnen (1985) cites a study in which rats initially had lowered glucose levels of the kind that normally result from food deprivation. The animals were then injected intravenously with 20 mg of glucose at their predicted time of meal onset. Such an

artificially induced increase in glucose level led to a delay in eating. Harris (1990) also cites data that show inhibition of food intake when glucose is chronically infused into selected areas of the brain.

Glucose is known to affect eating behavior, but the glucostatic hypothesis is not sufficient for explaining hunger and eating onset (or satiety and eating offset). Various peripheral sites, as in the intestines and liver, have receptors that affect the onset and offset of eating independent of glucose signals. Cholecystokinin, already discussed, is released from the gastrointestinal tract and from the duodenum in response to stretching as well as in response to the nutrient composition in the tract. In this way, independent of glucose, it induces satiety (Harris, 1990). Neuropeptide Y (NPY) is found in the intestines (Pinel, 1990), and receptors in the hypothalamus are sensitive to NPY. Increasingly, more neurochemicals are found that affect eating onset and offset, apparently independent of glucose. Not only NPY but norepinephrine, galanin, and several types of endogenous opioids have been found to be involved in stimulation of eating, and in addition to CCK, cessation of eating has been found in studies with satietin, bombesin, corticotropin-releasing hormone (CRH), oxytocin, and serotonin (5HT) (Rowland et al., 1996). These findings displace the once exclusive emphasis on the glucostatic hypothesis for explaining hunger and eating onset and satiety and eating offset.

Insulin

The interaction between glucose and insulin affects the way palatability of food can affect eating. The preabsorptive phase, at the beginning of eating, sets off chemical processes. Insulin is released by the pancreas as a conditioned reflex at the start of a meal. The more palatable the food, the more insulin is released. Insulin release is not related to the caloric or nutritional value of the ingested substance. For example, a saccharine solution, which is highly palatable but is not a nutrient, also elicits the insulin release. Insulin release is induced by stimulation of receptors in the mouth (Le Magnen, 1985) and by the sight and smell as well as the taste of food (Stricker & Verbalis, 1993). Because it is a conditioned response, insulin release also can become extinguished (Le Magnen, 1985).

The interaction between blood glucose regulation and insulin is an example of the feedforward regulatory process discussed by Ramsey and colleagues (1996). It permits negative feedback before there is homeostatic perturbation. Through learning from ingestive experiences, animals come to anticipate upcoming events. Foods high in absorbable sugars can cause a large increase in blood glucose level, and the rising level activates the negative feedback mechanism of increased release of insulin. Through learning, the animal anticipates the food-related increase of blood glucose level, and the postprandial increase of that level is attenuated through release of insulin *before* the absorption of glucose. This early insulin secretion (cephalic insulin) is mediated by neural connections between the brain and pancreas and that secretion is modified by learning. When an animal associates cues with foods that increase blood glucose level and the release of insulin, the cues alone can elicit insulin release even when there is no change in blood glucose level. Predictive cues lead to homeostatic regulatory responses, and these occur before an actual homeostatic disturbance. This permits the individual to stop eating (anticipatory satiety) long before the meal has a major caloric impact within the body. That is, anticipatory cues activate a negative feedback loop for offset of eating *before* a homeostatic disruption. Signals secreted when food initially enters the gut may provide the cues that mediate this feedforward satiety system.

Insulin release, as a conditioned response to the sight or smell of palatable food prior to eating, helps bring about eating because the insulin lowers the glucose level just before meal onset. Insulin release in response to the taste of food during eating helps keep blood glucose from attaining excessively high levels while the meal is being consumed. During the postabsorptive phase, after eating is complete and the stomach and intestines have emptied and nutrients are no longer in the blood, insulin is no longer released. At that time the fuels needed by the body are converted from energy stores (stored from carbohydrates and fats) into usable energy.

The interaction between glucose and insulin also is seen by the fact that when insulin is externally administered for a continuing period, glucose is pushed into storage at a faster rate, which leads to overeating that can lead eventually to obesity (Martin et al., 1991). As already noted, however, under normal circumstances insulin is released only for short periods of time, and body energy stores are created and utilized in a balanced fashion. Insulin is released not only prior to eating but also during eating (the absorptive phase). Insulin helps convert glucose to glycogen and to triglycerides, for energy storage in the cells (Stricker & Verbalis, 1993). Insulin receptors have been identified in brain tissue. Some researchers have suggested that insulin in certain brain regions, and not only in the blood, might serve to reduce food intake (Harris, 1990). Still another way in which insulin has been hypothesized to reduce food intake (Pinel, 1990; Woods & Gibbs, 1989) is by insulin receptors giving information about body fat.

Lipids

Carbohydrate storage involves glycogen (Martin et al., 1991), and fat tissue contains adipocytes (fat cells) that store energy as triglycerides. Triglycerides are large molecules that can produce the highest amount of metabolizable energy per unit of weight (Le Magnen, 1985). Although glucose has been thought to affect eating and short-term energy regulation (rather than long-term regulation), fats and fat cells have been thought to play important and varied roles in both long-term and short-term energy regulation.

Free fatty acids are at higher circulating concentrations after food deprivation. Hypothalamic centers have been found to be sensitive to such concentrations, and in this way to control eating onset when one is hungry and to terminate eating when one is satiated. What is known as the *lipostatic hypothesis* refers to the suggestion that the brain receives signals about body fat and uses this information to regulate food intake. Vertebrates possess fat cells throughout the body, and when the animal or human is food deprived, the fat stores are emptied. At that time the triglycerides are converted to free fatty acids (lipolysis). When food is ingested, the triglycerides are synthesized (lipogenesis) to provide the energy store. The autonomic nervous system is involved in various processes that mobilize the energy and empty the energy store.

Fat synthesis occurs when one's energy intake through eating is greater than one's energy expenditure. At that time the energy taken in is converted to adipose tissue store. When energy intake is less than expenditure, the fat is used as fuel for energy metabolism. In this way long-term energy balance is achieved and the animal or human has *body weight maintenance*. What is regulated is body fat mass. Body weight as such is not regulated in this process, because lean body mass and body water also contribute to body weight. Many studies with rats and humans have shown that over a 24-hour day there is a 12-hour cycle of fat synthesis that leads to an increase in body fat store, and this is followed by a 12-hour cycle of emptying the fat store. Thus, variation in body fat mass exists within a day in line with the sleep-wake cycle of rats and humans. This type of regulation also is involved when other temporary imbalances occur between energy intake and expenditure, such as occur with periods of exercise (Le Magnen, 1985). The lipostatic hypothesis, that regulation of body fat determines food intake, was used primarily to explain long-term homeostasis and weight regulation, and it explained some aspects of short-term eating onset and offset.

Some animal behaviorists suggested that, for free-living nonhuman animals in their natural territories, mammalian white fat stores have long-term survival functions, such as protection against the harsh winters, and in females, as signal to the reproductive system when the energy reserves are adequate for pregnancy. However, this assumption has been challenged by systematic studies of Bronson and colleagues (Bronson, Heideman, & Kerbeshian, 1991). They determined the length of time that fat reserves could be exhausted in peripubertal female house mice. The animals were subjected to food deprivation at different temperatures, and the data indicated that the animals could store only enough fat to protect themselves from short-term energy emergencies, lasting only a few hours or at most a few days. The animals lost fat rapidly when food deprived, even in temperatures that were not unusually severe. The researchers proposed that fat stores do not serve long-term regulation and that fat stores do not regulate puberty and ovulation in small mammals.

Precisely how fat stores function in nonhuman animals and in humans still remains an open question (Rowland et al., 1996). New findings continue to emerge. Glycoproteins, such as satietin and adipsin, have been identified, and these are currently under investigation for their role in long-term energy balance (Martin et al., 1991). Humans depend almost entirely on the liver for fatty-acid synthesis, yet rats, which have different mechanisms, have provided most of the data bearing on the lipostatic hypothesis. It is not known to what extent data obtained from rats are also valid for humans.

Total body fat, number of fat cells, and size of fat cells appear to affect the stability of weight over a long period. At one time a point of view known as "set-point theory" was thought to explain long-term weight stability. It was thought that the body has a mechanism that "sets" the weight of the individual (animal or human), and deviation from that point initiates behavior that leads to the required weight gain or loss, either through modulating food intake or by altering energy utilization and expenditure (Keesey & Powley, 1986). Contemporary researchers have replaced the concept of a set point and have focused, instead, on identifying the complex interacting processes that provide the continuity or maintenance of a stable weight over a long period. Research on specific protein molecules has suggested possible mechanisms, involving fat cells, to explain stable weight maintenance.

It is known that genetic factors may play a role in overeating and increase in adipose tissue (Flier, Cook, Usher, & Spiegelman, 1987; Price & Gottesman, 1991; Zhang, Proenca, Maffei et al., 1994). In mice, an obese gene (*ob*) has been identified. Mice (known as *ob/ob*) with two copies of the mutant *ob* gene regulate their weight at a high level, resulting in obesity, increased adipose tissue, and hyperglycemia. Research prior to the 1980s had suggested that fat cells release an OB protein which signals the brain and periphery about the level of fat cells. Research in the 1990s investigated whether the overeating of the *ob/ob* mice was due to a deficiency in such an OB protein. When the *ob/ob* mice were given treatments (intraperitoneal injections) of this protein, their metabolism and appetite were changed significantly and they lost body weight, percent body fat, and serum concentrations of glucose and insulin (Pelleymounter, Cullen, Baker et al., 1995). Wild-type mice injected with the protein also showed significant weight loss, decreased food intake, and reduction of body fat (Halaas, Gajiwala, Maffei et al., 1995). It is thought that a peripheral protein-based signal is generated in adipose tissue and acts on brain neuronal networks to regulate eating and energy balance (Campfield, Smith, Guisez, Devos, & Burn, 1995).

Contemporary research on the role of protein molecules released by fat cells may come to help explain the relationship between eating, metabolism, and weight stability. Clearly, obesity in humans is more complex than in mice. Humans may have a genetic predisposition to gain weight on a high-fat diet, but that predisposition is due to more than a single gene (Barinaga, 1995).

BIOLOGICAL PROCESSES IN THIRST AND FLUID LEVEL REGULATION

Parallel to what was said for hunger and eating, thirst is a motivation (an intervening variable) and drinking is the consummatory response. As was also described for hunger and eating, one can be thirsty and not drink (Ferguson, 1993b), or be satiated with liquids and still drink. As as with eating and hunger, drinking can provide a convenient measure to infer thirst, and humans can give subjective statements or make ratings regarding the internal state of thirst. As with hunger, ratings of thirst can be a valid reflection of the internal state of water deprivation, and thirst ratings have shown a positive relationship with the amount of water drunk subsequent to the ratings (Rolls et al., 1980).

Different Kinds of Thirst and Definitions

All cells of the body depend on water, which provides oxygen, circulates nutrients, and removes waste. The human body consists largely of water, with estimates ranging from 40% to 60% (Grossman, 1990) and even up to 70% (Rolls & Rolls, 1982). The required water volume needs to be

maintained within a narrow margin of deviation in line with homeostatic principles. If water is decreased below normal levels *within the cells* the condition is called "cellular dehydration," and if it is decreased *outside the cells* (either between the cells or in the blood plasma) the condition is called "extracellular dehydration." Most of the water in the body is within the cells. Of the fluid that is extracellular, only a small percentage is in the blood plasma. A large loss of blood plasma is fatal, however, and not only the cellular fluid but also the necessary extracellular fluid levels must be maintained. Thirst is induced by different processes when it is due to cellular dehydration than when it is due to extracellular dehydration.

Because drinking can occur for many reasons, physiologically oriented writers have distinguished between *primary* and *secondary* thirst (Fitzsimons, 1979). This is analogous to but not the same as the primary versus secondary distinction between biological and learned drives (e.g., Hull, 1951) already described in this chapter. The physiologically primary, or "regulated" (Verbalis, 1990), thirst involves homeostatic processes that reinstate the necessary water balance, which is not the case with the secondary or "unregulated" thirst.

Cellular Dehydration. Cells in the body have membranes. With reference to thirst, membranes can act as barriers between the cellular and the extracellular fluid compartments (Rolls & Rolls, 1982), and they can actively maintain the differences in concentration of sodium (in the extracellular compartment) and potassium (within the cells). These membranes are permeable to a solvent like water but not to a solute like sodium. Water tends to move across the membrane and establish an equal concentration of the sodium on both sides of the membrane. The term *osmosis* refers to such movement of a solvent (water) across a semipermeable membrane into the more concentrated solution. Pressure (called *osmotic pressure*) may be provided in the more concentrated solution, and this can be increased to a level that prevents the water from crossing the membrane.

The term *osmole* refers to the active particles in the water, and *osmolality* refers to the number of osmoles per kilogram of solvent. This term is used to refer to the activity of the particles in the solution. When water is lost through the skin or urine, the blood plasma osmolality increases, and after drinking occurs, plasma osmolality returns to normal. Drinking that is due to raised plasma osmolality is called *cellular dehydration drinking* (Ramsey, 1991).

Acute increases in plasma osmolality lead to decreases in cell size due to cell shrinking. In the *hypertonic* condition, when the solution outside the cell membrane has a higher osmotic pressure than the cell content, water will diffuse out of the cell and the cell shrinks. In the *hypotonic* condition, when the solution outside the cell membrane has a lower osmotic pressure than the solution inside the cell, water enters the cell and expands the cell. Tonicity refers to the characteristic of the solution with respect to the osmotic pressure across the cell membrane (Rolls & Rolls, 1982). In thirst, the increased plasma sodium concentration is the main reason for the increased osmotic pressure and the cellular dehydration (Rolls & Rolls, 1982). The increased osmolality of the blood plasma leads to cellular dehydration and to the state of thirst because of the change in osmotic pressure (the fact that the solutes in the plasma cause the withdrawal of water from inside the cells). The amount of plasma sodium concentration and of plasma osmolality are highly correlated, so cellular dehydration can be inferred by either one of these two measures.

Extracellular Dehydration. This complex process involves (a) amount of sodium in the plasma, (b) plasma volume, and (c) cellular volume. A deficit in plasma volume leads to an appetite for sodium, and when sodium is ingested, the extracellular volume is restored. A decrease of sodium in a diet changes the plasma osmolality, which leads to a decrease in the extracellular water, due to the cells becoming overhydrated.

Thirst in many species involves both extracellular and cellular dehydration, and sodium plays a role in both. Between periods of drinking, water lost through the skin or urine leads to a rise in plasma osmolality, and without water replenishment the blood volume falls. The amount of blood volume decrease depends upon the amount of sodium deficiency. The decrease in blood volume (extracellular fluid) is called *hypovolemia.* When plasma volume decreases by about 10%, hypovolemic thirst occurs (Fitzsimons, 1991). Extracellular and cellular dehydration drinking can occur independent of one another. This is seen by the fact that changes in extracellular fluid can lead to drinking even without a change in cellular volume. Many species of animals have been found to drink more water after sodium depletion, and the reason is the loss of extracellular water (Rolls & Rolls, 1982).

Receptors in the vascular system (in the heart and in the arterial system) are sensitive to hypovolemia. Stretch receptors are responsive to changes in blood volume and baroreceptors are responsive to changes in blood pressure. Loss of blood plasma decreases return of blood to the heart in the veins (venous return) and this reduces arterial blood pressure. Moreover, decreased blood pressure is sensed by receptors in the kidneys (renal receptors). Through action of the sympathetic nervous system, the kidneys secrete renin reflexly.

Renin is an enzyme that acts on an otherwise inert peptide (angiotensinogen) in the blood. The action of renin on the substrate in the plasma forms *angiotensin* I, which in turn is converted to angiotensin II. This has powerful dipsogenic effects (i.e., induces drinking) in animals. Angiotensin II is considered to be instrumental in hypovolemic thirst in animals. When injected intracranially, angiotensin II was found to induce a large amount of drinking (Rolls & Rolls, 1982). Although the evidence is not yet fully established, it has been suggested (Szczepanska-Sadowska, 1991; Thrasher, 1991) that, at least for nonhuman animals, angiotensin II plays a significant role in maintenance of body fluid homeostasis for normal thirst due to water deprivation. In nonhuman animals, it is also thought to play a homeostatic role for hypovolemic thirst.

The question has been raised whether in humans hypovolemia leads to thirst (Verbalis, 1990). Some researchers minimize the importance of hypovolemia for human thirst and drinking, although they recognize its importance for thirst and drinking in nonhuman animals. In line with the fact that hypovolemic thirst may not play a significant role for humans, some researchers also question whether angiotensin II is important for humans, either for hypovolemia or for normal thirst (Rolls, 1991). Rolls (1991) argues that normal thirst in humans is clearly due to cellular and not to extracellular dehydration. She proposes that no firm evidence exists for the dipsogenic effect of angiotensin II nor for hypovolemia as a normal source of thirst in humans, and she suggests that extracellular fluid volume depletion in humans is not likely to produce thirst except in severe dehydration or in certain types of pathological conditions (e.g., hemmorrhage). Further research is needed to verify the extent to which thirst in humans differs from that in nonhuman animals.

Some question remains whether angiotensin functions as a neurotransmitter or as a hormone (Rolls & Rolls, 1982) or as both (Szczepanska-Sadowska, 1991). Angiotensin has many properties, including that of being a powerful vasoconstrictor, so stretch receptors may be sensitive to it. A more potent form of angiotensin also has been identified, called angiotensin III (Oldfield, 1991). The locations of the significant angiotensin receptors in the brain and in the periphery, which in animals are presumed to mediate drinking in hypovolemic thirst, are still not fully confirmed (Oldfield, 1991).

Osmoreceptors, Vasopressin, and the Lateral Hypothalamus

Osmoreceptors are receptors that respond to cellular dehydration. Cellular dehydration is the crucial antecedent for thirst. Osmoreceptors are sensitive to the *effective* (relative) and not the *absolute* osmotic pressure. Sodium infusion into various brain sites, which changes the osmolality and the sodium concentration, increases cellular dehydration and subsequent drinking. Although increased sodium concentration leads to thirst and drinking, so does infusion of other types of hypertonic solutions. This provides strong evidence that for most animals (the possible exceptions being sheep and goats) there are only osmoreceptors, and not also sodium receptors, for thirst (Ramsay & Thrasher, 1990; Rolls, 1991; Rolls & Rolls, 1982). Saline injected into the bloodstream via the carotid artery can lead to cellu-

lar dehydration and drinking in dogs (Ramsay & Thrasher, 1990). In humans, intravenous injections of hypertonic sodium chloride were found to lead to verbal reports of thirst and to the release of an antidiuretic hormone (called *vasopressin*) that is normally released under conditions of thirst (Rolls, 1991).

Osmoreceptors are located in various brain sites as well as in the periphery. Details of these sites go beyond the scope of our present discussion but are described in several sources (e.g., Ramsay & Booth, 1991; Ramsay & Thrasher, 1990). Areas of the brain identified with thirst are the anterior ventral region of the brain near the third ventricle (organum vasculosum laminae terminalis, or OVLT) and other forebrain areas (such as the subfornical organ, or SFO), with a major role played by the anterior hypothalamus. Although the supraoptic nucelus has been identified as a site for osmoreceptors (Rolls & Rolls, 1982), the importance of this site versus other sites is still somewhat controversial (Ramsay & Thrasher, 1990). Additional areas involved in thirst due to water-deprivation may include the somatosensory cortex (Schallert, 1991). Peripheral receptor sites also have been identified in the stomach, intestine, and liver.

Our knowledge about how cellular dehydration leads to thirst and water intake can be traced back to the work of several investigators, most notably Verney (1947). He suggested that when cell volume decreases due to increased osmolality of plasma, receptors in the brain are excited and these stimulate secretion of an antidiuretic hormone (called ADH, or arginine vasopressin [AVP], or vasopressin). Diuresis refers to release of urine, and *antidiuretic* means the prevention of urine release. Normal drinking occurs irregularly throughout the waking hours, so regulation of internal fluid levels is as much affected by the excretion of urine as it is by water intake.

Investigations in the 1950s identified the hypothalamus as the brain area that contained the important osmoreceptors that led to thirst and drinking. Work by Malmo and Malmo (1979) revealed that neuron firing in the lateral hypothalamus and lateral preoptic area increased in proportion to the hypertonicity of saline or sucrose solutions injected into the carotid artery. Other areas (like the OVLT, described by Ramsay and Thrasher, 1990) also have been recognized as crucial for the onset of drinking under conditions of cellular dehydration. Once the osmoreceptors become sensitive to the cellular dehydration, vasopressin usually is released into the bloodstream by the posterior pituitary gland. This release acts on the collecting ducts of the kidney, called nephrons, and causes them to retain water.

Vasopressin secretion serves to conserve water as water deficit develops. Although water retention and drinking tend to occur together, they also may function somewhat independently. When osmoreceptors respond to cellular dehydration, vasopressin secretion conserves bodily fluid by decreasing the volume of urine that the kidneys produce, and ordinarily drinking is also initiated. The ability to concentrate urine serves to minimize, but does not prevent, water loss. In nonhuman animals that have access to food and water, urine osmolality is greater than is plasma osmolality.

Water deprivation typically leads to the sensation of thirst, the behavioral act of drinking, and vasopressin release. However, vasopressin release in animals need not always be linked with drinking (Pinel, 1990). How the osmoreceptors lead to drinking is not yet fully known, although in nonhuman animals this possibly occurs as a reflex (Musty, 1982). The suggestion that water retention and drinking may be independent in some respects is based on the fact that in nonhuman animals, hypertonic solutions injected into the brain that lead to vasopressin release do not always lead to drinking, and those that lead to drinking do not always lead to release of vasopressin (Pinel, 1990). Research with dogs has shown that after the dogs drink water, their plasma osmolality falls in about 9 to 12 minutes, but by 3 minutes their plasma vasopressin is significantly reduced (Ramsay & Thrasher, 1990). There is no rapid fall in plasma vasopressin if water is introduced directly into the dog's stomach, and this suggests that oropharyngeal monitoring that occurs with the act of drinking serves to inhibit vasopressin secretion.

In nonhuman animals, osmotically induced drinking has been said to occur when plasma osmolality increases around 2% above basal level. In humans a comparable magnitude of increased plasma osmolality seems to produce a sensation that is subjectively reported as thirst (Verbalis, 1990). Although humans often drink liquids following the sensation of a dry mouth, this is thought to be a learned and not a primary reaction. Oropharyngeal sensations (like a dry mouth) do not seem to control thirst and drinking but may have regulatory value for satiety and the cessation of drinking. In humans the main stimulus for unlearned regulatory thirst and drinking is the firing of osmoreceptors and the renin-pituitary activity involved in vasopressin secretion (Verbalis, 1990).

As already pointed out, circulating levels of vasopressin (or AVP) in plasma produces antidiuresis (retention of urine). The kidney in humans and nonhuman animals is extraordinarily sensitive to small changes in plasma AVP levels. Urinary concentration is directly proportional to vasopressin levels. Whereas hypovolemia and changes in blood pressure alter AVP secretion in animals, in humans it is thought that AVP response to decreased blood volume is muted or even absent (Verbalis, 1990). Even in animals, hypovolemia is considered at best to represent 30% of the antecedent of thirst, with 70% of thirst due to cellular dehydration and changes in osmolality, and there is general agreement that in humans hypovolemia does not play a role in normal water intake and renal (kidney) water conservation. Humans, like nonhuman animals, need sodium to ensure that a basal level of extracellular fluid volume is maintained. However, humans normally do not have a specific salt appetite nor an appetite for other nonnutritive solutes. Unlike humans, noncarnivorous animals normally do have a specific appetite for salt (NaCl). In humans as in nonhuman animals, there are specific mechanisms whereby the kidney excretes solutes, and these appear to be more complex than the fairly simple system of AVP-controlled water excretion (Verbalis, 1990).

Salt Appetite

A strong motivation exists in rats and other animals to obtain and consume salty-tasting substances. This motivation is innate and analogous to thirst. Aldosterone, which is a hormone secreted by the adrenal cortex, helps to preserve body sodium. Angiotensin not only leads to the secretion of vasopressin but also controls aldosterone secretion. Stricker and Verbalis (1990) point out the close relationship between hypovolemia and a sodium deficiency need in rats. Hypovolemic rats have heightened salt consumption as well as increased drinking. When rats have a loss of *body sodium,* they have increased aldosterone secretion, which preserves body sodium, and they have a heightened sodium appetite, which facilitates the animals' increasing their sodium intake. However, the loss of body sodium is not accompanied by a change in water excretion. In contrast, if they have lowered *plasma sodium* concentration as a result of excess body water, they excrete water into urine but do not secrete aldosterone (for preserving body sodium) nor do they develop sodium appetite. Stricker and Verbalis (1990) suggest that angiotensin (angiotensin II) provides an important excitatory stimulus for sodium appetite. When rats have a sodium-deficient diet for a long period, such as 8 days, they drink large volumes of salt solutions. Rats during pregnancy and lactation also consume sodium in larger amounts than normal.

Other hormones play a role in salt appetite and in thirst. The hormone oxytocin, secreted by the posterior pituitary, plays a role in both salt appetite and thirst. Plasma oxytocin level is thought to vary inversely with sodium appetite in rats (Stricker and Verbalis, 1990) and oxytocin secretion is thought to occur during cellular dehydration. Laboratory rats that are fed with a high sodium diet ingest water normally. Stricker and Verbalis (1990) suggest that when the animals are sodium deprived, however, neural signals that normally lead to drinking are directed instead toward salt intake and away from water intake. A complex relationship exists between salt intake and drinking, which includes inhibitory as well as excitatory signals. Both oxytocin and vasopressin are involved in these processes. In the past, the two types of consummatory responses of salt intake and drinking, and the two corresponding motivational states of salt appetite and thirst, were considered to be independent. They were thought to be controlled by separate neural and hormonal processes. Recently, however, some researchers (Stricker & Verbalis, 1990) have come to consider them as interrelated systems.

Drinking, Drinking Offset, and Nonprimary Factors

Drinking as a function of water deprivation is not common in humans. Humans drink a large amount of liquid with their meals and they often drink between meals. In many countries, tea and coffee drinking signify positive emotional and social occasions within the routine of daily life. Party drinking of alcoholic and nonalcoholic beverages is a frequent social activity but is unrelated to dehydration from water deprivation. Loss of both salt and water through sweating do occur in vigorous sporting activities and with exercise, but serious dehydration and salt loss are not common in the daily life of most people. Thus, thirst in humans is infrequently a major type of motivation. Estimates have been made that drinking occurs with meals in such a way that cellular dehydration is ordinarily not at an extreme level. Drinking of many kinds of fluids (milk, soda, tea, coffee) is common, so that water intake due to cellular dehydration is most easily observed in laboratory studies.

Studies with laboratory animals have found that the amount animals drink is linearly related to the length of deprivation time (Musty, 1982). Because thirst can be induced in many ways, some researchers (e.g., Epstein, 1990) have suggested there is more than one kind of thirst. For example, when angiotensin II is injected either into the brain or intravenously, thirst and drinking are very much increased. Also, when animals or humans eat dry food or are water deprived for long periods (48 hr), thirst and drinking increase and so do levels of angiotensin II in the blood. Additionally, the effect of gender and sex hormones has been found to play a role in rodents, not only in eating (Wade, 1975) but in water and salt intake. Female rats drink more salt solutions than do male rats, and adult female rats decrease water intake during estrus (A. N. Epstein, 1990).

Rats have been found to drink more at night, when they are doing many other kinds of activities like grooming, locomoting, and eating. Rats, like humans, also drink more when they ingest salty substances. The change in salinity is likely to be sensed by osmoreceptors. As water is consumed, the salinity in the blood and cellular fluid is decreased and water consumption as well as water retention in the kidney is decreased (Musty, 1982). Many kinds of environmental events can lead to drinking offset. The physiological events known to lead to drinking offset are a decrease in osmoreceptor firing and a change in firing of oropharyngeal receptors.

Researchers have found that animals drink different amounts according to whether their diet is high in proteins or carbohydrates, and that different amounts of drinking occur both *before* and *after* the meal consumption. Water and food intake can have other reciprocal influences. For example, water-restricted animals have been found to decrease their food intake (Collier & Levitsky, 1967), and if animals on a food schedule are suddenly not fed, they may drink inordinate amounts of water as a kind of compensatory "filling up" reaction (a schedule-induced polydipsia).

Early researchers believed that the sensation that signaled thirst and led to drinking was a dry mouth. Although the contemporary focus on brain centers and hormones (angiotensin and aldosterone) has replaced this earlier belief, subjective ratings of thirst do relate to the sensation of a dry mouth. In one study, in which human subjects were given hypertonic saline infusions, the subjects' thirst ratings increased in line with the increase in plasma sodium concentration, plasma osmolality, and plasma vasopressin concentration, and the experience of a dry mouth consistently related to these increases (Rolls, 1991). Subjects found the relief of the dry mouth satiating, and they drank until the plasma sodium level and osmolality, as well as the thirst ratings, returned to the preinfusion levels. A different study induced thirst by means of 24-hour fluid deprivation (Rolls et al., 1980), and, as was found in the above study with the hypertonic saline infusion, thirst was accompanied by a dry mouth. In the 24-hour fluid deprivation study, subjects stopped drinking before a significant plasma dilution had occurred, with subjects attributing the cessation of drinking to the experience of stomach fullness.

Several studies with humans have shown that drinking can cease before the baseline plasma levels are reached. Rolls (1991) explains this by suggesting that in addition to the cellular rehydration and plasma changes, gastric, intestinal, and oropharyngeal factors are likely to play a role in the offset of drinking. When humans live normal daily routines, in contrast to laboratory circumstances, it is probably the case that they drink fluid in anticipation of changed body fluid conditions. Rolls (1991) cites one study that tested subjects in their daily environment, and the subjects were found to start and stop fluid intake before noticeable changes occurred of the kind that are associated with cellular dehydration.

Taste receptors on the tongue, and other somatosensory receptors, elicit licking (drinking) in the rat and other mammals. At one time it was assumed that regardless of how thirsty the animal was (how long it had been deprived of water) the rate of licking in rats was a constant amount per burst of licking. Eating was known to vary in rate of intake as a function of strength of (hunger) motivation, but it was thought that licking rate (water intake) was not altered as a function of strength of (thirst) motivation nor as a function of how palatable the solution was. However, contemporary research has shown that the rate of licking will vary according to a number of environmental factors (Zeigler, 1991) and that the amount of licking is monitored by the animal. It is now also thought that nonhuman animals can exert anticipatory control over drinking just as humans can. The animal's prior experience appears to lead to learning the correlation between amount of licking and volume intake, and drinking ceases when the feedback signal from the monitoring matches a preset value that specifies how much should be drunk (Mook, 1990).

As with the consummatory response of eating, the consummatory response of drinking follows a circadian rhythm. More consuming occurs during the normally wakeful hours for the given species. For humans and nonhuman animals, drinking typically accompanies meals, and palatability of food and drink appears to be a major factor in normal fluid intake. Flavors of available fluids affect amount of fluid consumed (Pinel, 1990). It is clear from all of the above findings that many factors, and not merely cellular dehydration and "primary" thirst, lead to drinking.

THE ROLE OF CULTURE AND LEARNING IN HUNGER AND EATING

The biological, inborn, "primary drive" aspects of hunger and eating are important, but such aspects are only part of the total influences that shape food-related behavior. Food-related behaviors for humans and nonhuman animals are influenced by individualized learning experiences and environmental cues, and for humans, many facets of eating are strongly influenced by culture.

Taste and Appetite

Culture

Culture shapes a wide range of food taboos and food practices (see reviews by Rozin, 1996, and Rozin & Shulkin, 1990). Different countries and different religions prescribe different sets of food-related behaviors. What is considered disgusting and unappetizing by one group may be considered a delicacy by another group. Religious rules for fasting, of what foods to eat and not eat, are expressions of learned beliefs and behaviors adopted by large groups of people. For example, devout Moslems and Jews refrain from eating pork, and devout Hindus refrain from eating beef. Devout Catholics abstain from eating meat on Fridays and they observe special rules about food and fasting at the time of Lent.

Cultural variations exist in eating practices at the dinner table. For example, Americans, like Europeans, use their knives to cut their meat by holding their knife in the right hand and their fork in the left hand. If they are right-handed, Americans put down the knife after cutting the meat, transfer the fork to their right hand, and pick up the meat with the fork in the right hand. Europeans, in contrast, do not transfer the fork to the right hand but keep the knife in the cutting position and pick up the meat with the fork in the left hand. People in India eat food with well-washed hands. Chinese people use chopsticks to eat their food. Different styles of eating exist,

which are often unrelated to differences regarding what foods are eaten, what foods are taboo or considered delicacies, and how foods are prepared and cooked.

Cultural values of beauty also influence food-related behaviors. Societal definitions of "ideal body shape" can exert a strong influence on food consumption. Eating patterns differ for women than for men, in part because a slim body is considered ideal for women more than for men. Recent years have found a greater rise in eating disorders in women than in men, and these disorders can be traced at least in part to the values society has set regarding gender and body shape (Rozin, 1996).

The kinds of foods eaten in different societies may be determined by the availability of certain foods in different geographic areas, and traditions and beliefs also influence the kinds of foods eaten by people of various cultures. In a modern industrialized society, in which foods are flown in or shipped by refrigeration methods unheard of a century ago, changing beliefs as well as marketing practices can influence personal eating patterns. Pizza was not widely known at one time within the American culture, and today pizza parlors are found in large as well as small communities in the United States. Tacos, which were popular primarily in areas with a strong Mexican heritage, are now eaten in all parts of the United States. Cultural shifts occurred in other countries, also. Hamburger chains came into existence in former communist countries once political beliefs and practices changed, and eating at hamburger restaurants has even become a high-status symbol.

Immediate environmental demands also shape mealtimes. For example, in hot tropical climates it is functionally adaptive to eat a big meal relatively late in the evening and to have only a light meal followed by a "siesta" in the hot middle of the day. In such a society a large dinner at 9 or 10 p.m. is not unusual, whereas in cooler climates, as in most of the United States, the normal dinner hour is much earlier in the evening. In relatively cooler northern countries in Europe the big dinner usually is eaten at midday, with only a small and light meal eaten in the evening. Temperature, geography and availability of specific foods, and culture-based beliefs affect eating patterns, and so do unique and individual learning experiences. In various ways humans learn food preferences and aversions that guide *when* one eats, *what* one eats, and *how* one eats.

Learned Aversions

From the time of the 1960s, experiments revealed that *taste aversions* can be learned. Garcia and colleagues (Garcia, Ervin, & Koelling, 1966; Garcia, Hankins, & Rusniak, 1974; Garcia, Rusniak, & Brett, 1977), in studies sometimes described as "bait-shyness" research, found that if animals become ill after tasting a particular food they will avoid that food the next time it is encountered. This can occur with taste alone or when taste is accompanied by smell. The illness need not occur immediately. Even illness occurring after several hours can result in a learned taste aversion. Besides humans, rats, mice, cats, monkeys, birds, and fish have all shown this type of avoidance learning, and all kinds of illness can lead to it. If by chance, or as a result of chemical treatments, humans get sick following a particular food, that food becomes distasteful (Garcia et al., 1974), and this can happen even with food that previously was highly desirable, like ice cream (Bernstein, 1968).

Learned food aversion like bait-shyness is established in ways similar to the studies of Pavlovian conditioning of fear. Fear, discussed in more detail in a later chapter, is relevant to food aversions in that both can be acquired by pairing a neutral stimulus like a colored liquid (which after conditioning is called the CS, or conditioned stimulus) with an innately aversive stimulus like shock (the US, or unconditioned stimulus). The CS acquires the aversive characteristics of the US from such pairings. In operant conditioning, the individual can learn avoidance not only of the aversive US but also of a CS that has been paired with it. In learned food aversions, a neutral stimulus (food or some flavored liquid) is paired with a negative US. Illness (malaise) rather than a painful stimulus is used as the innately negative condition (US) in the bait-shyness procedure. In regular Pavlovian conditioning the CS-US interval is very brief (from half a second to

a few seconds), but in the learned aversion procedure the interval is much longer (possibly several hours). Of particular relevance in the training of learned food aversions is the use of nausea, which curtails eating. Compared with a painful stimulus as the US, nausea is more nonspecific. Learned food aversions thus involve a learned association between a neutral stimulus and an innately aversive condition, and the nonspecificity of the US and the long CS-US duration make food aversion learning different from the usual Pavlovian (classical) conditioning.

A broad approach to the question of food avoidance and taste aversion was advanced by Rozin (1989, 1996; Rozin & Fallon, 1987, 1988; Rozin & Schulkin, 1990). In studies with rats, Rozin and colleagues (Pelchat, Grill, Rozin, & Jacobs, 1983) found that even sucrose solutions would be avoided if the stimulus was paired with the experience of nausea, induced by lithium chloride, or with the experience of pain, induced by shock presentation. The animals' behavior with these acquired distastes, which the researchers called *negative palatability shifts,* differed according to whether the learned aversion was a result of association with nausea or with danger. Studies with humans and nonhuman animals have shown that foods paired with nausea evoke a negative affect and distaste of the food, whereas food paired with shock leads to avoidance of the food but without the negative affect (Rozin & Shulkin, 1990). The data show clearly that prior experience can lead to a variety of avoidances of foods and tastes. In describing *human* aversions and how these are learned, Rozin and colleagues integrated findings from animal research with data pertaining to individual human experiences as well as the role of culture.

The approach taken by Rozin and Fallon (1987) emphasizes three types of beliefs humans have that are bases for avoiding foods. One is called sensory-affective, which refers to the belief that the food tastes or smells bad. The second refers to the belief that harm follows the ingestion of the food, and this can be bodily harm (getting sick from the food) or social harm (criticism or shame being given). The third type the authors call "ideational," although if one defines ideation as a belief, all the above are, in fact, ideations. Rozin and Fallon (1987) refer to this third type as a belief about the item itself, not about its taste or about the consequence that will follow from its ingestion. This third type of belief refers to the item being either *inappropriate* as food (typically, because it is nonnutritive, like paper or sand), or the item being offensive, leading to the emotion of *disgust*. All three of the above types are learned beliefs. The first type of belief concerning taste as a sensory quality is a *belief* about a taste, not the direct sensory *experience* of a taste.

Taste can be innately pleasurable (like sweetness) or innately aversive (like bitterness). A young infant and young rat will show strong innate avoidance in response to bitterness. If a neutral-tasting substance (e.g., colored water) immediately precedes the presentation of an innately aversive taste (e.g., quinine) and this is repeated often, in time the previously neutral-tasting substance will also be avoided. This conditioned aversion can be found in animals, and it differs from the human cognitions Rozin and Fallon (1987) emphasized.

Beliefs, in general and about taste, are learned in many ways. For instance, a sensory-affective belief regarding the taste of an item could be learned without actual experience with the taste. If parents tell a child that something should not be eaten because it "tastes bad," the child can learn that belief without direct immediate experience. This differs from the avoidance of bad-tasting food either due to its innate aversiveness or because the item has gained bad-tasting qualities through Pavlovian conditioning.

Research has shown that by the age of 3 years, children can tell that a food that looks edible but has been contaminated should not be eaten (Siegal, 1995). Beliefs can help protect humans. Young babies may not avoid items that an older child would avoid. An infant with limited cognitive development may ingest items of all kinds, such as paper or sand as well as dangerous items. However, some beliefs that may have been protective at one time may not be needed at a later time. This is true for an individual's as well as for a group's belief. Avoiding pork, as is done by persons of Islamic and Jewish religions, would be protective for people living in the hot Middle East before the days of refrigeration, but with modern cooling and meat-inspection systems, a belief in the harmfulness and the offensiveness of eating pork, giving a strong emotional basis for pork avoidance, is no longer needed for protection. Beliefs and emotional reactions of disgust can be limited to items that have unique values for a culture or for a specific family, but some are universal, such as the disgust that feces elicits in adults (Rozin & Fallon, 1987).

Rozin and Fallon (1987) emphasized those beliefs that refer to the item itself (their third, "ideational," type) rather than the beliefs about the item's taste or the harmful consequences. Rozin and colleagues (Rozin, Millman, & Nemeroff, 1986) found that if items associated with unpleasantness are linked with a food, the unpleasant quality transfers to it. This is called "the law of sympathetic magic." For example, people have an aversion to consuming a favorite liquid that has been stirred by a brand-new comb or flyswatter. Another example the researchers found was that people had an aversion to drinking a palatable juice into which a dead and sterilized cockroach had been dropped and then removed. This so-called "contagion" contrasted with subjects' reaction toward drinking that same type of juice when a neutral object had been dropped into it for the same amount of time. A sweet-tasting substance is likely to be judged more pleasant tasting by a person told it was sugar than by a person told it was crushed-up cockroaches. Since at the age of 3 years children believe a liquid that had contained a cockroach is contaminated and should not be drunk, and the researcher considered that a correct response (Siegal, 1995), the question is whether a long history of believing in the unhealthiness of cockroaches can be mitigated by a single occasion of telling subjects that the cockroach had been sterilized, as done by Rozin et al. (1986). Some cases of "sympathetic magic" might be more appropriate than others.

The literature on food avoidance reveals that it can be learned in many ways. Many studies have shown that taste aversion and food avoidance can be learned through Pavlovian conditioning, through bait-shyness type of conditioning that involves illness, and through the cognitive learning that Rozin and colleagues described. One's culture and one's individual learning experiences, as well as innate taste biases, influence human taste aversions and food avoidances.

Appetite and Appetizing

If we say "this tastes terrible, I just lost my appetite," we are not referring to a state induced by food deprivation but to an intervening variable linked to the taste of an item of food. Taste has a motivational effect that concerns the *incentive value* of food and that has powerful effects on the consummatory response of eating. An *appetizing* taste is affectively pleasant, and *appetite* is an internal state, similar to hunger. The appetizing quality of food influences how much is eaten in the same way that taste aversion, which is affectively unpleasant (Rozin & Shulkin, 1990), influences how much is not eaten. Thus, in an inverse way, studies of taste aversion bear on appetizingness: that which is aversive and even disgusting is not at all appetizing. Animals and human infants need to learn not only which foods to avoid, but also which foods are safe and appealing.

Social Enhancement. In a broad review of the effect of social facilitation on food selection in rats, Galef and Beck (1990) showed that when infant mammals stop suckling, they need to learn which foods are safe. Although many people think that young animals and infants instinctively select the appropriate foods to eat to fulfill their nutritional needs, this is not so. Studies called "cafeteria feeding experiments" show that when weanling rats are presented with a wide selection of foods in the laboratory, their food selection is not adequate even to maintain their body weight, to say nothing about fulfilling their nutritional needs. Many weanlings in such studies have died because of failure to select life-maintaining amounts and kinds of food.

Beck and Galef (1989) found that when weanling rats were given choices of three diets that contained inadequate levels of protein and one diet with ample protein, weanlings without the presence of a knowledgeable adult rat did not select the diet

that would sustain them in good health. In contrast, animals were able to grow well when they were in the presence of an adult rat previously trained to consume the protein-rich diet. From this and other studies, the researchers concluded that social enhancement of dietary self-selection can occur in the laboratory, and that social learning is presumably the method by which animals in nature acquire the necessary information and skills for eating foods that are safe and nutritional. With rats, not only with humans, the presence of *conspecifics* (members of one's own species) is necessary to provide a large amount of social learning about food.

Social learning about eating in rats occurs as follows: (1) The presence of an adult rat at a site attracts young to the site, where they begin feeding. (2) Adult rats deposit olfactory cues at feeding sites, and this attracts weanlings to these sites for feeding. (3) A naive rat that interacts with and observes a "demonstrator" animal eat a certain diet will come to prefer that diet.

Galef (1989) tested the strength of the effect of social enhancement in rats. Is the power of such social influence, of naive animals learning which foods to eat through observation of experienced rats, so great that social learning can dominate the effect of individual experience? Experimental and control animals were given a bait-shyness type of avoidance learning experience (in which hungry animals ate a food and subsequently were made ill). The experimental rats were given prior experience either with one or with two "demonstrator" conspecifics, and the control rats had no "demonstrator" experience. On recovering from the illness, a large number of the experimental animals (that previously had been in the presence of one or two demonstrator conspecifics) ate the food that had been associated with their illness. They failed to exhibit an aversion to the food even though it had been followed by illness. In contrast, the control subjects showed the expected food aversion as a result of their bait-shyness type of learning experience. Galef and Beck (1990) concluded as a general finding that rats' social enhancement experience, which leads to food being sought, can mitigate an individual's learning of food avoidance. Because the animals showed large individual differences in the degree to which food aversion could be diminished as a result of learning from conspecifics, Galef and Beck (1990) concluded that variation exists between rats in how much they will be influenced by *social* compared with *individual* experience.

Galef and Beck (1990) suggested that food learning due to social enhancement gives an individual animal benefit from a broad base of food information. The animal can select needed nutrients of proven quality (as shown by the behavior of the demonstrator conspecifics) and is not limited by individual (and perhaps accidentally aversive) information. Social learning can augment individual experiences, thus widening information about nutritious and safe foods. If rats can benefit from such social facilitation in their selection of positive foods, a much greater benefit from social facilitation can be expected in humans, who have far more complex intellectual prowess and far more sophisticated means of social communication. Galef (1996) described many vertebrate species that show social learning of food preferences, and some show social learning of instrumental activities that will procure food for consumption.

Rather then addressing the question of how humans learn to seek desirable foods by means of social learning, Redd and de Castro (1992) assessed the role of social influence on the *amount of food* that is eaten. Does a person eat more food in the company of others? Data from a series of correlational studies showed that when one other person is present at a meal, compared with when one eats alone, on the average 28% more food is consumed. When four, five, or six persons are present, these averages rise to 53%, 71%, and 76%. To assess if such an increase in food consumption as a result of number of persons present would be found when subjects specifically set out to eat alone or with others, Redd and de Castro (1992) asked subjects to follow three 5-day plans for a total of 15 days. Undergraduate men and women filled out questionnaires for the 15 days. Order of conditions was randomly assigned to the subjects. The three 5-day conditions were for subjects to eat as they would normally (and if this included other persons, to indicate the number), to eat alone, and to eat with other persons. The results showed that when sub-

jects ate normally or in the with-people condition, subjects ate significantly larger meals and consumed more overall calories than in the alone condition. This social facilitation was also evident when subjects ate in the "normal" condition. That is, in the normal condition, when subjects ate with others they also consumed more than when they ate alone. The research also showed a surprising dissociation between eating and hunger ratings, because many significant differences were found between the three conditions in the *kinds* of foods and the *amount* consumed, but premeal and postmeal subjective hunger ratings were not significantly different for the three conditions.

Many variables are involved for humans regarding the social nature of eating and its effect on the amount consumed, and a strong emotional dimension is evident. Eating with others is a pleasurable activity for most persons, and the subjects in the above study reported feeling more depressed when eating alone than with others. The social nature of eating is complex. Food has symbolic value in most cultures, often with rituals involved in food consumption. Humans are a highly social species, and most persons think of a meal as an opportunity for social interchange rather than as a biological necessity. In this way, the social pleasures associated with a meal can alter the quality and quantity of food consumed. A meal for human beings has social symbolic value, and pleasure is gained not only in terms of the hedonic appetizing quality of the food but in terms of the social context of the meal.

Hedonic Factors. As Galef (1996) pointed out, the social aspects of food consumption tended to be disregarded in earlier research. This was evident in the work of P. T. Young (1948, 1949; Young & Chaplin, 1945). He approached the question of what makes food appealing or appetizing in a series of nonsocial studies with rats. Young showed that when rats taste, touch, and smell foods, they show affective arousal ("enjoyment") to some foods and not to others. Foods that are enjoyed he called "palatable," and they were preferred in taste tests over less enjoyable foods. This hedonic value was not related to nutritional need. Casein, a protein with high nutritional value, was not preferred in many taste tests, but saccharine, with no known nutritional value, was preferred in many such tests.

Young (1949) distinguished between *appetite* and *palatability*. He considered the former to be a specific hunger, based on the nutritional need of the individual. He considered the latter to be the positive hedonic attribute of the substance being ingested, and that relates to sensory qualities like taste and smell. What Young called palatability would be called "appetizing" by contemporary researchers. Hungry rats but not satiated rats increase their food consumption as a function of palatability, which means that palatability is not the only factor in increased food consumption. The amount consumed depends in part on an animal's overall state of hunger. Though satiated animals don't consume palatable foods, they will show preferences. The best test for palatability is if the food is preferred in a taste test, especially a brief-exposure test that involves a choice among several items (Young & Greene, 1953).

Later researchers have shown that palatability affects the amount and rate of eating at the start of a meal. Greater insulin release occurs at the start of a meal and a larger amount of food is consumed for foods of high versus low palatability (Le Magnen, 1985). As a meal continues, shifts in hedonic preferences are likely to occur, and food that is judged more palatable at the start of a meal may be less preferred as the meal progresses.

Young and Greene (1953) noted the possibility of such a shift. They compared sucrose solutions of high and low concentrations and concluded that satiation could be responsible for such shifts. Many investigators have observed a hedonic shift during the course of eating, both in humans and in animals. A shift that appears to be unambiguously due to a surfeit in the taste, and not due to loss of hunger that accompanies eating and a filling stomach, has been called *sensory-specific satiety* (Hetherington & Rolls, 1989, 1996; Rolls, Rolls, Rowe, & Sweeney, 1981). The word "satiety" here does not refer to loss of hunger in the way Young and Greene (1953) meant, as a result of eating and decreased food deprivation. Rather, it refers to a *sensory satiation,* of not finding a given taste as pleasurable after repeated exposure to that taste. Once eating begins,

and prior to postingestive absorption, sensory-specific satiety occurs, with the given food becoming less pleasurable. This was found in subjective pleasantness ratings, slowing of rate of eating, and various measures of food preference.

Young (1949) advocated that hedonic preferences in rats should be measured by having subjects choose between briefly presented substances. In studies with humans, the primary measure for assessing the palatability of foods has been pleasantness ratings. With sensory-specific satiety, foods eaten from the start of a meal are later judged less pleasant than at the start, and new foods introduced later in the meal tend to be judged as more pleasant than the prior food. Because newly experienced foods in a meal may be judged appealing, people given many foods may eat more than is nutritionally required. Hetherington and Rolls (1996) reported a study in which people reported their reasons for stopping eating after free access to cheese and crackers. Those who stopped for the reason of lowered pleasure or interest in eating the food were found to consume significantly fewer calories than those who stopped for the reason of feeling full. These and other findings showed that hedonic value is influential in the amount that people consume. Sensory-specific satiety could be advantageous in limiting a person's food intake, and the reverse also can occur. Even though food-deprivation hunger has been satisfied, people may find themselves eating for reasons of taste (*incentive value*). When this happens, they eat not because they have a physiological need (hunger), nor because they have a specific hunger of the type Young (1949) called "appetite," but because tasting the food is pleasurable.

Taste preference relates to the incentive value of a food substance, and the pleasure aroused by certain foods has motivational characteristics. This was demonstrated in many of the experiments Young (1949) reviewed. Rats in runways or mazes will *run faster* to preferred than to nonpreferred foods, and this is in line with what is known for a wide range of incentive variables studied with nonhuman animals and humans. The higher the incentive value of an item or event, the greater the output in performance (the faster one runs, the more responses one makes, the shorter the latency in one's response, and the larger one's effort). Contemporary researchers do not define *appetite* the way Young did, as a deprivation-induced state, but instead most contemporary writers use the term to refer to the internal state of incentive motivation. Appetite is yoked to *palatability* or appetizingness, which is a function of sensory cues like taste and smell (Bartoshuk, 1989).

Taste provides information as well as hedonic pleasure or displeasure, and this has important consequences. The information value of sensory or other events is called a "cue function." Events in the external environment provide many cues, such as when to be quiet or when to take an umbrella. The internal environment also provides cues, such as when to go to the bathroom, when to have a nap, or when to eat. Signals from the external and internal environments provide countless cues (information) that guide one's actions. Thus, researchers have asked whether people eat because of external environmental cues (such as the sight or smell of food) or whether they eat because of internal physiological cues, like stomach contractions and other bodily cues. Researchers addressing these questions did not relate their work to the fact that eating is a necessity for survival, but instead they explored in what way cues for eating are involved in "eating disorders" and "weight disturbances."

Weight Maintenance and Eating Disorders

Cues, Obesity, and Eating Restraint

Researchers seek to discover what signals animals and humans use to initiate and cease eating. One study, for example, showed that breakdown of starch in the mouth, which produces maltose, serves as an important cue. Detection of reduced concentration of maltose by sweet-sensing taste buds was thought to induce a hunger sensation, and detection of restored concentration at the same sensor in the mouth was thought to provide a satiety cue (Poothullil, 1992). This taste cue was hypothesized to signal hunger versus satiation more powerfully than the cue provided by glucose. Maltose may provide sensory information for onset and offset of eating that is not merely hedonic but involves homeostatic regulation of internal processes.

Sensory information is important for what is eaten and how much is eaten. How well food tastes to a person is in part genetically determined, but many other factors influence the pleasantness of taste. Because the sense of smell adds to the pleasures of taste, changes in olfaction, such as impairment of smell that often accompanies aging, can alter food preferences in older persons and lead to eating disturbances (Duffy & Bartoshuk, 1996).

External and Internal Cues. Overweight and underweight individuals differ from normal control subjects not only in the amount eaten but also in how much they use sensory cues. Some studies have found obese individuals, whose weight is significantly greater than that of normal-weight persons, to be hyperreactive to food tastes. Nisbett (1972) gave ice cream flavored with quinine (a bitter taste) and unadulterated ice cream to overweight, normal-weight, and underweight persons. The overweight ate a lot more of the unadulterated and less of the bitter-tasting ice cream than did underweight subjects, with normal-weight subjects between the two extremes. The underweight subjects in fact ate nearly the same amount of good- and bad-tasting ice cream, which revealed a hyporeactivity to food tastes. It is as if the overweight consume food on the basis of its taste, with good-tasting food overeaten and bad-tasting food undereaten; normal-weight subjects being next in taste sensitivity; and underweight subjects being least sensitive to taste. The inference is that the underweight subjects consume food amounts largely on the basis of internal hunger cues, normal subjects are somewhat influenced by taste and somewhat influenced by internal hunger cues, and overweight subjects are minimally influenced by internal hunger cues and very much influenced by the taste of the food.

Pleasurable focus on the sensory cue of taste can relate to overeating not just in obese persons. Hetherington and Macdiarmid (1994) gave laboratory subjects free access to greatly liked chocolate. Those who were known to overeat chocolate not only consumed more but showed *less sensory-specific satiety* than did control subjects who comparably liked chocolate. Overeaters gave higher ratings of the pleasantness of the taste and the pleasure of eating chocolate after consumption than did control subjects, whose ratings of pleasantness of taste and pleasure of eating chocolate significantly decreased after consumption. Nisbett (1972), Pliner (1974), and Rodin and colleagues (Rodin, Elman, & Schachter, 1974) concluded from a series of experiments that obese persons are overly reactive to all types of external cues. These include visual and taste cues of the food itself, and more cognitive cues like the face of a clock to indicate time of day (and thus whether it was time to eat). Reliance on external cues for the overweight subjects was evident also by situational cues, such as whether the food was within reach or hard to obtain.

Singh (1973) did a study with rats that found if they were trained to work to obtain food before VMH-lesioning surgery they continued to work after becoming obese, but if they had no presurgery training to work for food, then they did not work to get food as much as did normal rats. On the basis of that study, Singh and Sikes (1974) used human subjects to assess two hypotheses: whether overweight and normal-weight subjects differed in their food consumption because of a difference in reliance on external cues, or instead, whether their difference in eating was due to a difference in willingness to exert effort and to work for their food.

College students were assigned to one of four conditions: (a) wrapped chocolates and wrapped cashews, (b) wrapped chocolates and unwrapped cashews, (c) unwrapped chocolates and wrapped cashews, and (d) unwrapped cashews and unwrapped chocolates. Subjects first received the test for chocolates and then for cashews. Hershey Kisses, which are normally encountered in a wrapped condition, were used for the chocolates. Each subject was given two bowls, each with 75 chocolates, and told the study involved a taste test. The person was to eat as many chocolates as needed in order to determine the difference in taste between chocolates in the two bowls. Half the subjects received the chocolates in a wrapped condition, and half in an unwrapped condition. Following a questionnaire and water consumption, each subject received cashews. For half the subjects these were wrapped in aluminum foil and for half the subjects the cashews were un-

wrapped. Unlike the chocolates, which normally come wrapped, the cashews normally do not come wrapped. Again, subjects had to eat from two bowls to compare the taste of the contents. Comparison of overweight and normal-weight subjects was based on measurement of subjects' triceps skinfold. This measurement had been used in other research as a basis for judging whether individuals were overweight or of normal weight.

The findings showed that chocolates were consumed in equal amounts by both groups of subjects, and that wrapping had no significant effect. However, for the cashews, wrapping was a significant variable for the overweight subjects. They consumed more if the cashews were unwrapped than wrapped. Wrapping had no effect on cashew eating of normal-weight subjects. An interaction occurred, with overweight subjects eating more unwrapped cashews and less wrapped cashews than did the normal-weight subjects. Consumption of the cashews could be interpreted to reveal the pattern reported by Nisbett and Rodin and others, that the wrapping provided an external cue and thus altered the food consumption of overweight but not of normal-weight individuals. However, why was the effect not found for the Hershey Kisses? Singh and Sikes (1974) reasoned that the study with college students showed data analogous to those obtained in the rat study. That is, people are used to unwrapping Hershey Kisses and thus have been trained to work for them, while for the wrapped cashews there was no prior training. Overweight rats ate less of a food that required work if they had not had prior training to work for getting food, and in an analogous way, the overweight college students were less willing to work to eat the cashews, for which they had not previously been trained to work (to unwrap).

The concept of "work" is different from the concept of sensitivity to external cues, and it may be relevant in some cases of eating behavior. However, it does not explain why obese persons would respond to cues about time more than do normal-weight persons, that is, regardless of the length of time since they last ate, obese persons were found to eat when they believed it was time to eat. Possibly the variable of "expectation" and not "work" separates overweight from normal-weight subjects.

That is, overweight subjects consume food in terms of prior expectancies, and this relates to unwrapped versus wrapped cashews, eating when the clock face indicates the normal mealtime, eating normal-tasting but not bitter ice cream, and eating food placed close by (which is the normal place for food to be consumed) versus food placed far away. Expectation is a major factor in differences in eating behaviors in various groups of individuals.

Expectation can influence eating behavior also with nonhuman animals. Weingarten (1985) reported that if rats are under a state of deprivation and a neutral stimulus is always associated with a specific food, the stimulus through conditioning becomes a CS or signal for the presentation of that food. When subsequently the CS is presented to the food-deprived animals, the rats wait for that specific food and eat it when it is provided, rather than eat the same kind of food that is continuously present in another place in the cage. Other explanations also have been offered to explain why people with weight and eating disturbances eat differently than do people in the normal range of weight and eating. In addition to altered sensitivity to cues, "expectation," and "work," the variable of endogenous opiate peptides may be related to obesity (Drewnowski, 1996). Researchers have suggested that food reduces stress by means of opioid receptors, although conclusive data are not yet available.

Genetic predisposition for obesity has been identified for certain groups (Drewnowski, 1996) whose metabolism genetically makes them especially susceptible to obesity. Dietary and nutritional variables, which are important for normal-weight persons, are especially critical for people with genetic predisposition to obesity. Obese men and women eat a diet that is rich in fat, but obese men and women differ in their food preferences. Steaks and french fries seem to be preferred by obese men, and foods high in fat and sweetness (ice cream and chocolate) seem to be preferred by obese women. Preference of calorie-dense diets appears to be due to many factors, including an individual's learning history and genetic, dietary, and sociocultural factors.

Subjective Reports of Cues Associated with Hunger and Eating. Eating as a consummatory response

needs to be distinguished from hunger as an internal state not only for researchers but also for individuals in their daily life. Moreover, in daily life people do not always differentiate between hunger (a deprivation-induced state), due to length of time since last eating, and subjectively "feeling hungry." One can "feel hungry" when one is bored, unhappy, or tired, and thus subjective hunger can be dissociated from the physiological cues that normally accompany the deprivation-induced state of hunger.

Stunkard and Koch (1964) inserted a gastric balloon into the stomach of obese subjects, which permitted recording of gastric contractions. During the observations, subjects were asked if they were hungry or had a desire to eat. These verbal measures were correlated with measures of gastric motility. Although the correlations were different for men and women, the overall finding was that, compared with nonobese subjects, the obese subjects were less sensitive to cues from their stomachs. That is, obese women tended to report not feeling hungry (even when gastric contractions were taking place), and obese men reported either feeling hungry all the time (even when there were no gastric contractions) or not feeling hungry (even when there were gastric contractions). Nonobese subjects did not show these types of biases and insensitivies to gastric motility. Griggs and Stunkard (1964) suggested that obese subjects' nonnormal sensitivity to cues from stomach motility was due to these individuals having experienced a different type of learning, in how they associated verbal statements and gastric motility, compared with nonobese subjects. The researchers suggested that new learning can change the obese subjects' responsiveness to such cues.

Hull (1943, 1951) had distinguished between the energizing aspect of motivation, called drive (D), and cues, called drive stimuli (S_D), which are associated with the energizing aspect of motivation. In discussing hunger, one can say that for normal eaters the drive stimuli coming from gastric motility provide reliable cues that become associated with the verbal response of "I am hungry," and certain obese persons may need to learn such cue-response relationships. Whereas for normal eaters the state of hunger triggers sensations (internal cues) that become associated with verbal responses of "I am hungry," for nonnormal eaters external rather than internal cues may become associated with subjective reporting of "I am hungry." Individuals with eating disorders are likely to have learned atypical patterns of associations between cues and food-related responses.

People consume food for a variety of reasons that include cultural factors, like sociability at parties, and individual factors, such as wanting to reduce boredom or to "get even" with a parent or spouse who is nagging that one is "too fat" and one should go on a diet. Griggs and Stunkard (1964) found that people differ in their sensitivity to stomach cues, and they also differ in the degree to which they modulate their eating behavior by evaluations of subjective hunger. Additionally, Hetherington and Rolls (1996) found that people's subjective reports of taste pleasantness is not always precise. Many persons do not distinguish between the pleasantness of the taste of food (as a characteristic of the taste) and the pleasure of eating (as a characteristic of the intake response). Subjective descriptions as learned verbal responses may be relatively unreliable indicators of a wide range of processes involved in hunger and eating.

Dietary Restraint. At one time the focus for research on eating disorders was devoted to the study of obese persons, who were thought to represent a homogeneous group. Recent evidence, however, suggests that obese people represent a heterogeneous population (Dresnowski, 1996), and the earlier research focus has shifted to include people with various eating and weight disorders. Stunkard and Messick (1985) developed a three-factor eating questionnaire to measure how people differ with respect to their eating behavior. The measure identifies "restrained eaters," or individuals who restrict their food intake as a means of controlling their body weight. The researchers made use of a concept from the conditioning literature that is called "disinhibition." Inhibition means holding back a response, and *disinhibition* refers to releasing the inhibition. If dieters who restrict food intake are in a state of disinhibition, will they stop inhibiting (stop restricting) their eating and consequently increase their food intake? Studies have shown that normal

eaters do not increase food intake after ingesting alcohol (a known disinhibitor), but restrained eaters will be more likely to increase food intake.

Using the eating questionnaire, Stunkard and Messick (1985) found that restrained eaters who score high on a disinhibition factor on the test are likely to eat more when they are depressed, but restrained eaters who score high on a factor related to cognitive control do not show this eating pattern. Dieters differ in their methods to restrain eating, and they are also vulnerable to different reasons for why they stop their dieting. The scale reveals why some, but not all, underweight persons are especially sensitive to taste cues. For example, restrained eaters scoring high on the disinhibition factor say, "Sometimes things just taste so good that I keep on eating even when I am no longer hungry." However, other restrained eaters would say, "I often stop eating when I am not really full as a conscious means of limiting the amount that I eat." Depending on the means by which individuals maintain their dieting, they also will react differently to stress, to internal cues, and to external cues.

Weight Instability. Many people have been on a diet at some time, and some persons go on diets often. Because subjective hunger and acts of eating are influenced by many variables, a large number of people have periods of gaining weight, followed by dieting. In one study (de Castro & Elmore, 1988), subjects kept records for 9 days, and hunger ratings were found to correlate only moderately with meal size. In another study (Mattes, 1990), 12 men and 12 women kept hourly records during their waking day for 7 days. Although the group as a whole showed a significant correlation between hunger ratings and computed energy content of the subjects' eating ($r = .50$) Monday through Friday (weekdays), on weekends the correlation was not significant, not were correlations significant for any individual subject. When the correlations were based on frequency of eating rather than computed energy content of eating, 6 of the 24 subjects showed a significant correlation between eating occurrences and hunger ratings. Of special interest is the finding that eating when not subjectively hungry, and not eating when subjectively hungry, occurred 31.6% of the time; over 20% of the time that subjects initiated eating they were not subjectively hungry. If one eats without being subjectively hungry, and if subjective hunger is only poorly correlated with caloric intake, it is easy to understand why many people gain unwanted weight. Griggs and Stunkard (1964) found a similar pattern in their 1-year work with an obese subject. At the end of the year the subject said that gastric contractions did not affect how much he ate. He indicated that the act of eating was hardly ever prompted by feelings of hunger, and he gained 3 pounds during the year in spite of efforts at weight control.

To lose weight it is helpful but not sufficient to change eating behavior and alter one's response to cues, and merely restraining food intake is also not sufficient. Caloric intake has different effects, depending on whether the calories are obtained from a high-fat or a low-fat diet. As Van Itallie and Kissileff (1990) pointed out, when fats, proteins, and carbohydrates are metabolized in the mammalian body, equal amounts of calories are not interchangeable as energy sources. Different foods have different thermic effects (an energy conversion described in layperson language as "burning off" calories). Carbohydrates are readily broken down into glucose (Rosenzweig, Leiman, & Breedlove, 1996), whereas excess calories consumed by eating fat will lead to increased adipose tissue. Details of how food and fat stores are related are still not fully clear, but it is thought that excess carbohydrate calories are more likely dissipated as heat whereas excess fat calories are more likely to be deposited as body fat (Drewnowski, 1991). Storage from excess fat consumption does not only lead to more total weight gain but also leads to higher percentage of body fat compared with lean body tissue.

The amount of stored fat compared with lean body tissue affects the basal metabolic rate. This is the rate of energy used for maintaining bodily heat and other resting functions. Restricting caloric intake lowers basal metabolism as well as weight, and severe eating restraint affects metabolic rate much more than it alters body weight (Rosenzweig et al., 1996). For this reason, dieters who restrain from caloric intake may find it difficult to lose weight, since the body "burns" calories at a slower rate. Ex-

ercise, however, helps by "burning" calories and by increasing lean body tissue, and lean body tissue, in turn, contributes to a higher basal metabolic rate. Because metabolic rate determines how many calories the body burns, the presence of lean body tissue is advantageous for keeping one's weight down.

Dieters may lose weight, regain it, lose again, and in this way go through many cycles. A graphic name for this is "the yo-yo effect." Each time a person goes through such a cycle, weight gain is easier and weight loss becomes more difficult. This is because in each period of lowering food intake a compensatory decrease occurs in metabolic rate, and when the rate of burning off calories is decreased, fat storage increases (fat cell size and fat cell number). From an evolutionary perspective, it is as if the body compensates for reduced energy intake by converting more energy for storage, for later use in a time of low food consumption. For weight-conscious dieters, unfortunately, cycles of dieting make weight loss increasingly more difficult with each round of curtailed eating. This has been found by people who go on "crash diets" for short-term purposes, including wrestlers who seek to lose weight only to get into a lower category in an upcoming meet.

Weight loss entails losing both lean and fat body mass, so weight loss induced by restrained eating alone is not as effective as consummatory restraint coupled with exercise for keeping weight down. With exercise lean body mass is retained while body fat is lost. Long-distance runners who have very little body fat can eat large quantities of food without weight gain. Research has shown that exercise has beneficial effects not only on humans but also on rats. Rats trained to swim or to run for a number of weeks were found to have significantly lower resting levels of blood glucose compared with untrained rats (Tan, Morimoto, Sugiura, Morimoto, & Murakami, 1992), and exercise appears to alter insulin sensitivity to blood glucose.

Restrained eating taps into controversy among researchers with regard to the concept of "set point." Some (Keesey & Powley, 1986; Stunkard, 1982) argue that long-term weight regulation follows a set point, and overeating and short-term weight gain are compensated subsequently by undereating, thus returning animals and humans to their normal (set-point) weight. They contend that only with severe changes in eating patterns or with drugs and hormone changes will a new set point be reached. Other investigators (Harris, 1990; Van Ittalie & Kissileff, 1990) challenge the set-point theory, rejecting the idea that the body has a preset level or point to which weight adjusts. Van Ittalie and Kissileff (1990) emphasize that body energy dynamics modulate weight in line with specific adaptive processes of the individual. For example, in nonhuman animals, those that hibernate have different energy dynamics, reflected in altered metabolism and body fat stores just before (compared with during or after) hibernation. Unresolved issues remain on the question of whether a preset level adjusts weight or metabolism.

Anorexia, Bulimia, and Obesity: Disorders and Disease

Diagnoses that involve deviant weight and eating behavior date back to the early days of psychiatry, with *anorexia nervosa* noted in patients who were hospitalized with severe, even fatal, weight loss. The disorder involves extreme restraint in eating. Although very much below normal in weight, such individuals think of themselves as heavy and fat. A different disorder is known as *bulimia nervosa*. It involves binge eating, in which as many as 20,000 calories can be consumed in a single binge, followed by purging, either through self-induced vomiting or by other means of eliminating the ingested food. Bulimic patients are not likely to have severe and fatal weight loss, but their health can be impaired in many other ways. *Obesity* can severely injure health, due to the strain imposed on the heart and other organs by the individual's excess body weight. Some obese people are also binge eaters (Drewnowski, 1996), but binge eating combined with purging often results in normal weight and normal appearance. Although the three clinical groups differ in outward appearance, researchers have asked whether these groups nevertheless share certain psychological similarities. For example, do these individuals deviate in their sensitivity to stimuli associated with eating? Do they have comparable histories of conditioned flavor experiences?

The liver provides cues relevant to ingestion, and some researchers have hypothesized (Friedman, 1990) that hepatic metabolism of ingested fuels produces unconditioned stimuli that can lead to the conditioning of flavor preferences that involve hedonic as well as aversive conditioning. Questions arose whether the clinical groups differ in such conditioning, or instead, whether they differ in their learning of symbolic and social-cognitive values concerning food, eating, body weight, and body appearance.

Comparisons. Booklets distributed by medical centers give estimates that up to 25% of adolescent females have an eating disorder, and data show that there is a rise in such disorders in males (Maude, Wertheim, Paxton, Gibbons, & Szmukler, 1993). Some individuals with eating disorders do not have aberrant weight or appearance, and many keep their disorders secret even from family members, so that accurate estimates are not readily available. At one time bulimia and anorexia were classified together in a grouping, but contemporary researchers identify bulimic patients as a separate group. Bulimic patients are known to have distinct psychiatric symptoms, such as depression (Hinz & Williamson, 1987), and some have been hospitalized as users of psychoactive drugs (Wilson, 1992). Estimates of frequency of bulimia in the adult population vary, but it is known to be more prevalent in women than in men. Some estimates are that up to 5% of women have this eating disorder (Hinz & Williamson, 1987), and among college-age students the percentage is presumed to be much higher. Anorexia is less frequent than bulimia but similarly occurs more in women than in men and in younger (under age 25) than in older women. Although depression can be found in persons with anorexia, this disorder is more closely linked with denial and with obsessive and compulsive characteristics.

Weight in bulimic individuals may be in the normal range, but anorexic persons may drop weight to as low as 60% of normal, with injurious consequences for growth (stunting, if it occurs in adolescence) and menstruation (amenorrhea, with infrequent and irregular menses). It can lead to infertility and in extreme cases to death. With proper treatment given in time, the various deficiencies can be reversed. The frequency of bulimia and anorexia in young women increased in many countries between the 1930s and the 1980s. Recent evidence, however, shows there may be a decline in eating disorders in the 1990s (Heatherton, Mahamedi, Striepe, Field, & Keel, 1997).

In contrast to the restrained eating disorders, in which individuals severely curtail normal food ingestion, obesity involves excess food ingestion. Body mass index (BMI) has been used as a measure to identify obesity. It is computed by the ratio (in kilograms) of a person's weight over height (in meters, squared), and it correlates well with measures of adiposity such as skinfold thickness (McHugh, 1990). A ratio of 30 would be considered obese, compared with a ratio of 20 in a lean normal-weight person.

Anorexic individuals verbalize that food is distasteful, but bulimic and obese individuals state they crave food. Anorexic and bulimic individuals seek to reduce weight and body size. Cultural, psychodynamic, and genetic factors have been identified as leading to the different types of eating disorders. Beliefs about control as well as beliefs about one's own body weight have been found to play important roles. For example, women who believe themselves to be overweight and who show perfectionism (striving for high standards of being perfect, including perfect body shape and weight) are at risk for developing bulimic symptoms (Joiner, Heatherton, Rudd, & Schmidt, 1997). How parents and children interact in the family also is likely to play a role. Some efforts have been made to observe families and their modes of interaction, in order to identify if the type of disorder is related to family interaction patterns.

In one study (Humphrey, 1989), 74 family triads were observed. Family discussion dealing with the daughter's separation from the family was videotaped, and ratings were made of the interactions between the daughters, average age of 18 years, and their biological parents. The clinical groups consisted of underweight bulimics, normal-weight bulimics, and anorexic subjects. Their family patterns were compared with those of normal nonpatient subjects. The normal subjects' family patterns re-

vealed significantly more mutual support and a higher percentage of approach and helping behavior, and there was more evidence that the family members enjoyed one another. The family pattern of the anorexic subjects revealed on the one hand parental efforts to keep the daughter too dependent on her parents, and on the other hand the parents were nonsupportive of her feelings and her need for self-expression. Nurturing affection, control, and emphasis on "good appearance" were characteristics of families in which the daughter had an anorexic disorder. The bulimic families did not show affection, and much hostility and mutual belittling was evident. Research of this type can lead to improved understanding of the different clinical groups and can help explain why certain individuals in the population develop severely debilitating eating disorders.

Societal processes and not just the immediate family are important factors. Cultural variables have significant effects on eating disorders. For example, in economically wealthy nations anorexia seemed to be more prevalent in the upper socioeconomic classes and obesity more prevalent among the lower classes. In contrast, in economically less well developed nations, obesity was more prevalent among the well-to-do whereas poorer persons tended to be thin to the point of emaciation (McHugh, 1990). The thinness of poor persons is not to be confused with that of anorexic patients, however. Anorexic persons achieve extreme thinness by self-selected purposive restraint in food intake, whereas external pressures (lack of available food or excessively hard labor) determine the excessive thinness in many lower-class persons. The possibility of genetic factors has also been raised, with obesity and anorexia possibly having a genetic predisposition (McHugh, 1990; McHugh, Moran, & Killilea, 1989).

Group Differences in Taste and Eating. Clinical observations have yielded two major findings. One is that taste preference and food consumption are not always highly correlated. The other is that obese and bulimic individuals, who have similar food preferences, have preferences opposite those of anorexic persons. Obese women tend to prefer food that is rich in fat, and anorexic women like sweet tastes but not the oral sensation of foods that are high in fat (Drewnowski, 1991). When bulimic persons in a clinical population go on eating binges, they seem to prefer consuming high-fat foods, whereas anorexic persons find high-fat foods aversive.

Laboratory experiments examined the way individuals in the different groups respond to various cues. Hetherington and Rolls (1989) assessed sensory-specific satiety for five groups of subjects: normal-weight controls who were not on a diet, normal-weight dieters, overweight dieters, normal-weight bulimics, and low-weight anorexics. Subjects came to the laboratory one time after an overnight fast and another time after having their usual breakfast. On both occasions subjects rated feelings of hunger and fullness as well as pleasantness of taste of nine foods. After the ratings they were offered low-fat cottage cheese, with instruction to eat as much as they wished. Following this, subjects again made ratings of hunger and pleasantness of tastes for the same nine foods and they did so repeatedly at various times, up to 60 minutes following the cottage-cheese eating. After that, subjects could eat a variety of high-calorie foods.

As would be expected, anorexic and normal-weight dieters had significantly less food energy intake than the other groups of subjects (see Figure 8.4), both after deprivation and following a normal breakfast. The anorexic subjects rated hunger very low and fullness very high before the test meals, whereas rated hunger was high and fullness low for the other groups. Sensory-specific satiety (of lowered pleasantness ratings for cottage cheese as a result of consuming it, relative to ratings for the uneaten foods) was present for the anorexic and control subjects but not for the bulimic and dieting groups. Thus, significant differences were evident. The bulimic and anorexic clinical groups differed from each other in their evaluations of the palatability of foods and of their hunger/fullness, the anorexics differed markedly from the normal controls in hunger/fullness evaluations, and the bulimics differed markedly from the normal controls in sensory-specific satiety.

One would hypothesize that in a laboratory setting anorexic subjects would take in less food en-

FIGURE 8.4

Total energy (kcal) consumed in both first and second courses after a standard breakfast (no-deprivation condition) or after overnight fasting (deprivation condition). Intakes for the anorexic (anorex), bulimic (bulim), control (norm), normal-weight restrained (nwtr), and overweight restrained (owtr) subjects are shown.

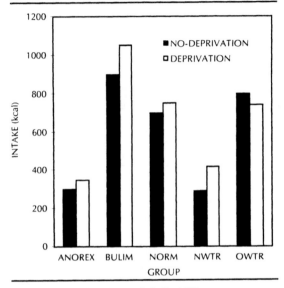

Source: From Hetherington & Rolls, 1989.

ergy than normal control subjects and that obese subjects would take in more. This was found for anorexic subjects but not consistently for obese subjects. In reviewing a number of studies on food intake of obese compared with normal control subjects in a laboratory test, Kissileff (1989) found that sometimes the obese subjects do eat more and at other times they do not. What does occur in laboratory studies of obese subjects is that their response to taste cues is different from that of normal subjects, even though they do not consistently consume more than normal subjects.

Research that compared obese and normal subjects (Hill & Blundell, 1989) had the subjects ingest a glucose solution, and for 60 minutes they repeatedly sampled a sucrose solution which they rated for pleasantness. They also repeatedly rated their hunger levels. Normal control subjects reduced both hunger ratings and pleasantness judgments of sucrose, whereas obese subjects reduced hunger ratings but showed no loss of judged pleasantness of sucrose after ingesting glucose. In a second study, in which obese and normal control subjects ate small lunches, the hunger ratings again decreased for both groups but ratings of pleasantness of food during eating remained high for the obese subjects while they dropped (sensory-specific satiety) for the normal control subjects. Thus, like the bulimic subjects in the Hetherington and Rolls (1989) study, the obese subjects continued to find food highly palatable rather than decreasing in pleasantness as a function of ingestion. Obese and bulimic subjects have marked overeating outside the laboratory, and this may be due to the fact that food continues to taste good to them, regardless of how much they eat. Many studies consistently have found that bulimic subjects do not decrease their judgment of pleasantness for food after finishing a meal, and their judgment of hunger and satiety is colored by their general urge to continue eating.

To assess if the continued pleasantness of food for bulimic persons reflects a general hypersensitivity to external sensory stimulation or is related only to the taste of food, an interesting study (Faris et al., 1992) gave bulimic and normal control subjects tactile stimulation tests. Touch thresholds (to measure how much stimulation is needed before the stimulus is felt) were obtained by using fine fibers in a standardized test for this purpose. The bulimic and normal subjects were found to have comparable thresholds for touch. Pain thresholds also were obtained, by applying pressure to the finger tip until subject indicated first feeling pain (pain detection) and then indicating pain as too uncomfortable (pain tolerance). For pain detection and pain tolerance, bulimic subjects had significantly higher thresholds: more pressure was needed before subjects indicated they felt pain and before they rejected pain as too uncomfortable. This study shows that bulimic subjects are not generally hypersensitive to all types of external stimuli. They have normal sensitivity to neutral stimuli (touch sensation), and they are *less* sensitive to pain from pressure stimulation on their fingers compared with normal subjects. Their higher sensitivity to pleasantness of foods

during the course of a meal is, therefore, not a generalized hypersensitivity. It is possible that bulimic persons have a sensitivity bias toward positive (versus neutral and negative) hedonic stimuli of all kinds, and not only a hypersensitivity for pleasant taste. More research is needed on this topic.

Food can affect an individual's state in many ways. For example, research with infant rats (Blass, Shide, & Weller, 1989) has shown that milk can quiet crying pups and elevate their pain thresholds. Other studies have shown that fat and sucrose also have calming effects to counteract stress. These antinociceptive effects are thought to depend on opioid pathways in the nervous system. Whereas the calming effect of milk, fat, and sucrose are quite long-lasting, tactile calming effects (infant rats touching a conspecific or human infants sucking a pacifier) disappear as soon as the touch contact is removed. One possible reason for people to be hypersensitive to taste could be due to an association acquired from early childhood, when food ingestion calmed the discomforts of stress. Much more research is needed to provide firm answers on issues involving the effects of eating, taste, and hunger signals.

Is There an Ideal Figure and an Ideal Weight?

Dieting in adolescent girls became more frequent and occurred at an increasingly younger age between the 1960s and 1980s. In Europe and North America, dieting in girls under age 15 was on the rise, and overeating in dieters, as compensation, was also increasing, thereby making bulimia more evident.

Cultural and Societal Factors. Underlying the restrained food intake in preteens and in adolescents was the desire to be more attractive, which was defined as being thinner. Dissatisfaction with one's body appearance was involved in this process. A study in England (Hill, Oliver, & Rogers, 1992) explored attitudes of 9-year-old and 14-year-old girls, who were asked if they were on a diet and how satisfied they were with their body shape. The restrained eaters had a significantly greater discrepancy between their ideal and their actual figure, and this was true for the younger as well as older girls. Dissatisfaction with body appearance and body build was high in the restrained eaters, even though almost 50% of the dieters were within normal weight limits for their age. In the 9-year-olds a significant negative correlation was found between dieting and body esteem. The 14-year-old dieters were especially dissatisfied with their hip and thigh sizes. The researchers concluded that adult values regarding the aversiveness of obesity and the attractiveness of thinness are adopted already by children 6 to 9 years of age, and this forebodes dangers regarding the likelihood of young adults acquiring eating disorders. The subjects were from middle-class homes.

In economically developed nations, the inverse relationship between socioeconomic status and obesity became increasingly significant as girls became women. In middle-class families a motivation to avoid being overweight was strong for girls and women. This relationship was not found as clearly for boys, although longitudinal studies, which assessed how college students fared 10 years later, showed that men gained weight after college and therefore became more concerned about dieting after their college years (Heatherton et al., 1997). Binge eating and purging behavior increased in adolescent males in the 1980s (Whitaker et al., 1989), and by the 1990s young males were at increasing risk for eating disorders.

The values set by a society are relevant to the relationship between socioeconomic status and incidence of obesity. Socioeconomic status and obesity are related differently for economically underdeveloped nations than for developed ones (Sobal & Stunkard, 1989). In societies with severe food shortages, "being fat" may come to represent an ideal of beauty, especially for women. Brown and Konner (1987) note that in some societies, adolescent daughters in wealthy families are given special fattening experiences before marriage. "Fat is beautiful" is believed in some cultures today, and it certainly was believed in parts of Europe in past centuries. Portrayal of voluptuous women in the paintings of the 16th- and 17th-century Dutch masters provides ample evidence. Chubby cherubs and sensuously overweight women in paintings of

Rubin and others give a vivid image of the positive regard given to obesity in a different era.

Societal attitudes have changed in modern times in Europe and North America, especially gender specific attitudes. Contemporary beliefs about the ideal body shape are gender specific and differ according to socioeconomic status. Whereas in developed nations a strong inverse relationship exists between socioeconomic status and incidence of obesity in women, that relationship is not found for men. Sobal and Stunkard (1989) reviewed many studies, which show that a shift toward a thinner ideal body shape for women has occurred since 1960. Self-esteem, perceived weight, and body satisfaction tend to differ for boys and men compared with girls and women. Girls and women are far more likely than boys and men to believe they are too heavy. For women in contemporary developed nations "thin is beautiful," and thus women would be likely to underreport their weight on a survey. Data from one study (Smith, Hohlstein, & Atlas, 1992) with 101 women college students supported that prediction. The subjects generally underreported their weight, and this was as true for subjects with normal eating patterns as for persons who had a tendency toward bulimia or anorexia.

Women far more than men in contemporary society believe their build, weight, and appearance are significantly inferior to their ideal. This is already evident in adolescence (Maude et al., 1993). For example, in one study with college students (Zellner, Harner, & Adler, 1989), men showed no significant differences between how they rated their present figure, their ideal figure, or the figure they thought women would find most attractive. In contrast, mean ratings for women differed between their present figure and the figure they considered ideal and that they thought men would prefer. Women's self-critical reactions were not realistic in terms of men's thoughts about attractiveness in women. The men rated as attractive the same figure that women without eating disorders rated themselves presently to be, and this figure the women considered to be heavier than their ideal. Women with eating disorders had more exaggerated reactions, rating their ideal figure significantly thinner than did women without eating disorders.

The data on underreporting of weight (G. T.

Smith et al., 1992) is congruent with the extreme wish for thinness in women. Such underreporting appears to be a way to hide information considered to be socially undesirable. In studying college students, Fallon and Rozin (1985) found results similar to Zellner et al. (1989): (1) Women but not men judge their current appearance as significantly heavier than their ideal figure; (2) womens' perception of what men consider to be the ideal female figure is far thinner than the figure men pick as the ideal. In some studies, women's ideal figure was significantly thinner than women's perception of the men's ideal female figure (Fallon & Rozin, 1985; Zellner et al., 1989), but other studies found no difference between the women's ideal figure and the figure that women thought men considered attractive (Rozin & Fallon, 1988). Rozin and Fallon (1988) assessed to what degree parents and their college student offspring agreed on judgments concerning ideal figures. Judgments could be compared for father and son and mother and daughter. The results showed that both the mothers and daughters showed significant disparity between ideal and actual figures. Also, both generations of women exaggerated men's preference for thinness. The men misjudged women's preference for the ideal male figure, but did so in the opposite way from how the women distorted what men prefer. Whereas women believed that men prefer *thinner women* than the men in fact did prefer, the men distorted female preferences by believing that women like *heavier men* than the women actually did prefer.

Similarities between mothers and daughters, and between fathers and sons, were striking. The women more than the men reported major concerns about weight, and they reported more dieting and eating restraint than did the men. The majority of mothers and daughters said they ate more when depressed, but less than a third of the fathers and sons said they did so. The researchers concluded that gender is a more potent factor than generation in the types of cognitions and emotions people have with regard to weight and body ideal. How the mothers and fathers thought at the time they were of college age was not assessed. Cultural values have deep effects, and societal emphasis on thinness leads people to accept "thin is beautiful."

Different explanations have been proposed for beliefs regarding ideal weight and body shape. For instance, attractiveness for thin figures in women has been explained in evolutionary terms. Women with a low waist/hip ratio were said to be attractive because of the suggestion of youth (Singh, 1991) and fertility, and sociobiological implications were noted for ideal figures in terms of reproduction and continuity of the species (Buss, 1989). A more cognitive perspective is taken by many psychologists, who point to learned values regarding the ideal figure. Most psychologists agree that the cultural concern with thinness leads to dangerous consequences of eating disorders.

Eating Disorders and Their Change. Persons with eating disorders tend to have disturbed cognitions, with more anxiety and lower self-esteem, and they have other disturbed beliefs compared with normal control subjects (e.g., Mayhew & Edelmann, 1989). Gender differences may be decreasing, as shown by data on Australian youths (Maude et al., 1993) that revealed that disturbed cognitions and disorders of eating behavior may be more prevalent in males than previously believed. Beliefs about self-value (self-esteem) can have strong effects on eating behavior in adolescent girls and boys.

Depression is often associated with eating disorders. The best predictor of binge eating in adolescent girls was found in one study to be the exaggeration of one's body size and the intense desire to be thinner (Wertheim et al., 1992). Because eating binges typically include high-fat foods, cognitions about foods also are important with regard to eating and its disorders (Drewnowski, 1991). Moreover, food can lose its incentive value, as already described for experiments with rats (Balleine & Dickinson, 1994; Balleine et al., 1995), which showed that the incentive value of food decreased with the presentation of cholecystokinin (CCK, which induces satiety).

Certain experiences can heighten the incentive value of food and eating and other experiences can decrease these incentive values. In early childhood, experiences with food and eating shape long-term eating patterns (Birch & Fisher, 1996). Eating also may be more disturbed at some times than at others. For example, in some persons with SAD (seasonal affective disturbance) excessive eating occurs in the months of winter darkness but not in other seasons. Even in nonhuman animals, different stressor circumstances lead to different effects on eating. Stress has been found to decrease food consumption and body weight in rats. In one laboratory investigation it was found that different schedules of reinforcement and stressor intensities had contrasting effects, with mild shock overall increasing food consumption and more severe shock in some cases decreasing it (Dess, 1997).

Behavioral treatment for children (e.g., L. H. Epstein & Wing, 1987) and adults (Baell & Wertheim, 1992) and various forms of psychotherapy have had success in treatment of eating disorders, and such success depends on many factors (Brownell & O'Neil, 1993). Large amounts of social support are significant in altering pathological eating patterns, when the support is given by family or friends, weight-control groups (e.g., Weight Watchers, which is international and has groups in many countries), or therapeutic treatment groups (Olmsted et al., 1991; Wertheim, Gaab, Coish, & Weiss, 1989; Wilfley et al., 1993). Social support has been a key factor in helping people make significant changes in their eating patterns and in their resultant overall health.

EFFECTS OF HUNGER, THIRST, AND GLUCOSE ON RESPONDING AND INFORMATION PROCESSING

Satiation tends to lead to lethargy and slow activity, and moderately strong hunger and thirst lead to vigor, persistence, and strength of responding for normal-eating nonhuman animals and humans. This is seen at feeding time in a hospital nursery with newborn infants, which is a noisy time compared with the period soon after the babies have been fed. Parents of a young child in its first few months easily identify the quiescence of a satiated and satisfied infant in contrast to the agitation shown by a hungry child. The energizing aspects of hunger and thirst affect strength of responding, and the *directional* aspects of hunger and thirst affect *selectivity* of responding. Hunger and thirst also affect "sensitivity."

The Directional Effects of Hunger and Thirst

Sensitivity to Cues

Internal Signals Associated with Hunger and Thirst. People can tell when they are very, rather than slightly, hungry or thirsty, and they can distinguish when they are hungry from when they are thirsty. People and nonhuman animals can discriminate between amounts and types of motivation. They show behavior appropriate to the state, such as seeking food when hungry and liquid when thirsty. Kendler (1946) demonstrated this with rats. He trained them when they were both hungry and thirsty over many trials in a T-maze. At the end of one arm the animals found food and at the end of the other arm the animals found water. Later, when the animals were only hungry (and not also thirsty) they made the correct choice of running down the arm that had contained the food, and likewise, when the animals were only thirsty (and not also hungry) they made the correct choice of running down the arm that had contained the water. This directionality, of selecting an action that is appropriate to the internal state, stems from the motivation cues ("drive stimuli") becoming associated with specific responses and with specific rewards or other external stimuli.

Whereas in the Kendler study the training occurred under both food and water deprivation and the appropriate reward was chosen under a single deprivation condition during testing, other studies trained animals under only one type of deprivation but with two kinds of rewards. When under testing the subjects were switched to another type of deprivation (e.g., from thirst to hunger, or hunger to thirst), the animals selected the reward appropriate to their motivation under testing (such as selecting a sucrose solution rather than food pellets when thirsty). Not only was an appropriate choice made, but in these studies the subjects also showed more instrumental responding (more lever pressing) for the appropriate reward (Dickinson & Ballein, 1990; Dickinson & Dawson, 1989).

What internal signals provide the cues for hunger and thirst are not yet fully understood. Stunkard (Griggs & Stunkard, 1964; Stunkard &

Koch, 1964) used a modification of a less valid ear-lier method by Cannon and Washburn (1912) to measure internal hunger signals, and, as already discussed, gastric motility as a peripheral signal provided reliable hunger cues for normal control subjects. In contrast, Malmo and Malmo (1983, 1988) identified central rather than peripheral cues in their study on thirst. They sought to identify the relationship between specific brain cell activity and sensitivity to external stimuli relevant to thirst. These researchers recorded multiple cell fir-ing in the dorsal midbrain and in the lateral preop-tic area of the brain in freely moving animals. In-creased firing was evident following intracarotid hypertonic saline injections or intraventricular an-giotensin II injections. Increased firing also oc-curred when distinctive odors of a solution were presented that in the past had been repeatedly asso-ciated with drinking. Even if the animals had not been deprived of water (were not thirsty), the odor of the external stimulus elicited increased activity in these brain cells, and the odor-induced firing was very much increased when the animals were de-prived of water for two days. This was *selective sensitivity,* because such increased cell firing did not occur when the animals smelled stimuli that in the past had not been previously associated with drinking.

The increased brain activity was not due to the fact that the thirsty animals were generally more ac-tive. Although the amount of brain cell firing tended to increase with head and body movement, when general body activity was not increased, the dorsal midbrain cell firing nevertheless did increase for thirsty animals, and this increase was magnified when the animal encountered specific stimuli that had been associated with water intake. Malmo and Malmo (1988) emphasized that the interaction of internal signals and external cues is important for understanding the directionality of thirst. Thirst as an antecedent *pushes* the animals, and they are *pulled* in the direction of an olfactory stimulus that represents an acceptable source of water. Once the consummatory response is activated (drinking be-gins), oral rather than olfactory sensations become predominant, but prior to the consummatory re-sponse, odors play a dominant role.

Stimuli Have Activating Effects. Stimuli are im-portant for learning (Houston, 1991; Roberts, 1998) and for the way motivation affects behavior. Whereas Malmo and Malmo (1988) showed that environmental stimuli can selectively direct the be-havior of motivated nonhuman animals, stimuli also activate behavior in an energizing fashion. The dynamic or alerting effect of stimuli was noted by Hull (1951), who indicated that the stronger the stimulus was, the more it arouses or alerts, and he called this "stimulus-intensity dynamism." The stronger a neutral stimulus is for becoming a CS (conditioned stimulus), the more it will increase the response strength of the CR (conditioned response), and strength of the US (unconditioned stimulus) produces both more response strength and in-creased learning (associative strength) of the CR (Hovland & Riesen, 1940; Kimble, 1961, pp. 342–345; Spence, 1953, 1956).

Hunger or thirst can interact directionally with external stimuli, as Malmo and Malmo (1988) found, and they can also interact with stimuli non-selectively to increase general activity. Campbell and Sheffield (1953) explained the increase of ac-tivity with hunger on the basis of a general and non-selective heightened sensitivity to stimuli. They proposed that animals are more active when hungry because an increase in motivation leads to a greater sensitivity to environmental stimuli, and it is this sensitivity, not an energizing characteristic of moti-vation, that leads to increased activity. Other re-searchers also tested this "heightened sensitivity" hypothesis, and Hall (1956) concluded that al-though motivation on its own does energize behav-ior (increases response output), environmental stimuli will magnify this effect.

Students of the writer of the present book tested this sensitivity-activation hypothesis in an ingen-ious study (Kocher & Berry, 1982). They used mu-sical selections for the environmental stimulation. Previous studies had shown that nonhuman animals as well as humans were responsive to musical stim-ulation (Bates & Horvath, 1971; Corban & Gou-rnard, 1976; Cross, Halcomb, & Matter, 1967; Lan-dreth & Landreth, 1974; Lundin, 1967). Before data collecting began, a panel of eight judges rated vari-ous musical selections, and the final choices were sedative music (*Nobilissima Visione* by Hindemith) and arousing music (*Miraculous Mandarin Suite, Opus 9* by Bartok). Each musical selection was played via a tape player at 80 db in 2 minute segments. Six adult female Sprague-Dawley rats, whose predeprivation weight ranged from 264 to 343 g (mean of 313 g), were placed on a food-deprivation schedule (with water constantly present). They were maintained at 80% of their predeprivation weight for 21 days. The last 10 days of pretesting the animals received operant conditioning training with continuous reinforcement in a Gerbrands conditioning chamber. By the end of the 10 days the subjects attained about 120 operant bar press responses in 20 minutes, or about 12 bar presses for an average 2-minute segment.

Following the pretesting, in the main experiment the testing occurred without reinforcement and all the subjects were given three different stimulation conditions. They were tested at three different body-weight levels in a counterbalanced within-subjects design. They were tested at levels of 80% (high deprivation level), 90% (medium deprivation level), or 100% (low deprivation level) of their predeprivation weight. At a given body-weight level each animal was exposed to a stimulus sequence consisting of three environmental stimulus conditions, and the sequence was repeated three times. Stimulus conditions were: no music (control condition), sedative music, or arousing music. For the experimental days of testing, on a given day each animal was placed for 1 minute into the operant conditioning box, followed by nine 2-minute testing segments (three repeated sequences of the three stimulus conditions). Each testing day was under a different deprivation (weight-loss) condition. Order of stimulus condition and order of body-weight level were counterbalanced across subjects. For example, subject number 4 on the day of testing at 100% body-weight received the following sequence three times: 2 minutes of sedative music followed by 2 minutes of arousing music followed by 2 minutes of no music. Under 90% and under 80% body weight, different stimulus sequences were presented, and different animals received different combinations of deprivation and stimulus sequences.

The results are presented in Table 8.1. The data show that for high and medium hunger (80% and 90% body weight), *type* of stimulation (sedative versus arousing music) had no effect on activity, with comparable bar pressing for the two types, but *presence of stimulation* had a marked effect, with far more bar pressing under the two music conditions than under the no-music condition. The interaction of musical stimulation and weight loss had a significant effect, seen by the fact that under high hunger the animals had many bar presses under music (compared with no music), but when the animals were minimally hungry (100% body weight), stimulation did not alter activity, a low and similar number of bar presses occurring for the three stimulus conditions. The interaction confirmed the conclusion of other researchers who found activity to be an interactive function of both the external stimulation and the hunger (or thirst) motivation. As expected, the energizing effect of hunger motivation also was evident. The hungrier the subjects were (the more body-weight loss they had) the more bar presses occurred, and this was true for the control

TABLE 8.1
Effect of Environmental Stimulation and Hunger Level on Mean Number of Bar Presses per 2-Minute Sessions

Percentage of normal body weight	Control (no music)	Stimulating music	Sedative music
80%	29.00	37.17	42.67
90%	21.67	31.17	32.33
100%	12.17	13.83	13.83

Source: Data from a study by Kocher and Berry (1982).

condition (no stimulation) as well as for the two conditions of music stimulation.

Thirst and hunger clearly increase generalized reactivity to external stimulation, and that effect may be influenced by additional factors. Animals that have undergone surgical procedures show that preoperative conditions affect postoperative behavior. Schallert (1989) found that the type of deprivation schedule given to preoperative animals affects the way animals later orient to sensory stimulation. Restricted food or water intake normally makes animals more reactive to sensory stimulation in general, and Schallert (1989) found that in addition to generalized sensitivity, the thirsty animals in his research were especially reactive to stimuli that were water associated. Rats exposed to an intermittent schedule of water deprivation oriented persistently to the drinking spout and even followed the spout as it was pulled from the home cage. However, this reactivity to external stimuli occurred only when the animals had received deprivation intermittently. When the animals preoperatively did not have intermittent deprivation schedules but only fasting or water deprivation, they did not show the hypersensitivity, presumably because without intermittent deprivation they had not attended to the differential cues provided by the different deprivation states.

The Interactive Effects of Hunger and Food

Deprivation and Desirability of Food. The attractiveness of food can be altered according to how hungry the nonhuman animal or human is. With increasing food deprivation, a nonhuman animal or human gains increased sensory pleasures (from taste, smell, texture, or appearance) from the food as long as there is no prior negative experience with the food (Heatherington & Rolls, 1996). When one is hungry food is desirable early in the eating process, and it becomes less desirable later when one is more satiated (Booth, 1989). Several neurochemical processes have been found to mediate this relationship (Hoebel, Hernandez, Schwartz, Mark, & Hunter, 1989). An application of this principle is that if one does not want to buy a lot of food items in a grocery store, a good precaution is to go shopping when one is well fed (satiated) rather than hun-

gry. The hungry shopper is likely to find many foods appealing and thus is likely to buy a lot more food items than one would buy if not hungry.

Studies of *contrast effect* reveal that food deprivation increases sensitivity regarding the desirability of food. Brazier (1996) used a reward-shift procedure similar to one used by Crespi (1942). This is a procedure often used to assess the interactive effects of deprivation and food magnitude, and in this the animals are first trained under one reward magnitude and then tested under a different magnitude. Brazier (1996) used lick rate to study whether animals that were shifted from a low to a high sucrose concentration showed a positive contrast effect (PCE) of more licking than unshifted subjects receiving only the high concentration. She also assessed negative contrast effect (NCE), of lesser licking in animals shifted from a high to a low sucrose concentration, compared with nonshift animals receiving only the low concentration. Deprived rats received only limited feeding in their home cage, which gave them 90% body weight at time of testing, while nondeprived subjects were given ad lib food in their home cage. On test days, some nonshift control subjects in each condition were given 4% sucrose solution, some nonshift control subjects were given 32% sucrose solution, and the experimental subjects were shifted between the high or low sucrose solutions every 2 days. Experimental subjects received five upshifts (from low to high) and five downshifts (from high to low), starting with the high 32% sucrose solution. Total number of licks and time spent at the drinking tube within the 5-minute test sessions were recorded on each of 22 test days.

Several results occurred. Predictably, the deprived animals (controls and experimental) gave more licks than did the nondeprived. There was more overall licking of the 32% than the 4% sucrose solutions by nondeprived as well as deprived unshifted subjects, and the difference in licks between the 4% and 32% sucrose solutions was much larger for the deprived than for the nondeprived unshifted subjects. These findings, of more licking under high than low motivation, of more licking of high than low sucrose concentration, and of a greater difference in licking between high and low sucrose concentration for the hungry compared with nonhungry control subjects, show the predicted effects of hunger and food. However, it is the contrast effect for the experimental subjects that provides strong support for the fact that under hunger the animals are more sensitive to the desirability of food.

Both the nondeprived and deprived experimental subjects showed NCE, of markedly decreased licking after downshifts from 32% to 4%. That is, nondeprived and deprived downshifted experimental animals gave far lower numbers of licks than the control animals run nonshifted under the 4% sucrose solution. Crespi (1942) had called this excessive low responding, when animals are shifted from receiving something more positive to something less positive, a "depression effect" to indicate what he assumed was a negative emotional reaction like disappointment or depression. Contemporary researchers use a less emotionally loaded term and call it a "negative contrast effect." The NCE, nevertheless, is assumed to reflect hedonic value. The NCE in the study by Brazier was evident for both the deprived and nondeprived subjects, revealing the undesirability of low compared with high sucrose concentrations.

The data for PCE, however, were different for the deprived than for the nondeprived subjects. Just as Crespi called NCE a "depression" effect, he called PCE an "elation" effect, implying a positive emotional reaction when an animal receives something more positive after something less positive. Brazier found the PCE only for the deprived animals and *not* for the nondeprived animals. As seen in Figure 8.5, deprivation was significant for PCE but not for NCE. This points to the high sucrose concentration being more desirable for the hungry subjects. Studies of learned flavor preferences involving saccharin and sucrose (Capaldi, Owens, & Palmer, 1994) showed that deprivation enhances the reinforcing value of sweetness because of its caloric content. Had calories alone led to increased licking for the 32% versus the 4% solution in the experimental deprived subjects, the experimental animals on the upshift days would have licked the same amount as the nonshift high control subjects. The upshifted and nonshifted deprived subjects would have reduced hunger equally by licking the

high sucrose solution, and no PCE would have been found. The fact that the deprived experimental subjects licked *more* than the nonshift high controls on upshift days (they demonstrated PCE), and the fact that the nondeprived experimental subjects did not show PCE, points to hunger increasing the desirability of food at high concentration.

Interaction of Hunger and Food Activates Instrumental Responding.   Not only is a larger amount of food concentration more appealing when one is hungry, but does it also activate (energize) performance more when one is hungry? Many studies have shown that hunger or thirst, compared with a nondeprived state, lead to increased instrumental responding, and also that when rewards (also known as positive reinforcements) are large, more response output occurs than when rewards are small (Osborne, 1978; Pubols, 1960; Zeaman, 1949). In animal studies, *large rewards lead to increased performance* in terms of more bar pressing, faster running, and shorter response latency than do small rewards. This is generally known as the "reward magnitude" effect.

Since hunger and food magnitude each increases performance, does increased hunger lead to a heightened impact from a larger food reward? To answer this, Ehrenfreund (1971) measured rats' running speed in the center of a straight runway. If increased hunger makes animals more responsive to a large reward, then very hungry animals given six pellets (at the goal area in the end of the runway) should run a lot faster than very hungry animals given one pellet, whereas the less hungry animals should not have as big a difference in running speed as a function of reward magnitude. Ehrenfreund (1971) did a shift study similar to the one of Brazier (1996), only he assessed the interactive effect of hunger and food on *instrumental responding* whereas Brazier's study used *consummatory responding*. Ehrenfreund (1971) found hunger and reward magnitude interacted more after the shift than before the shift.

As seen in Figure 8.6, before the shift the more hungry subjects (85% body weight) ran faster than the less hungry subjects (98% body weight), and those with the large reward (six pellets) ran faster than those with the small reward (one pellet). Each

FIGURE 8.5
Deprived (a) and nondeprived (b) subjects and reward shifts. Mean number of licks as a function of sucrose concentration in subjects shifted every 2 days between a high-sucrose (32%) and a low-sucrose (4%) solution (AD and AN), and in unshifted subjects (4D and 4N, and 32D and 32N) during Phase 1. (Deprived is D, nondeprived is N.)

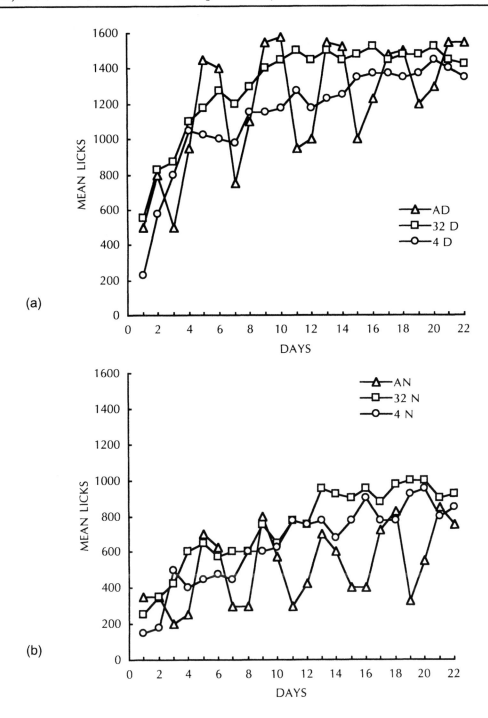

Source: From Brazier, 1996.

FIGURE 8.6

The effect of deprivation-induced drive (hunger) and magnitude of reward (food) on running speed scores over the middle 2 ft of the alley before reward shift (*top*) and after reward shift (*bottom*). The preshift scores (*top*) are for the four main groups, and the postshift scores (*bottom*) are presented separately for the two high-drive (*left panel*) and the two low-drive (*right panel*) groups. Note the way drive and reward magnitude interact, and the Crespi-type "depression" effect in the high-drive group shifted from high to low reward magnitude, in the post incentive-shift speed scores.

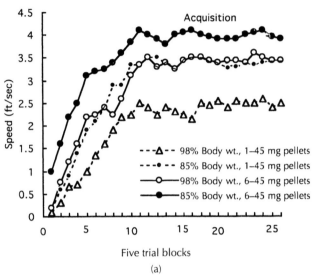

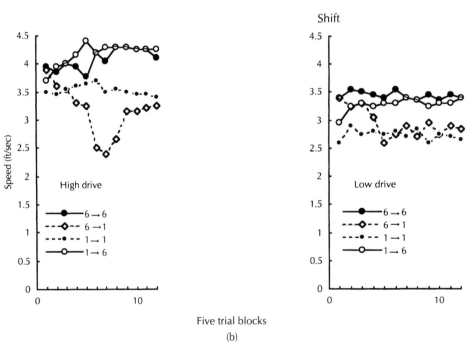

Source: After Ehrenfreund, 1971.

variable, motivation and reward magnitude, had a significant effect on running speed scores over the middle 2 feet of a straight alley. The two variables had an additive effect in the preshift running speed, but motivation and reward magnitude had an interactive effect in the postshift running-speed data. After the shift, the high hunger groups showed a small positive contrast effect (PCE) and a very large negative contrast effect (NCE) in running speed, with less effects in the low hunger groups. The instrumental response data of Ehrenfreund (1971) reveal in part what Brazier (1996) found with consummatory responses. Unlike PCE, the NCE data of Ehrenfreund were somewhat different from those of Brazier. Variation in results of contrast effects have been found in different studies in part because of the complexity involved in this type of investigation. Issues involved in contrast effect and shift studies have been ably discussed elsewhere (Dachowski & Flaherty, 1991).

Information Processing and Learning in Nonhuman Animals

The studies reviewed so far show effects of deprivation on sensitivity to external cues and they show complex interactive effects between deprivation and rewards on both consummatory and instrumental responses. Another type of study shows that the interactive effects involving motivation can also affect *information processing* and hence *learning.* Water-deprived and nondeprived rats received inescapable foot shocks in a series of studies (Maren, DeCola, Swain, Fanselow, & Thompson, 1994). Amount of immobility in body movements elicited by fear (freezing) was measured. The animals were given either one or three presentations of foot shock in a chamber, then returned to their home cages and given free access to water. One day later they were returned to the chamber in which foot shock had been given, and the amount of freezing was recorded. Overall, three foot shocks, compared with one, led to significantly more freezing. The amount of freezing was comparable for the deprived and nondeprived animals given three foot shocks, but for those given one foot shock, the

water-deprived animals had significantly more freezing than did the nondeprived animals.

Fear was conditioned in the present experiment by the association of the chamber and the shock, and the researchers explained the results to mean that thirsty animals require fewer aversive experiences to learn to associate the footshock with the contextual cues of the chamber. In one study of this series the researchers used EEG recordings and found that the thirsty animals had significantly more hippocampal theta waves in a narrow frequency band of 4.0 to 7.9 Hz, which the researchers considered to be related to contextual information sensitivity. They suggested that thirst increases hippocampal information processing, and this helped facilitate encoding of the contextual cues of the chamber. Thirst and hunger had been shown to affect hippocampal activity also by other investigators, and the researchers proposed that thirst increases information processing of contextual cues in a wide range of circumstances besides the present experiments.

Human Information Processing

Early Studies: The "New Look." A large literature on the "New Look in Perception" in the 1940s and 1950s sought to demonstrate that motivational or emotional states have a selective effect on people's information intake. This predated the 1980s and later "mood congruent" studies. Many of the early researchers hypothesized that motivation and emotion bias the individual's perception such that hungry, thirsty, or angry subjects would be selectively sensitive to stimuli relevant to a specific motivation or emotion. The New Look studies attempted to examine perception and intake of information, but methodological difficulties undermined the conclusions. Their work has been described in several reviews (e.g., Saugstad, 1966).

The New Look researchers studied the need for achievement (McClelland & Liberman, 1949) and also emotions (see a review by Jenkin, 1957), as well as hunger and thirst. Although the studies sought to evaluate how hunger and thirst alter subjects' *information intake* (*perception* of stimuli), the methods often used *response production*, like projection or response generation. This led later researchers to conclude that motivation does not alter perception, or in the language of signal detection, that motivation does not alter d' (sensitivity to stimuli as signals) but alters only response bias, which in the language of signal detection is beta, the measure of response criterion.

For example, a study by McClelland and Atkinson (1948) used *projection, not perception.* Young Navy men who were deprived of food for 1, 4, or 16 hours looked at a blank screen or at a screen with smudges. The experimenters, pretending that actual pictures were being shown that were hard to perceive, had the subjects tell what items were being shown, and the number of food responses were tallied. As expected, the 16-hour deprived subjects gave significantly more food responses than the 1-hour deprived subjects (although not significantly more than the 4-hour deprived subjects). A study by Postman and Crutchfield (1952) used *response generation,* in which college student subjects were given a preliminary task for inducing a food-relevant set. In contemporary cognitive psychology that would be called a "priming" task (Houston, 1991), with food words being primed so as to be more accessible. The subjects were given zero, one, two, three, or five skeleton words, with letters missing from actual words, for subjects to fill in to make into food words. Then subjects received the test of other skeleton words that had a high, medium, or low probability of being completed to make food words, and the number of food words actually produced was the dependent variable. Subjects were classified into three food-deprived groups according to when they last ate (0–1 hour, 2–3 hours, and 4–6 hours). The researchers found an interaction between hunger and other variables, but not a significant main effect for hunger.

The above studies showed that food deprivation has some effect on response production, but they did not provide data to show in what way hunger motivation affects perception (information intake). Other studies did collect data to show how hunger alters perception, and some predicted an overall energizing effect (Taylor, 1956) and others predicted a selective effect (Wispé & Drambarean, 1953). Neither prediction was clearly supported. The stud-

ies used a tachistoscopic procedure to establish perceptual thresholds, with a high threshold indicating that the stimulus is not readily perceived (a low threshold indicating the stimulus is readily perceived).

A tachistoscope presents stimuli very briefly, and researchers found a subjects' perceptual threshold by varying, for example, the duration or the brightness of the presented stimulus. Stimuli may be pictures (Lazarus, Yousem, & Arenberg, 1963) or words (Wispé & Drambarean, 1953). Many methodological problems arose with these studies. For example, Gilchrist and Nesberg (1952) presented pictures of food items at a prescribed illumination, and after the stimulus presentation the stimulus was turned off and the subjects had to adjust the new illumination level (set above or below the prior level) to match the brightness of the presented stimulus. In this case, *memory* of *brightness* was measured, not actual perception of the pictures. Other problems were lack of control over what stimuli were used and what categories were used. Whether the stimuli are good exemplars of a category is very important (Oden, 1977). A test of the selective effect of hunger on perception of food-relevant versus non-food-relevant stimuli requires a comparable size of category and comparable exemplar status for the two types of stimuli. If food words are exemplars of a food category (like "bread") and nonfood words are simply random words that do not belong to a prescribed category, stimulus identification will be biased. Wispé and Drambarean (1953) believed their findings confirmed the selective effect of hunger and that the motivation-relevant words were more readily perceived (lower thresholds for correct naming), but the nonequivalence of the word categories and of the exemplar status of the words prevents this conclusion. The overall conclusion from studies in the 1940s and 1950s is that hunger and thirst did *not* lead to differential or selective perception of motivation-relevant stimuli, and hunger and thirst did *not* lead to a general energizing effect, of overall improved stimulus perception.

Recent Studies. The threshold procedure used to assess the effect of motivation or emotion on perception required that the stimulus be presented repeatedly. If a stimulus is presented initially at too dim a level for recognition, and the threshold is determined by repeating the stimulus at increasingly brighter levels until the subject can correctly identify the stimulus, not only is brightness altered but the stimulus itself is shown repeatedly. The same is true for obtaining a duration threshold in which the stimulus is presented at increasingly longer durations until it is correctly identified. Studies have shown that mere repetition of a brief stimulus tachistoscopically, without change in brightness or duration, increases the likelihood that the stimulus will be correctly identified (Haber, 1967; Standing, Haber, Cataldo, & Sales, 1969). Increase of brightness or duration was a confounding factor in the earlier studies, and a more sensitive measure of information intake was required.

In the procedure devised by Erwin (Erwin & Ferguson, 1979) and employed by the present writer in a series of studies (Ferguson, 1983b, 1988, 1989b), words were presented very briefly and repeatedly without any change of duration or brightness until they were correctly identified. The dependent measure was not a threshold but the number of presentations or trials that were required for correct word naming. This procedure, called "information purchasing" (Ferguson, 1992a, 1993a), required the subject to "purchase" more information (another stimulus exposure) for correct word naming. No new word was shown until the previous one was correctly identified. Studies using this procedure presented words of different emotional and motivational content to college student volunteers. In the first study of the series (Erwin & Ferguson, 1979), before testing the subjects were told either to abstain from food for 12 hours (hungry) or from water for 12 hours (thirsty), or to eat a big meal within the hour prior to testing (food satiated) or to drink a lot of water within the hour prior to testing (water satiated). Two additional groups of control subjects received no eating or drinking instructions and they entered the laboratory with whatever level of hunger and thirst they ordinarily would have for an experimental session. Five of the groups worked on mazes in the hour before the experiment. The four motivation-instructed groups did so in the belief that the study concerned the way hunger (or thirst, or satiation, depending on the condition to which the sub-

ject had been assigned) affected maze performance. The one control group believed the study concerned maze performance (but not that it related to hunger or thirst). The subjects of these five groups brought their mazes to the laboratory and only at the end of the study, during debriefing, realized this was a decoy procedure. The sixth group was a pure control group, and had no previous involvement, the subjects coming to the experiment in the usual fashion of studies in psychology.

If the selective (directional) effect of motivation altered perception in terms of decreasing the amount of information needed for motivation-relevant words, then hungry subjects should recognize the eating words soonest (requiring fewer stimulus presentations) and thirsty subjects should recognize the drinking words soonest. This did not happen. On the other hand, if the energizing effect of motivation altered perception in terms of decreasing the amount of overall information needed for correct word naming, then all categories of words would be recognized sooner by the hungry and thirsty subjects compared with the control and satiated subjects. This *did* happen. Table 8.2 provides the data for amount of motivation and word categories, and Table 8.3 provides the data for type of motivation and type of category.

As seen in Table 8.2, the fact that the deprived subjects required fewer trials (less information) to correctly recognize the words than did the control subjects, and the control subjects took fewer trials than the satiated subjects, reveals the energizing effect of motivation. Moreover, the fact that both the food- and water-deprived subjects (hungry and thirsty) recognized the drinking-relevant words sooner than the eating-relevant words, and that the same was true for the satiated subjects (food satiated and water satiated), as seen in Table 8.3, means that the selective hypothesis was not supported at all. Instead of a selective motivational effect, a significant category effect was found, with neutral words recognized more readily than drinking-relevant words and the eating-relevant words being the least readily recognized stimuli. Analysis of the types of words used gave evidence of how important category breadth is and how important the exemplar status of the words is. The neutral words were animals (cat, cow, hen, dog, and fox). They

TABLE 8.2
Effect of Motivation and Word Category on Mean Number of Trials Required for Correct Word Naming

| | Word category | | |
Amount of motivation	Food	Water	Neutral
Deprivation	12.00	8.03	5.03
Control	16.82	13.53	8.55
Satiation	19.18	17.90	13.52

Source: Data from Erwin and Ferguson (1979).

TABLE 8.3
Mean Number of Trials Needed for Correct Word Recognition as a Function of Type of Motivation and Type of Words

| | Word category | | |
Motivation type	Food	Water	Neutral
Deprivation			
Food	8.97	5.87	4.73
Water	15.03	10.20	5.33
Satiation			
Food	17.97	16.07	12.30
Water	20.40	19.73	14.73

Source: Data from Erwin and Ferguson (1979).

belonged to a more clear-cut category than did the words of the other categories, and they were the most readily recognized. The food-eating words (ate, egg, fig, eat, and fed) and the water-drinking words (wet, cup, tea, sea, and icy) represented more fuzzy categories and the words were not as potent exemplars of their categories.

To control for these factors, additional studies were conducted with clear-cut categories and well-defined exemplars. The same kind of results occurred. One study (Ferguson, 1983b) tested hungry and satiated subjects with food words (bun, yam, pie, oat, cob, and sip), negatively emotional words (hag, flu, pus, foe, sin, and rot), and neutral animal words (elk, emu, pup, fox, cow, and doe). The words of the three categories were matched on the basis of associative variables known to affect word learning and tachistoscopic recognition. These vari-

ables were word frequency (Thorndike & Lorge, 1944) and a measure of associativeness in interletter contiguities, called "Generated Value" (Underwood & Schulz, 1960). The results of the study showed that, in interaction with these associative variables, hungry subjects recognized words sooner than did satiated subjects. Due to the study using different words than used in the prior study (Erwin & Ferguson, 1979), food words and not animal words were recognized soonest. Figure 8.7 presents the findings, which show that hunger motivation had an energizing effect in facilitating word recognition. Another study in that investigation (Ferguson, 1983b) tested subjects according to their anxiety without regard to hunger or satiation. Highly anxious persons were compared with persons with low anxiety. Word categories had a significant effect for these subjects in the same way they had for

FIGURE 8.7

Mean number of presentations to first correct word recognition for each level of interletter associativeness. (GV is generated value—see text.)

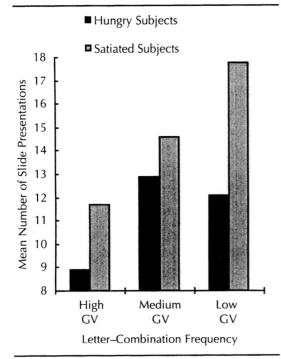

Source: From Ferguson, 1983b, p. 261.

the subjects who had the food manipulation (hungry or satiated), with food words recognized soonest and negative emotional words recognized the slowest. The same significant word-category effect occurred in the two separate studies, one with anxiety and the other with hunger, which shows that one must be careful in interpreting significant word-category effects. Without knowing that anxious subjects also recognized the food words soonest, one would be likely to draw the *wrong* conclusion, that the earlier food-word recognition by hungry and satiated subjects reflects motivation-relevance, with hungry and satiated persons being more preoccupied with food and therefore able to recognize the food words soonest.

Although sensitivity was not selective for the motivation-relevant words, the *energizing* effect of hunger yielded perceptual sensitivity. Later studies

with different words (e.g., Ferguson, 1988) confirmed that hunger can heighten general sensitivity but does not lead to selective sensitivity. Other types of studies assessing the relationship between food deprivation and food-word processing, using different techniques (M. W. Green, Elliman, & Rogers, 1996), found category of word to have a significant effect and that persons with a high rating of hunger did not have differential responses to food words compared with neutral words.

Several conclusions emerge from studies with nonhuman animals and humans under hunger and thirst motivation. One is that subjects have higher response output (Ferguson, 1982), and they also show more exploratory behavior (Bolles, 1975). Hunger and thirst also have a selective *response-generating* effect, as evident from some of the early New Look studies and from later studies (e.g., Schallert, 1989). Hungry human subjects are more likely to think about or to emit eating-related responses, and hungry or thirsty animals are likely to make selective responses to food or liquid according to which motivation the animal is experiencing. Hunger and thirst motivation do not seem to have a selective *perception* effect; rather, these two motivations increase overall sensitivity to external stimuli. They have an energizing effect on intake and processing of information. What mechanisms are responsible for this heightened sensitivity is not yet clear. A number of physiological explanations are likely to be involved. One, hippocampal long-term potentiation, was identified in the study of water-deprived rats given foot shock (Maren, et al., 1994). From an adaptive point of view, it is an advantage for hungry or thirsty humans or nonhuman animals to take in and process environmental information, because such intake and processing would increase the likelihood of finding food or water that leads to consummatory responding.

Effects of Sweets and Hunger on Measures of Memory

Sugar Can Enhance Memory Performance

Gold and colleagues (Gold & Stone, 1988; Lee, Graham, & Gold, 1988; Manning, Parsons, Cotter,

& Gold, 1997; Ragozzino, Unick, & Gold, 1996; Stone, Rudd, & Gold, 1990, 1992) have assessed if sugar can enhance memory performance of nonhuman animals and of humans. Their focus has been on the aging process. As nonhuman animals and humans age, they experience memory losses, with some memory processes declining more than others. Gold (1991) reported that high blood glucose increase after glucose ingestion shows poor glucose control, and in older individuals (rats and humans) this is correlated with poor memory scores. The researchers consistently found with older individuals that glucose administered by ingestion or injection enhances memory performance, and they sought to identify which brain sites are most crucially involved (Parsons & Gold, 1992; Stone et al., 1992).

A different approach from that of Gold and colleagues was used by White (1991, 1996). In a variety of learning tasks with rats, White found that glucose and fructose enhance memory. The major effect is from glucose, and it facilitates memory for young as well as older animals. This facilitating effect may be mediated through the liver, with the liver sending signals to the brain by means of the autonomic nervous system. Possible brain sites affected by the memory-enhancing effect of glucose are certain hypothalamic cells and the caudate nucleus (White, 1991). Additional brain areas have been identified by Gold and colleagues (Ragozzino et al., 1996) in the septohippocampal system. Research with rats (Ragozzino et al., 1996) showed that anticipation of a liquid reward enhanced hippocampal release of acetylcholine (ACh), and the researchers found in different studies that injection of glucose during behavioral testing increases ACh output in the hippocampal formation. Glucose did not alter ACh release in animals kept in their home cages, which suggests that glucose augments ACh output only when cholinergic neurons are activated. The glucose enhancement of memory and the ACh release both had their effects in an inverted-U dose-response manner (low and high doses did not have the noted effects but medium doses did).

Over many studies involving verbal memory in humans and various types of instrumental activity and avoidance conditioning in animals, Gold and

colleagues found that older animals and humans show sleep impairment and memory performance losses, both of which can be reversed with glucose intake (Arankowsky, Stone, & Gold, 1992). In young animals the glucose intake (ingestion in humans, injection in nonhuman animals) does not improve sleep and may not improve memory performance, but glucose does improve sleep and memory in individuals with impairment of sleep and memory (amnesic animals, humans with senile memory losses, and Alzheimer patients). The possible reasons for this are still being explored. Various neurotransmitters appear to mediate the loss and the improvement with glucose. Because recognition memory in normal aging decreases less markedly than does recall memory, the emphasis in aging studies is on storage and retrieval processes in memory. It is thought that the brain may lose its capacity for normal glucose uptake in old age, thus leading to sleep and memory performance losses. Glucose given exogenously appears to improve certain aspects of memory performance, activity level, and sleep.

Gold and colleagues tested a wide range of possible interactive neurochemicals (morphine, norepinephrine, and amphetamine), which have varying effects on young and old animals. These neurochemicals affected memory and, though the researchers did not implicate it, also have a potential impact on arousal. The memory enhancement of epinephrine appears to be mediated by glucose (Gold, 1991). Increased epinephrine level is complexly associated with arousal, so it is possible (although not discussed by the glucose researchers) that the relationship between arousal and memory enhancement involves glucose. Arousal may stimulate release of endogenous glucose, and exogenous intake of glucose may also increase arousal. In aging there is a loss in arousal as well as a loss in sleep and memory performance, thus an increase in arousal from various sources could improve sleep and memory performance in ways that at least partly are similar to the improvements with glucose ingestion. In addition to the glucose-induced changes that occur in animals of all ages (such as hippocampal ACh release), some glucose-induced improvements in memory storage and retrieval are likely to be related to increased arousal and activity level.

Event-related Brain Potentials and Memory Performance

The effects of satiation and hunger on nonhuman animal learning has been the subject of a great deal of behavioral research, yet relatively little is known about what physiological processes are associated with these effects. Moreover, the effects of satiation and hunger on memory performance in human subjects have received only minimal empirical investigation. Studies by Geisler and Polich (1992) are relevant to these issues.

The P300 or P3 event-related brain potential (ERP) is sensitive to metabolic conditions, and P3 latency refers to a highly specific parietal lobe brain potential change following target stimulus presentation. If glucose levels are drastically reduced, for example through increases in insulin level, the P3 latency is lengthened. Glucose changes also have been found to alter ERPs in other specific areas of the brain. Relationships between P3 activity and memory performance were found by a number of researchers (e.g., Ladish & Polich, 1989). Several researchers found the P3 amplitude to be larger and the latency shorter for good versus poor memory performance.

In the first of two studies by Geisler and Polich (1992), subjects who had eaten within 3 hours of testing were compared with others who had not eaten for at least 6 hours. Data showed a significantly larger P3 amplitude for the low hunger subjects, but no significant P3 latency differences were obtained. In the second study, all subjects refrained from eating for at least 15 hours. The ERP measures were taken before lunch, immediately after lunch, and again after another 30 minutes following the postlunch measures. Three different word lists were used for the memory performance measures. For each test the subjects had to write down as many words as possible immediately after 20 words of a list were orally presented one at a time by the experimenter. Subjects' glucose levels, temperature, and heart rate also were measured.

Although overall memory performance did not differ for the three test sessions, specific word positions showed significant effects. Recall of the last block of items is on the basis of short-term memory (STM) and recall on the early word blocks represents long-term memory (LTM). Performance on the early word blocks decreased in the postlunch testings and recall performance on the last word block rose, thus LTM recall suffered and STM recall improved as a result of subjects' eating lunch.

Following food consumption, the P3 amplitude increased significantly from before lunch to both of the after-lunch sessions, and the two after-lunch sessions showed similar P3 amplitudes. Other brain sites also showed increased amplitude of ERPs after lunch. P3 latency effects were not as strong as the amplitude changes found as a function of eating. Glucose levels and heart rate increased significantly, with a steady rise across the three testing sessions, but body temperature showed no marked changes. Because the change in the STM recall across all three sessions was very similar to the P3 amplitude change across the three sessions, the researchers suggested that a rise in generalized arousal affected both the P3 and the STM recall in a comparable fashion. The continued rise in heart rate and glucose levels following lunch contrasted with the STM and P3 amplitude leveling off between the two postlunch measures so that more than one process took place. These data bear on the findings of Gold and colleagues. Eating lunch in the Geisler and Polich study significantly increased the blood glucose levels of the subjects, STM memory performance, and P3 amplitude. These subjects were young graduate students and not older persons with memory losses. A gain in memory performance due to food consumption, presumably due to the rise in blood glucose levels, reveals a sensitive effect from sugar on memory. Geisler and Polich attribute the gain in memory performance to a rise in arousal, with the heart rate measure providing an independent basis for this conjecture.

The above findings provide a paradox. On the one hand, Ferguson and colleagues (Erwin & Ferguson, 1979; Ferguson, 1983b) found *hunger* to facilitate information intake, yet studies on the memory enhancement of glucose and studies by Geisler and Polich (1992) show that memory performance is better right after eating than when subjects are hungry. Possibly different types of arousal are involved, and each may have different effects, depending on the nature of the task and the performance being measured. The Ferguson studies involve encoding of new information as well as LTM, of word codes being retrieved from long-term lexical memory. Clearly, further studies are needed to relate the effects of hunger and glucose to memory performance for various kinds of tasks.

Task demands have been found to be relevant in some glucose studies. For example, on verbal performance in which young and older persons did not differ significantly, glucose administration did not facilitate the performance of the older persons, yet for recall, in which young and older subjects did differ, glucose improved memory performance of the older but not the younger persons (Manning et al., 1997). It is reasonable to assume that both hunger and glucose level alter information processing and memory, yet hunger and glucose level are likely to have different effects for different task demands. Geisler and Polich (1992) obtained a significant LTM-STM by glucose interaction, with STM performance rising and LTM performance dropping after lunch when blood glucose levels rose. The extent to which task performance involves STM versus LTM may be important in comparing effects of glucose and hunger. Different sources of arousal are likely to facilitate performance in distinctive ways. In reviewing how motivation affects hippocampus long-term potentiation, Maren and colleagues (1994) concluded that a variety of motivational states, including fear, lead to specific changes in hippocampus activity. These researchers noted that emotional reactions involved in fear conditioning also depend on the amygdala, and these two brain areas have different effects on contextual cue learning and discrete cue learning. Other researchers also found these two brain areas to have different effects on learning. Instead of water deprivation and fear, the study by McDonald and White (1995) involved discriminations regarding food and no food. The results showed that under some task conditions the learning was hippocampus based and

under other task conditions the learning was amygdala based. Future research may find similar differences in the interaction of arousal and task demands when studies compare hunger as a source of arousal, and glucose as a source of arousal.

SUMMARY

Thirst and drinking have characteristics also found for hunger and eating. Consummatory responses of eating and drinking can occur without hunger or thirst motivation. Hunger and thirst are "primary" motivations that help keep the organism alive. For hunger and eating and thirst and drinking, specific brain areas and peripheral sites are crucial. For both eating and drinking, taste plays a significant role.

Neural circuitry and hormonal factors provide ways for the individual to regain homeostatic balance after food or water deprivation and after food or water are used for bodily functions (metabolism).

Learning plays a large role in the way hunger and thirst are modified by the environment and in the kinds of behaviors the individual displays when hungry or thirsty. Homeostasis refers to the equilibrium that living organisms seek in order to keep constancy in their internal environment relative to changes in the external environment. Negative feedback mechanisms maintain the stability of the internal environment. Feedforward systems, represented by learning to anticipate internal changes, permit negative feedback mechanisms to occur *before* homeostatic perturbations. A feedforward system involved in eating is illustrated by the interaction between glucose and insulin.

Previously held assumptions about simple hunger and satiety centers controlling eating onset and offset are no longer tenable. The belief that the body has a simple set-point for weight, to which short-term eating behavior adjusts, also has been challenged. Many kinds of processes are involved in both short-term and long-term energy regulation. The hypothalamus is crucial for food and water consumption, and additional brain areas as well as peripheral sites outside the central nervous system play significant roles in onset and offset of hunger and thirst motivations.

Emphasis is increasingly directed toward understanding the interaction between peripheral and central processes, and on identifying the complexities underlying both short-term and long-term energy regulation at many levels, ranging from the behavioral to the anatomical to the molecular. Action of the liver and of peptides in the gut and brain are important for onset and offset of eating. Cholecystokinin and neuropeptide Y have been found to play significant roles.

Water is needed by cells, and cellular and extracellular dehydration are identified as sources of thirst. Osmoreceptors respond to cellular dehydration. Vasopressin secretion leads to retention of water by the kidneys. Loss of blood volume (hypovolemia) leads to extracellular dehydration and release of renin by the kidneys. The action of angiotensin II leads to drinking and is important in hypovolemic thirst.

Hunger and thirst function within constraints of the circadian rhythm for the sleep-wake cycle, with more eating and drinking taking place during the "awake" hours. During the individual's normal waking time, length of deprivation is linearly related to the strength of the consummatory response. The longer the time of deprivation of food or water, the larger is the amount eaten or drunk.

Culture shapes what, how, and when we eat, as well as values and beliefs regarding food, body weight, and desirable body characteristics. Some of these values and beliefs relate to religions and to gender.

Culture as well as individual learning experiences lead to taste aversions and taste preferences. Garcia showed how bait shyness can be learned in nonhuman animals through methods that are similar to, yet different from, Pavlovian fear conditioning. Rozin showed that learned aversions differ if the distastes are learned by experiences with nausea rather than with danger. Aversion learned with nausea leads to strong negative emotional reactions.

Food can have positive incentive value, as when it is *appetizing*. An internal state, *appetite,* is related to this positive incentive value of food. Social enhancement in nonhuman animals has been demonstrated, with young rats learning food preferences by observing adult rats' eating. In humans, an additional type of social enhancement occurs, in that more food is consumed when one eats with others compared with eating alone.

Young explored the hedonic aspects of eating and referred to the *palatability* of food. He found that strongly preferred foods lead to greater amounts of instrumental responding to attain the food. With increased food-deprivation (hunger), nonhuman animals and humans show heightened sensory pleasure from food. At the start of a meal, even nonhuman animals eat more and at a faster rate when food is highly palatable.

Sensory-specific satiety was studied by Rolls, who found that once eating begins, the food being eaten, compared with novel food, becomes less pleasurable. This is a normal occurrence. However, persons with an eating disorder, compared with normal-weight and normal-eating persons, have been found to show significantly less sensory-specific satiety for highly palatable foods like chocolate. Overweight persons, especially, tend to be highly sensitive to the taste of food.

Persons with eating disorders do *not* relate subjective characteristics of "feeling hungry" in a reliable way to physiological internal cues (like gastric motility) that accompany food deprivation. Obese persons may rate themselves as hungry most of the time, and persons with anorexia nervosa, who are extremely underweight, are likely to rate themselves as not hungry even after many hours of food deprivation.

Dieting, or being a *restrained* eater, is likely to lower basal metabolism (the rate of "burning" calories). Thus, losing weight may be difficult when reduction of caloric intake is the only method used for weight reduction. To ensure that restrained eating leads to weight loss, the dieting person also needs to engage in exercise, which increases lean body tissue, and this, in turn, increases basal metabolism.

Persons with eating disorders of anorexia, bulimia, and obesity have been compared on a number of variables like responsiveness to food cues, food consumption, and personality characteristics. The groups have been found to differ in certain cognitions, in early childhood experiences with food and eating, and in personality dynamics. In some individuals a genetic predisposition may contribute to the eating disorder.

Socioeconomic factors influence which body size and shape are considered to have high value. In wealthier nations, the cultural emphasis on "thin is beautiful" has led to a growing incidence of eating disorders in adolescence and even childhood years. Girls more than boys, and women more than men, have shown eating disorders, but in recent years boys have shown an increase in eating disorders. Beliefs about one's body are related to self-value (self-esteem), and in adolescent girls and boys, low self-esteem has been found to be associated with disturbed eating behavior. A variety of therapeutic treatment methods have been found to be effective in treating eating disorders.

Hunger and thirst alter the hedonic value of food or water, and they influence instrumental responding and information processing. Hunger and thirst provide internal cues that can be used for learning about a reward of food or water and about instrumental responses associated with obtaining the reward. Hunger and thirst *push* the organism, and environmental cues related to the reward *pull* the organism.

Appetitive motivations like hunger and thirst heighten sensitivity to environmental cues. When an individual is hungry or thirsty, more than when satiated, environmental stimuli can lead to increased *activity* in a generalized way and in selective ways.

An interaction between hunger and food magnitude occurs for both consummatory and instrumental responding. Contrast effects have been found when animals receive shifts in magnitude of food reward, with negative contrast effects being stronger than positive contrast effects.

Under water deprivation and fear conditioning animals may show improved learning and information intake. Studies with human subjects show that appetitive motivation increases *information intake* in a general and energizing way, not selectively. Experiments using a high-speed tachistoscope and an information purchasing procedure found information processing is more likely to be facilitated as a function of the energizing rather than the directive effects of hunger and thirst. Hungry subjects do not *perceive* food words sooner than nonfood words, although response generation studies show that hungry subjects *generate* more food words compared with nonfood words.

Studies with nonhuman animals and with humans show complex effects of glucose level on activity, sleep, and memory performance. The relationship between the effects of arousal and glucose, and how glucose compared with hunger affects learning and memory, are still not fully clear. The way hunger and glucose affect learning and memory depends in part on the characteristics of the task and on the performance being measured. Physiological recordings concomitant to behavioral measures help to provide a better understanding of how motivation and glucose affect performance on memory tasks.

Rewards, Incentives, and Goals: Addictive Processes, Extrinsic Incentives, and Intrinsic Motivation

GENERAL THEORETICAL ISSUES

The term *reward* ordinarily means that a pleasurable event follows a specified behavior. Philosophers, theologians, poets, and educators have known that rewards can have a strong impact on behavior, and hedonism, or the seeking of pleasure and the avoidance of pain, was given prominence by writers over many centuries (Wertheimer, 1987). However, modern researchers have found that rewards and hedonism do not have as simple and easily predictable effects as early writers envisioned. Pleasurable outcomes may lead to *learning* of new *responses* or to altered *motivation* (*seeking* pleasurable or satisfying *outcomes*), and various cognitions also may be involved.

Many questions have arisen about rewards. How and why do they affect behavior? Do principles of conditioning apply to all behavior, or are cognitions and volition also important? The first part of this chapter reviews studies from a noncognitive perspective, with mice, rats, and pigeons providing much of the data and theories being discussed that pertain to such data. A noncognitive perspective characterized the way reward, goal, and incentive were conceptualized by the early learning theorists. For example, for Hull (1951) "goal" had no cognitive meaning and was synonymous with reward. A rat was said to run to a goal box, which referred to a place at the end of a runway where the food was located, and no cognition or internal representation

was implied. With the exception of Tolman (1948), the early behaviorists for the most part were concerned with how reward noncognitively affected learning and performance.

In What Ways Has the Effect of Reward Been Studied?

Notable early psychologists who studied reward were Thorndike (1911), Skinner (1938), and Hull (1943). Although pleasure seeking was a basic component of Freud's writing (Freud, 1920/1938), he did not specifically address issues of reward. Thus, Freud is identified with hedonic theories but not with theories of reward.

Instrumental and Operant Conditioning: A Brief Historical Overview

Animal Studies. Early psychologists realized that responses can be learned not merely as a result of practice (the principle of repetition or of frequency) but greater learning can occur if, during practice, the responses lead to satisfying outcomes. Using chickens, cats, dogs, and monkeys, Thorndike (1898, 1911) found that animals learn by trial and error to make the responses that lead to satisfying outcomes. These "satisfiers" in time became known as "rewards." By the early 1920s, studies of animal learning showed that behavior can be modified significantly if rewards are provided in a timely and consistent fashion. Thorndike's work had far-reaching influences. Psychologists found that rewards had beneficial effects on learning not only for animals but also for children and adults. Thorndike (1933) stated a famous *Law of Effect,* which described the powerful effect of rewards on learning. Initially this "law" stated that responses followed by a satisfier (reward) will tend to be increased on the next occasion, and responses followed by an "annoying" state of affairs (punishment) will tend to drop out. Thorndike initially believed punishment had as strong an impairing effect as reward had a facilitating effect, but later the weakening effect of punishment was dropped from the Law of Effect. Many studies showed that punishment led to questionable and variable results, so the law was changed and became known as the "truncated" Law of Effect, referring only to the benefits of reward and not including any statement about punishment. This reward-oriented Law of Effect had a powerful influence on psychology (Postman, 1947, 1962; Thorndike, 1935). For many years, psychologists believed that the single most important variable that affected behavior was that of reward. Their concern, like that of Thorndike, was primarily with the effect of reward on *learning,* not with the effect of reward on motivation. The *fact* that a reward followed the correct response was said to lead to learning, and the *amount* of that reward was said by some psychologists to alter motivation and performance (Black, 1965; Hull, 1951; Spence, 1956).

Although before the 1970s most psychologists considered reward necessary for learning to occur, a few did not believe it to be necessary, believing that contiguity between stimulus and response was sufficient to establish learning (Guthrie, 1935). Others, like Tolman, emphasized the motivational importance of rewards, believing that reward affected performance but not learning (Tolman, 1932; Tolman & Honzik, 1930). Tolman posited that without reward a nonhuman animal or a human can learn what to do in a situation, but subsequently the learned behavior is likely to be performed only when a reward is presented.

The early investigators (Hull, 1943; Thorndike, 1935) considered the effects of reward on learning not to involve conscious awareness. The effects of

reward for many early behaviorists were postulated to be simple and direct. Thorndike (1913) considered the reward to "stamp in" the association between the preceding stimulus and response, and in later learning trials the response would be repeated in the presence of that stimulus. Similarly, Hull (1943) and Skinner (1938) denied any role for intentionality or awareness, and, like other behaviorists of that time, assumed that an automatic-like process increased the probability of responses if these were followed by reward. This approach contrasted with the cognitive theory of Tolman (1932), who posited that animals and people formulate plans and expectancies and that animals, like people, purposively make responses that lead to reward. This conceptualized the effect of reward in motivational terms, based on the animal's intentions.

A typical early experiment used a puzzle box (Thorndike, 1898). After many tries a cat would make the appropriate response (like pushing a lever) that opened a door, thus enabling the cat to leave the box. Following a series of rewarded trials the cat easily made the correct response. Other experiments used mazes, in which a rat after many trials would learn to find the food at the end of the maze without entering blind alleys that delayed receipt of the reward (Hull, 1932; Hunter, 1930). Preferring single-response measurement techniques rather than mazes, Skinner (1938, 1969) developed a box that was known by his name (the Skinner box), in which a rat pressed a lever that led to the delivery of a food pellet. Thus, various experimental approaches assessed the way reward altered learning (Hull, 1943; Thorndike, 1913) or response probability (Skinner, 1969). Most experiments with puzzle boxes, mazes, and the Skinner box tended not to assess the way reward altered motivation, with notable exceptions being the studies of Tolman (1932) and the reward-shift work of Crespi (1942), already described.

Puzzle-box and maze learning were called "instrumental learning," in that the response was instrumental for obtaining the consequence of the reward (Hilgard & Marquis, 1940). Under the influence of Skinner, in later years the term *instrumental learning* was dropped in favor of *operant conditioning*, which did not imply intentionality (as might the term *instrumental*) but rather emphasized in objective terms that the behavior operates on the environment (Ferster & Skinner, 1957; Skinner, 1938, 1969). In Skinnerian language, the "satisfying" consequence was no longer called a reward but, instead, a reinforcement. When the response led to a positive outcome, the term *positive reinforcement* was used. This was distinguished from the term *negative reinforcement,* in which the outcome was removal of discomfort or pain and not the presentation of something positive. If an animal learned to escape from a puzzle box without food being present outside the box, the "reward" was escape from confinement, which is a negative reinforcement. This contrasts to positive reinforcement, which occurs when an animal receives food subsequent to making the correct response.

Many types of schedules of reinforcement were developed in operant conditioning studies. Variable and fixed reinforcement schedules were used, in which the reinforcer was presented either in variation around a mean or on a fixed basis, and the reinforcements also could be in terms of elapsed time or in terms of number of responses. These schedules were called fixed ratio (FR), variable ratio (VR), fixed interval (FI) and variable interval (VI). Thus, an FR 5 schedule meant that the individual (nonhuman animal or human) had to make five designated responses before a reinforcer was presented and a VI 2 schedule meant that on the average a reinforcer was given every 2 minutes, provided a designated response occurred in that interval. Skinner (1962, 1989) rejected the distinction between learning and performance and instead focused on the effects of reinforcement schedules on behavior.

Reinforcers provide information and can increase associative strength, but reinforcers also provide hedonic or motivational enhancement, thus increasing performance but not learning. These dual functions were assessed behaviorally by early researchers like Tolman (1932; Tolman & Honzik, 1930). Contemporary neuropsychological researchers found that reinforcement involves more than one system and has a number of effects (Evans & Vaccarino, 1990; Vaccarino, Shiff, & Glickman, 1989; White, 1991). Vaccarino, Schiff, and Glick-

man (1989) described two ascending dopamine systems that serve two different functions of positive reinforcers: a mesolimbic system that involves *motivational* properties, and a nigrostriatal system that involves memory consolidation properties involved in *learning and retention* of responses. Neuropsychological studies on opiates showed that food can have motivation-inducing properties, with morphine increasing eating. Studies of brain pathways show that opiates act on taste and thereby on the affective/motivational properties of food (Evans & Vaccarino, 1990). White (1991) found that different brain sites were involved in hedonic satisfaction than were involved in reinforcement for learning and memory (associative process). Review of a number of studies indicated that certain brain sites exist for which reinforcement affects learning and memory, and others exist for which reinforcement affects only performance but not learning and memory. Behavioral as well as physiological data show the importance of distinguishing between these two functions of reinforcement.

The reinforcer of food can alter memory and not only provide hedonic satisfaction. In one study (White, 1991) mice were on a platform, and when they stepped off they received a foot shock in a passive avoidance task. Some animals were fed immediately after their first foot shock experience and some were not. On the next day of testing, the mice that had been fed right after they stepped down and received shock showed more passive avoidance, that is, they stayed longer on the platform than did the unfed animals. Had the food been hedonically satisfying, the fed mice would have stepped off the platform more quickly rather than staying longer on the platform, because stepping off led to food plus shock, compared with the unfed mice that received only shock when stepping down. The greater avoidance learning by the fed mice revealed their better association and memory about stepping down and getting shocked.

Human Studies. The type of positive reinforcers that were used in animal studies tended to be related to "drive reduction" (Hull, 1943), like food given to a hungry animal. However, positive reinforcers could also be merely pleasant-tasting substances, like saccharin (Sheffield & Roby, 1950), that did not involve reduction of deprivation. Human studies used the same type of positive reinforcers as were used in animal studies, but additionally they used praise, gifts, or other kinds of satisfiers. For example, one study (Schwartz & Johnson, 1969) assessed whether positive reinforcers can increase spontaneous changes in GSR (galvanic skin response) by presenting slides depicting nude females to college student men each time they showed a spontaneous GSR. The reinforced responses were significantly more frequent for the experimental subjects in contrast to the spontaneous GSR of subjects in a control group, who were shown the slides but never after spontaneous GSR.

Similar to the animal studies, many studies with humans focused on the effect of reward on learning. Immediately after a given response was made, the person received reinforcement, and the response increased in strength or probability after many trials or many experiences over time. These types of studies were done in the laboratory to assess the way operant conditioning can lead to acquisition of new responses. Outside of the laboratory, applying the operant conditioning model of Skinner, researchers adopted reinforcement methods in numerous field settings with a large variety of individuals. Studies of this kind were identified as *behavior modification,* in which the focus was on increasing response probability according to specific schedules of reinforcement. Praise, tokens, or food were often used as reinforcers. In one study (Ferster & DeMyer, 1962), three autistic children were trained to press a key, and a token coin served as positive reinforcer. The coin could be traded for a variety of pleasurable activities (such as playing with an electric train, receiving trinkets from a machine, looking at TV). Once the key-pressing behavior was learned, more complex behaviors were developed, again using token coins as reinforcers. With training, the children learned to match simple figures by pressing a correct key.

Behavior modification programs have taught schoolchildren to increase their cooperative behavior (Azrin & Lindsley, 1956) and to decrease their disruptive behavior in the classroom (Hall, Lund, & Jackson, 1968). The procedure involved identifying a specific behavior that the experimenter, teacher, or parent sought to alter. Many behavior modification studies have used tokens, which could be exchanged for desired objects, activities, or candy. Although behavior modification techniques have utilized additional variables and not only positive reinforcers, a wide range of behaviors have been altered solely on the basis of such reinforcers. A review of many years of work, involving a whole community in a housing project and the use of reinforcers, was provided by Greenwood et al. (1992).

Praise as a Verbal Reinforcer

Praise is a commonly used positive reinforcer in behavior modification programs and in laboratory studies. It has been used with psychiatric clients (Fuoco, Lawrence, & Vernon, 1988), with schoolchildren (Mills & Grusec, 1989), and with college students (Baumeister, Hutton, & Cairns, 1990). One study with college students (Phillips, 1968) sought to evaluate the effectiveness of vicarious reinforcement compared with the direct experience of receiving a reinforcement. Subjects listened to a tape of another person, whose responses alternated with the subjects' responses. Subjects in the direct reinforcement condition received the reinforcement word "good" every time they gave a response belonging to a preselected class of words (such as human words, or weapon words). Subjects in the vicarious reinforcement condition received no reinforcement following their *own* responses, but on the tape they heard the praise of "good" after each time the other person said the correct response word. Phillips (1968) found that with the word "good," direct reinforcement was more effective than vicarious reinforcement. Some researchers believe that vicarious learning, with another person obtaining reinforcement after the correct response, is as effective as when reinforcement is received by the individual directly, but most psychologists advocate that when possible, direct rather than vicarious reinforcement should be given.

Praise does not affect all individuals in a similar manner. Praise more than tokens has been found to relate complexly to motivation, possibly having a greater effect on motivation than on learning. Praise may maintain appropriate behavior in some individuals and in some situations, but it may not be effective for others. Praise has symbolic and social meaning. Thus it cannot be used in the same way that food is used for a rat in a maze, as merely another type of reward to increase specific responses. Compared with tokens or food, praise has far more complex motivational characteristics.

Praise is used often to alter behavior in daily life as well as in scientific experiments. When one gives praise as a positive reinforcer, the specific words one uses can make an important difference. What sounds reinforcing to one person may not sound that way to another. One person may interpret the statement "your car looks good" as praise, another as insult, by interpreting the words to mean that the speaker was surprised and expected a bad-looking car. Words have different meanings according to the circumstances, the persons involved, and the way they are said.

Praise has cultural meaning. Words that are effective at one time in history or in one community need not be effective in another era or community. For example, studies in the 1950s and 1960s (Douvan, 1956; Zigler & Kanzer, 1962) showed that the verbal reinforcer of "good" was more effective in altering behavior for children of lower socioeconomic families and the verbal reinforcer of "correct" was more effective in altering behavior for children of middle-class families. Such results would not be likely in the 1990s. The connotative meaning of words can be measured by a test called the "semantic differential," and this was used by Komorita and Bass (1967). With statistical analysis the researchers found three factors for words like "kind," "good," "nice," and "trustworthy." Two of the factors were affective-emotional and moral-ethical. Thus, words of praise do not all communicate the same meaning. In experimental work as well as in everyday situations, praise and other types of verbal reinforcers are frequently used with the assumption that different verbal rewards are interchangeable. The complexity of praise as a positive reinforcer is often underestimated. Because of its symbolic and social meanings, praise more than tokens or food rewards, can have a wide variety of effects on behavior. Although contemporary reinforcement theorists consider far

more complex processes than did the early behaviorists (e.g., Gewirtz & Pelaez-Nogueras, 1993; Heyman & Tanz, 1995; Ho, Wogar, Bradshaw, & Szabadi, 1997) and some make use of utility functions related to economics and decision theory (e.g., Rachlin, 1997), they still explain "mental" acts in a noncognitive way and in terms of environmental factors. They conceptualize the effects of reinforcers on the basis of mechanisms or processes that preclude volition, awareness, conscious choices, or deliberative decisions.

Reward Variables That Affect Learning and Performance

Rewards have potentially *informational* as well as *satisfaction-providing* aspects. A reward can increase the likelihood of a person's responding because it gives feedback (information) regarding the quality or quantity of one's performance, with the focus being on the *action*. The reward in this case serves to give direction to the person's behavior. Rewards also can increase responses because people seek outcomes that gives pleasure or satisfaction. In this case, the reward has motivational characteristics. It is sought to provide either immediate hedonic pleasure (like that given by candy) or a more cognitive and symbolic satisfaction (such as a high mid-term grade or a job promotion). In such a case, *obtaining the rewarding outcome* becomes the focus, and the action is merely a means to that end.

Unlearned and Conditioned Rewards and Motivations

A reward like food for a hungry animal or human has different qualities than a reward like tokens that can be exchanged for a prize or for the opportunity to watch television. Chapter 8 described the distinction between primary and secondary, with some motivations, such as food-deprivation hunger, being biologically determined and called *primary motivations* and some rewards, such as food, having a biological basis and being called *primary rewards*. For some time the term *secondary rewards* was used for learned rewards, but the contemporary term is *conditioned rewards*.

Rewards can be motivating, and this differs from deprivation-induced motivations in the sense of "pull versus push" already discussed. Motivation from reward, the pull motivation, is called incentive motivation, and differs from the push motivations. For many years psychologists assumed that learned push motivations can only be established for aversive motivations, like fearing a person who has abused one in the past, and that conditioned push motivations could not be established for appetitive motivations like hunger. However, an ingenious study by Segal and Champion (1966) did establish a secondary or conditioned appetitive motivation.

The procedure for establishing secondary motivations consists of pairing a neutral stimulus with a primary motivation, a procedure comparable to that for establishing secondary rewards by pairing a neutral stimulus with a primary reward. This procedure is like classical conditioning, already described with regard to little Albert's learning to fear a white rat and as discussed with regard to taste aversions. The essential part is to pair a neutral event with a primary one, and then, depending on the way the pairing occurs, the neutral stimulus will take on either motivational or rewarding characteristics. If the neutral stimulus is paired only with hunger and not with food, it is a conditioned appetitive motivation, and if the neutral stimulus is paired with food, it is a conditioned reward.

Segal and Champion (1966) deprived rats of food for 24 hours in a cage that had vertical black and white stripes on the paneling of the cage. The animals were never fed in the striped environment. On alternate days the animals were fed in their regular home cages. Control group animals also were fed and deprived on alternate days, but their feeding and deprivation occurred in the striped environment. Thus, control animals had no selective training for learning to associate the striped environment with hunger, because stripes were associated with both hunger and food. After 20 days of exposure to the striped environment, a bar was introduced into the testing cage and all the animals were tested in a nondeprived (low hunger) state. The question was how soon bar pressing would occur. If pairing the striped environment with the hunger

motivation had led to that environment becoming a conditioned appetitive motivator for the experimental animals (the animals experiencing a motivational arousal akin to a hunger state), these animals when tested in a striped environment should press the bar significantly sooner than when tested in a different environment. Also, they should press the bar significantly sooner than control animals tested in the striped environment, because the control animals would not have developed a conditioned motivation in the striped environment.

To assess these possibilities, control and experimental animals were divided into two groups, with half the control and half of the experimental animals tested in the striped environment and half tested in an all-white environment that had never been paired with either food or hunger. As predicted, the experimental subjects that were tested in the striped environment pressed the bar significantly sooner than did those tested in the white environment, and no such significant difference occurred for the control subjects. The mean bar-press latency for control animals and for the experimental animals tested in the white environment was long and the three subgroups had comparable long latencies. In contrast, the experimental animals tested in the striped environment had very fast latency for bar pressing, and this was true on the first trial before any outcomes occurred for bar pressing. Their motivation on the first trial was clearly a learned appetitive motivation based on hunger and not an incentive motivation, because no reward had been paired with the environment.

If familiarity with the striped environment were the reason for short latency in bar pressing, the control subjects tested in the striped environment also should have shown the short latency, but they had a long latency. The procedure of pairing a neutral environment with primary motivation has been used in many studies of conditioned aversive motivation, in which the testing environment has been paired with aversive stimuli, but the above study is notable because the learned motivation was based on hunger.

In contrast to the above procedure for establishing a *learned motivation,* pairing a neutral stimulus with a primary reward leads to a *learned reward.* Other terms used for such rewards are *conditioned reinforcement, conditioned reward,* or *second-order conditioned reinforcement.* In a study with hungry rats trained and tested in a Skinner box, Brown (1956) trained experimental animals by presenting a light and buzzer sound along with a food pellet. No bar was in the Skinner box, and at preset intervals the light and sound occurred, followed a second later by a pellet in the food cup for the experimental animals. Light and sound were on for 2 seconds for experimental as well as control animals, but the control subjects received food pellets in the cup only at a considerably later time following the offset of the light and sound. Following 30 trials of the above procedure, a bar was put in the box. All the animals were still hungry, and each animal was left in the box until 20 bar presses occurred.

For both experimental and control animals, each bar press was followed by a 2-second light and buzzer sound. The question was whether pairing a neutral stimulus with a primary reward would lead to a conditioned reward, whereby this stimulus provides reinforcing properties for acquiring new responses. As predicted, the experimental rats made their 20 bar-pressing responses significantly sooner than the control animals when no food was present and only light and sound were presented after each bar press. The neutral stimuli (light and sound) had taken on conditioned reward characteristics because of their pairing with food for the experimental animals. The control animals also had received the neutral stimuli but these were never paired with food. Consequently, the light and sound served to reinforce the bar pressing of the hungry experimental animals, by taking on food-substitute value, but these same stimuli did not have such reinforcing properties for the hungry control animals.

The conditioned reward value in the above study came from pairing the neutral stimuli with food during training, but the animals were also hungry. Bar pressing with only light and sound during testing would have been different for the experimental animals had they been nondeprived (satiated) during training. The conditioned reward value of the neutral stimuli was thus derived from the fact that

the food and neutral stimuli had been presented when the animals were hungry. In a variety of studies, including deprivation shift studies, the value of a conditioned reward has been shown to be dependent on the motivational state of the subjects at time of training and testing (Lopez, Balleine, & Dickinson, 1992).

In many studies of conditioned reward, the neutral stimuli and food both follow an instrumental response. This has led to disclaimers that the conditioned reward is based on conditioned value, and controversy has arisen regarding the role of instrumental responding in establishing a conditioned reward (Williams, 1994a, 1994b). As noted above, the conditioned reward training in the Brown (1956) study was not connected with any instrumental response. Thus, data support the view of Williams (1994a, 1994b), and show that conditioned reward value can be acquired by association between specific neutral stimuli and the primary reward without any association between instrumental response and reward.

Delay and Magnitude of Reward

Two variables that are known to affect the way reward alters learning or performance are delay of reward and magnitude of reward. Studies of *magnitude* have included both the quantity and the quality of the reward. Studies in chapter 8 already described that when one is hungry, food is more appealing, and the larger the magnitude of the food reward the greater the increase in responding. The study by Ehrenfreund (1971) showed that rats run faster when presented a large compared with a small amount of food reward at the end of a runway. Formulations of Hull (1951), Spence (1956), and Kimble (1961, p. 123) stated that reward magnitude affects only performance and not learning. Larger or more appealing rewards of all kinds increase performance speed or output (Osborne, 1978), that is, they increase effort and not learning of new associations.

The postulation that quality and quantity of reinforcement affect only performance and not learning was challenged by research on the effect of saccharin on memory. Stefurak and Van der Kooy (1992) assessed whether saccharin improves memory for place conditioning. Chapter 8 cited studies that showed glucose but not saccharin improves memory, but the research by Stefurak and Van der Kooy (1992) approached the role of saccharin from a different perspective. They gave saccharin as a reinforcer following training in both aversive and appetitive taste conditioning and in place conditioning, and they found improvement in memory, which leveled off at a maximum consumption of saccharin of about 140 mg per rat. This was not like the effect of glucose, because only the consumption, not the injection, of saccharin enhanced memory, whereas the effect of glucose occurred also with injection. The researchers proposed that the memory enhancement of saccharine was due to the motivational aspect of the sweet taste, and that this involves different brain processes than are involved in the memory enhancement of glucose. If further studies like this demonstrate that certain kinds of learning and memory are enhanced by increased quantity and quality of reinforcement, this will force abandonment of the previously held belief that reward magnitude affects only performance and not learning.

The question of how magnitude of reward affects performance and learning differs from consideration of *delay* of reward. Delay of reward refers to the interval between response and reinforcement. The shorter the delay that follows a response, the more readily the response is learned (Kimble, 1961, p. 140). This has been called the "delay-of-reinforcement gradient." With animals or small children it is readily observed (Richards & Marcattilo, 1978). In testing whether delay of food reinforcement affects the strength of a neutral stimulus becoming a conditioned reinforcer, Mazur (1995) gave pigeons a red key or a green key to peck with red or green houselights turned on during the delay for food, and he used various conditions of reinforcement and delay of reinforcement. He found that the lesser time during the delay of food in the presence of the neutral stimulus and matching environment led to increased strength of the conditioned reinforcer. Other research has shown, however, that under some circumstances the loss with

long delays can be overcome. Whereas normally a long delay of reinforcement weakens or even prevents learning, *marking* the correct response each time it occurs can overcome the effect. Presenting a brief tone or light immediately after a correct response is made, or in other ways marking the response with a salient event, enables the animal to learn even with delays as long as 60 seconds. The memory of the response seems then to be associated with the reinforcer, enabling the animal to learn even with long delays between response and reinforcer (Lieberman, Davidson, & Thomas, 1985).

Because large and immediate rewards are preferred, researchers have investigated to what extent nonhuman animals and humans will choose a delayed large reward over an immediate small reward. The above studies describe the effects of reinforcement on performance and learning as direct and not mediated by complex cognitive processes. Older children and adults, as well as macaque monkeys, can bridge long time gaps and they can regard rewards in cognitive and symbolic ways. They can and do select large delayed rewards over small immediate ones (Logue, Forzano, & Tobin, 1992; Tobin, Logue, Chelonis, Ackerman, & May, 1996). For older children and adults, rewards often do not have the same simple and direct effects that are found with pigeons, rats, and small children. Nevertheless, studies with pigeons, rats, and small children have helped increase understanding of the effects of reinforcers on behavior and learning, and have also helped provide methods that can be effective with special-needs populations with limited development of cognitive and symbolic processing. These issues concern aspects of reinforcement that are closely related to the topic of motivation. More complete descriptions of the effects of reinforcement are provided by Domjan (1998) and Roberts (1998).

BRAIN STIMULATION, REWARD SYSTEMS, AND DRUG ABUSE

For many years researchers have assessed the ways that reward can affect motivation, and they also have investigated the neurophysiological bases that underlie the action of rewards.

Reward Systems

Which brain areas and pathways are involved in the action of rewards was investigated by means of brain stimulation studies. Following the dramatic findings of Olds and Milner (1954), many studies sought to understand how brain stimulation in certain regions can provide highly intense "pleasure" or excitement that exceeds the reward value of natural reinforcers like food.

When electrodes are placed in brain regions like the septal area and the hypothalamus, rats typically press a bar at a high rate if responses are followed by bursts (trains) of electrical stimulation. The early researchers were astonished to discover that electrical stimulation of specific brain areas provided a very strong reward. The pulse frequency in different studies varied between 20 and over 200 pulses per second, and pulse duration typically was 0.1 or 0.2 milliseconds, although it could go far longer. Number of pulses in each burst of stimulation could vary, as could train durations. In a Skinner box, rats pressed the bar and received stimulation for many hours. The rate of such self-stimulation was found to increase (up to a point) with the intensity of the current and with the pulse frequency, pulse duration, and train duration. In addition to rats, cats, and monkeys, even occasionally human subjects for special medical treatment were found to show high rates of intracranial self-stimulation, and in experiments with animals, self-stimulation was tested with many kinds of instrumental responses, like shuttle box or maze running (Kling & Schrier, 1972).

The potency of such self-stimulation reinforcement was found to be very high, possibly because it occurred immediately after the overt response. For example, Routtenberg and Lindy (1965) found that if two bars are available in the Skinner box, one to deliver food and one to deliver bursts of electrical stimulation to specific brain regions, some of the hungry animals starved to death. They neglected to press the bar that delivered food reinforcement and instead continuously pressed the bar that delivered

the electrical stimulation. The highest rates of self-stimulation were found if the electrodes were placed in the hypothalamus. A number of studies found that rats would press the bar for self-stimulation even for periods of as much as 24 hours, until they were exhausted, and after rest they would resume bar pressing.

Intracranial self-stimulation seemed to have primary reinforcement properties, because when neutral stimuli were paired with rewarding brain stimulation bursts the neutral stimuli became conditioned reinforcers. In one study (Stein, 1958) rats had electrodes implanted in the "reward" areas of the septum or hypothalamus. First, the animals learned to associate one lever in a Skinner box with a tone delivery and the other lever with no consequence following lever pressing. Then, without levers present, over 4 days they received the tone and, half a second later, a half-second train of brain stimulation. This occurred with 100 pairings a day. When subsequently the animals were tested again with the two levers and no electrical stimulation, they pressed the lever that delivered the tone far more after the conditioned reinforcement training than before the training, and they pressed that lever far more than the lever that produced no effect.

At one time the hypothalamus was thought to be a "reward center" of the brain, but in time researchers came to believe that multiple reward sites exist and that stimulation of the hypothalamus excites one or more diffuse interconnected neural systems (Wise, 1996). The self-stimulation studies suggested that, in seeking "pleasure" even to the detriment of health and survival, animals behave as though addicted. Some of the patterns animals displayed were akin to intoxication (R. K. Siegel, 1989). Under ordinary conditions, rats mostly find alcohol aversive, although rats can be bred to have an alcohol preference. In general, animals do not tend to show addiction from drugs the way humans do (Wise, 1996). Nevertheless, in psychopharmacological experiments, when drugs were injected into animals, the drugs heightened the effects of self-stimulation rewards. This permitted studying the rewarding role of drugs by means of self-stimulation experiments.

Magnitude of reward was evident in self-stimulation, with high intensity leading to increased lever-press responding. The interpretation of this effect was that high intensity stimulation is most likely to reach additional and distant reward areas and not merely the site of stimulation. At low doses of stimulation, Skinner box lever pressing tends not to occur beyond chance levels, but when a threshold of stimulation is reached, lever pressing exceeds chance level. As stimulus intensity increases beyond threshold, rate of lever pressing sharply increases until some maximum is reached. Excess stimulation beyond a given amount then leads to decreased lever pressing. The intensity of the stimulus that is required for specific rates of lever pressing for self-stimulation can be compared with the amount of stimulus intensity required to bring about that rate of responding when drugs are injected. In this way, drugs have been evaluated in terms of the way they alter the maximum response rate and in terms of the way they negate or enhance the rewarding impact of the stimulation.

Addiction and Substance Abuse

Since the 1950s a variety of definitions of addiction have appeared, according to the World Health Organization. For some time addiction was considered in terms of *habit,* but that tended to obscure the idea that addiction is not merely learned and repetitive behavior but highly motivational in its origin and manifestation. Drug dependence, evidence of withdrawal symptoms when the drug is removed, and action of psychoactive agents are often linked with the term *drug addiction.* However, all of these characteristics need not be present in order to identify drug taking as drug abuse or addiction. In cases of drug abuse, however, the reward or reinforcement of taking the drug is present, and there is a strong compulsive pattern in self-administration and drug ingestion behavior.

Data from Self-Stimulation Studies. Self-stimulation studies reveal that many rewarding effects of drugs of abuse involve activation of the dopamine system of specific brain regions, especially the mesocorticolimbic system (U.S. Congress, Office of

Technology Assessment, 1993). Figure 9.1 shows important areas of the brain identified as part of the drug reward system. The brain reward system involves various structures, a key part being the mesocorticolimbic pathway (MCLP). It consists of axons of neurons in the middle part of the brain, the ventral tegmental area. These axons project to the front part of the brain, that is, to the nucleus accumbens, which is a collection of cells in the limbic system, and to the medial prefrontal cortex. Ventral tegmental neurons release dopamine to regulate activity of cells in the nucleus accumbens and the medial prefrontal cortex. Other connections occur between the nucleus accumbens and limbic structures like the amygdala and hippocampus. The nucleus accumbens sends signals back to the ventral tegmental area. Additional neuronal pathways that contain various neurotransmitters regulate the activity of the mesocorticolimbic dopamine system. Different drugs of abuse involve different structures, and all drugs do not involve the dopamine system.

Addictive drugs that increase the potency of self-stimulation, as measured by response rate, tend to heighten dopamine activity (Wise, 1996). However, drugs of abuse differ with regard to the critical neurotransmitters activated. Alcohol affects several neurotransmitter systems in addition to that involving dopamine. Because drugs of abuse for humans are also the types of substance that heighten the rewarding effect of self-stimulation in animals, such self-stimulation studies have provided much of the contemporary biopsychological knowledge about human substance abuse. Injection of these drugs in animals leads to a lower stimulus intensity in electrical brain stimulation that is required for a given rate of responding.

As in humans, differences exist in animals. Selective breeding, for example, has led to animals of one breed freely choosing ethanol consumption of a large amount and another breed consuming hardly any alcohol in a free-choice situation. Rats bred for alcohol preference, compared with those bred to abstain from alcohol, show very different responding in mazes (Colombo et al., 1995) and in self-stimulation conditions (Gatto, McBride, Murphy, Lumeng, & Li, 1994). However, if alcohol is injected

FIGURE 9.1

(a) The mesocorticolimbic pathway from the ventral tegmental area to the nucleus accumbens and the frontal cortex. (b) Schematic drawing of the brain reward system for drug reinforcement.

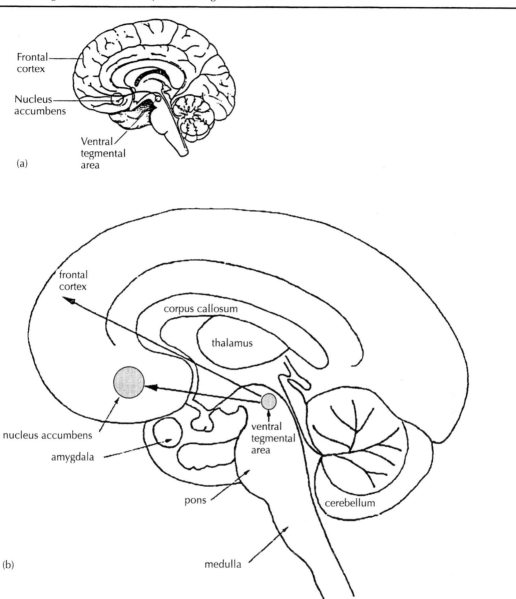

directly into specific brain areas, such as the ventral tegmental area, even rats bred not to prefer alcohol show some lever press responding for ethanol injection rewards, though they do so significantly less than do alcohol-preferring rats (Gatto et al., 1994).

Data have been reported about animals in the wild eating plants that cause some type of intoxication (R. K. Siegel, 1989). However, free-living animals ordinarily do not seek drugs for reward effects. Thus, self-stimulation laboratory studies provided unusual opportunities for examining the effects of drugs. Self-stimulation studies have investigated the actions of drugs, located their neurochemical pathways, and identified the site of maximum reward. Such studies found that amphetamine, morphine, cocaine, nicotine, and cannabis (marijuana) all have heightened rewarding effects, although at somewhat different sites.

Many drugs abused by humans act on brain areas that are identified as rewarding with measures of self-stimulation and response rates in animals. Dopamine is involved in many of these drugs. For example, when adult rats over an 8-week period were given low doses of ethanol (alcohol) intake, which did not induce ethanol tolerance or dependence, a significant increase in number of specific dopamine receptor sites were found (Lograno et al., 1993). Even though some drugs, such as cocaine and amphetamine, have their most rewarding effects in nonidentical brain areas, many drugs have been found to activate the mesolimbic dopamine system (Wise, 1996). Not all addictive drugs show comparable effects, and questions still remain about areas of action of a number of drugs. Caffeine, nicotine, and alcohol (ethanol) have rewarding pathways that differ from each other and from those of other addictive drugs. The drug nicotine involves neurotransmitters like acetylcholine in addition to dopamine. Release of acetylcholine from neurons in the cerebral cortex may be responsible for the EEG activation that occurs after nicotine intake (Henningfield, Cohen, & Pickworth, 1993), and many differences exist in the action of nicotine compared with other drugs.

Overall conclusions from self-stimulation studies are: (1) specific brain areas and neurochemical reward pathways in the brain mediate the effects of drugs abused by humans, (2) dopamine is implicated in brain reward pathways, (3) in addition to similarities, differences exist between drugs in their areas of effect and their neurochemical actions.

Controversy exists whether specifically the dopamine reward system plays a role in all drugs of abuse and whether drug abuse can be explained generally in terms of reward properties of drugs. For example, Pavlovian conditioning has been found to affect drug dependence (MacRae & Siegel, 1987; MacRae, Scoles, & Siegel, 1987), and various researchers indicate that many factors are involved in drug dependence and drug abuse. White (1996) pointed out that rewards have many effects, some but not all being tied to pleasure and some but not all involving learning. The association of environmental cues with pleasure, and the learning of specific responses to conditioned rewards, have been identified by many researchers as reasons to suggest that substance abuse cannot be tied to a simple reward system nor to a single reinforcement process.

Human Drug Use and Abuse.   One way for studying drug abuse and relapse is to investigate the strength of *urge* to continue drug ingestion. Differences exist between people in how strong urges are to resume ingestion after abstinence. Urge can be considered a motivational state analogous to hunger, especially in the case of smoking. Nicotine is considered a weak reinforcer compared with cocaine and amphetamine because the dopamine release with nicotine is weaker, but the urge to smoke can be very strong. Nicotine activates one of the receptor subtypes for acetylcholine, and this provides a strong biological basis for the urge to smoke. When these "nicotine receptors" are activated, dopamine neurons in the ventral tegmental area are activated. In addition to this, activation of nicotine receptors stimulates release of norepinephrine from neurons in the locus ceruleus and reduces serotonin activity in the hippocampus (U.S. Congress, Office of Technology Assessment, 1993). The biological basis for smoking urges are augmented by subjective factors.

Urges very in intensity and frequency. A number of studies found that individuals who experience more intense urges after abstinence are also more likely to relapse and return to smoking. To identify the relevant variables, one study (Shiffman et al., 1997) required research volunteers (long-time smokers with a high motivation and commitment to quit) to monitor their reactions for a number of weeks. Baseline data were obtained for 2 weeks of smoking and further data were obtained for up to 4 weeks after cessation. Many subjects had lapses, resuming smoking after at least 24 hours of abstinence. Temptations and urges to resume smoking were recorded about five times daily. The results showed that the best prediction for lapses was the urge intensity upon waking. Because at time of waking the environmental cues for smoking were minimal, waking urges reflected strong internal pulls. Theories of drug abuse that focus on withdrawal symptoms, and that postulate that stronger craving occurs during abstincence than during the period of ingestion, were not supported. The present study found that, overall, urges were not as strong after cessation as during the period of ad lib smoking. Individual differences proved to be important for frequency of lapses, and a wide range of motivational and cognitive variables were related to smoking urges.

Some practitioners working with drug-abusing persons speculated that drug addiction, especially alcohol abuse, has a strong genetic basis. The assumption was that for some individuals, a genetic disposition for certain brain activities would increase likelihood for the addiction. Contemporary researchers are studying the role of genes, by studying some strains of mutant mice and their withdrawal reactions under drug removal compared with other strains. These researchers also identify molecular and cellular changes that relate to gene expression (Nestler & Aghajanian, 1997). The issues of drug abuse are broad and complex, and a full discussion of this topic is not possible here. Only a few relevant points are considered.

Why humans use and abuse drugs is still not known fully, although it is increasingly known how various drugs alter neurophysiological and neu-

roendocrine functions. Increasingly, research is targeting molecular and cellular adaptations that occur in specific neuronal cell types in response to chronic drug use (Nestler & Aghajanian, 1997). Many drugs have similar effects on animals and humans in their arousing or their sedating qualities. Not all drugs of abuse lead to withdrawal symptoms, and controversy exists to what extent withdrawal and accompanying negative emotional and motivational states are crucial for addiction. One perspective that focuses on negative motivational states describes the development of addiction in terms of hedonic homeostatic dysregulation (Koob & Le Moal, 1997). The researchers distinguish between *substance use, substance abuse,* and *substance dependence,* with dependence being *addiction.* Koob and Le Moal (1997) postulate that addiction involves progressive dysregulation of the brain reward system. Small lapses in self-regulation of substance use can bring small distress. Spiraling distress may occur with some individuals, with small distress leading to larger regulation failures, which lead to further distress and negative emotion, and a spiraling process with progressive dysregulation then possibly leading to addiction. Increasing reward thresholds (which means less reward from the drug), indicating sensitization, contribute to the spiraling process.

Other researchers place emphasis more on the rewarding, not the distressing, processes that lead to drug dependence. Regardless of their emphasis, all contemporary researchers agree that drugs of abuse are artificial sources of pleasure or reward, are taken externally and put into the body, and that they significantly change nervous system activity. This process can lead to a key sign of addiction, compulsive-like behavior (behavior that leads to the obtaining and ingestion of the drug). Many psychologists think that a "reward" outcome occurs in the initial phases of drug use and this initial pleasure begins the course of drug abuse, but some (e.g., White, 1996) doubt that all drug abuse begins with an initial experience of pleasure.

Family background, childhood experiences that affect personality, cultural variables, physical and emotional stressors, and level of skills in coping with stress and anxiety have been identified as relevant to the use and abuse of drugs (Finn et al., 1997; Morgenstern, Langenbucher, Labouvie, & Miller, 1997). Controversy abounds regarding what circumstances lead to drug abuse and for what reasons therapeutic methods do or do not succeed in removing the drug abuse. Whatever specific view psychologists and mental health workers take, however, they generally believe that in some way the use and abuse of drugs involves reinforcing or pleasurable experiences. The reinforcement may be positive, in that the person feels more relaxed or cheerful with selected drugs or the person feels more energetic and active with certain drugs. Negative reinforcement may also occur, with the drug leading to a removal of an aversive state (like anxiety or stress).

In addition to the physiological pleasure-providing aspects of drugs, many cognitive reasons exist for drug *use*. Even animals have been found to use drugs in a social or gregarious manner (Ellison & Potthoff, 1983), and humans have been known to use drugs for seeking peer approval and heightening a sense of personal power without the effort normally required for obtaining power. Less clear are the reasons for drug *abuse*. The opponent process formulation of Solomon (1980) has offered one explanation regarding the process of addiction. The formulation states that in the early stages of drug use the pleasurable components (such as relaxation or euphoria) are strong, and the aversive components (like withdrawal symptoms or craving) are weak. In the early stages, the drug use is primarily rewarding and pleasurable and brings positive reinforcement. Gradually, the aversive aspects become stronger, and the person seeks an increased dosage and more frequent drug ingestion to reduce displeasure (negative reinforcement). Other explanations, that are more cognitive than the opponent process formulation, emphasize that ingesting drugs can involve a wide range of social and symbolic meanings, so that an individual may abuse drugs as an act of rebellion against family or authority figures, or as an effective method for social or activity withdrawal. Drugs can affect one's judgment and attributions, and use as well as abuse of drugs can be directed to bring about such cognitive changes.

Researchers have pointed out the strong interactions between drugs and various motivations. Drugs can heighten and satisfy, or diminish and negate, various motivational states. For example, hunger and drugs have been linked, with humans as well as animals. In one study with rats, morphine was found to have replacement value for food in hungry animals (Nader & van der Kooy, 1994), and in another study morphine was found to increase the speed of eating in food-deprived rats (Noel & Wise, 1993). In humans, interactive effects also have been found between drugs and sexual motivation, drugs and affiliative motivation, and drugs and the need for power. For example, McClelland (1973) found that individuals who have a high need for *social* power tend to drink alcohol only to a small extent, in contrast to individuals with a high need for *personal* power who tend to be heavy drinkers. Aggressive behavior in human beings is altered according to amount of alcohol consumed. Depending on the dosage, alcohol can inhibit or exaggerate aggression. Because a large dosage of alcohol can lead to aggressive behavior, one way to explain McClelland's (1973) finding is that heavy drinking facilitates aggression and this aids in attainment of a goal of personal power.

The relationship between amount of alcohol consumed and aggressive behavior was investigated in a laboratory study by Taylor and Gammon (1974), who gave college student men over the age of 21 either a high or a low dosage of alcohol (bourbon or vodka). These men then competed in an experiment in which, unbeknown to the subjects, a confederate of the researchers participated. After each trial in what was presumably a reaction-time experiment, the winner was to give shock to the loser. Wins and losses were preprogrammed by the researchers. The question was, what levels of shock would the subjects use to administer to the confederates? One finding was that at the start of the study, subjects under the high alcohol dosage gave the confederates significantly higher shocks than did those under low dosage. Moreover, once the trials proceeded and the subjects themselves received shock, those with the high alcohol dosage became even more aggressive than did the low-dosage subjects. The effect was greater for subjects ingesting vodka than for those ingesting bourbon. Relevant to the finding of McClelland (1973) concerning individuals with a high need for *social* rather than personal power, was that the low-dosage subjects (for either vodka or bourbon) gave much lower shock intensity than did control subjects who ingested no alcohol. Because drinking a small quantity of alcohol can inhibit aggressive behavior, individuals with a high need for social power, who are concerned with facilitating socially constructive behavior in others, may ingest a small amount of alcohol as a method to increase social sensitivity and facilitate social interaction. Persons high in need for social power would have learned this fact from their own life experiences with alcohol ingestion.

That we learn what to ingest from others in our social group has already been discussed in regard to eating behavior; it was pointed out that young rats learn where and what to eat by association with their elders. This learning has also been observed with other animals and with other types of behaviors. Of special relevance to the topic of addiction is the observation reported by R. K. Siegel (1989, pp. 44–45), that koala bears become addicted to the bitter-tasting eucalyptus plant as a result of early and long exposure to the plant by close association between the infant and mother. The koala is an Australian marsupial that lives during infancy in its mother's pouch, and the months of association with the smell and taste of the eucalyptus during infancy appears to lead to an irreversible addiction to the plant. Animals exposed to the plant since earliest infancy will not eat any other food and die if not supplied with the plant, although koalas exposed in early infancy to another diet have been conditioned to eat and survive with foods such as cow's milk, bread, and honey.

Various drugs have been shown to mask the discomforts of hunger, anxiety, and depression. Humans as well as animals have been found to use, and abuse, drugs according to the effects of the drug and the circumstances of the individual at the time of use and abuse. For example, nicotine and caffeine have effects different from those of alcohol or the opiates. Of special interest is the effect of nicotine. Not only the lethal effects but also the addictive effects of nicotine have been observed in many animal species

(R. K. Siegel, 1989). Nicotine acts on specific receptors in the brain and periphery and affects nearly all components of the endocrine and neuroendocrine system (Henningfield et al., 1993). Nicotine ingestion has been found to be both relaxing and arousing. In humans, nicotine ingestion (whether by means of gum chewing, injection, or cigarette smoking) has been found to assist in weight control and to heighten learning and memory performance. To what extent the age of the smoker and the length of time of smoking influences these effects is not fully clear. It is known, however, that the initial use of tobacco and the development of nicotine addiction typically occur in adolescence (Heishman, Kozlowski, & Henningfield, 1997).

Learning plays an important role in the way nicotine affects human behavior. As with other drugs, in which external environmental cues can become associated with withdrawal effects, environmental cues can induce cigarette cravings (Hatsukami, Hughes, & Pickens, 1985). Moreover, with many drugs, environmental cues can become associated with the rewarding effects of ingestion. This has been found for nicotine intake and other addictive drugs, and the environment can provide powerful cues for stimulating cigarette smoking (Fisher, Jr., Lichtenstein, & Haire-Joshu, 1993; Lando, 1993; Niaura et al., 1988).

Complex neurophysiological, experiential, and symbolic processes lead both to drug use and to addiction (Goodwin, 1994). Multiple therapeutic measures are most effective for decreasing addiction (Fisher Jr. et al., 1993). As has been demonstrated with therapy for alcohol and heroine addiction, therapeutic methods for nicotine addiction can use blocking agents (Jarvick & Henningfield, 1993), which contain a pharmacological antagonist of the addictive drug. Other methods involve giving a mild form of the drug. For example, help to stop smoking has involved use of a nicotine gum that reduces the craving for cigarettes. It also dissociates the relieving aspects of nicotine with the instrumental responses of smoking behavior.

Additional effective strategies to stop nicotine addiction use training for stress management. This is important, for if stressors and their removal were initially associated with the early onset of nicotine ingestion, the alleviation of stressors in other ways would remove the need for a person to rely on nicotine for stress reduction. If nicotine or alcohol ingestion reduces the feeling of displeasure created by stressors, the cigarette smoking or alcohol drinking will have led to negative reinforcement. Removing stress by other means would curb the necessity of smoking or drinking as sources of reinforcement (stress removal). Stress management techniques also can help people cope with the distress created by withdrawal symptoms. A major aspect of therapeutic treatment for all effective substance abuse and substance dependence programs, not just for those involving nicotine or alcohol, is helping the individual learn effective coping and stress management skills.

For addiction treatment, self-help groups have been found to be effective. Some are based on the 12-step program for alcohol abuse, with a comparable program existing for nicotine abuse (Hurt, Eberman, Slade, & Karan, 1993). Therapy also can help the person know the ways that conditioning and motivation affect drug abuse behaviors. A wide range of learning techniques can be helpful that involve conditioning and training of alternative responses (Fisher Jr. et al., 1993). Because the action of rewards in addictive behavior has far-reaching consequences, effective treatment of drug abuse requires replacing the rewards that were provided by drugs with satisfactions that are more long lasting and that facilitate meaningful relationships and heightened self-regard (Bandura, 1982; Dreikurs, 1972). Facilitative social support systems can provide powerful social and cognitive rewards that replace the neurophysiological and neurochemical rewarding effects of drugs abused in addiction. Several successful intervention strategies have been described by Ward, Klesges, and Halpern (1997).

INTRINSIC MOTIVATION, EXTRINSIC INCENTIVES, AND ACHIEVEMENT MOTIVATION

Incentive and Incentive Motivation

Contemporary neurophysiological researchers have shown that food can have motivation-inducing characteristics. Not only food but also other reinforcers are known to have motivating characteristics. As shown in the discussion of addiction, *incentive* is reinforcement that *induces* motivation. When reinforcement *reduces* motivation, like food reducing hunger in a learning experiment, the term incentive is not appropriate. An incentive is sought in its own right, such as when nonhuman animals seek electrical self-stimulation of specific brain areas.

Humans are strongly motivated by incentives. In older children and adult humans, incentives have cognitive and symbolic value. Incentives may be inner satisfactions or externally provided events, and they may be positive or negative. A positive incentive is something one seeks and a negative incentive is something one avoids. For one person a large potential payoff when playing the slot machines may serve as a strong positive incentive to continue playing, whereas for another person the realization that one can lose large amounts of money may serve as a strong negative incentive that leads to cessation of playing. The present chapter is devoted primarily to positive incentives. Negative incentives, of events one seeks to avoid, are more appropriately considered in the chapter dealing with fear and anxiety (chapter 13). The term incentive usually implies a positive outcome, so unless the word "negative" is designated, the word "incentive" should be understood as a positive event.

Incentives like bonuses or prizes are concrete (not abstract) and tied to selected actions or responses. Getting a bonus after a number of months of a special work assignment can be a strong incentive that provides the motivation for working hard on the assignment. *Incentive* is similar to *goal,* but the two variables refer to different characteristics. A goal is a cognitive representation of a destination (in terms of a cognitive map) toward which one strives, and an incentive is a reward to be obtained on performance attainment. Incentives may be extrinsic outcomes, like money or a prize for outstanding work, or they may be intrinsic, like feelings of satisfaction following good work. An incentive can be provided by an external source, like a promise of a bonus by one's boss, or it can come from an internal belief, like "I will be so relieved when this job is done" and the relief is the anticipated hedonic outcome. Incentives goad (motivate) the individual, in that the motivational pull occurs *before* the performance. Regardless of whether one eventually obtains the desired job or money, the anticipation (in the here-and-now) of the future reward provides the motivation. Although the incentive refers to a future event, the motivation that energizes and directs effort and behavior is in the present. In this way, incentives "pull" and motivate a person. Incentive motivation in nonhuman animals has been studied with conditioned reinforcers (neutral stimuli paired with food) or with sucrose, but in humans the incentives involve rewards that have value as a result of social and cultural experiences, like money, gifts, or awards.

Intrinsic Motivation and External Rewards

Incentive motivation that involves internal outcomes is called intrinsic motivation and that which involves external outcomes is called extrinsic motivation. *External* describes events or objects provided from outside the individual, and *internal* refers to thoughts or emotions generated within the individual. The term *intrinsic motivation* covers a wide range, from anticipation of inner satisfaction following some action to intrinsic pleasures derived from an activity (Staw, 1976).

The intrinsic motivation of enjoying a specific activity may lead a person to spend many hours in practice at a sport or practicing a musical instrument. Alternatively, the person may pursue an activity due to the extrinsic motivation of seeking to obtain money or public honor. Many educators advocate the advantage of intrinsic motivation, and they recommend that students should study and work hard on projects because of the joy of learning and not because of prizes, honors, or high grades.

Intrinsic motivation is typically considered to refer to interest in the task itself (Amabile & Hennessey, 1992), with the emphasis on enjoying or gaining pleasure in doing the task. However, some theorists relate intrinsic motivation to other basic human needs or motivations, like satisfaction in meeting challenges or promoting the well-being of others. Some theorists tie intrinsic motivation to the need for competence (DeCharms, 1968), self-effi-

cacy (Bandura, 1991), self-determination (Deci, 1980), and to personal growth as well as the advancement of the common good (Dreikurs, 1995).

Does Intrinsic Motivation Decrease with Extrinsic Rewards?

Writers who advocate that humans should rely on intrinsic rather than extrinsic sources of motivation differ from those who emphasize behavior modification through reinforcements and other extrinsic factors. Researchers who emphasize cognitive and motivational processes rather than conditioning procedures have found that extrinsic incentives may decrease intrinsic motivation, as, for example, when a person believes the extrinsic incentive is the reason for doing an activity (Lepper & Green, 1978).

General Considerations: Why Is Intrinsic Motivation Important?   Many reasons exist for advocating the importance of intrinsic sources of motivation. One reason is the fact that, especially for adults, external rewards in everyday life are given in an unpredictable way with unreliable frequency. Without consistent and frequent reinforcements, people are likely to stop taking actions and doing what is required of them. A Skinnerian, who advocates the use of extrinsic behavioral control by reinforcers, would counter this by saying that unpredictable and infrequent external rewards need not diminish actions as long as the person has received prior training with various schedules of reinforcement, particularly those schedules in which reinforcement is given after long intervals or only after a large number of responses. For example, animals have persisted in steady bar pressing even when food occurs only once in over 5,000 bar presses (Collier, Hirsch, & Hamlin, 1972). However, theorists from a human and cognitive-motivational perspective would argue this is not a pertinent analogy, since human action in everyday life is not motivated by hunger and behavior is not maintained by reinforcement of food. It is not the case that environmental factors are unimportant, but rather that extrinsic rewards do not play the role that a Skinnerian would advocate.

A cognitive-motivational theorist would counter

the Skinnerian argument by saying that prior training on reinforcement schedules will not maintain behavior over long periods of sporadic rewards, because humans form expectancies and these alter motivation and behavior. If on many occasions the rewards that one has anticipated as outcomes following actions do not occur, the person will decrease his or her expectation of external rewards, and this will lead to decreased motivation. If the person relies on extrinsic incentives for motivation and energy for actions comes primarily from extrinsic rather than intrinsic motivation, decreased expectation of rewards will decrease motivation and the person will be less productive and exert less effort. In time the person can become listless and withdrawn. This can happen to adults but is especially likely in children, if they have been trained to rely primarily on extrinsic incentives. From this cognitive-motivational viewpoint, prior training in reinforcement schedules does not inoculate the person against feelings of discouragement and lowered motivation for action, and therefore it is preferable to train children to rely on intrinsic motivation.

A different advantage for training people to rely on intrinsic motivation is that reliance on extrinsic motivation is not conducive to problem solving and creativity (Amabile & Hennessey, 1992). From the perspective of human cognitive-motivational theory, reliance on inner satisfactions, which are self-generated, is always possible even when extrinsic incentives are absent. Intrinsic motivation provides a continuing source of motivation, enabling the individual to continue to exert effort and take actions even in the absence of external incentives. Moreover, intrinsic motivation is considered by many to heighten self-esteem. Some specific theoretical formulations regarding the advantages of intrinsic motivation are discussed next.

Adler and Dreikurs. The theory of Adler (1930), already mentioned in a previous chapter, is a cognitive, social, motivational, and developmental theory of personality. A younger colleague of Freud, Adler at first embraced Freud's theory, but by 1914 he rejected many tenets of that theory and established his own school of thought. Adler's theory emphasizes social motivation, subjective appraisal, goal direction as the source of motivation, and holism. The theory postulates that human beings are decision makers, who make choices and set goals on the basis of subjective appraisal of events occurring in their lives. According to Adler, the fundamental motivation of humans is to belong and to contribute to the community (Ferguson, 1995). This motivation in German is called *Gemeinschaftsgefühl*, which translates loosely into English as "social interest" (Adler, 1929/1969, 1933/1964). From the point of view of Adlerian theory, social interest is an innate potential that is brought forth by appropriate upbringing experiences. When children are raised with democratic and encouraging methods and are stimulated from early years to contribute to the well-being of the family, the children feel they belong and they want to contribute as equal members. They will contribute in the family in preschool years and later in school, and then increasingly in the larger human community. In this way, children with strong social interest help with chores and exert effort in many prosocial ways for largely intrinsic satisfactions and not because they seek to receive external rewards.

Rudolf Dreikurs, a younger colleague of Adler's, wrote books that detailed child-training methods so that parents and teachers can help children to develop into effectively functioning individuals. In these books, Dreikurs (1992; Dreikurs & Cassel, 1990; Dreikurs, Grunwald, & Pepper, 1998) pointed out that rewards and punishments were not effective, because they diminished internal (intrinsic) motivation. According to Dreikurs, inner motivation is necessary for prosocial, responsible, and self-reliant behavior. Giving money or prizes or other rewards that had no intrinsic relationship to the actions will only diminish an appreciation for the action. For example, when the child sets the table, that action contributes to the family meal. The child gains a sense of value and believes he or she is an equal with other members of the group. The child who helps with family work gains self-respect through contribution. Washing the dishes after dinner helps provide clean dishes for the family. When the child contributes to a happier family life, that leads to inner satisfaction, which is far more effective than are arbitrary rewards like money or special presents.

In advancing Adlerian theory, Dreikurs (1969, 1992) pointed out that for children to behave in constructive and cooperative ways they need to be educated to develop high social interest. Social interest involves shared responsibility and mutual respect in democratic social relationships that are based on social equality. Persons with high social interest experience healthy functioning under conditions of success as well as adversity. Social interest is both a cognition and an emotion, which strengthens people's belief in a fair and reasonable world and a belief that they are capable individuals. People with such beliefs are more likely to focus on the well-being of the group and not only on possible personal gains. Effective parenting and teaching methods help children to believe they are valued and contributing members of the community rather than that they are inferior to others.

Dreikurs disavowed rewards and extrinsic incentives, in that these do not teach a child to make effective choices, to take responsibility for his or her own actions, or to be concerned with the welfare of other persons. Rather, rewards signify an arbitrary consequence given by a controlling external agent. Rewards teach the child to depend on outside agents instead of on his or her own inner resources. They teach an individual that control for actions come from external rather than internal sources, and they minimize a sense of responsibility for the consequences of one's actions. Rewards may strengthen outward behavior but they do not prosocially direct goal setting and choices, nor do they heighten internal resources and inner strengths. Effective living requires internal (intrinsic) motivation that is based on a strong belief in one's own strength and a commitment to democratic problem solving (Dreikurs, 1971/1992). The raising and educating of children require methods that focus on strengthening the child's self-concept and that foster the child's contributing to the welfare of the community of which she or he is a part. External rewards and punishments fail to accomplish these ends and they often undermine such processes.

Alternatives to externally administered rewards and punishments are *natural* and *logical consequences* and the use of *encouragement*. Rewards do not teach the child the appropriate values or cognitions, but natural and logical consequences do (Dreikurs & Grey, 1992; Dreikurs & Soltz, 1992). Within democratic group processes, learning from the consequences of one's actions enables an individual to accept, and to learn from, the realities of social living. If the child puts toys away after playing with them, she or he later will find them, and they will be in good shape the next time the child wants to play with them. Having the adult put the toys away, or the adult nagging the child until the child puts them away, prevents the child from learning to be responsible. Logical and natural consequences allow the child to learn from his or her mistaken actions.

Adults experience natural consequences daily, and Adlerians advise that under normal circumstances this is the best way for children to learn. The college student who attends parties instead of studying is likely to experience the natural consequence of impaired performance on an upcoming test. The adult who plans ahead and leaves for the store with adequate time will be able to make wanted purchases, whereas the person who waits until the last minute before leaving the house to go shopping is likely to find the store closed. In adult living the individual needs to function adaptively with problem-solving skills rather than constant external monitoring or controls, and within limits of safety, children also should learn from the realistic consequences of their actions. Many specific techniques are recommended as alternatives to rewards and punishments.

An important Adlerian concept is that of *encouragement,* which is advocated as an alternative to praise and criticism (Dinkmeyer & Dreikurs, 1963; T. B. Evans, 1989, 1996; Meredith & Evans, 1990). Encouragement enhances the person's self-esteem, whereas praise is directed toward specific behavior. Encouragement focuses on future actions, whereas praise refers to specific actions done in the past. Praise often pits a child competitively against peers (such as "you finished your work before anyone else") and this is likely to diminish social interest and to decrease cooperative relationships with peers. In some situations praise may benefit the person, and because of its social quality praise is preferable to material rewards like money or prizes, but praise should be used sparingly so as to prevent the child from acquiring an inappropriate self-oriented focus. Praise involves extrinsic motivation, and the aim of encouragement is to increase the child's intrinsic motivation (Pitsounis & Dixon, 1988). Encouragement heightens self-confidence for future actions.

Too many times praise results in the child's belief that although past actions led to external acknowledgment of success, future actions aren't going to be acceptable. When that happens, instead of praise leading to motivation that energizes future-directed effort, praise may discourage the child and leave the child with lower motivation for those same actions that were the focus for the praise. Adlerian theory points out that motivation derived from internal processes (intrinsic motivation) provides an advantage over motivation based on rewards (extrinsic motivation). External incentives have no intrinsic or logical relationship with one's actions. Motivation derived from such external incentives is likely to be fragile, to foster competitive rather than cooperative values, and to lead to cognitions and goals that do not help meet the demands of social living.

Empirical tests of these postulates are not easy to accomplish, because the advocated methods refer to long-term patterns of social interactions and not to immediate and specific task behaviors. Clinical case studies verify the Adlerian model, and numerous case illustrations are provided in books by Dreikurs (Dinkmeyer & Dreikurs, 1963; Dreikurs, 1992; Dreikurs & Cassel, 1990; Dreikurs & Grey, 1992; Dreikurs et al., 1998). These differ from brief experimental tests with performance conducted in less than an hour. One experiment, in which college students performed a simple reaction time task under praise, encouragement, performance feedback, or a control condition, found no significant performance differences between the conditions (Hunt, 1995). The lack of significant effects occurred apparently because this kind of simple performance on an unchallenging task did not arouse either extrinsic or intrinsic motivation.

Studies that use more long-term behaviors and that also compare parental behaviors with children's school performance provide more suitable tests. A study of fifth graders (Ginsburg & Bronstein, 1993) measured family patterns and parental style. Children from overcontrolling and undercontrolling family styles had an extrinsic motivational orientation in school and lower academic performance than did children whose family style involved encouragement and autonomy support. The latter group of children had an intrinsic motivational orientation in school and higher academic performance. The aim of that investigation was not to test the Adlerian approach, but the data nevertheless support Adlerian theory.

Deci's Approach. Unlike the Adlerian approach, which was derived from clinical data and personality theory, the work of Deci (1975) began with laboratory studies of college students. In one experiment (Deci, 1972), one group of participants was given no external reinforcers while persons in other groups received money and/or verbal reinforcement (praise, congratulations) for successfully solving puzzles by using cubes. Intrinsic motivation was measured by the amount of time the participants spent on the puzzle activity when they did not think the experimenter was observing them. The results showed that awarding money for correct solutions significantly decreased the amount of free-time activity when the participants thought they were not observed. Praise slightly decreased the activity for women but increased (although not significantly) the activity for men. The effects of praise were thus somewhat ambiguous, but the effect of money was clear, in showing that external reinforcement decreased intrinsic motivation for task performance. A 1973 study by Deci, Cascio, and Krusell (cited in Deci & Ryan, 1991) further tested whether men and women differ when receiving verbal reinforcement, and the results were significant, with women decreasing their intrinsically motivated activity after receiving verbal positive feedback and men increasing theirs.

Early in his work on intrinsic motivation Deci

(1975) formulated what he called a "cognitive evaluation theory." Because in a real-world field setting as well in laboratory studies Deci found that extrinsic rewards can decrease intrinsically motivated activities, he suggested that this is due to a change in appraised locus of causality. At the outset, participants engage in certain behaviors because of internal rewards, like feeling competent. But if the individuals later receive money and further engage in the activity, they will come to believe they are doing the activity (the locus of causality) for external and not internal reasons, and this diminishes the previous intrinsic motivation. Thus, Deci proposed that a person's evaluation of the cause or source of the action affects how external rewards alter motivation and action.

The way Deci conceptualized intrinsic motivation was related to but not the same as the way Adlerians conceptualized it. Dreikurs (1992; Dreikurs et al., 1998) emphasized inner satisfactions, such as interest in the task or activity itself (like the joy in learning or playing music), pleasure in the belief that one can contribute, or satisfaction in the act of helping. In contrast, Deci (1975) did not focus on the prosocial dimension, but instead he considered a sense of "competence and self-determination" as the basis for intrinsically motivated activities. Deci posited that extrinsic rewards will decrease intrinsic motivation activities due to a change in locus of causality when the *controlling* aspect of rewards is most salient. Because rewards provide information as well as signify external control, when the *informational* aspect is most salient, as in many cases of positive feedback or praise, the person's sense of competence will increase, and in that case the intrinsically motivated activity will not be decreased by the extrinsic reinforcement.

In his later writings Deci (Deci & Ryan, 1991) was more concerned with self-determination, actual as well as subjectively appraised self-determination. Going beyond a mere emphasis on inner sources, he noted that a *self-determining inner source* was the basis for intrinsic motivation. Intrinsic motivation was not activated merely because inner sources were involved. According to his later conceptualization, if internal pressures or compulsions, or "socially acquired introjects" (Deci &

Ryan, 1991, p. 238), rather than well-integrated self-determination led to the motivated behavior, the action would not be intrinsically motivated. Studies on the effects of self-determination have found social context and cognitive variables to affect internalizing processes (Deci, Eghrari, Patrick, & Leone, 1994). With this emphasis on self-determination, how much the person feels controlled is the most important issue. In Deci's later writings, the point is made that if the person feels an internal necessity or duty rather than a sense of free choice or self-determination, this does not signify what is meant by intrinsic motivation.

Empirical Tests of Deci's Theory. A number of studies tested Deci's cognitive evaluation theory with field as well as laboratory experiments. Some studies supported the theory and others did not.

Variations in procedure can create problems for verifying Deci's theory. For example, in an important early study, Deci (1971) introduced an extrinsic incentive for the experimental participants after an initial no-reward session, by telling them before their *second* session that they would get money for correctly solving the puzzles. Both the control and experimental groups spent considerable time working on their puzzles in the free period that immediately followed the first no-reward session. This indicated considerable intrinsic motivation in both groups. Following the second session, the experimental participants spent far more time working on puzzles in the free period than did the control participants, which would suggest that extrinsic incentives heightened rather than diminished intrinsic motivation. However, the reverse was true. When in the *third* session both groups were given puzzles without an extrinsic incentive, the control group worked a long time on puzzles in the free period whereas the experimental group markedly dropped their postsession free-period puzzle work. Table 9.1 reveals the different free-period puzzle times. It is evident that giving the experimental subjects an extrinsic incentive led to their increasing their free-period activity only when they believed they were going to receive an external reward. When later they had no extrinsic incentive, they decreased their free-period activity, falling below the activity level

TABLE 9.1
Mean Number of Seconds Working on the Puzzles in the Free Period

	After 1st session	After 2nd session	After 3rd session
Experimental group	248.2	313.9	198.5
Control group	213.9	202.7	241.8

Source: Based on data from Deci, 1971.

of the control group. The control group that never received an extrinsic incentive maintained a steady level of intrinsically satisfying activity.

Had the second-session free-period puzzle work been used as the critical measure of intrinsic motivation in this study, one would have concluded that an extrinsic incentive increases intrinsic motivation. One would not have known that later when the extrinsic incentive is absent, intrinsic motivation (measured by free-period puzzle work) was markedly diminished by the second-session extrinsic incentive. Thus, to test whether an extrinsic incentive decreases intrinsic motivation, the critical response measure is not the one taken in the free-choice period during which the extrinsic incentive is offered. Care must be taken to use the appropriate measures.

Studies continue to assess if external rewards diminish intrinsic motivation. In one investigation the researchers (Overskeid & Svartdal, 1996) assigned participants to do a task in one of six conditions. These differed according to whether the participants were simply told to do the puzzles or were given a choice about doing the puzzle, and whether they received a high, low, or no monetary reward for doing the puzzle. All groups had 20 minutes to work on the puzzles. Then they had a free period in which their puzzle activity was observed. They also were asked to rate on a visual analog scale from 0 to 100 to what extent they felt it was their "own choice" whether to do the puzzle during the experiment. A high rating for this item would represent a strong subjective feeling of self-determination or autonomy. Figure 9.2 shows the mean subjective autonomy ratings for the six groups.

Overskeid and Svartdal (1996) conducted two

FIGURE 9.2
Subjective autonomy as a function of choice and reward.

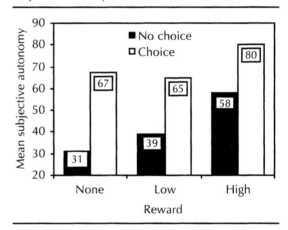

Source: From Overskeid & Svartdal, 1996, p. 327.

experiments. The data overall showed that (a) autonomy ratings and ratings of interest in the task were not correlated significantly, (b) interest ratings were not significantly affected by reward, and (c) the groups with the high reward gave high subjective autonomy ratings. The researchers concluded that the data did not support Deci's formulation. What is not known is how the participants would have reacted following a later nonrewarded session, comparable to Session 3 in the Deci (1971) study. Would the rewarded participants have markedly reduced autonomy ratings, interest ratings, and free-period activity if later these individuals were to do the task *without* an extrinsic incentive? Although reward led to high ratings of autonomy during the reward session in the above investigation, this session was analogous to Deci's (1971) second session. How people react if nonreward follows reward is a crucial question, especially when they are compared with individuals who perform tasks without any offer of extrinsic incentive. Advocates who point out the negative effects of reward (e.g., Dreikurs, 1992) argue that one of the noticeable impairing effects of reward occurs at a later time when the person is to perform a task without any extrinsic incentives.

Deci's intrinsic motivation hypotheses were supported by some laboratory studies and by some field investigations. One field study that found support for them (Jordan, 1986) gave workers a job survey that measured internal work motivation similar to Deci's intrinsic motivation. Over a period of a few months, a significant difference was found between groups: Workers who received a monetary bonus incentive that was contingent on job performance showed decreased intrinsic motivation; workers who received a promised bonus that was not tied to job performance showed an increase in intrinsic motivation.

A laboratory study by Koestner, Zuckerman, and Koestner (1987) with college students varied test conditions and also the kind of praise that was given. The concern here was to assess if different kinds of praise had similar effects, and the answer was "no." Subjects received one of two test conditions, either ego involvement or task involvement. In the former, participants were told the test measures creative intelligence, and in the latter they were told only that they would be working on a puzzle, with no reference made to intelligence testing. Under each test condition there were three groups. One was a control group who received no praise, one group received praise that focused on the participant's ability, and another group received praise that focused on the participant's effort. Following their completing a hidden-figure puzzle task, the participants were left alone in the room, just as was done in Deci's studies, with reading material available and also additional puzzle tasks similar to the one they had just completed. The participants were unobtrusively observed, and the number of seconds they spent working on unused puzzles in the free-choice period provided the measure of intrinsic mo-

tivation. Several results were obtained. One was replication of the gender differences in intrinsic motivation noted already (and cited in Deci & Ryan, 1991). Women tended to show more free-choice puzzle activity when not given praise and men showed more free-choice puzzle activity when given praise.

Of importance to the Deci formulation were the other findings. The control subjects under both ego- and task-involving conditions spent on the average 120 seconds on the puzzles in the free-choice time. Persons who received ability-focused praise spent a mean of 270 seconds under the ego-involving, and 295 seconds in the task-involving conditions, and the group given effort-focused praise spent little time (mean of 52 seconds) under the ego-involvement condition but spent quite a long time (mean of 229 seconds) under the task-involvement condition. As predicted by theories that emphasize the efficacy of intrinsic motivation (both Adlerian theory and Deci's cognitive evaluation theory), task involvement, overall, led to more intrinsic motivation than did ego involvement. Ability-focused praise enhanced intrinsic motivation under both task- and ego-involvement conditions, whereas for subjects given effort-focused praise, the test conditions were crucial, intrinsic motivation dropping markedly under ego involvement but not under task involvement. Thus, a significant interaction was found between the kind of praise the subjects received and the kind of task conditions in which they thought they were engaging. The researchers considered this finding to support Deci's postulation, that when persons feel themselves to be competent they are more likely to be intrinsically motivated. Unfortunately, the problem of appropriate measurement prevents a firm conclusion. Praise for ability could be detrimental, after all, because intrinsic motivation could still drop if the participants later were to perform the task without praise. The Koestner et al. (1987) study provided no data on that point. Theorists like Dreikurs (1992) would predict that if the persons in both types of praise groups were to perform the task later without praise, their intrinsic motivation would decrease relative to the control group.

Additional Perspectives

An issue that arises with predictions about extrinsic incentives and intrinsic motivation concerns the relationship between motivation and performance. Changes in performance do not necessarily mirror changes in motivation. Another issue is whether different measures of motivation are related to one another. Some studies questioned whether interest in a task and a free-choice activity mirror the same underlying motivation. As found in the investigation by Overskeid and Svartdal (1996), ratings of interest and autonomy that had been presumed to be related were in fact not significantly related. How various measures of motivation are related to one another and to performance are crucial issues explored by many investigators.

Relationship Between Motivation and Performance.

Some studies found that when interest in a task is improved, so also is performance. For example, an investigation of computer-based learning with schoolchildren (Lepper & Cordova, 1992) found that performance and learning were significantly increased when intrinsic motivation was heightened. Questions remain, however. Do extrinsic incentives have a different effect on intrinsic motivation than they do on performance? Also, are the effects of intrinsic motivation on performance different than the effects of extrinsic incentives on performance?

An investigation of preschool children (McCullers, Fabes, & Moran, 1987) provides useful findings. An extrinsic incentive (a promised toy) had an adverse effect on immediate drawing performance, but when the children were shifted back from reward to nonreward their performance again improved. One interpretation of these data is that performance reflects various motivational factors, only one of which is intrinsic task motivation. Although performance dropped, intrinsic motivation could have remained high. Another interpretation, which is not congruent with Deci's original formulation but still plausible, is that a temporary lowering occurs for both intrinsic motivation as well as performance during the time when extrinsic incen-

tives are given. Already by preschool age, children have well-developed beliefs about the relationship between extrinsic incentives, effort, and memory. O'Sullivan (1993) found in one study that 4-year-old children believe that recall increases with effort and that a strong incentive compared with a weak one leads to higher effort and to greater recall of learned material. In a related study, she found that children of this age make more effort and pay more attention to the stimuli they are to remember when the extrinsic incentive is desirable versus when it is a nonfavored prize.

Because high effort is required for effective performance on many tasks, the way extrinsic incentives relate to beliefs about effort and task requirements is likely to have an important bearing on whether extrinsic incentives improve motivation and performance. Although young children believe that a desirable versus low-value incentive leads to high effort and to better recall and performance, by the time of adulthood an individual may have different (possibly cynical) beliefs. For example, if a person believes that for easy tasks rewards are more attainable and that low payoffs are given for performance on easy tasks (versus high payoffs for difficult tasks), then the person may exert more effort for a task that offers a low, compared with a high, extrinsic reward. This was found to occur in one investigation with university students. The researcher (Svartdal, 1993) suggested that because people learn incentive-effort beliefs, these will mediate the amount of effort people exert on tasks offering external incentives.

Factors that alter motivation need not alter performance, and vice versa. The processes by which extrinsic rewards can alter motivation and by which they can affect performance depend in part on the immediate context of the task, the individual's motivational dispositions and overall state, and the total circumstances in which the performance occurs. For example, Miller and Hom (1990) gave college students either solvable or unsolvable tasks and then anagrams to unscramble. Extrinsic rewards minimized performance decrements after failure on tasks that were given under high ego-involving conditions but not on tasks given under low ego-involving conditions. The authors suggest that extrinsic incentives can reduce ego involvement and preoccupation with personal esteem and thus can increase approach motivation after failure on ego-relevant tasks. These authors suggest that for persons who feel threatened or have other maladaptive motivational states, extrinsic incentives may be useful to maintain performance and to maintain the motivation to approach rather than avoid tasks.

To perform well on tasks, individuals need to have an adequate grasp of task demands and to pay sufficient attention to relevant cues (Derryberry, 1993). They also need to have appropriate memory strategies. Extrinsic incentives can alter what one attends to and what one remembers. For example, Derryberry (1989) found that when participants played a video game in which pretarget cues were presented, attention to cues differed for positive and for negative incentives as a function not only of the immediate incentive on a given trial but also of the outcome of the immediately preceding trial.

Praise Can Have Many Meanings. Various writers have argued that extrinsic reinforcements, especially praise, are disruptive and decrease constructive effort for task accomplishments. From that perspective, individuals would be advised to seek internal rather than external rewards for incentive motivation. Several studies have been presented so far to show that one needs to consider the meaning that praise has for an individual. The Koestner et al. (1987) study showed that praise for ability has different effects than does praise for effort. The way people appraised the task (whether it does or does not signify an important personal characteristic, like intelligence), and thus how they appraised performance, altered the way praise affected intrinsic motivation. Other researchers have shown additional ways that the meaning persons give to praise is important. For example, if a person receives praise for an action, the person may believe that the individual giving the praise had low expectations regarding her or his accomplishments. This was found in research by Meyer (1992), who found that praise can have this paradoxical effect.

A different point of view was proposed by Baumeister and colleagues (Baumeister et al., 1990; Baumeister & Showers, 1986). They suggest that praise can make a person self-conscious and thus disrupt performance, especially on tasks requiring a high level of skill. Praise can exert pressure on a person, who may believe after receiving praise that subsequently only high levels of performance are acceptable. In one investigation (Baumeister et al., 1990) subjects received a task that required either effort or skill, and subjects received either praise ("good job") or no praise. The results showed that praise had opposite effects on performance, depending on whether the task involved primarily effort or primarily skill. For effort-relevant tasks praise improved performance, but for skill-relevant tasks performance was impaired following receipt of praise. In this study the task demanded effort or skill, and that is not the same as the effort-based or ability-based praise described in the Koestner et al. (1987) study. It is important to note that what is demanded by the task can be very different from the qualities for which one is praised.

Whether praise improves performance is a different question from whether praise increases or decreases intrinsic motivation. When praise increases a person's efforts, praise nevertheless may impair performance if increased effort interferes with task requirements. Moreover, praise has many possible meanings, and the incentive value of praise will not be the same for all persons and for all circumstances. How praise is given, what words are used to convey the praise, and who gives the praise are important considerations. When incentives, including praise, are given as rewards following actions, they can serve to affirm one's self-concept. They can also give information about one's performance independently of self-concept. That is, rewards can alter one's self-esteem or merely give performance feedback. Because money, praise, and various other rewards have diverse symbolic meanings, these meanings will alter in complex ways how extrinsic incentives become sources of incentive motivation. What can be interpreted as praise in one situation can as readily be interpreted as criticism or even insult in another situation. Moreover, praise coming from someone who is not esteemed or who is not considered to have good judgment will have very different meaning from praise given by an esteemed person whose judgment one respects. Thus because many factors affect both motivation and performance, simple conclusions about the effectiveness of extrinsic versus intrinsic incentives, or about the usefulness of praise, are not possible.

Incentive Value Learning.   The meaning that incentives have was shown to be important for both children and adults. Learning of incentive values and of incentive-action sequences is not limited to human beings, however. In a simple way, incentive learning can be demonstrated for animals. According to Dickinson and Balleine (1994, 1995), two processes mediate the way internal motivation directs instrumental actions in rats, and incentive learning is one of these processes. The incentive learning in rats occurs by associating a given reward, which follows instrumental responding, with an internal motivational state. The more the reward is appropriate to the internal state (like sucrose solution to a hungry animal), the more incentive value it has and the more the animal will make instrumental responses for that reward. Less instrumental responding occurs when the reward is not appropriate to the internal motivational state.

For human motivation, one needs to consider the symbolic nature of the reward, the experience one has had with the reward (e.g., Maki, Overmier, Delos, & Gutmann, 1995), the conditions under which the reward is sought, and the many beliefs the person holds that affect the meaning of the reward (e.g., Longstreth, 1972). When human actions are rewarded, what is involved is not only the reward but the social interaction between "giver" and "receiver." The rewarding process thus involves human interactions and thereby also human relationships. For many psychologists, close relationships involving extrinsic rewards are not ideal. Dreikurs (1971/1992) pointed out that rewards belong to an autocratic mentality and are not appropriate in democratic and egalitarian relationships, and Kohn (1993) considered that rewards rupture relationships.

For humans, incentive learning is enormously complex and may differ for praise, money, or gifts.

The social context and social symbol of an incentive affects a person's behavior in a significant way (Dougherty & Cherek, 1994). In one study (Ferguson & Schmitt, 1988), strategies of cooperation or competition determined the amount of points a player gained in a simulated marketing game. College students played against a presumed person, though in fact the "person" was a computer. The study demonstrated that how many points were won was significantly dependent on whether the players believed the other person was a woman or a man.

The social and emotional meaning of money or how a gift is given has a bearing on its motivational and behavioral consequence. Because of the symbolic and social learning associated with praise, money, prizes, or other extrinsic incentives, predictions of how extrinsic incentives alter motivation and performance in humans requires knowledge of many additional variables that go beyond the simple reinforcers or incentives studied with nonhuman animals.

Incentives, Success and Failure, and the Achievement Motive

Many incentives are not concrete objects or verbal messages from others. Some incentives already discussed regarding intrinsic motivation are emotional outcomes, like feeling happy that one could help another person. Others are tied directly to action, as action outcomes.

Success and failure on a task refer to performance levels, but the concepts of what is success and what is failure are based on comparisons with some standard or ideal. A given score on a test, for example, can indicate successful performance when it is the maximum score possible, or if far from the maximum, when 95% of other test takers score far lower. Somewhat similarly, inner satisfaction or its absence can be related directly to the way performance compares with a specific standard or criterion. The 5-year-old riding a two-wheel bicycle, who falls off on the first attempt but after a half hour of practice manages to stay on the bike for some minutes, is likely to evaluate staying on the bike without falling as a great success. In contrast, a person who has ridden for many years would think that if she or he was able to stay on the bike for only a few minutes this would be a decided failure.

Success and *failure* represent judgments about performance outcomes in achievement situations, and as judgments they are influenced by objective criteria as well as subjective evaluations. A judgment of successful performance for a 5-year-old is likely to be evaluated as failure for a 25-year-old. The college student in an introductory-level foreign language class may consider the translation of a paragraph to be a success, but after 4 years of foreign language classes, if this were the student's maximum performance it likely would be judged a failure. In the same way that many factors contribute to the judgment of success and failure, so do many factors contribute to the *incentive value* of success and of failure. One person may judge that having many friends represents a valued attainment, whereas another person would not consider this significant and instead values success in high work achievement.

A group of researchers between the 1950s and the 1980s studied motivational dispositions toward success and failure in achievement tasks. The motivational disposition was construed to be like a trait, remaining stable throughout a person's lifetime. This area of research was initiated by McClelland (1961; McClelland, Atkinson, Clark, & Lowell, 1953; McClelland, Clark, Roby, & Atkinson, 1949), whose work on the relationship between the power motive and alcohol drinking (McClelland, 1973) was presented in a previous chapter. Although McClelland studied the power motive extensively, he is best known for his work on the achievement motive.

Achievement Motivation Theory: McClelland and Atkinson

The theory of achievement motivation sought to explain the relationship between society, individual motivation, and behavior in achievement situations (McClelland, 1955, 1961). Individuals with a high achievement motivation disposition are likely to have been trained as children to be independent. Their parents are likely to have set moderately high standards and to show confidence in the child's ability to succeed. High achievement motivation dispositions are established by the time the children enter school, and such children are more optimistic and have a more realistic appraisal of their own performance than do children with a low achievement motivation disposition.

What Is Achievement Motivation? A former student and later colleague of McClelland, Atkinson (1964) distinguished between an active motivation and a motive, saying that a learned disposition to achieve is the "achievement motive." A person with a high achievement motive takes pride in accomplishments and seeks and enjoys success. This stable disposition is learned from the way parents raise the child, and the disposition remains through adulthood. Although the achievement *motive* is a tendency for the individual to seek success in achievement, the tendency becomes aroused into an *active motivation* only in certain types of situations. These involve (a) moderate, rather than high or low, likelihood of success, (b) the success must be a result of the person's own efforts, and (c) feedback regarding successful performance is given promptly.

Certain characteristics identify the person with a high achievement motive. The person is a moderate risk taker and prefers medium risks over extremely high or extremely low risks. Because the person with a high need to achieve is seeking successful performance by means of his or her own effort, this person is motivated more intrinsically than extrinsically. Important for the person with a high achievement motive is performance feedback, not extrinsic incentives.

The original theory of achievement motivation was based on the personality theory of Henry Murray (1938), who developed a well-known projective test known as the Thematic Apperception Test (the TAT). The theory of Murray covered various needs, of which achievement was one. The latter was designated *nAch,* and for this reason "nAch theory" is the way achievement motivation theory is sometimes described.

The achievement motive was originally measured by the number of achievement themes occurring in stories a person tells about pictures like those used in the TAT. Other types of measurements based on self-report were developed later, but they were found to measure different processes than the original nAch studied by McClelland (McClelland, Koestner, & Weinberger, 1989). McClelland et al. (1989) identified the achievement motive studied on the basis of projective test stories as an *implicit* motive, which is related to spontaneous behavioral trends over a long time period. The long-term behavioral trends occur because pleasure is derived from the achievement activity itself.

Success-seeking Versus Failure-avoiding. Atkinson (1964) distinguished between success seeking and failure avoiding. Although in later years Atkinson (Atkinson & Birch, 1970, 1978) developed a dynamic action theory that differed from his early formulations, his earlier focus on the difference between success seeking and failure avoiding helped to identify an important difference between achievement motivation and test-taking anxiety. In situations of challenge and testing, some individuals thrive while others are very anxious. He considered it important to assess individuals on both the achievement motive projective test and the test-anxiety paper-and-pencil test, and then he compared two kinds of persons. One kind was the person who scored *high* on the nAch projective test and who scored *low* on test-taking anxiety. The other kind was the person who had low nAch and high test-taking anxiety. The two groups differed significantly in the way success and failure served as incentives. Whereas the first group was found actively to seek success, the second group was found instead to *seek to avoid failure*. The first group was not motivated to avoid failure.

Atkinson (1964) postulated that to predict a person's behavior in an achievement situation one needs to measure both opposing tendencies, of failure avoidance and success seeking, and to subtract one tendency from the other, which yields a net or resultant tendency. The resulting tendency determines how the person behaves in an achievement situation. The tendency to seek success (T_s) is a function of the success-seeking motive, the probability of success, and the incentive value of success, and this is described by the equation $T_s = M_S \times P_s \times I_s$ (Atkinson, 1964, p. 242). The tendency to avoid

failure (T_{-f}) is a function of the failure-avoiding motive, the probability of failure, and the incentive value of failure, and this is described by the equation $T_{-f} = M_{AF} \times P_f \times I_f$. The motive is measured by scores on either the achievement test (M_S) or the anxiety test (M_{AF}), P is the expectancy or probability estimate of either success (P_s) or failure (P_f), and I is the incentive value of either obtaining success (a positive outcome, I_s) or of avoiding failure (a negative outcome, I_f). Atkinson (1964, p. 244) suggested that $I_f = -P_s$, which means that the tendency to avoid failure has a relationship to task difficulty. A difficult task (that is, one with a low P_s) also has a low negative incentive value of failure, so that failing at a difficult task is less humiliating than failing at an easy task.

Although the original research defined probability and incentive values in objective terms, like a roll of dice determining probability and money defining the value of the incentive, it became clear that probability and incentive are also defined subjectively. Individuals differ in how they subjectively interpret objective probabilities of success and failure (Atkinson, 1957, 1964). For example, individuals with a high resultant achievement seeking are likely to interpret an objective probability of success of .5 more optimistically as a subjective probability of .67, whereas individuals with a high resultant fear of failure would be likely to interpret that more pessimistically, as a subjective probability of success of .33.

Many studies found support for the main principles outlined by Atkinson and McClelland, and later studies amplified and clarified the theory (Covington & Omelich, 1991; Humphreys & Revelle, 1984). Support was found especially for the postulation that performance differs for success-seeking compared with failure-avoiding persons. Many kinds of performance measures have found differences between these types of individuals, including risk taking and academic performance, and these types of individuals also differ in the way they make attributions about successful and failing performance. Risk-taking differences are described here, and attributions are discussed in the next chapter.

Early research (Atkinson, 1958) found that children in a ring-toss game differed in where they stood to play according to their achievement motive. Those with high achievement motivation (wanting to do well by means of their own effort in a challenging task) stood about midway from the peg, whereas those with low achievement motivation either stood very far from the peg (thus making the task inordinately difficult and making failure less humiliating) or very close to the peg (thus minimizing the probability of failure). Medium risk taking has several benefits. One is that the task is challenging, with success not assured, yet when it occurs it is due to one's efforts and not the result of the task being too easy. Another benefit is that one is realistic and does not court failure, as happens when one consistently tackles very difficult tasks whose probability of success is low. Later research confirmed that success-seeking and failure-avoiding individuals differ in their risk taking, their responsiveness to external incentives, and their preference for which types of activities they undertake (Blankenship, 1987; Covington & Omelich, 1991).

Covington and Omelich (1991) extended the success-seeking and failure-avoiding conceptualization by showing that these two tendencies are sufficiently independent to justify a quadrapolar rather than a bipolar model. By assessing individuals in terms of being high or low on each dimension, these researchers discovered, for example, that persons who are high in both approach and avoidance tendencies have unique characteristics. They are both highly anxious and highly achievement oriented in their strivings. Covington and Omelich call them "overstrivers" and indicate that these individuals have considerable intrapsychic conflict. Persons who are low in both approach and avoidance tendencies are called "failure acceptors." As students they tend to have poor study skills which, however, do not make them anxious. These researchers found behavioral and attitudinal patterns that strongly support the Atkinson-McClelland formulation for resultant success-seeking (high nAch and low anxiety) and resultant failure-avoidance (high anxiety and low nAch) individuals.

Achievement Performance, Achievement Motivation, and Beliefs About Achievement. Two important points are that *achievement motivation* is not the same as *achievement performance,* and in some situations persons with a high achievement motive may not have achievement motivation aroused, so that they do not exert strong effort to achieve successful performance. An example of the second point was found in a study by Raynor (1970). He gave college students in an introductory psychology class an nAch test, a test-anxiety questionnaire, and a questionnaire that asked the students to indicate the degree to which they considered a good grade in the course to be important for their future career. At the end of the semester, when grades were analyzed for the students in terms of achievement motives, interesting results were obtained. Those whose motive to achieve success was greater than their motive to avoid failure ($M_S > M_{AF}$) had higher grades in the course than did students with the opposite motives ($M_{AF} > M_S$), but this occurred only for students who considered a good grade in the course important to their future career. For students who did not consider a good grade in the course important for their future career, the achievement motive orientation did not have a significant effect. Thus, a significant interaction was found between the student's achievement tendency and degree to which the task (the course and course grade) was instrumental in attainment of long-range success. The conclusion is warranted that achievement motivation was aroused for the ($M_S > M_{AF}$) persons who considered the course important for future success but was not aroused for those with a different belief about the instrumentality of the course. This confirms a view proposed by Raynor (1969), that the motivation to strive for success in a task is a joint function of immediate and future events.

Regarding the distinction between achievement motivation and attained achievement in performance, a study by Atkinson and O'Connor (1966) is relevant. These researchers demonstrated that extrinsic incentives can alter immediate motivation and achievement performance for persons with a resultant tendency for failure avoidance. Extrinsic incentives led to their having high achievement, even though their achievement motive was low. Atkinson and O'Connor found that for persons with a *low* achievement motive and low resultant tendency to seek achievement success, extrinsic motivation provided by strong extrinsic incentives like money or social approval help them attain high performance. The high achievement of these individuals is not due to high achievement motivation but to extrinsic incentives raising immediate motivation and effort output.

This bears on the work of Miller and Hom (1990), whose study (described earlier) showed that when failure was experienced under ego-involving conditions, extrinsic incentives can increase performance by counteracting the withdrawal that otherwise would occur after ego involved failure experiences. For a wide range of circumstances, actual high achievement may occur in the absence of achievement motivation as defined by activated high nAch. Both extrinsic and intrinsic incentives need to be considered when predicting performance involving actual achievement, and this is especially so under challenging circumstances (Atkinson, 1983, see pp. 147–163).

There are a wide range of circumstances under which nAch and performance may not be congruent. For example, persons with a *high* achievement motive may not attain high achievement performance due to lack of talent, lack of experience, or characteristics of the task and other handicapping situational factors. Equally, persons with a *low* achievement motive may attain very high achievement performance due to high talent, vast experience, or facilitating characteristics of the task and other enabling situational factors. Thus, actual achievement and achievement motivation need to be distinguished. One can have high achievement as performance and not have high "need for achievement" and, likewise, one can have a high "need for achievement" yet not achieve a high performance in a given situation.

The Atkinson-McClelland theory of achievement motivation had a far-reaching influence on studies of achievement motivation and achievement performance. Contemporary research provided additional considerations, particularly emphasizing various kinds of cognitions and how these alter achievement strivings after the person has encountered success or failure experiences. For example, Dweck (1991; G. D. Heyman & Dweck, 1992) emphasized that people differ in terms of a *mastery*

compared with a *helpless* orientation, and they differ in terms of a *learning* goal versus a *performance* goal. Learning goals are associated with intrinsic motivation, and performance goals, which emphasize the evaluation of being competent, tend to diminish intrinsic motivation. Thus strivings for success and reactions to failure will differ, depending on the person's self-concept and goal.

The traditional Atkinson-McClelland achievement motivation theory identified individual differences in motive disposition concerning striving for success in achievement situations. The theory also described some of the situational variables that arouse achievement motivation in persons whose motive disposition was for a high achievement. Later writers sought to identify individual differences concerning people's reaction to success and failure in achievement situations. Emphasizing cognitive processes, later formulations focused on the types of causal reasoning or attributions people use when they encounter success or failure in achievement situations. The relationship between the motive disposition to achieve and cognitions about achievement continues to be an important area of research.

Expectancy-Value Theory and Success and Failure

The Atkinson-McClelland theory began with a focus on learned individual differences in motive disposition, and *expectancy* (probability of success or failure) and *value* (incentive of success or failure) constructs were added later. What then finalized as the Atkinson-McClelland achievement motivation theory related motive disposition with situational factors that involved the probability and the attractiveness of incentives, and for this reason the theory sometimes is identified as *expectancy-value* theory. Other expectancy-value formulations were derived from the Atkinson-McClelland theory, and the work of Feather illustrates one of these. Formulations that refer to expectancy about incentives, such as *locus of control* of reinforcement (Rotter, 1966) and *attribution* theory (Weiner, 1986, 1991), are presented in the next chapter.

For many years, Feather (1961, 1965, 1988, 1991, 1992, 1995) has studied expectation and value. The variables of expectation and value bear on the relationships among incentives, motivation, and performance. A person's expectation for successful or failing performance is partly dependent on the motive disposition of the person. In an early study, Feather (1965) found a difference in estimates of the likelihood of successful anagram solving between those persons who were high in nAch and low in test anxiety and those who were low in nAch and high in test anxiety. When subjects were given anagrams that they were told were moderately difficult, persons with a high achievement motive and low anxiety gave higher estimates of successful task completion than did individuals with the reverse motivational dispositions.

In another study (Feather & Simon, 1971) subjects worked on anagrams in same-sex pairs, and they were to make a number of ratings and estimates about their own performance and the performance of the other person in the pair. Difficulty of the task was manipulated by the experimenters so that half the subjects would experience success and half would experience failure on the task. There were many findings regarding reactions to one's own performance and reactions to the other person's performance. A main finding concerned the way a person's success or failure affected her or his own satisfaction ratings. The researchers anticipated and found that satisfaction with one's performance was much higher after a success than after a failure experience. However, contrary to what the researchers anticipated, the subjects' *expectation of success or of failure* did not alter their satisfaction ratings. The ratings were not higher for success when it was unexpected (versus when it was expected), nor lower for failure when the failure was unexpected. Other studies had found that satisfaction with one's performance was affected by whether success (or failure) had been expected. The researchers hypothesized that when expectations and satisfaction ratings are based on several experiences, as occurred in the Feather and Simon study, actual task performance could mask the way expectancy of success or failure affects satisfaction with one's performance attainment.

In later studies, Feather (1988) was not only concerned with the relationships among achievement motive, success and failure experiences, and performance expectations, but he focused increasingly

on subjective values and how they affect action. In his earlier work Feather focused on values of incentives in line with the studies of Atkinson. In his later formulations Feather conceptualized values far more broadly, as beliefs of what is important and of what ought to occur. He theorized that values function as motives. For Feather, values can be verbalized and are an important part of one's self-concept. Values represent how good or desirable, or bad and undesirable, an object or circumstance is, and from such values the person develops specific valences. *Valence* is a term coined by a famous phenomenological and social psychologist, Kurt Lewin (1936), and the term designates how attractive or aversive an event or object is.

Feather conceptualized expectations broadly, to pertain either to subjective probabilities of success or failure for performance or to the outcome or incentive that follows the performance. In one study that assessed how values, valences, and performance expectations relate to decisions made by university students about their enrollment in course areas, Feather (1988) gave students questionnaire items. Some measured self-concept of ability in mathematics or English, others measured specific valence of mathematics and English, and some dealt with value about these two areas. For example, value items asked how important it was for the person to do well in mathematics, how much the activity gave enjoyment, and how much the activity was instrumental to reaching both long-term and short-term goals. More general and personal values were also measured. Feather found that mathematics ability and valence predict course enrollment in mathematics and science, and that mathematics ability and mathematics valence measures relate to each other positively. Certain general values also were found to relate to mathematics valence. English valence and English ability were less clearly related and not as dramatically predictive for course enrollment as was mathematics valence and ability. Overall, general *values* influenced specific *valences*. Feather (1988) also found that assumptions about one's ability (and thus likelihood of successful performance) in conjunction with valences influence actions, in this case, selection of course enrollments by university students.

Other studies have shown dramatic relationships

among general values, specific valences, and expectations about actions. For example, in one study a general expectancy variable called "control-optimism" represented expectations of unemployed people about finding a job (Feather, 1992). Job valence represented the attractiveness or desirability of finding a job. Job-seeking behavior was found to be positively related to job valence but unrelated to control-optimism. Values linked to the work ethic (measured by test items concerned with the work ethic) were positively associated with job valence, thus revealing that general values bear on specific valences and these affect specific actions.

From many sources, the cumulative evidence is that to some extent the expectancy of success or failure of one's action or performance bears on whether one takes an action or performs on some task. One's beliefs about the attractiveness (valence) of either the action or the consequence of the action also affects one's action or performance. The later work of Feather (1992, 1995) has pointed out that specific valences relate to more general values, and that these values are not only cognitions (beliefs or attitudes) but also have motivational consequences. Like needs, such as nAch, values can also be motivating because they can involve commitment and volition for specific actions.

One can make the following conclusions about rewards, incentives, motivation, and performance. Incentive motivation can be directed toward outcomes following one's actions, and these can be extrinsic or intrinsic incentives. How values relate to these is not yet fully clear. Most contemporary researchers in the field of intrinsic motivation advocate the advantages of intrinsic incentives for learning and they advocate that intrinsic incentives increase self-confidence. However, some researchers believe that the distinction between "extrinsic" and "intrinsic" is not always straightforward or dichotomous (Condry & Stokker, 1992). Expectations of whether one will succeed or fail in one's actions, the motive disposition one has about seeking success or avoiding failure, the attractiveness or aversiveness of the outcome following one's actions, and one's overall values (which include short-term and long-term events) are likely to shape one's motivation and actions at any given moment, and one's motivation and actions will vary in terms of the specific situation and specific task.

SUMMARY

Reward has potent and complex effects on behavior. Rewards can lead to learning of new behaviors, and they also can provide changes in performance and motivation without involving new learning. The Law of Effect of Thorndike stated that responses followed by a satisfier (reward) will tend to be increased on the next occasion and those followed by an annoying event (punishment) will tend to drop out, but this has been "truncated" so that the "Law" now refers only to the response-increasing effect of the reward.

Skinner based his theory and research on the effect of reward but replaced that term with *reinforcement*. Positive reinforcement refers to the way reward was used in the Law of Effect, and negative reinforcement refers to the removal of something painful or uncomfortable. Both positive and negative reinforcement are presumed to increase response probability. Skinner and colleagues used schedules of reinforcement that led to various types of response patterns. Reinforcement procedures were used in real-life applications and were called *behavior modification*.

Studies of the hedonic versus the associative aspects of reward showed that different brain areas mediate the rewarding (hedonic) effects on performance compared with the associative effects on learning and memory.

Praise does not have the same meaning or the same effect on behavior for all individuals, because cultural, symbolic, and personal experiences alter the way praise is interpreted by the individual.

Learned motivation based on hunger (deprivation) can be developed, but many more learned motivations are based on aversive pushes and on reward pulls. Although controversy exists whether a neutral stimulus gains reward value and becomes a conditioned reinforcer by pairing the neutral stimulus with a primary reinforcer like food, or whether instrumental responding is also necessary, considerable evidence indicates that instrumental responding is not necessary for the previously neutral stimulus to gain reward value and function as a conditioned reinforcer.

In studies with pigeons, rats, and small children, the magnitude of reward was shown to alter performance but not learning, whereas delay of reward was found to alter learning and memory. The delay-of-reinforcement gradient refers to the fact that shorter delays lead to stronger learning (and longer delays impair or prevent learning), but delays of up to 60 seconds have been found to lead to learning if the correct response is immediately marked with a neutral stimulus like a tone. Moreover, studies of the effect of strong concentrations of saccharin suggest that magnitude of reward may lead to learning and memory as well as to performance changes. For certain nonhuman primates and older humans, reward and its magnitude have cognitive and symbolic meaning, so that the effects are not comparable as they are for small children and nonprimates.

Self-stimulation studies with animals showed that rewarding effects of drugs involve activation of certain brain structures, a special one being the *mesocorticolimbic pathway.* The dopamine system plays an important role in the rewarding effects of many drugs of abuse. Not all drugs are abused or lead to addiction. It is important to distinguish substance use, substance abuse, and substance dependence. The dependence (addiction) may result from dysregulation of the brain reward system due to distress, and withdrawal symptoms may be a major source of distress, or the dependence may be more due to nervous system and brain reward changes that occur in addiction. Genetic, cellular, and molecular variables in substance abuse and dependence are being investigated.

Relief from stress (negative reinforcement) may instigate drug use and lead to drug abuse and addiction. Therapeutic methods that help the person develop improved methods of coping with real-life problems and learn effective stress management skills, as well as provide emotional and social support, have helped individuals overcome drug abuse and drug dependence.

Psychologists use the term *incentive* when reinforcers have motivational effects. Whereas some reinforcement theorists describe the effects of reinforcers in terms of mechanisms that preclude voli-

tion, conscious choices, or deliberative decisions, other researchers consider *cognitive* and *volitional* factors in the way reinforcements affect behavior and choices.

Internal outcomes can provide internal incentives, and incentive motivation of this type is called *intrinsic motivation.* When external outcomes provide external incentives, the incentive motivation is called *extrinsic motivation.* Practicing a musical instrument can involve intrinsic motivation, of seeking to obtain pleasure from the music, or extrinsic motivation, of seeking to obtain an award or money.

Many reinforcement theorists indicate that environmental controls and thus extrinsic factors, including reinforcement schedules, are all that are needed to maintain high levels of responding, and that internal processes are not important for high performance. In contrast, many social psychologists and personality theorists emphasize that humans need to have self-confidence and the appropriate motivation for attaining high levels of performance. The importance of relying on intrinsic factors was advocated by Adler and Dreikurs, Deci, and many others.

Deci proposed a *cognitive evaluation theory,* which stated that a person's evaluation of the source or cause of her or his action affects how external rewards alter motivation and action. When control is important, external rewards can diminish intrinsic motivation. Then, if a person believes the external rewards are responsible for some action, this can lessen intrinsic motivation and lower performance.

Deci focused on self-determination in his later writings. Whereas in his early work intrinsic motivation represented a wide range of inner causes for the motivation, in his later conceptualization intrinsic motivation occurs only when the inner source is self-determined without compulsion. Free time spent on a task has been used as a measure of intrinsic motivation; it has been found to be greatest when no external reward is provided. Problems of measurement can arise if the person believes that later an external reward will be offered. For a valid test of intrinsic motivation, the person needs to have no knowledge or belief about an external reward. Length of free time on a task would then show the strength of intrinsic motivation.

The relationship between effort and performance is important. In some circumstances, increased effort is not sufficient to raise performance. Thus, whether external rewards, like praise or money, do or do not improve human performance depends on many factors. If the task requires skill, praise may impair performance. This may be because the person focuses on increasing effort, which could interfere with task requirements. If the task requires effort, praise can improve performance.

As occurs in animal conditioning, with reward value depending on how closely the reward matches the ongoing motivation of the subject, external rewards can have low reward value if they don't match a person's intrinsic motivation. Mismatch can also lead to the external reward decreasing an incongruent intrinsic motivation. When a person strives to master a skill for the inner satisfaction of pride in accomplishment, external control by means of promise of money represents a mismatch with the intrinsic motivation. If the person does not have strong self-confidence, for example, such a mismatch can diminish the intrinsic motivation.

Success and failure in achievement situations are determined by both objective and subjective factors. Developed by McClelland and colleagues, achievement motivation theory has generated many studies, which show that some persons strive for success and others strive to avoid failure. Atkinson distinguished between the *motive* to achieve, which is a disposition, and the *motivation* to achieve, which is a motivational state activated in a given situation. The incentive value and the probability of success on a task were found to determine the strength of motivation in a given situation. Persons with high test-taking anxiety, by seeking to avoid failure, differ from persons with a high achievement motive, who strive to attain success.

The word *valence* is used to designate the attractiveness or aversiveness of an incentive. Feather, a former student of Atkinson, studied a person's *values* and considered them broader than the valences of incentives. The strength and type of value a person has can affect incentive valence, and Feather found that for out-of-work persons with a strong belief in the value of work (strong work ethic), the valence of looking for a job was positive and high.

Specific task characteristics, subjective and objective meanings of an incentive, motivational disposition, and expectations all affect the type and strength of incentive motivation and the way incentive motivation affects performance.

CHAPTER 10

Goals and Success-Failure Beliefs

The present chapter considers how goals, expectations, and beliefs about reward and success influence motivation and performance. One explanation for why incentives improve performance is that the promise of a reward prompts one to alter one's aspirations concerning the performance. Without a promised reward, one "may not care" how well one performs on a task. The performance standard toward which one strives may be fairly low. A reward that is contingent on attaining a high level of performance can prompt a person to raise her or his performance standard. Thus, the anticipation of reward in itself may not be the basis for improved performance, but the *link* between a *high performance standard* and the *reward* may be the reason for improved performance.

The promise of a reward merely for doing a task has generally been found not to lead to high levels of performance. However, when the promised reward is given only upon attaining a given performance standard, performance tends to be raised to meet that standard. Research has assessed whether the offered incentive changes the person's own aspiration for how well the person wants to do. Studies have also examined whether raising one's aspiration leads to increased effort and more effective task strategies.

GOALS, LEVEL OF ASPIRATION, AND LEVEL OF EXPECTATION

The Work of Kurt Lewin and Colleagues

Psychologists have long assumed that human goals are complex. For example, there are easy and hard goals, and short-term and long-term goals. Also, there are desirable goals that we do not expect to attain and desirable goals that we believe we can reach. As reviewed by Austin and Vancouver (1996), the term *goal* has many meanings. *Content* of goals refers to sought outcomes. Outcomes can be internal, like gaining knowledge or feeling healthy, or they can refer to one's relationship with the environment, like getting approval or advice from another person, or mastering a task or gaining fame. Goals also have *structure*, which refers to the interrelationships among one's goals. People have dominant goals and less important goals, and the interrelationships follow some pattern or structure. Goals also involve *planning and striving*. Overall, goals are cognitive representations of what one seeks to reach, obtain, or attain.

Conceptualizing goals in a different vein, Kurt Lewin and his colleagues (Lewin, Dembo, Festinger, & Sears, 1944) focused on performance goals, on what level of performance a person wished or anticipated. These researchers studied performance and goals while the person did the task. Goals were differentiated according to different levels. Researchers do not all agree on how best to label or conceptualize the different levels (e.g., Locke & Latham, 1990), but most agree that one level refers to wish or hope, usually called "level of aspiration." It is the performance we would *like* to attain. Another is "level of expectation," which is the performance we realistically *expect* to attain. Early researchers, like Preston and Bayton (1941), asked subjects to identify three levels of attainment: the most they hoped to attain, the least they expected to perform, and the performance they thought they would in fact do.

Goal levels can vary between the highest possible or maximum performance to the lowest performance level, which would represent deep failure if one were to perform that poorly. A highest level might be a fantasy or dream level, although this was not included by Lewin et al. (1944). For example, when small children say they want to be an astronaut or movie star or Hall of Fame home-run champion, they are describing such a fantasy or idealized performance level. A more probable level of wish or hope is what Lewin et al. (1944) called the level of aspiration (LA). The aspiration of "I wish to run the 3-minute-mile" would not be a fantasy for a fast runner who has a reasonable possibility of attaining that speed. LA represents what one might anticipate attaining with 25% to 10% probability. A lower performance level but one with a higher probability of attainment is called level of expectation (LE). Lewin et al. (1944, p. 364) identified this level as having approximately a 50% subjective probability. For example, "I wish to run a mile in 3 minutes, but realistically, at this stage of readiness, I expect to run a mile in 3.3 minutes" would represent a statement of expectation rather than of hope or wish for a runner.

Research on LA and LE examines the performance goals people set on specific tasks or for specific trials on a task. Various levels can be studied, including LA, LE, and lower levels (Locke & Bryan, 1968). For each goal level there is a certain objective as well as subjective probability for the attainment of that level of performance. Lewin et al. (1944) showed that levels of aspiration and expectation regarding upcoming performance represent combinations of valence (or desirability) and probability of attainment. A wished for LA has a higher valence but a lower probability of attainment than does an expected LE.

People do distinguish between level of aspiration and expectation. Even young children (e.g., Ferguson, 1958) can make the distinction between a *desired* (LA) and an *anticipated* (LE) performance attainment. Because LA represents a wish or hope of a desired performance attainment, one that is wanted but not very likely to occur, LA is char-

acteristically higher than is LE. Moreover, LA and LE change according to the level of one's actual performance. Although various relationships have been found between LA, LE, and performance, a typical pattern is that LA and LE rise when performance improves and drop when performance declines. Both LA and LE are sensitive to changes in performance over trials, but the reality-based LE is overall more sensitive to changes in performance, rising with success and falling with failure. Defensive patterns are also possible and have been observed (Greenberg, 1985), in which goal levels rise or fall inversely with performance.

When performance is determined by skill, LA and LE are likely to be influenced by performance, but when performance is determined by effort, performance is likely to be influenced by LA and LE. The relationship between goals and performance is reciprocal, with goals altering performance and performance altering goals. Factors like task variables are likely to affect the goal-performance relationship.

Other Research on Level of Aspiration and Level of Expectation

Researchers following up the work of Lewin et al. (1944) related LA to decision making (Siegel, 1957) and gave support to the view that aspiration level was a joint function of valence and probability. The formulation of Atkinson (1964), described in the previous chapter regarding the incentives of success and failure, was influenced by Lewin's conceptualization about the interaction of valence and probability.

To relate LA or LE to performance, a measure of goal discrepancy is sometimes used as an indicator of motivation. That measure compares the level of performance on a given trial with the LA or LE for the subsequent trial. For illustration, a person is told that 100 simple arithmetic problems will be given and the person is then asked to rate or verbally state an LA ("how many problems I would like to finish") and LE ("how many problems I think I can finish"). Then the person works on the problems for a preset time. Following that performance, the person is asked again for LA and LE for the next trial.

The comparison of performance on the first trial with the LA or LE for the second trial describes the _goal discrepancy_. Goal discrepancy indicates the motivation for the next trial, of how much the person seeks to improve on the next trial. Another measure compares the LA or LE with the subsequent performance. One can compare the pre-performance Trial 1 LA or LE with the actual performance on Trial 1. This represents a _performance discrepancy_ (called by Lewin et al. [1944] an "attainment discrepancy") measure, and it identifies how much the performance reaches the prior aspiration and expectation levels. Discrepancies have been used in many measures that study the motivational characteristics of goal setting, and controversy exists whether goals or goal discrepancies better measure motivation (Pervin, 1992).

Some individuals have a disposition to have a high positive goal discrepancy, of setting aspiration and expectation far ahead of actual performance, and others tend to have a low positive goal discrepancy, in which LA and LE are only slightly ahead of actual performance. Some people do not follow a characteristic pattern, but instead vary the amount of goal discrepancy according to the task and situation. The majority of individuals have a positive goal discrepancy (desiring and expecting to perform better on a subsequent than on a previous trial), but some people show a negative goal discrepancy, in which their LA and LE for future trials are lower than their actual performance on prior trials. That is not typical. A negative goal discrepancy can indicate an apparent "not caring" or can reveal a more deep discouragement. Whereas young adults tend to have a low positive goal discrepancy, among older adults, especially those over age 70, the patterns are somewhat different. Older adults are likely to be less optimistic and less sure of their ability to control events in their lives, and negative goal discrepancy scores, have been found (Gerrard, Reznikoff, & Riklan, 1982).

Although Lewin et al. (1944), Preston and Bayton (1941), and other early researchers distinguished between levels, more recent investigators unfortunately tend to use the terms _aspiration_ and _expectation_ interchangeably. Published studies may have one term in the title or in the abstract of the ar-

ticle, yet the procedure that was used actually pertained to the other term. To know whether a given study has assessed aspiration or expectation, one has to read the details of the method of the study and not rely merely on the descriptive words the author uses.

The specific type of rating or question that is asked of the subjects determines whether the person describes aspiration, expectation, or some quite different motivational variable. For example, in one investigation (Ferguson, 1962) college students were asked either to give an LA (how many items the subject would like to complete within the time limit) or a different kind of measure that indicated the subjects' amount of ego involvement in the task. The measure, called EI_R, asked subjects how interested they were in doing well on the task. Whereas LA was a specified desired level of attainment, EI_R was a self-disclosure regarding the strength of the desire to do well, without identifying exactly what the subject thought "doing well" was. Both motivational measures tapped into an overall aspiration regarding future performance, but one (LA) specified the performance level and one (EI_R) did not. The subtle difference in wording was significant, and the data likewise revealed a significant difference.

The subjects in that investigation were given either success or failure conditions by being allowed enough time to finish approximately 70% or only enough time to finish 40% of 50 digit-substitution items. Half the individuals in each group also received high ego-involvement instructions (that the task is an intelligence test and indicates likelihood of career success) or low ego-involvement instructions (that the task is only just being developed and individual scores cannot be adequately evaluated). The subjects made their initial ratings after the ego-involvement instructions but before they performed the task, and they made ratings again after they worked on the task and had experienced either success or failure. The results showed that persons in the success condition raised their LA slightly and those in the failure condition greatly dropped their LA from preperformance to postperformance ratings, and the difference between success and failure was highly significant. In contrast, the EI_R measure did not show a significant increase or decrease as a function of success and failure, and what EI_R difference occurred between success and failure was opposite to the LA measure. The EI_R increased slightly rather than decreased when subjects experienced failure.

Another study in that investigation (Ferguson, 1962) used only the failure condition and subjects were tested just prior to taking a course examination. As in the other study, LA dropped significantly after failure, compared with preperformance level, but EI_R remained relatively stable. Thus, when aspiration is measured as an explicitly stated desired level of attainment (LA), actual performance influences the subsequent desired attainment level. However, when aspiration is measured in a more global way (EI_R, or how interested one is in doing well) and "success" is not explicitly defined, ratings are not altered markedly by prior performance. Within limits, regardless of how well or poorly one does, one's interest in doing well on the task remains fairly stable. Table 10.1 presents the mean ratings for LA and EI_R for scales in which subjects rate LA as well as EI_R from 0 to 50, and 50 is the maximum possible performance on a trial.

Data from the above study show that the type of question subjects are asked makes a significant difference in terms of what aspect of aspiration is tapped. Aspiration is complex, and the precise words used to define it play an important role in measuring it. A study with 5- to 10-year old children showed that already at age 5 children reliably can give LA and LE and can distinguish the difference. The study (Ferguson, 1958) tested Adlerian principles regarding sibling relationships, and LA,

LE, and performance measures were obtained. The data illustrate some of the general findings regarding LA and LE reported in the literature.

Two siblings were tested in separate rooms and each child was shown a paper with 40 pairs of dots. The investigator showed how the dots could be connected and then told the child a fictitious norm. That is, 20 dots allegedly could be connected within 1 minute by children in the age range of the child and his or her sibling. In addition to receiving the fictitious norm, half the children were told that the sibling was fast and could connect 30 pairs of dots and half were told the sibling was slow and could connect only 10 dots. Before doing the task, the children were asked how many dots they would *like* to connect (LA) and how many they *think* they can connect (LE). Thus, preperformance LA and LE were based on information concerning performance of a fictitious same-aged normative group and an alleged performance of a sibling in a nearby room. The children had no other basis for making LA or LE judgments, because it was a novel task and they had no previous performance to rely on for their goal setting. Two samples of children provided the data. Table 10.2 presents the means of the children's LA and LE, with 10 sibling pairs in each experimental condition.

Notable is the fact that the mean LA was generally high, being between the maximum possible (40) and the fictitious norm (20), and that the mean LE was overall far lower than the LA. This difference between LA and LE is typical. Overall, LA was not affected by information about how the sibling allegedly performed, but LE was. When the

TABLE 10.1

Effects of Ego-Involvement Instructions and Failure Performance on Mean Level of Aspiration (LA) and Ego-Involvement (EI_R) Ratings When Experiment Occurs Just Before Course Exam

	EI_R		LA	
	High instruction	**Low instruction**	**High instruction**	**Low instruction**
Preperformance	39.8	39.1	42.0	43.4
After 1st failure	38.8	41.0	36.0	32.4
After 2nd failure	37.5	39.4	33.4	28.4

Source: From Ferguson (1962) Table 5, p. 413.

TABLE 10.2
Mean Level of Aspiration (LA) and Level of Expectation (LE) of Children Aged 5 to 10 Years

Response measure	Group I		Group II	
	Sib was "fast"	Sib was "slow"	Sib was "fast"	Sib was "slow"
LA	28.95	28.25	32.25	28.20
LE	24.50	18.20	28.95	22.05

Source: From Ferguson (1958), modified from Table 2, p. 217.

children were told that the sibling did better than the normative group, their LE was significantly higher than when they were told their sibling performed less well than the normative group.

In the absence of information about their own performance, the children's LE was related to peer information in two ways: LE in comparison with LA was closer to the performance of 20 dots completed by the fictitious normative group, and LE but not LA was significantly affected by information about how well the sibling allegedly performed. This kind of realism occurred for *expectancy* but not *aspiration*. Already by the age of 5 to 10 years, children have a clear distinction between what one can expect to attain compared with what one would like to attain in one's performance. Without their own experience on which to base their expectations, the children's use of information about how others perform illustrates an anchoring effect or frame of reference that also has been observed repeatedly with adults (Chapman & Volkman, 1939; Festinger, 1942).

Other data in the above investigation showed what is generally found, that performance affects LA and LE, and in turn LA and LE can influence performance. With children as well as with adults, a wide variety of patterns have been observed that relate performance and goal levels. In young adults, goal-setting patterns relate to feelings of adequacy and self-acceptance (Cohen, 1954). Researchers have found "neurotic" versus "normal" patterns (Himmelweit, 1947), and unattainable goal levels have been identified as a possible self-handicapping strategy (Greenberg, 1985). Beliefs about oneself bear on motivational processes and strongly alter goal setting, as was found by Sears (1940) with

children who had a history of discouragement and anticipated school failure. In another study (Hilliard, Fritz, & Lewiston, 1982), asthmatic and diabetic children were compared with healthy children. The lowering of goal levels after success, which is not the "normal" pattern, was found more often in the chronically ill compared with the healthy children. Extreme goal discrepancies, of setting LE far from actual performance, have been found in many studies to be related to discouragement and feelings of low satisfaction. In contrast, realistic goal setting, in which LE and performance tend to be in close proximity, is related to a wide range of indicators of self-confidence, optimism, and high satisfaction (e.g., Bills, 1953; Gerrard et al., 1982).

Various tasks have been used to measure LA and LE. One favorite laboratory task is a simple game-like wooden board that uses a small ball and grooves, called the Rotter Form Board (Rotter, 1942). To be an effective laboratory task for studying LA and LE, the task needs to permit a subject to obtain different scores on discrete trials that can be presented fairly quickly. Measures of LA and LE have been obtained with persons from a wide range of ages. Goal-setting levels are affected by immediate performance (Bayton & Whyte, 1950; Wenar, 1953) and by various situational variables, like payoffs, nature of task, and social variables (Feather, 1964; MacIntosh, 1942; Sutcliffe, 1955). Social variables are especially powerful. For example, Hilliard, Fritz, and Lewiston (1985) found that when performing a task with their parents, asthmatic and diabetic children set higher goal levels than did healthy children, but when performing alone, the ill and healthy children did not differ significantly in their goal levels. In addition to immediate and situational factors, long-term personality variables and stable motive dispositions, like anxiety, desire to control, and the need to achieve, also have been found to relate to goal-setting levels (Burger, 1985; Hodapp, 1989; Yamasaki, 1992).

Researchers have sought to understand how people set goals and what factors influence their goal levels, and a number of psychologists have theorized that goal levels play a large role in decision making and in bargaining negotiations (Komorita & Ellis, 1988; Lopes, 1987; Ostmann, 1992; Schneider, 1992). A number of researchers have posited that the level of aspiration or expectation that people have affects the kinds of concessions they make in bargaining situations and the kinds of coalitions they are likely to form in bargaining settings. Also, the extent to which people seek or avoid risks when confronted with positive and negative outcomes in risky decisions is thought to be affected by their goal levels. For example, some people may prefer risks entailing small gains (and small losses) over large gains (and large losses). The kinds of decisions they make when confronted with risky alternatives will be influenced by their goal levels for negative (loss) as well as positive (gain) outcomes.

Goal levels reflect motivation at a given moment. Although for many years researchers neglected to use measures like LA, LE, and goal discrepancy, more recent investigators have rediscovered that these measures provide reliable and important ways to assess motivational states. Moreover, investigators have explored how long-term motivational dispositions affect the way individuals characteristically set goals. Thus, goal setting has been found to vary according to momentary factors and it reflects long-term values and dispositions.

INDIVIDUAL DIFFERENCES IN GOAL SETTING

Goal Setting and the Achievement Motive

Achievement motive researchers in the early years of their investigations found that the need to achieve (nAch) strongly affects goal setting. Children with a high need to achieve were found to set goals that were difficult enough to be challenging but not so difficult that failure would be likely. Such children were taught to be independent at an early age. Parents of high nAch children showed high confidence in their children. They showed this in laboratory testing by expecting fairly high levels of performance for their children, whereas parents of low nAch children set lower goals. Also, the former type of parents, but not the latter type, tended to give their children considerable independence training, letting the children make their own decisions about a number of daily activities or events. This type of goal-setting training seemed to have effects later in life. As was found with children, in young adults achievement motivation affects goal setting. Levels of performance attainment and task selection as a form of goal setting differ according to the person's motive disposition to achieve, and nAch affects goal-setting choices following success and failure experiences (Moulton, 1965).

The literature on the achievement motive showed that goal setting is influenced by long-term dispositions, and additional dispositions, learned in childhood, have been identified by other researchers. These dispositions also can affect the way an individual reacts to success and failure on achievement-related tasks.

Dweck: Performance Goals Versus Learning Goals

Long-term dispositions pertaining to self-concept were found to affect the kinds of goals children set in achievement-related tasks. Dweck (1992) identified two kinds of goals: seeking to *prove* that one is competent, and this focuses on one's ability, versus seeking to *improve* one's competence, and this focuses on long-term effective functioning. She conceptualized these as different kinds of personal goals in the face of achievement-related challenges. The former are called "performance goals" ("How well am I doing, as an indication of how able I am?") and the latter are called "learning goals" ("What can I learn from my performance so that I can improve on the next occasion?").

The *performance goal* has a defensive quality. It involves testing oneself and seeking to confirm one's adequacy as a person on the basis of performance at a given occasion. Dweck (1991) related this defensiveness to a quality of "helplessness." In contrast, the *learning goal* does not tie performance to testing one's adequacy. Task performance is appraised as offering an opportunity to learn, not as a threat to one's self-concept. This quality Dweck (1991) calls a "mastery" orientation. Dweck (1991, 1992; Elliott & Dweck, 1988) found that when children experience failure, children with these two kinds of aims react very differently. Those with a performance goal show three reactions: to attribute their failure to low ability, to show negative emotion regarding their performance, and to show poorer subsequent performance. Those with a learning goal are oriented toward mastery, look for solutions or ways to improve, and do not focus on their failure or assume it to reflect low ability. Also, those with a learning goal have more positive emotional reactions and tend to improve their subsequent performance. When children encounter failure, those with a performance goal react in a somewhat helpless manner, whereas those with a learning goal react with a more solution-seeking and task-mastery orientation.

By the time children are in preschool, and certainly by first grade, they show dispositions toward a defensive or mastery approach (Dweck, 1991). When working on puzzles, children were found to differ in terms of being persistent and seeking new challenges or being nonpersistent and repeating puzzles they already solved. When their LE was measured prior to a second task of building a tower, the two types of children did not differ. They expected to build towers of comparable height. However, once the towers toppled, nonpersisters had significantly lower expectancies than did persisters for later trials of tower building.

According to this formulation, children entering first grade bring to their school experience a set of existing biases and dispositions. These in turn shape the way the children react to failure experiences. Moreover, performance versus learning goals can also be experimentally induced in preadolescent children. In one investigation, Elliott and Dweck (1988) gave fifth-grade children a pattern recognition task consisting of geometric forms. All the children received both "performance" and

"learning" task instructions. The former presumably would not let the subjects learn anything but, instead, would show the experimenter "what kids can do." The "learning" task presumably permitted the subjects to learn "new things" and also would lead to mistakes. Approximately half the subjects were then given instructions to induce a performance goal (the children would be filmed and their performance evaluated by experts) or a learning goal (no mention of filming, and instead an emphasis on the fact that the learning task would help in school and help "sharpen the mind"). The children then "chose" one of the two tasks, but in fact they worked on the same pattern recognition task.

Some children were led to believe they had high ability on the task, others that they had low ability on the task. During the task activity, failure experiences were presented to *all* the children. The results showed that children who received the "learning" emphasis significantly more often selected the learning task and those who received the "performance" emphasis significantly more often selected the performance task. Additionally, children in the "performance" condition who were led to believe that they had low ability on the task showed a significant drop in problem-solving strategies after failure. These subjects also made many statements that attributed their failure experiences to personal deficiency. The other groups of subjects rarely made such statements. Thus, regardless of what bias or disposition the subjects brought into the testing situation, when performance versus learning goals were experimentally induced, and when ability beliefs were experimentally induced, fifth-grade children in a laboratory setting were found to show positive or negative, productive or nonproductive, reactions following failure trials. Thus, during preadolescent years, children still can modify their reactions according to situational factors. Their reactions and performance are not yet shaped exclusively by long-term dispositions. The findings from the study also suggest how children might acquire their long-term "helplessness" versus "mastery" orientation. If over a number of years they consistently are presented with performance versus learning goals and consistently receive low versus high ability information, such experiences are likely to lead to the helplessness orientation and to the performance goal disposition.

Dweck does not refer to Dreikurs, but the literature on the importance of performance versus learning goals nevertheless is congruent with the writings of Dreikurs. Dreikurs (1971/1992) pointed out that by the time people reach adulthood, it is essential for them to believe in themselves, rather than look for evidence of being worthwhile. Unless one believes in one's value as a person (in one's adequacy and ability), behavioral evidence will not persuade the person: Whatever success the person attains, she or he will interpret the success in a way that does not change the fundamental self-concept, and in a wide range of situations the person will seek to "prove" his or her value or adequacy. For such an individual, failure in performance will be interpreted as personal failure ("I am a failure as a person"). In contrast, the person whose self-concept is one of adequacy and value is likely not to link task performance with self-adequacy. This individual is not likely to interpret failure in performance as an indication of being a personal failure. A person with a self-demeaning self-concept will be defensive and will use performance failure as verification of self-failure and will not use success in constructive ways. In contrast, a person with a self-adequacy self-concept will use both negative and positive performance feedback in a constructive fashion. Studies reported by Dweck and her colleagues (1992, 1991; Elliott & Dweck, 1988) provide empirical support for Dreikurs' conceptualization.

Dreikurs and his students extended Adler's principles and techniques of encouragement (Dinkmeyer & Dreikurs, 1963; Evans, 1989, 1995, 1996) to help children and adults, and in particular to dissociate the link between immediate task performance and belief regarding "Am I good enough?" Encouragement methods were designed to help individuals form a self-concept of value, ability, and adequacy.

Dweck related her conceptualization of learning versus performance goals to intrinsic motivation (Heyman & Dweck, 1992). She considered that learning goals heighten intrinsic motivation. This occurs because involvement in challenging tasks and persistence in the face of obstacles, which are

characteristics found when individuals pursue learning goals, are likely to increase intrinsic motivation. In contrast, performance goals can decrease intrinsic motivation if, in order to prove competence, the individual sought only short-term incentives and low-risk outcomes. However, Dweck does not assign a one-to-one relationship between learning goals and intrinsic motivation, because other factors and other goals are also important in determining the relationship between beliefs, goals, and intrinsic motivation.

Further investigations are still under way to discover whether findings with children apply to adults. For example, one study (Hayamizu & Weiner, 1991) with college students aged 18 to 26 revealed two kinds of performance goals, one for gaining approval and one for advancement in school. Just as the work of McClelland and his colleagues showed different motive dispositions tied to various "needs," not just the "need to achieve," it is possible that adults seek various performance goals, including power, achievement, approval, affiliation, and various categories that have been identified in the "need" literature. Overlapping cognitive and motivational issues are involved in the study of goals, motives, and beliefs. How goals alter motivational states and in turn are affected by them, and the relationship between goals and long-term motive dispositions, remain important areas for further study.

Other Goal-Expectancy Approaches

Eccles has explored questions similar to the ones reviewed above by Dweck: In what way do individuals differ in their self-beliefs, beliefs about tasks, and goals for task performance, and to what extent do these differences occur in childhood? Eccles (1993) has shown that school and family expectancies and actions play a large role in the expectancies of children and adolescents with respect to school achievement and peer relationships. Eccles and Wigfield (1995), in a large study that assessed expectancies and beliefs, gave questionnaires to over 500 adolescents over a 2-year period. The researchers found that by fifth and sixth grade, stable beliefs and expectancies have been formed regarding task values, self-assessment of ability, and assessments of tasks. Task values include beliefs regarding the importance of doing well on a task and the usefulness of a task for achieving future goals, as well as intrinsic interest in the kinds of tasks the researchers investigated (e.g., interest in mathematics).

Competence beliefs were found to be related to performance expectancies on a task. Moreover, on the basis of the questionnaire data, Eccles and Wigfield (1995) found that adolescents tended to value an activity in which they thought they could do well. Thus, competence judgments influenced task valence. This shows the reciprocity between task valence and success probability in a way somewhat different from the valence-probability hypothesis proposed by Lewin et al. (1944).

As described earlier, Lewin et al. (1944) proposed that levels of attainment that are less probable have higher valence (a person would more desire attaining that level): A score of 100% correct answers is less probable but more desirable than a score of 80% (on a test of moderate difficulty). Both relationships between valence and success probability are likely to be correct. The Lewin et al. (1944) valence-probability prediction concerns within-task comparisons, and the Eccles and Wigfield (1995) findings concern comparisons between tasks. People are likely to value tasks in which they excel, and within those valued tasks, very high performance that is not assured (has moderate or even low probability) is going to be more valued (has higher valence) than a lower performance attainment with a higher probability of occurrence.

Goal levels within a task may be altered by different variables than are goal choices that represent selections between tasks. In many studies, Eccles (1984; Eccles & Wigfield, 1995; Eccles [Parsons], 1983) found that task performance related to self-concept of ability, and task choices were more related to task values (such as intrinsic interest and belief about the future utility of the task). In her work, Eccles showed that many variables pertain to task-related goals, and goal setting can be defined and measured in various ways.

Goal characteristics can be measured by questionnaires, as used by Eccles and Wigfield (1995),

and they can be measured by self-report of daily activities. The latter procedure was used by Emmons and Diener (1986), who had college students keep daily records of various situations they encountered for 30 days. "Having dinner" or "talking on the phone with my parents" would be examples. These situations were then classified according to various goals, such as "caring for others" or "convey information to others." Goals were rated for importance and whether the goal was attained. The researchers found that the amount of time spent in various situations was a function of *goal importance* and *goal attainment.* In some situations the actual amount of time spent on an activity was related to success in goal attainment, but in other situations it was more related to goal importance (value). Thus, for adults who have not only freely chosen activities but also have demands imposed on them, performance attainment in situations or activities, goal expectancies (what one seeks to attain), and goal choices (in terms of which activities one selects) are likely to be complexly determined.

Another approach to goals was taken by Cantor (1990; Cantor & Fleeson, 1994). The word "task" commonly refers to an activity or apparatus in which specific performance occurs, like the task of "clearing the table" or the Rotter Form Board apparatus used to measure LA and LE. Cantor uses the word "task" far more broadly. She refers to task as an age-appropriate life task, like the task of "being independent" when a young adult leaves home and goes to college. In this larger framework, of defining tasks and goals within a developmental perspective that focuses on life pursuits, Cantor conceptualized goals in relationship to a wide range of situations and in regard to life satisfactions. The goals and tasks that Cantor described are at a conscious level but may involve aspects of personality and culture of which the person is not aware. For example, a task of "independence" may become translated into a conscious goal of "I'll do my own laundry rather than bring it home to my parents on weekends." However, the person may be less sharply aware of other aspects of the task or goal.

The issues raised by Cantor relate tasks, goals, and strategies to age-related life demands. During childhood one faces certain types of tasks and goals, in adolescence one needs to relate to other tasks and goals, and in young, then older, adulthood one must face still other tasks and goals. Individual differences in goals thus can be studied from the perspective of trait-like dispositions, like the achievement motive or "helpless" versus "mastery" orientation, and they can be studied in terms of certain ages and life events.

The meaning Cantor gave to "tasks" involves a similar broad perspective that was used decades earlier by Adler (1932, 1933/1964) in his description of "life tasks." Adler described three main life tasks that confront every adult: friendship, work, and love (Dreikurs & Mosak, 1966). The mental health of a person can be ascertained by how well the individual deals with these three tasks, that is, how well the person functions in close social relations, in the domain of work, and in an intimate love relationship. Overall, Adler's are broader "tasks" than Cantor's, although she also describes tasks of friendship and intimacy, which mirror the "tasks" described by Adler.

A more important difference between Adler and Cantor is that she conceptualizes "goals" not on the basis of individual differences in personality but on the basis of specific "tasks." Although Adler, like Cantor, considered goals to be directed toward "tasks," the fundamental aspect of goals in Adler's theory is that goals are shaped by and reflect the core of personality, called "lifestyle" (Dreikurs, 1995; Ferguson, 1995). According to Adler, goals pertain to all of a person's actions, with all behavior being goal directed, and the uniqueness of each person is expressed through the individual's unique lifestyle.

For Adlerians, goals may be situational, in the way Emmons and Diener (1986) described, and they are also a reflection of personality, especially the individual lifestyle. Thus, Cantor and Adlerians have similar perspectives on life tasks, but they differ in their conceptualization about goals. Moreover, for Adler, goals need not be conscious: a person's goals occur on the basis of beliefs and choices, but neither the goals nor the beliefs and choices need to be in awareness. For Adler and Dreikurs, as for Cantor, the important aspect about goals is that they reveal the transactions between an

individual and life events. Neither formulation seeks predictions of performance goals over trials on tasks defined in the more traditional way, that is, a specific apparatus or test. In that sense, neither Adlerians nor Cantor would predict specific goal measures like LA, LE, and goal discrepancy. Other psychological theories, however, like those of Lewin et al. (1944) and Atkinson (1964), are concerned with such predictions, because they are concerned with achievement tasks and performance, not with life events and general human relations. The word "goal" thus refers to many levels of behavior. Some theories focus on goals in terms of individual differences (long-term dispositions or personality). Others focus on developmental differences, and still others seek to assess how goal setting relates to performance in achievement tasks. With regard to goals and performance, other theorists emphasize the role of beliefs regarding success and failure.

BELIEFS REGARDING SUCCESS (VERSUS FAILURE) AND REINFORCEMENT

Do some people generally expect to have success on tasks of achievement, and do they face any achievement task with a high success expectation? In part this question was addressed by the theorists already discussed, but the question has been more directly tested by another group of researchers.

Beliefs About Success and Failure on Tasks and Self-Efficacy

A test devised by Motowidlo (1979), called an Estimate of Self-Competence scale, measured a person's belief in task-related competencies. The scale was found to be a reliable measure of a person's general belief about ability. It did not reflect actual ability or belief about specific abilities (on specific tasks). Some people generally expect success on tasks because they believe themselves in general to be competent. An example of a question on the Motowidlo (1979) scale is, "When you try to reach important goals of any kind, what percent of the time do you feel you have really succeeded?" Data reported by Motowidlo (1979) show what many clinical psychologists have found and what Dweck (1991) reported, that even though people may in fact have high ability, they do not necessarily believe they have high ability, and they may face tasks without a general expectation that they will be successful.

A similar concept to the one measured by Motowidlo (1979) was described by Bandura (1977, 1986, 1989, 1997; Bandura & Jourden, 1991). He named the beliefs people have about their own competencies "self-efficacy." Bandura (1991, p. 96) conceived of self-efficacy as "self-beliefs of capability." Whereas *Motowidlo measured a general belief in competence* and thus a general expectation of success, the *self-efficacy beliefs of Bandura are specific* regarding a given skill or task, like a belief in memory capacity or belief in one's persistence. Bandura pointed out that a self-belief in specific competencies leads to better performance, like a belief in memory capacity leads to better memory performance and a belief that one can persist in a challenging task leads to greater persistence in reaching one's goal in a challenging task.

Self-efficacy is evaluated for each task or in each situation. Confidence ratings in this type of study usually are made on a 10-point scale, with the high point measuring "extremely confident." For example, studies were conducted in which subjects were hypothetical managers of simulated organizations and the task involved production attainments (Bandura & Jourden, 1991; Cervone, Jiwani, & Wood, 1991). The subjects had to make complex organizational decisions, and their self-efficacy was measured by confidence ratings made for each of nine levels of production attainments. A different study involved physical exercise (Lerner & Locke, 1995). Subjects performed a sit-up endurance test, and their self-efficacy was measured by ratings of how confident they were in being able to do sit-ups. Ratings in this study were for each attainment level in increments of 5 sit-ups, from 10 up to 75 sit-ups per minute. The sum of the person's confidence scores provided the measure of self-efficacy for that person.

In most instances self-efficacy refers to confidence regarding performance attainment and reflects appraisal of one's abilities. However, it also

may include a belief that one can exert influence over events that affect one's life. A belief in one's efficacy has been shown to help people cope with stressors, to persist in activities even in the face of repeated failure, and to tackle challenges. Self-evaluation of *inefficacy* has been shown to lead to anxiety, high levels of physiological stress responses, and reduced effort in reaching challenging goals. The value of the self-efficacy construct is that self-appraisal of ability is not necessarily related to actual ability, and reactions to failure as well as to success are often related to self-efficacy beliefs rather than to actual ability.

When people judge themselves to be capable in a task they are more likely to set higher goals for themselves and they remain committed to their goals. Although ordinarily in a simple task people set their level of expectation slightly above their preceding attainment (a positive goal discrepancy), people who judge themselves to be inefficacious may lower their goals following a high attainment, based on the belief they cannot repeat the success, whereas people with a *high self-efficacy* are likely to set more challenging goals (Bandura, 1991).

Locus of Control of Reinforcement

The Work of Rotter. Beliefs about "good things that happen" were examined by Rotter (1966). He measured a general belief about *outcomes* that follow actions or performance. His "locus of control of reinforcement" concept was more general than the "self-efficacy belief" described by Bandura (1989), and Rotter's scale did not directly measure belief about one's competence. Motowidlo (1979) approached success expectations by measuring general belief about one's *competence* in actions or performance, and Rotter approached success expectations by measuring people's belief regarding the likelihood that their actions will lead to *reinforcement.*

Rotter stated that individuals differ in their beliefs about "why good things happen." Some people believe that the occurrence of good things follows something they have done, that is, the good things occur as a result of their own actions. They believe they have control over the occurrence of the good things. This belief is called a "belief in internal control" of reinforcement (Rotter, 1966). If a reinforcement or good outcome occurs but the person does not believe it is due to his or her own action, it is called a "belief in external control" of reinforcement (Rotter, 1966). Rotter, Seeman, and Liverant (1962) showed that people differ in their belief in "locus of control of reinforcement."

Rotter (1966) developed a 23-item Internal-External Locus of Control scale (with 6 additional filler items) to evaluate whether a person believed in external or internal locus of control of reinforcement. The items on the scale came in pairs, and the person answering the test chose which of the two statements fit his or her belief. Although the items refer to outcomes that follow performance and do not directly measure self-belief in competence for doing a task, some items do include appraisal of effectiveness in task performance. The items cover a broad range of events. For example, for the two statements dealing with planning, one states, "When I make plans, I am almost certain that I can make them work," and the other states, "It is not always wise to plan too far ahead because many things turn out to be a matter of good or bad fortune, anyhow." For each item the person picks the best fit, and a total score then reveals whether the answers are more in the direction of a general belief in "internal" or "external" control.

The general belief in internal or external locus of control of reinforcement has been found to be a stable and long-term disposition. It biases the way a person reacts in a wide range of situations. It has been found to relate to other important dispositions (Rotter, 1990, 1992). Many researchers have sought to relate the locus of control belief to other dispositions, traits, values, and motives. For example, people with high self-efficacy beliefs tend to have a belief in internal locus of control of reinforcement. A belief in internal locus of control means that one expects one's actions to determine the course of environmental events. If one does well and exerts effort, success and positive outcomes are expected to occur, and if one's skill or effort is deficient, positive consequences are not expected to occur. People with high nAch tend to believe in internal locus of control. In contrast, people with an "external" belief view the world in terms of environmental events occurring independently of one's actions. One's actions are not responsible for *either* good *or* bad things happening. This belief is more likely to be found in people with low nAch.

How parents raise their children has been found to bear on the children's developing either external or internal control beliefs. Children raised to believe that they are responsible for outcomes are likely to have an "internal" orientation, but this is not the case if "feeling responsible" refers mainly to negative outcomes and punishments.

The "locus of control of reinforcement" scale measures primarily how responsible one believes one is for positive reinforcements, or good things following one's actions. If children are raised to feel responsible mainly for bad things that result from their actions, this would not lead them to have a positive view of the consequences of their actions. They would not be likely to have an "internal" belief. Katkovsky, Crandall, and Good (1967) found that 6- to 12-year olds who did not acknowledge responsibility for their own actions (had an external belief) had domineering, rejecting, and critical parents, whereas children with a belief in internal locus of control had parents who were warm and praising. Developmental changes in belief have also been investigated (Carton & Nowicki, 1994). In particular, a study of over 500 children from first to sixth grade (Skinner, 1990) showed that from ages 6 to 8 years, a fairly simple set of beliefs existed regarding causes for school success (and failure), but by ages 9 to 10 years the children revealed a larger variety of factors in their beliefs. By ages 9 to 10 years they had a clearer separation of internal and external factors, and this became even more detailed by ages 11 to 12 years.

The Work of Others.   One may fail to place locus of control internal to oneself because one believes the world is chaotic, that chance events or fate determines what happens. One can also believe the world is orderly yet fail to believe in an internal locus of control of reinforcement, because one believes that powerful others are in control. The order in the world is believed to be due to their control, and one's "external" belief is not related to a belief in fate but to others being powerful and undermining one's own control. Many studies have sought to identify whether, as Rotter (1966) indicated, a single external-internal dimension represents people's belief about locus of control of reinforcement, or whether more than one dimension is involved. These studies showed that the locus-of-control variable represents more than one dimension.

Levenson (1972, 1974a, 1974b) found that "external" beliefs were either a belief in powerful others or a belief in fate or chance. Inmates at a large prison were given "internal," "Powerful Others," and "Chance" scales, each scale consisting of eight items that could be rated for strength of agreement. Inmates who had been in prison for more than 5 years showed a belief in being controlled by powerful others significantly more than did inmates who served less than 6 months, but no significant differences were found for the "internal" or "chance" scales. Other researchers in many countries have validated the work of Levenson, and their studies show that in addition to an external belief in "chance," the concept of "powerful others" needs to be included for identifying a person's external belief in locus of control (Brosschot, Gebhardt, & Godaert, 1994).

Collins (1974) found that the "external" belief could be represented by four types of *world* beliefs, namely, that the world is: difficult, or unjust, or governed by luck, or politically unresponsive. Corresponding beliefs about reward or *reinforcement* were: rewards are given in complex and difficult ways, or effort and ability are unrewarded, or reward is based on luck, or those who provide rewards (especially the government) are unresponsive. Paulhus and Christie (1981) developed a different multifactor approach to internal versus external beliefs. These researchers had a "Spheres of Control" scale with statements that the subjects rated from 1 to 7 for amount of agreement. The scale combined beliefs in one's competence with beliefs in outcomes, and it measured locus of control beliefs according to three areas: personal efficacy ("I can learn almost anything if I set my mind to it"), interpersonal control ("If there's someone I want to meet I can usually arrange it"), and sociopolitical control ("This world is run by a few

people in power and there is not much the little guy can do about it").

Many scales based on the content of the Rotter (1966) scale have been developed. Lefcourt (1992) indicated that at least 18 scales have dealt with locus of control beliefs. Many of these are more specific than the original generalized approach of Rotter, insofar as they refer to specific content areas (e.g., marital satisfaction), are geared to specific age groups, or are relevant to certain types of concerns. Generally, beliefs in locus of control of reinforcement have been found to relate to coping styles, health, achievement motivation, and academic achievement. In particular, people with a belief in *internal* locus of control of reinforcement tend to have lower anxiety than those with a belief in *external* locus of control (Volkmer & Feather, 1991; Watson, 1967), and this in turn affects other issues, such as coping with stress.

Immune responses have also been linked to locus of control beliefs. In one study (Reynaert et al., 1995), natural killer (NK) cell activity was significantly lower in depressed hospitalized patients compared with normal control subjects. A lower internal belief was associated with lower NK cell activity within the depressed patient group. The less the patients believed in their own control, the more their cellular immunity was decreased. A number of studies have shown that anxiety and depression are linked with external rather than internal locus of control belief. Because anxiety and depression in turn lead to other debilitating effects, it is not surprising that a person's belief regarding locus of control of reinforcement has far-reaching consequences.

Cultural variations have been reported, with people in different countries showing different kinds of response patterns. For example, in sampling from 43 countries, over 9,000 responses to the Rotter scale were analyzed, and cultural variations were found (P. B. Smith, Trompenaars, & Dugan, 1995). Countries with similar cultures, like Holland and the United States, were found to show similarities in locus of control responses (Brosschot et al., 1994). Because locus of control beliefs are learned, differences in belief could be expected between widely different cultures, and differences can be expected within a culture across time. Some studies reported that a change had occurred within the United States, with beliefs becoming more "external" in the years following Rotter's 1960s work, but careful analysis of relevant data negated this. Especially among women, no major shift has occurred in locus of control beliefs (H. L. Smith & Dechter, 1991).

Generally a belief in internal locus of control leads to more adaptive and effective behavior, but this is dependent on specific situations. In some circumstances, a belief in external locus of control may lead to more effective behavior. It is important to understand this interaction between locus of control beliefs and the nature of specific situations. A study by Watson and Baumal (1967) provides a good illustration of this interaction. Women college students were given nonsense syllables to learn. Some were led to believe that how they performed on a first list would help prevent their receiving shock on a second list to be learned later ("skill" orientation). Others were led to believe that the first-list performance would not prevent shock on a second list because the shock in the later list would occur by chance ("chance" orientation). The dependent variable was the number of errors made on what subjects believed to be the first list. (In fact the subjects did not receive shock nor a later list.)

The mean number of errors made by the subjects was a function of both their locus of control beliefs and the instructions about control or noncontrol of subsequent shock. As shown in Table 10.3, those with an internal belief learned the list much better under the "skill" orientation and those with an external belief learned the list much better under the

"chance" orientation. Whereas "internal" subjects did better when they believed their performance controlled the subsequent outcome, "external" subjects did better when they believed the subsequent outcome was not controlled by their performance. One's stable disposition regarding locus of control beliefs can benefit or hinder performance according to one's expectations about a given situation.

GOALS AND PERFORMANCE ATTAINMENT

Performance and goals are affected by subjective and objective variables, including the type of task and the nature of the situation. When goal setting is used to measure how motivated the person is on achievement tasks, goal level serves as the *dependent* variable. When the goals are preset, either by the person or by an external source (like a teacher or a production manager), goal level is the *independent* variable, and how well the person performs relative to the preset goals is the dependent variable. The effects of preset goals are evident in school performance and in work-place productivity. In school and the work place, success is judged according to how well performance reaches or exceeds preset goals.

Locke and Goal-setting Theory

When goals are preset, either by oneself or by another person, these preset goals have a strong effect on subsequent performance. An early study by Locke (1966) illustrates this. Four groups of college students were given a simple task in which they had to state uses for objects, like an ashtray, and the experimenter stated different goals for the four groups as standards for success. One group was given an easy goal, of providing four correct responses for each trial (of 1-minute duration). Another group was told to get better than 14 uses for these objects per trial. For a third group, the subjects were asked to set their own standard of number of uses that should be exceeded, and a fourth group was given a progressive rise of difficulty over the 20 trials. The progressive rise began with beating the easy goal of 4 correct responses and ended with beating the goal of 15 correct responses, which was one more cor-

TABLE 10.3
Mean Number of Verbal Learning Errors Made by "Internal" and "External" Persons as a Function of "Skill" or "Chance" Instructions

	"Skill"	"Chance"
Internal	46.5	65.9
External	60.5	49.2

Source: Data from Watson and Baumal (1967).

FIGURE 10.1

Performance increase in a simple verbal response task as a function of an increase in the standard set for performance.

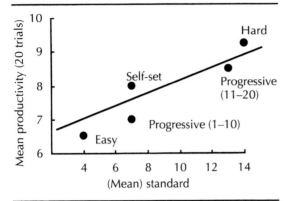

Source: After Locke, 1966.

rect response than even the hard goal. As seen in Figure 10.1, the actual performance of the four groups differed markedly over the 20 trials.

Of interest is the fact that the mean self-set goal was about 7 responses, and the subjects in the self-set goal group had a mean output of about 8 responses. That compared with a mean of about 6.5 responses for the easy-goal group and about 9 responses for the hard-goal group. The progressive-goal group's performance mirrored the effects of the "easy" and "hard" goal groups: during the early trials when the goal was easy, subjects gave about 7 responses, but in the later trials when the goal was hard, these same subjects gave a mean of over 8 responses per trial. The groups differed significantly in their output of responses, and the differences were in direct relationship to the goal level (set either for them by the experimenter or set by the subjects themselves). Because this was a simple task in which accuracy was not an issue but speed was involved, response output was dependent on the amount of effort the subjects expended. *Speed* of performance is a good measure of *motivation*, whereas accuracy measures are sensitive to learning and cognition as well as motivation. The data show that preset goal levels influence subject's motivation, both when self - set and set by the experimenter. Effort, or "how hard I try," depends on

"what standard I strive for," and higher goals lead to more "trying." The study also shows that individuals do not necessarily set their own goals to "try" at the maximum level. Goals set by another person may be higher and more effective than self-set goals for high levels of performance output.

Many variables affect the relationship between performance and preset goals, but the most important, according to Locke's goal-setting theory (Locke & Latham, 1990), is the actual goal level: if the goal is within reason of the person's ability, performance is a positive function of goal level (the higher the goal, the higher the performance attainment). Additional important variables in Locke's formulation, which affect performance, are goal specificity, commitment to the goal and its attainment, and goal intensity. The latter refers to the amount of thought the person gives to conceptualizing the goal and to planning actions to attain the goal. Cognitive effort devoted to the goal is likely to make the goal more attainable. High goals that are specific lead to higher levels of performance than high goals that are ambiguous. Instructions to "do your best" are ambiguous in that they do not specify the level to be attained. Goal commitment is important, because when a person is committed to attaining a goal, he or she is more likely to exert effort and to be persistent in reaching the goal.

Research by Others on Goal Setting and Goal Striving

People usually are more committed to goals they themselves set than goals that others set. In part this is related to the question of implicit and intrinsic versus explicit and extrinsic motivation. It is also related to issues of autonomy (Koestner & Zuckerman, 1994) and self-efficacy (Bandura, 1977, 1997). Individuals who are confident in their abilities and in goal attainment (self-efficacy) and who function in autonomous ways that rely on implicit or intrinsic motivation are especially likely to be persistent in their effort to attain self-set goals, even in the face of failure. To use goal-setting procedures effectively, managers and other leaders need to understand the motivation of their workers or associates. When people are asked to set their own goals and to persevere in efforts to attain these, managers need to be aware of who is likely to persist in the face of failure and who is more likely to be discouraged and to withdraw. To help managers and employees, goal setting in a real-life organization can be evaluated by a goal-setting questionnaire (Lee, Bobko, Early, & Locke, 1991).

A problem that managers need to consider, however, is whether management desires persistence for self-set goals. Some organizations welcome autonomous persistence, but not all do. In some organizations, management seeks docile rather than persevering behavior, and the preference is for control by managers. Thus, the management philosophy plays a crucial role in how much self-set versus manager-set goals are sought in the organization (Ferguson, 1996).

Goals that are set for a person by others can be strongly accepted if the goal seems to be reasonable and attainable. How strongly committed a person is to a goal set by another can be measured by ratings of commitment and by the extent to which a person, when given a free choice at a later time, self-sets the same goal that previously was set by someone else. For example, a student may consider a teacher's goal for performance to be too high, but if after working effectively the student comes close to the goal or actually attains it, at a later time the student may self-set the same goal. Sometimes self-set goals are higher than goals set by another, and sometimes self-set goals are lower. Many factors, including personal dispositions, affect the relationship between goals one sets oneself versus goals that are set for one by another person. Self-chosen goals tend to have more goal commitment than do assigned goals, and self-chosen activities tend to be remembered better than assigned activities (Kuhl & Kazen, 1994).

Whether performance is better under self-set or assigned goals, and whether it is better under high goals or moderate or low goals, in part depends on the strategies one utilizes and the abilities one brings to the task. Kanfer (1994; Kanfer & Ackerman, 1989) pointed out that merely identifying what goal levels one works toward is not enough to predict one's performance, because performance also depends on what resources one brings to the

task and how these resources are allocated in one's task performance.

At times and under some circumstances, participating in the decision about a specific goal helps people to meet high goal levels (Latham, Erez, & Locke, 1988; Locke, Latham, & Erez, 1988). Also, the way one attributes failure or success to one's performance (attainment) discrepancy can affect how one reacts to goals (Mone & Baker, 1992). Making goals public, rather than keeping them private, has been found to affect goal commitment (Locke & Latham, 1990). Especially for difficult goals, making them public tends to increase commitment to such goals (Hollenbeck, Williams, & Klein, 1989), and a high need to achieve also can increase goal commitment for difficult goals.

The disposition of an individual to choose certain types of goals does not necessarily mean the individual is inflexible about goal selection or about goal-committed actions. The literature on the achievement motive has shown that although high nAch individuals tend to choose goals of intermediate level, once high (difficult) goals are adopted (either as self-set or assigned goals), high nAch individuals tend to be effective (exert effort and remain persistent) in attaining the goals. One explanation is that high nAch individuals tend to have a mastery rather than a helpless orientation, as these orientations are described by Dweck (1991).

Many people conceptualize motivation to involve both goal setting and goal action. For some theorists, intention refers to goal action and thereby motivation includes intention. For example, Adlerians consider all intentions (setting and carrying out goals) as motivational (Dreikurs, 1950/1992), with intentions referring to action-oriented goals and not to wishful aspirations. However, Heckhausen and Kuhl (1985) and Heckhausen and Gollwitzer (1987) distinguished between motivation and intention. They considered motivation to be a state that occurs prior to a goal-setting decision, and motivation to differ from volition. They considered volition to be a cognitive and intentional process that follows the goal-setting decision. From their conceptualization, *motivation* biases a person's choices, and *intentions* (volitions) enable a person to act upon and carry out the choices. Klinger (1992) based his ideas in part on those of Heckhausen and Kuhl (1985), and he suggested that self-chosen goals in real life are usually preceded by mental exploration of possible goal pursuits. He considered that environmental cues that are emotionally arousing can translate motivation into goal actions.

The literature on humans thus shows that goal level, goal valence, and goal commitment are complexly related to motivation. Dispositional, cognitive, and environmental variables affect goal setting and goal action. Different aspects of goal setting and goal striving are complexly determined, and multiple factors affect how goal setting and goal striving shape effort, performance, and persistence.

SUMMARY

Incentives may alter the performance level toward which a person strives. Lewin and others described various performance levels that are part of a person's goal structure. Level of aspiration (LA) refers to performance we would like to attain but which we have a relatively low probability of attaining. Level of expectation (LE) refers to performance we expect to attain and which we have a moderate (50%) probability of attaining.

LA and LE tend to change with performance over trials, rising with success and falling with failure in the typical pattern. Even young children can distinguish between LA and LE. A measure of goal discrepancy indicates how much future aspiration and expectation differ from prior performance. An optimistic person has moderately high positive goal discrepancies, whereas pessimistic persons may show negative goal discrepancies.

When success ("doing well") is not explicitly defined, past performance does not seem to affect individuals' ratings of how interested they are in doing well. However, a specific desired level of attainment (LA) is altered by the person's prior performance. This suggests that a subjective definition of "well" or success shifts according to an individual's performance at a given time.

Knowledge of how one's peers perform on a task influences one's LE when one has no prior experience with a task. Comparison norms become less influential when one has experience on which one

can base one's expectations. Goal setting varies according to momentary factors as well as long-term dispositions. The need to achieve, and mastery versus helpless orientation, are two kinds of long-term dispositions that have been found to affect goal setting and performance.

Dweck described performance goals, in which one seeks to *prove* one's competence, and learning goals, in which one seeks to *improve* one's competence. When children experience failure, their reaction is different if they are striving in terms of a performance goal rather than a learning goal. Children with a performance goal tend to drop their performance and to withdraw after a failure experience, whereas those with a learning goal are likely to persevere and even improve performance after a failure experience.

Dreikurs noted that a person's self-concept plays a major role in how the person interprets success and failure in performance. He extended Adler's methods of encouragement, and showed that encouragement is important in helping individuals cope effectively with failure experiences.

Eccles studied task values and their relationships to goals and performance. Cantor also did such studies, but she conceptualized tasks in a broader sense than those usually referred to, like a puzzle task. Cantor described tasks in terms of developmental and life demands, like the task of being independent in young adulthood. Goals were shown to relate to such life tasks. The way Cantor described tasks is somewhat like the conceptualization of Adler, although he considered life tasks in even broader terms. For Adler, the three main life tasks for an adult were work, love, and friendship, and specific goals shaped an individual's motivation in terms of these life tasks.

Bandura and others studied a person's belief in specific competencies. Self-efficacy referred to a self-belief of being capable in a task. Persons with high self-efficacy persist in activities even after failure, and they are more likely to set high goals for themselves.

Rotter developed a scale to measure belief in locus of control of reinforcement. Persons with an "internal" belief think that positive reinforcement will occur as a function of the person's own actions, whereas those with an "external" belief do not think that. Studies have shown that the internal-external beliefs do not represent a single dimension. Rather, one can have external beliefs in a number of ways, such as believing events occur by chance or believing that powerful others control what happens.

Coping responses and even illness and health have been shown to be related to one's beliefs regarding locus of control of reinforcement. Long-term beliefs about locus of control can interact with momentary circumstances in affecting performance. If a person has an "external" belief, the person may perform better than an "internal" person in situations that involve chance punishers, whereas the reverse may happen in situations in which the person's performance has control over punishers.

When goals change as a result of performance, the goal setting can be studied as a dependent variable. When goals are preset and the study assesses how goals alter performance, the goal setting is the independent variable. Both types of studies have been conducted. Much of the work of Locke has focused on goal setting as the independent variable, and the data show that performance is strongly influenced by goal level and goal commitment.

Whether goals are self-set or not also affects performance, as does goal valence. Managers can help improve performance by various methods of goal setting, although management philosophy also has important effects on goal setting and performance. With high goals individuals tend to have high motivation, in terms of effort, and they tend to show high performance, but this largely depends on goal valence and goal commitment. Various psychologists have different definitions for goal and intention, and they differ in how they relate goal, intention, and motivation.

CHAPTER 11

Aggression and Anger: Attribution, Mastery, Power, Competition

The last chapter considered how certain expectations regarding oneself and task characteristics relate to goals, and the present chapter extends this perspective. The literature on locus of control of reinforcement has shown that what one expects in the future is related to how one explains events in the past, and some theories of goal setting tie cognitions about the past to anticipation of future events (Karniol & Ross, 1996). Other approaches relate goal setting to self-evaluation (White, Kjelgaard, & Harkins, 1995). Self-assessment is related not only to motivation in achievement tasks but also to beliefs and motivation involved in conflict and antagonism. The present chapter discusses goals in regard to anger and considers *explanations of causes* for one's own and others' actions. Research on explanations of causes, of one's own and others' actions, is the concern of *attribution theory*.

Attributions shape emotions, and attributions are complexly related to motivation. Suppose a person slips on a banana peel. How the person reacts is very much influenced by the kind of causes the person attributes to the event. Emotions and actions differ if one believes (a) one is clumsy and should have noticed the peel before falling, (b) one's kid brother put the peel there intentionally, to cause harm and hurt, (c) life is dangerous and one can never feel safe, even walking in one's own house. Thus, whether one has the emotion of anger, and whether one lashes out against another person in an aggressive manner, in part are determined by one's attribution of the cause of the incident.

People have many kinds of thoughts, emotions, and actions in confrontational or antagonistic transactions or in goal-blocking circumstances. When the actions and reactions involve initiation of attack they are likely to be defined as aggression, but when they involve attack as a defensive counteraction, other labels such as fear may be used. Antagonistic reactions are varied, and so are methods of peaceful coexistence. Selye described two bodily reactions to stress, and he identified one as attack on the disturbance. He called it "catatoxic response" and meant by that "attacking and not giving in" (Selye, 1976, p. 408). The other reaction was nondefensive or refraining from counterattack, which Selye called "syntoxic response." In confrontational circumstances, individuals can move toward attack and become angry, or they can refrain from attack and follow a peaceful rather than antagonistic course.

Studies on anger have explored various modes of reaction. The present chapter focuses on "normal" rather than pathological circumstances, and thus it is not concerned with extreme attributions as in paranoia nor with extreme emotions of rage or other forms of pathological anger. Although psychologists need to understand pathological attributions and extremes of anger, these topics are outside the scope of the present chapter.

ATTRIBUTION AND ACHIEVEMENT

Humans try to explain actions in their daily life, in order to understand life events and also to help predict events. Valid causal explanations of past events provide the bases for good predictions of future events, in science as in daily life. Needless to say, causal explanations often are not valid, in daily life as also in science. Many explanations or attributions can be given about one's own and others' successes and failures. The literature on attributions gained momentum in relationship to the achievement motive and to performance on achievement tasks. Early researchers found not only that many factors shape whether one succeeds or fails in a task, but that many explanations are given by people for why their or others' prior successes or failures occurred.

If a friend studies diligently for an exam and gets a high mark, we may explain the successful performance as due to a large amount of effort or to high ability ("my friend would have done just as well without so much studying, because my friend is smart"). If someone we don't like studies as diligently and gets a high mark, we may explain the successful performance as due to good luck or an easy test. Many kinds of explanations are possible, and our biases from the past are likely to influence specific attributions. Explaining behavior to ourselves can help us formulate testable hypotheses ("next time I won't study so much, and we'll see if I still get a good mark") or to plan more effective coping strategies. Credit for the initial formulations that led to later attribution research is given to Heider (1958), who theorized that causal reasoning and social judgments fit into an equilibrium of beliefs.

Weiner and Attribution Theory

According to an early formulation by Weiner (Weiner & Kukla, 1970; Weiner et al., 1971), attributions for success and failure are made in terms of two dimensions. One relates to internal versus external causes, in the way conceptualized by Rotter (1966). That is, a person can attribute the cause of a high mark on a test to ability or aptitude (internal locus) and not to the task being easy (external locus). Another dimension relates to stable versus unstable causes. That is, one can attribute the cause of a high test mark due to effortful studying (unstable, because on another occasion one might not

TABLE 11.1
Two Dimensions of Attribution for Success or Failure in Achievement

	Internal	External
Unstable	Effort	Luck
Stable	Ability	Task difficulty

exert effort in studying) and not to aptitude (which is stable). Table 11.1 illustrates these dimensions.

In this type of model, if success and failure were explained as due to effort or ability, the attributions would be for internal causes, with effort being unstable and ability being stable. External causal attributions would be used if success and failure were explained as due to luck or task difficulty, luck being unstable and task difficulty a stable attribution. The early research by Weiner and colleagues (e.g., Weiner & Kukla, 1970) focused on attributions the person made regarding her or his *own* prior successful or failing performance. The researchers found that attributions about one's own success or failure experiences are different for high and for low nAch individuals. Individuals with a resultant high achievement motivation are likely to make internal stable attributions (having high ability) for success in achievement situations, and to make internal unstable attributions (not having exerted enough effort) for failure. In this way, self-confidence would be strengthened with success experiences, and effective coping strategies (such as using greater or more strategic effort) would be utilized to reverse the likelihood of continued failure experiences.

Although considerable support was found for these two dimensions, in time Weiner (1985) suggested the need for more dimensions. Weiner (1985, 1991) recommended three dimensions, adding controllability to internal-external and stable-unstable. Control refers to responsibility, intention, or volition. For example, one can control effort but, under usual circumstances, one cannot control aptitude. This 3 × 2 model was especially useful in understanding the way people made attributions about *others'* actions. Weiner, Perry, and Magnusson

(1988) found that whether help is given to people in distress is in part a function of the "controllability" attribution, of whether the other person could control or was responsible for the distress.

Controllability describes an action, and responsibility refers to a characteristic of a person (Weiner, 1993). People who are thought to fail in some action because of uncontrollable factors are likely to be given sympathy and help rather than anger or rejection. An attribution that failure occurs due to lack of effort, which can be controlled, is likely to lead to more negative social consequences than if the failure were attributed to lack of ability, which is not as easily controlled. Attributions in terms of these three dimensions, especially the dimension of controllability, appear to have consequences in the way others react to a person. This was found in terms of liking a person or being willing to help the person (Juvonen & Weiner, 1993) and with regard to emotional reactions people have to political leaders (Feather, 1993), and it was found to affect whether failing grades in school are punished (Weiner, 1994a, 1994b). Controllability attributions also influence whether people with illness are censured or assisted (Weiner, 1993).

Other Research Approaches

How one attributes success or failure in achievement situations involves a number of issues. Attributions made about one's own performance may differ from those made about others' performance. Evidence from the literature on nAch and locus of control of reinforcement has shown that individuals with high achievement motivation are likely to make causal attributions that lead to persistence rather than to "giving up" after failure performance. Especially in children and youths, attributions concerning their own ability is likely to influence their subsequent performance in achievement situations (Eccles [Parsons], 1983). However, in adulthood this may not be the case. In one study, only achievement motivation, and not attributions independent of achievement motivation, was found to predict whether performance improved after a failure experience (Covington & Omelich, 1979).

Relatively few data exist to show whether individuals with a high achievement motive make the same types of attributions about the performance of others as they make about their own performance. However, indirect evidence suggests that people with high nAch may indeed make attributions that credit rather than discredit others. Spence and Helmreich (1983) used the Work and Family Orientation questionnaire (WOFO) to identify persons with high and low achievement motivation. These researchers found that persons with high achievement also are high in the achievement motive. Those with high grades as well as high career success had high scores on scales of mastery and hard work, but they did not score high on a scale of competitiveness. Those who scored high on competitiveness as well as high on mastery and on hard work had less success in grades or career. Although high scores in motivation of mastery and hard work were associated with high success in achievement, this was true only for individuals who did not also score high on competitiveness. The study by Spence and Helmreich (1983) did not test for attributions, but indirectly it suggests that persons with high achievement motivation not only make positive (facilitative) attributions about their own performance but also make positive attributions about the performance of others (not competitively "putting down" others).

Originally, Weiner's two attribution dimensions concerned the way individuals explained specific successes or failures in achievement. Although Weiner's later three attribution dimensions extended to broader classes of behavior, the study of attributions nevertheless tended to continue to focus on specific events. In contrast, Seligman and his colleagues (Nolen-Hoeksema, Girgus, & Seligman, 1986; Seligman, Nolen-Hoeksema, Thornton, & Thornton, 1990; Seligman & Schulman, 1986) studied attributions in terms of dispositional, long-term tendencies, called "explanatory style." Seligman showed that people's characteristic style for explaining or interpreting events had significant consequences in a wide range of situations. Whereas Weiner's three attributional dimensions were stability, locus, and controllability, Seligman's were the first two and a third dimension called global-specific. The explanatory style dimensions of unstable-stable, internal-external, and global-specific were derived from his model of "learned helplessness" (Abramson, Seligman, & Teasdale, 1978). Seligman's model predicted that in achievement situations persons with a pessimistic style for explaining events would do worse than persons with an optimistic explanatory style. A pessimistic style was hypothesized to lead to negative expectations, which in turn would lead to lowered response output (or more passivity) and thus to lower achievement following failure experiences.

To assess whether the pessimistic explanatory style altered performance in achievement situations, one study (Peterson & Barrett, 1987) obtained freshmen's responses on a number of questionnaires. The researchers found that a pessimistic explanatory style, of internal, stable, and global explanations for bad events, was related to poorer college grades. The students with the pessimistic style did worse in college courses than did students who gave external, unstable, and specific causal statements for bad events.

In one investigation, Seligman et al. (1990) used an Attributional Style Questionnaire (ASQ) to measure explanatory style of highly ranked men and women varsity swimmers. This questionnaire yields a composite score as well as explanatory style scores separately for negative events and for positive events. In the first study, after each competitive swim during the season, the coaches rated each swimmer's performance, and the findings showed a significant relationship between explanatory style and rated performance. In the second study, after the end of the season, when the swimmers were preparing for Olympic trials, each swimmer was asked to swim her or his best event. Then, in order for the researchers to assess how the swimmers reacted to disappointment and failure, the participants received a false failure feedback. Following a rest pause, they again swam the event, and the coaches rated performance. The results showed that swimmers with an optimistic explanatory style for *negative* events swam faster in the second than the first event, and swimmers with a pessimistic explanatory style for such events swam slower in the second than the first event. The difference between the two groups was nearly significant and represented time differences that could lead to a win or a loss in an actual swim event. Explanatory style for *positive* events did not relate to swim times on the second compared with the first swim. The overall conclusion was that swimmers with a pessimistic explanatory style were more likely during the season to perform below expectations than were swimmers with an optimistic style (as shown in the first study), and (as in the second study) swimmers with a pessimistic explanatory style for negative events, but not those with an optimistic style, would show poorer performance after an apparent defeat. One's attributions about failure clearly affect how one copes with a failure experience. Talent did not account for the difference between the optimists and the pessimists. Rather, explanatory style led to success and failure in that investigation, and it is likely to affect achievement in a variety of other circumstances.

Attributions have been studied in many ways. Attributions have a bearing on many types of behaviors. Attributions relate to how well individuals regulate their everyday activities. This was found in achievement situations, like those involving course grades (Roney & Sorrentino, 1995), and also with regard to friendships (Higgins, Roney, Crowe, & Hymes, 1994). Cognitions that serve to protect self-esteem (Josephs, Larrick, Steele, & Nisbett, 1992) following decision making also reflect attributional processes. Individuals who have a tendency for low self-esteem are likely to rely on self-protective attributions.

Decision making about risk taking plays a crucial role in many aspects of adolescent life, with some decisions, like unprotected sexual activity and various kinds of drug use, having possibly stark long-term consequences. Numerous studies have evaluated adolescents' decisions whether to begin cigarette smoking. Adolescents consider health hazards as well as peer influences, and they often make incorrect attributions about smoking, which then lead to nicotine ingestion. For example, in their inference about the number of their peers who smoke, adolescents tend to overestimate that number (Hine, Summers, Tilleczek, & Lewko, 1997). People's explanations relate to self-concept, to assessments of their task skills, and to many long-held beliefs about themselves and about the safety or danger of the world at large.

How and to what extent a person strives for success, and how a person copes with success and failure, are closely intertwined with many of the individual's beliefs and attributions. Attributions may be for specific events or for global characteristics. Whether people withdraw after experiencing failure and difficulties, or whether they attempt to overcome failure and surmount hurdles, is related to the way people explain the failure or bad events. Attributions are learned in childhood and from imitation of family members ("I hurt myself because I was careless," or "I hurt myself because others weren't taking good care of me"). Wider cultural factors also shape attributions and beliefs (Coleman, Jussim, & Isaac, 1991; Schuster, Forsterling, & Weiner, 1989). Certain commonly held attributions are likely to be shared within a society or community and not shared by strangers. Actions by a member of one's own group are likely to be explained differently than are actions by people of other groups. Social symbols attached to self and others (such as high or low status, friend or foe) inevitably will influence the attributions a person makes about the actions of self and others.

ANGER

Attributions are complexly interrelated with emotions and actions. As suggested by Weiner (1991), one can react with emotions of pity or anger, depending on how one explains the cause of the event. In addition to attributions, many other factors play a role in anger.

In contrast to the way Ekman (1989, 1994a) and Lazarus (1991) define anger (as "basic" or "pure" emotion), Averill (1982) provided a contrasting *social psychological* perspective. He suggested that anger be conceptualized not in terms of biological evolution but as a product of social evolution. Anger has meaning primarily within a social context. Anger both stems from and has consequences for social interactions. Anger can lead to effective problem solving, improved harmony, and ultimately to greater mutual understanding and mutual respect. However, anger also can have opposite ef-

fects. Anger can help a person become energized to overcome obstacles, and it can also exaggerate rather than resolve problems. Anger can lead to impaired health, and it can interfere with effective coping strategies. This is in line with Selye's (1976) description of the ways the body defends itself and copes with stress, disease, or injury: sometimes it is more effective to defend oneself against stressors by an active attack (catatoxic reaction), and sometimes a peaceful response (syntoxic reaction) is more health providing.

As Lazarus (1991) indicated, anger occurs when a person feels demeaned, with injury or offense to identity (which is experienced as a harm or loss), and when the offense is blamed on someone. When the blame is on another person, anger is directed outwardly; when the blame is on oneself, anger is direct toward oneself. The attribution involved is *controllability,* that others or oneself could have acted differently and had control over the harm or loss. In addition to feeling demeaned or not treated in the way one believes one should be treated, one becomes angry when one makes an appraisal that the offense can be undone or eased by an attack (Lazarus, 1991). If attack would not ease or undo the offense, another emotion, not anger, would occur. Thus, anger involves the action tendency for an attack on whoever one blames for the offense.

Similar to the formulation of Lazarus (1991), Dreikurs (1992; Dreikurs & Cassel, 1990; Dreikurs & Grey, 1992; Dreikurs, Grunwald, & Pepper, 1998; Dreikurs & Soltz, 1992) stated that anger occurs as part of a social transaction, specifically when a person is engaged in a power contest. Such a contest involves a struggle over "who is boss." When interacting with a child, parents and teachers need to recognize their own emotions, and by doing so they gain insights about the goal of the child. If the parent or teacher experiences anger as a reaction to the child's behavior, that likely indicates the child's goal is to have power, with a power contest occurring between the child and adult. Many examples from case material attest to this process, not only from the writings of Dreikurs but from others, as well. For example, Saylor and Denham (1993, p. 106) describe the case of Lana: "The most frequent objects of Lana's anger were her children. The anger was usually triggered when she was 'tired' coupled with the children 'being exceedingly difficult' or failing to 'do as they're told.'"

Dreikurs advised that the best way for adults to help children is to understand mistaken goals that lead the child to misbehave or to act in ways that are not constructive or responsible. Adults who work with children need to understand the child's goal. If the child's goal is power, this typically leads to the adult's emotion of anger, and the adult's awareness of the anger provides a useful diagnostic clue. If the child's goal is not power, the adult is likely to react to the child's misbehavior with an emotion other than anger. For example, if a child's goal is attention (shown by behaviors that prompt the adult to give inordinate attention), this is likely to lead to the adult's emotional reaction of irritation rather than anger. Both Lazarus and Dreikurs, as well as many others, separate *anger* (as *emotion*) from *aggression* (as *action*). Anger need not lead to aggressive behavior, and aggression can occur without the emotion of anger.

Anger in Everyday Life

Anger as part of human emotion has been studied from various approaches, such as: biochemically; situationally, in terms of what situations give rise to anger; in terms of facial expression; culturally and behaviorally, in terms of actions taken when angry; and in terms of rules for expressing anger.

Neurochemistry and Neurophysiology. Early researchers (Ax, 1953; Funkenstein, 1955) suggested that specific and different neurotransmitter secretions are involved in anger compared with fear, with the adrenal gland secreting epinephrine in anger and norepinephrine in fear. Later researchers failed to verify this distinction (Smith, 1974), although norepinephrine is considered to be important in the emotion of anger. Norepinephrine is linked to increased cardiac output and blood pressure. Whether high norepinephrine signifies anger or, rather, more generalized tension and stress, is still unclear. In one investigation (Frankenhaeuser, Lundberg, & Fredrikson, 1989), men and women

managers were assessed at work and at home. Whereas men's norepinephrine levels dropped when they came home, the levels continued to rise for women, presumably because they, compared with men, were more involved in coping with family matters and household chores. Overall stress could be implicated in this type of finding.

Anger activates the sympathetic nervous system. When this system is activated, depending on the nature of the activation, neurochemicals are secreted from the adrenal gland (the medulla, which secretes epinephrine and norepinephrine, and the adrenal cortex, which secretes cortisol). Anger leads to sympathetic activation in ways that also occur for other emotions, but anger also has unique effects. One measure that has been found to distinguish anger from fear is skin temperature. When Ekman, Levenson, and Friesen (1983) measured heart rate and finger temperature and asked individuals to perform facial expressions associated with various emotions, the rise in skin temperature under anger simulation was highly significant. Figure 11.1 shows the findings. The underlying concept was that when people make facial expressions of anger, other components of anger, including autonomic nervous system activity, are also heightened. The way anger affected skin temperature differentiated it in comparison with other negative emotions like fear, sadness, and disgust.

The relationship between neurochemistry and anger has led to a wide range of studies involving anger and disease, discussed in a later section, and the question of how anger can be diminished has been explored both behaviorally and neurophysiologically. Does anger reflect a biological process as part of an innate "fight" versus "flight" reaction? Is anger-tension the opposite of peaceful-calm? Considerable controversy exists around these questions. Many physiological reactions appear to have an "afterreaction," based on the manifestation of an opponent process. Although many affect-arousing states have their opponent process, Solomon (1991) suggested that anger does not.

Cognition Versus Automatic Processes. Whereas the formulation of Solomon (1991) was based on

FIGURE 11.1
Changes in (A) heart rate and (B) right finger temperature during a directed facial action task (see text).

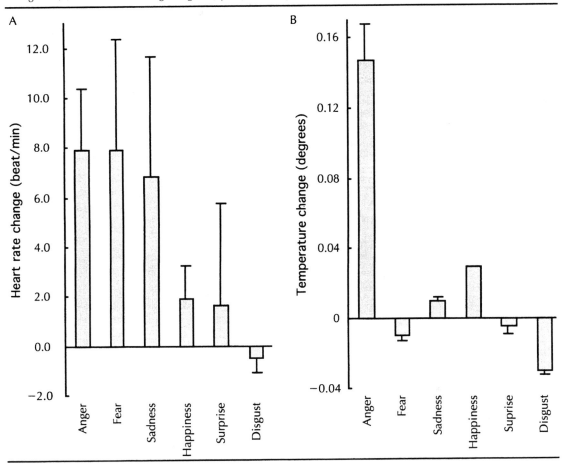

Source: From Ekman, Levenson, and Friesen, 1983, p. 1209.

automatic and physiological processes, a state opposite to anger could be proposed from a cognitive
perspective. A person in an antagonistic person-environment interaction is likely to appraise the circumstances as threatening and thus be aroused to
anger, which contrasts with "peaceful coexistence"
interactions that lead to opposite appraisals and to a
tranquil state. In many circumstances, individuals
with effective cognitive problem-solving and coping skills can maneuver a circumstance from one
involving threat and anger into one that leads to

peaceful coexistence and contentment. Insofar as
such skills can be implemented, emotions pertinent
to safety can replace emotions pertinent to threat.
    The concept of an automatic opponent process
indirectly is considered by psychoanalytic theory,
which posits that venting of tension brings *catharsis*, a kind of tension release. Some therapeutic
methods for reducing anger have used this cathartic
approach, of having the angry person punch a bag,
yell, or scream, in the belief that venting anger
brings tension release and a more calm state. The

results of research on this are not consistent. In some cases active expression of one's anger reactions has been found to release tension, but in other cases active anger reactivity leads to heightened (not diminished) anger arousal. Venting anger can become a reinforcing process rather than bringing calm and problem-solving strategies, and anger venting can spiral rather than lead to release.

Green (1990) reviewed studies that evaluated whether anger expression reduces anger, and the evidence is that rather than reducing anger, the display of anger may in fact increase it. Physiological arousal and aggressive behavior are likely to increase rather than decrease after display of anger. The most effective way to decrease anger seems to involve cognitive restructuring combined with a directed relaxation (through relaxation training). Relaxation reduces the physiological and emotional arousal of anger whereas venting in many cases increases anger. Programs that train people to relax and to develop suitable cognitions to counteract anger help people to become less angry and to show less physiological arousal associated with anger (Deffenbacher, 1988; Novaco, 1975). Thus, a process opposite to anger does exist, but it seems to require direct training. The kind of opponent process Solomon (1991) described is automatic and does *not* require direct training, so in that sense research indirectly supports his suggestion that there is not an opponent process for the emotion of anger.

Situations Giving Rise to Anger.   Various theorists have focused on identifying the types of circumstances that give rise to anger in everyday life. Situations that threaten personal values, self-esteem, and personal goals will lead to anger. The circumstance does not have to involve the direct actions of another individual, since threat to one's values, goals, and self-esteem can occur symbolically in many ways.

Dreikurs (1967a, 1967b, 1992) identified the goal of "getting one's own way" and "I am boss" as the basis for anger. He also included threat to one's self-esteem beliefs as important for anger arousal. In contrast to other theorists (Berkowitz, 1990; Weiner & Graham, 1989), Dreikurs (1992; Dreikurs & Cassel, 1992; Dreikurs & Soltz, 1992) drew a distinc-

tion between annoyance or irritation and anger. A goal of power is central for anger but not for annoyance or irritation. A parent or teacher will experience annoyance or irritation when interacting with a child whose goal is "attention," but the emotion of anger occurs when the adult and child interact with goals of "power." Although Dreikurs focused on social transactions, in symbolic terms impersonal events also could lead to anger. That is, if impersonal events challenge one's goal of being "boss," the impersonal events also can lead to anger. For example, if a person is studying for an exam and a storm cuts off the electricity, the individual may have an emotion of fear, or anger, or any other emotion, depending on how the storm relates to the immediate goal. If the private logic or internal script is, "How dare this happen, to interfere with my plan," and the goal is, "I must control events right now," then the emotion is likely to be anger. If the private logic or internal script is, "Unless I get a test score of 95 I'll not get an A," and the goal is, "I have to cover 100 pages in order to get the test score I need," then the emotion might be fear, or anxiety, and not anger. One can envision various scenarios, including an emotion of relief or even joy (and private logic of "Now I can go to bed and not be bothered with studying," "Now I have a good excuse for not doing well on the test").

From the perspective of Dreikurs (1967a, 1967b), emotion is a function of one's goal and the goal invariably has personal-social meaning even if the situation involves inanimate objects. As a hypothetical example, the toaster breaks just as one is about to make toast for breakfast, and three different individuals encounter this type of situation. One person has a goal of being boss of events, another person has a goal of "keep peace," and a third person has a goal of being a hero. When the toaster breaks, the one person is likely to react with anger and have an internal script of, "How dare the dog-gone thing not work when I want it to," the other is likely to eat cereal and without anger think, "I'll fix the toaster later when I have time," and the third person may emotionally react with satisfaction, roll up her or his sleeve, and immediately start fixing the toaster.

Anger directed to a door that won't open, to a car that won't start on a cold morning, or to an alarm that failed to go off on time, is directed toward an inanimate object that has become personalized by the angry individual. It is as if the door, the car, and the alarm are "supposed to do what I tell you to do." According to Dreikurs, only those barriers or attributions that are relevant to one's goal have a bearing on the type of emotion one experiences.

Research by Klinger (1992; Klinger, Barta, & Maxeiner, 1980) on "current concerns" has examined how people's thoughts, emotions, and actions relate to the valence, intensity, and commitment of goals in everyday life. College students described the content of their thoughts, emotions, and goals during the course of a day, and the kinds of emotions and thoughts they had were significantly related to their goal commitment, goal valence, and the intensity of that valence. Most of their waking thoughts and emotions dealt with their current concerns of the most salient and immediate goals. Klinger (1992) proposed a goal-generated "protoemotional" and emotional model that is congruent with the formulation of Adlerians. According to Klinger, commitment to a goal leads to a disposition to react emotionally to facets of the goal pursuit. This disposition occurs because environmental cues relevant to the goal set off arousal reactions. Progress toward the goal leads to a reaction of joy, and negative emotions arise when progress is blocked. Cues in the environment arouse rapid and weak emotional reactions at a nonconscious level (protoemotional reactions). If further cue processing occurs, arousal intensity increases and the reaction is a conscious emotion. As the emotional reaction becomes stronger, the person is able to translate intention (goal) into action.

Weiner (1985, 1993; Weiner & Graham, 1989) did not focus on a person's goals as the basis for emotion, but instead placed emphasis on attributions, especially attributions of others' intentionality and controllability. For example, anger is experienced when negative events occur to the person and the attribution is that others could have prevented the negative outcome. Thus, when others cheat or lie to a person, the emotion of anger is aroused. Annoyance or irritation is experienced when the negative event occurs to others and they could have prevented the negative outcome. Thus, when another student asks to borrow class notes be-

cause he or she "went to the beach" (presumably a controllable and avoidable action), annoyance is the likely emotion.

Berkowitz (1990, 1993) broadened the kinds of situations that give rise to anger beyond those referred to by Lazarus, Dreikurs, and Weiner. Personal threat, power, or controllability play a role but are not crucial in his formulation. His formulation emphasized the relationship between anger and aggression, and included both automatic and cognitive processes. In his cognitive-neoassociationistic theory, Berkowitz (1990) posited that any unpleasant occurrence, or any circumstance that leads to a person's "not feeling well," can lead to anger. Although attributions of injustice, controllability, and intentionality may increase anger, any kind of aversive event can lead to the emotion of anger. When individuals are uncomfortable or distressed, anger is more likely to occur.

According to Berkowitz (1990), whenever a negative affect or discomfort occurs (due to excessive heat or cold, pain, anxiety, and even sadness), two kinds of automatic and simple reactions are set in motion. One is an escape-associated or rudimentary fear reaction, and the other is an aggression-associated or rudimentary anger reaction. Each has an appropriate physiological, motor, and cognitive component. By a network of associations, in line with the network formulation of Bower (1981), negative reactions trigger a wide range of thoughts, memories, and action tendencies. Either the escape tendencies or the aggression tendencies will become dominant when negative reactions are triggered. Once the automatic reactions arise, cognitive elaboration follows. During this later cognitive stage the coping strategies and attributions will either heighten or diminish anger. Research by Berkowitz and colleagues has shown that being physically uncomfortable can lead to angry emotion and thought, to hostile memories, and to aggressive inclinations. The automatic level of reaction is associative in nature, in line with network theory, and the cognitive level of reaction involves attributions and other forms of thought. Thought can modify the rudimentary anger reaction and does so in normal everyday life.

In support of the formulation of Berkowitz, a

number of studies have shown that frustration leads to anger, and belief about the source of the frustration only in part plays a role. That is, when a person is blocked from an action or task, a belief that the blocking is intentional and avoidable (controllable) does lead to heightened anger, in the way predicted by attribution theorists like Weiner (1985, 1993), but the attribution alone is not the decisive factor. Even when individuals believe the blocking is unintentional and unavoidable, evidence of anger occurs.

This was found in a study by Dill and Anderson (1995), in which three groups of subjects received either intentional, unintentional, or no blocking. The experimenter presumably showed subjects how to do a paper folding (origami) task the subjects were to do on their own after the demonstration, but the instructions for the "frustration" subjects were given far too quickly to be effective. Some subjects were given an explanation that the experimenter could not help the speed, it was outside his/her control ("unintentional" frustration group). Other subjects received an explanation that the experimenter wanted to hurry because the experimenter's "boy/girlfriend is coming soon to pick me up and I don't want to make him/her wait" ("intentional" frustration group). Later, the subjects were asked to give ratings about the experimenter. The "unintentional" subjects gave less anger-associated ratings of the experimenter than did the "intentional" subjects, but subjects in both types of frustration gave significantly more anger-associated ratings than did subjects in the control condition, in which the experimenter slowed down the demonstration upon request to do so.

How one measures anger is important. The above study illustrates this, because self-reported anger in the Dill and Anderson (1995) study was *not* significantly different as a function of frustration. Only indirect measures of anger, like ratings of likeableness and ability of the "experimenter," were found to show the effect of frustration on anger. Thus, not only is it important to consider what *situations* arouse anger, but how the anger is *measured*.

Facial Expression. As already noted, Ekman (Ekman, 1992, 1993; Ekman, Friesen, & Ellsworth, 1972) and colleagues (Levenson, 1992; Levenson,

Ekman, Heider, & Friesen, 1992) have shown that directed facial actions produce autonomic nervous system reactions that are similar to those found with relived emotions. In several ways the facial expressions for surprise, fear, and anger differ from those of happiness, disgust, and sadness. Heart rate and skin temperature provide unique patterns for anger compared with fear, sadness, and disgust. According to Levenson (1994), anger and fear involve a natural "fight" or "flight" response. Data generally show unique patterns for anger, both for when anger is observed in others and when it is experienced directly. For example, Johnsen, Thayer, and Hugdahl (1995) presented to men and women subjects various facial expressions used in the research by Ekman. Heart rate was recorded along with ratings of how much the subjects experienced various emotions. Heart rate acceleration occurred when subjects viewed the happy facial expressions and deceleration occurred when subjects viewed the angry facial expressions. In a study of theater students who had learned to express different emotions in prototype fashion (Block, Lemeignan, & Aguilera, 1991), anger provided unique respiratory patterns, in terms of rate, amplitude, and duration of pauses in expiration (compared with unique inspiratory patterns found in emotions like sadness and joy). Thus, physiological responses differ markedly for anger compared with other emotions.

Although Ekman (1994b) stressed that facial expressions for specific emotions occur universally, facial activity and body expression in emotion involve far more than the specific muscle actions considered to be universal. The full constellation of muscle activity in expression of emotions varies across cultures. Averill (1994) enumerated many cultural differences in the circumstances that lead to anger and in the way anger is expressed. An extreme example is the head-hunting behavior of the Ilongot of the Philippines and their exhilaration when taking a head, which has characteristics of anger but is not at all similar to anger experiences in other social groups. For Averill, anger could involve various circumstances, such as an impulse toward aggression, an attempt to enforce social norms, or a response to frustration. Different social groups express these types of angers in different ways.

Cultural Variation. In reviewing how humans distinguish emotions from nonemotions and how they categorize emotions like anger, happiness, and fear, Russel (1991) found evidence for some common characteristics but also quite specific characteristics that differed across cultures.

Many studies have shown that variations in outward expression of anger is related to a complex array of social dimensions. For example, there are social groups in which members live in very close physical proximity, in which hierarchical patterns of status are sharply defined, and in which stable living patterns exist. Expressions of anger for such groups are likely to be very different from those for social groups in which fairly large domestic living space is available (fairly large homes or other open spaces), in which relatively fluid status distinctions exist, and in which considerable mobility is found (people moving away from each other and moving their dwellings). One might expect people who fit the former pattern to inhibit displays of confrontational emotion, both because such inhibition prevents intrusion into one another's personal space and because quite strict rules of conduct delineate actions. Traditional Chinese families fit the former pattern, and data show that they do teach their children that strong and negative feelings should not be expressed openly (Rawl, 1992). This contrasts with tales of emotional expressions in "the wild West" of U.S. frontier settlements and of reported anger expression in contemporary American households. American family life fits the pattern of the latter type of group, and one might predict that this group permits, if not condones, open expression of negative feelings, including anger.

Contrary to findings with traditional Chinese families, research with Chinese American women showed that their outward anger expression was higher than that of both African American and Caucasian American women (Thomas, 1993). The researchers reasoned that the freedom the Chinese Americans found after their immigration (as adults) to the United States led them to a pattern of anger display that was "overwesternized" (Thomas, 1993).

Anger is displayed according to rules set by the culture. Tavris (1989) and Averill (1982) described ways that different cultures permit or condone outward displays of anger. Thomas (1993) reviewed historical changes reported in American culture, with Victorian manners in the last century giving way to anger ventilation in contemporary society. Anthropological accounts have long provided data to show variation in cultures for anger expression, varying between peaceful groups and warring groups across the globe. Australian aboriginals (Berndt & Berndt, 1952; Simpson, 1951) had cultures very different from those of other groups in the South Pacific and the Europeans who migrated to Australia, and these differences included all aspects of life, including different patterns of anger expression.

Rules for Expressing Anger. Ekman (1972) separated universal facial expressions from those that differ between cultures. He pointed out that cultural differences exist in terms of the events that elicit particular emotions, the rules for controlling facial expressions in specific social settings, and the consequences for emotional displays. Interpersonal elicitors are socially learned, and children learn at an early age when and how emotional displays are permitted in their culture and what the consequences are when one does display emotion.

Far more variable than patterns of facial and bodily expressions of emotion are overt behaviors that signify emotion. In some cultures or subcultures anger is displayed by loud vocalizing, in others the anger is expressed by means of "cold silence." Overt actions and body language can express anger. We learn about anger from members of our family, from the ways that people interact in a neighborhood, and from the rules taught us by the wider culture. How we display our anger is learned from family, friends, school, and the larger society. Bodily and facial expressions, vocalizations, and ritualized overt behaviors reflect the rules we learn about expressing anger. We learn when anger is sanctioned and when prohibited. Subtle or explosive methods may be advocated by different groups.

Stories are many and varied about cultural differences regarding rules of conduct and occasions for anger. In one ethnic group, watching a poker player cheat may be an impetus for anger that remains unexpressed and then without warning the angered observer knifes the cheater to death. In another ethnic group the anger might not be felt as a moral outrage by an observer but only by other players, and killing over the cheating would be unthinkable. Subtle facial or bodily expressions expressing anger may be understood only by members of the group. Social learning, often without our own or others' awareness, is the key to this variation.

Because in animals anger can be inferred only from a display of overt action, how animal and human anger compare is not well understood. Amygdala stimulation of cats leads to "affective attack" (Kalat, 1992), with bodily behaviors and facial expressions resembling the expression of the emotion of anger experienced by humans. Although this type of display suggests a "hard wired" or biologically preprogrammed basis for anger expression, direct stimulation of brain centers can give rise to processes that differ fundamentally from those evoked by provocative environmental inputs. As Kalat (1992) points out, damage to the amygdala does not lead to an emotion but rather changes how animals interpret information. In general, emotional expression in humans has both subtle and varied form, and in many respects the display of anger in animals and humans is dissimilar.

Social learning in how humans display anger is seen in developmental changes. Rules of anger expression change for children compared with adults. Rules may differ for men and women, and for persons of different ages and social status. For example, data show that women are more likely than men to cry when angry (Thomas, 1993). Because factors of dominance and submission pertain to anger experience and to anger expression in humans, how and when people experience and express anger is shaped by a wide range of complex social variables.

Measurement of Anger

Anger has been studied as a state and as a trait. Tests have been developed to assess individual differences in momentary experiences of anger (as a state) and as a long-term tendency toward anger (as a trait or disposition). One scale that has been used widely for research is the Spielberger (1988) State-Trait Anger Expression Inventory. Another is the Anger Expression Scale (Spielberger, et al., 1985), which measures tendencies to *suppress* anger, to *express* anger *outwardly*, and to *control* anger. The first measures inhibition of anger display, the second refers to active anger expression in socially debilitating ways (cursing, throwing objects), and the third refers to calm or patient types of behavior.

People tend to have relatively stable anger tendencies. Some people become angry easily and often and express their anger in a wide range of circumstances. Others rarely experience or express anger. Individuals with high compared with low trait anger were found to have more frequent anger experiences, to have more intense emotional anger experiences, and to have these provoked by a wider range of circumstances (Deffenbacher, 1992). The "outward expression" scale tends to correlate positively and significantly with scores on the trait anger scale of the State-Trait Inventory, whereas the "control of anger" scale tends to correlate negatively and significantly with the trait anger scores. Anger-related physiological arousal was shown to differ in intensity between high and low trait anger individuals, although both types of individuals experience anger in similar kinds of situations (Deffenbacher, 1992).

Various anger scales tend to reveal common as well as unique characteristics. A scale that focuses on anger in specific situations is the Subjective Anger Scale of Knight, Ross, Collins, and Parmenter (1985). It asks individuals to indicate reactions to certain types of situations. Other scales focus on modes of handling or expressing anger, like the Spielberger et al. (1985) scale, the Framingham scale (Hayes, Levine, Scotch, Feinleib, & Kannel, 1978), and the Multidimensional Anger Inventory (Siegel, 1985). The "Anger-In" scale of the Framingham anger measure reveals a person's anger suppression. The "Anger-Out" scale measures anger expression that involves attack or blame, and the "Anger-Discuss" scale measures whether the person discusses the anger or the angry incident.

When scores on these scales were intercorrelated the scales were found to have common characteristics. The scales also showed high correlations with anxiety measures and with indices of illness. The majority of findings are that high Anger-Out, measured either by the Spielberger or the Framingham scale, is related to anxiety and lowered self-esteem, that high Anger-In is related to illness, and that Anger-Discuss (measured by the Framingham scale) is positively related to health (Thomas, 1993). Being able to talk about anger appears to have beneficial consequences. It helps the person and her or his relationships with others. Venting anger, and attacking or blaming others, have been found to be destructive to self-esteem, to one's health, and to relationships with others. Theorists do not agree, but data do show that rather than anger being eased after episodes of venting or attacking, the outbursts produce further distress, both for the person and for others. Theorists do agree that anger suppression is not beneficial. Because anger can help to pinpoint problems in daily living and in relationships, suppression of anger prevents the person from recognizing and resolving problems. Anger suppression not only prevents adequate problem solving but also is likely to lead to poor health.

The fact that Anger-Discuss is an effective mode of coping with anger can be understood when the dynamics of anger are considered. From the point of view of Lazarus (1991), anger occurs because of appraised offense encountered by an individual. From the Adlerian theory of Dreikurs (1967a, 1967b), anger like any other emotion has a *purpose*. In a constructive way it can provide energy and tactics for undoing a problem. If the coping strategies are solution focused, anger can lead to benefits for the individual and for others. Thus, from the perspectives of Lazarus and Dreikurs, discussion of anger can permit solutions and thus be a healthful and effective means of anger expression. This contrasts with venting, blaming, attacking, and suppressing anger, which are modes of anger expression that are not likely to lead to productive solutions.

HOSTILITY, ANGER, AND TYPE A PERSONALITY

Anger has been distinguished from aggression and from hostility. Both anger and hostility have been

found to relate to illness, especially cardiovascular disease. Research from the time of the 1970s has sought to clarify the way anger, hostility, and disease are related.

Hostility

As with the emotion of anger, considerable disagreement exists regarding what is meant by *hostility*. Generally, one can say the term covers an attitude of ill will, negative beliefs about others, anger emotion, and behaviors that are aversive to others. As Barefoot and Lipkus (1994) point out, hostility involves beliefs (like cynical attitudes and suspiciousness about others), emotions (such as anger, disgust, and contempt), and behavior. The behavioral aspects include verbalization of anger, emotionally laden expressions of negative feelings, rudeness, condescending behavior, and uncooperativeness. Interview-based measures of hostility utilize not only the content of what a respondent says but also behavioral indications, of how the respondent acts if confronted or challenged. Behavioral indicators in an interview have been found to be good predictors for disease outcomes. For example, ratings for hostile behavior would be given if in an interview the respondent is evasive or uncooperative in answering a question, displays a hostile tone of voice (demeaning or antagonistic tone), implies that the interviewer's question is pointless, and openly challenges the interviewer. Several interview methods have been used that provide a hostility score or index.

Self-report measures of hostility have been used for many years. A well-known scale is the Cook-Medley Ho scale (Cook & Medley, 1954), which is part of a famous personality scale (Minnesota Multiphasic Personality Inventory) called the MMPI (Meehl, 1954; Schmidt, 1945; Welsh & Dahlstrom, 1956). The Cook-Medley Ho scale was first developed to allow the identification of teachers with good, compared with bad, rapport with their students. The scale measures cynical beliefs and mistrust of others. Another scale, called Factor L, measures suspiciousness. It is part of another general personality inventory, the 16 PF test (Cattell, Eber, & Tatsuoka, 1970). Scores on the Factor L test have a high correlation with scores on the Ho scale. Another well-known self-report test is the Buss-Durkee Hostility Inventory (Buss & Durkee, 1957). It measures characteristics similar to those measured by the other self-report scales but also deals with irritability, resentment, assault, and verbal hostility. Factor analysis of scores on this test found two factors, the experience of hostility and its overt expression. This is analogous to the distinction made for anger, between anger experience and anger expression.

The Buss-Durkee test measures "neurotic hostility" (resentment, suspicion, experience of anger and irritability) and "reactive hostility" (display of anger and annoyance). Neurotic hostility refers to a constellation of anxiety, neuroticism, and hostility, and reactive or "expressive" hostility refers to behaviors that are harmful or aversive to others. In comparison with anger, which is an emotion, *hostility involves emotion, cognition, and behavior.* Thus, it is possible for one person to be hostile but not display anger (suppress anger expression) and for another person to be hostile and actively express anger (Helmers, Posluszny, & Krantz, 1994). Hostility can be shown in a wide variety of ways. Moreover, a face-to-face interaction involves different hostile processes than does formalized hostility between groups. When the cognitive component of hostility involves mistrust and suspicion, the hostility either explicitly or implicitly implies a belief in the antagonist being an enemy.

In one study, college students were interviewed about their conceptualization of an enemy (Holt, 1989), and hostile actions were cited as reasons for labeling both a known person and a group or nation as an enemy. Interviewees characterized a group or national enemy as having different beliefs and values from their own, but the subjects indicated that beliefs and values could differ between themselves and someone whom they know, without the other person being considered an enemy. Qualities for being a personal enemy are different from qualities for being a group or national enemy. Beliefs about what is a hostile act and who is an enemy are shaped by many variables: personal dynamics, situational characteristics, and norms of one's group and culture.

Type A Personality and Coronary Heart Disease

On the basis of clinical work done in the 1950s, cardiologists Friedman and Rosenman (1959, 1974) identified a set of psychological risk factors for coronary heart disease (CHD). They labeled the factors as being a "Type A coronary-prone behavior pattern" consisting of ambition, competitiveness, impatience, aggressive and hostile behavior, and time urgency. Individuals labeled as "Type A personality" tended to place themselves under unnecessary time pressure, to be unusually aggressive and hostile, and to have high achievement strivings. People with "Type B personality" in many cases also had high achievement strivings but they were less hostile and aggressive and had less time urgency than did Type A individuals. However, the pattern for Type B was not as clear-cut as the pattern for Type A, and the label "Type B" tended to be assigned to persons with high achievement motivation who lacked the characteristics of Type A persons. Of importance to the cardiologists, persons with Type A personality were far more likely than were Type B individuals to have cardiovascular illness, either coronary artery disease (CAD) or CHD.

The findings regarding the Type A pattern led to many psychological as well as medical studies. The original measure of Type A was based on interviews (Rosenman, 1978), but later studies used objectively scored self-report measures. The best known of these is the Jenkins Activity Survey for Health Predictions, or JAS (Jenkins, Zyzanski, & Rosenman, 1971). A form of this test was also developed for college students as subjects (Krantz, Glass, & Snyder, 1974). Research on Type A patterns was pursued not only for practical reasons concerning diagnosis and prognosis of disease and health, but also for basic science knowledge, to find out how positive and productive factors (like striving for achievement) relate to negative and destructive consequences in the Type A person. The ambition and hard-driving achievement striving of Type A persons appeared to lead to success in work or study, yet Type A persons also had impaired health. The question was, what aspects of the Type A pattern led to the productive outcome and what led to the destructive outcome.

In studies of college students and of academic psychologists, Spence, Helmreich, and Pred (1987, 1988) found some answers to the above question. Using the JAS, these researchers found that two factors make up the Type A pattern: one is achievement strivings, and the other is impatience-irritability. Academic and career successes were significantly related to the achievement striving scores of Type A persons but they were not related to scores on impatience-irritability. The latter but not the former were significantly related to measures of impaired health of students (Spence et al., 1987). Thus, achievement strivings were not the predictors of disease, but irritability and impatience were a predictor. Different aspects of the Type A pattern led to different effects. The researchers likened this two-faceted pattern to their findings about achievement motivation as measured by the Work and Family Orientation Questionnaire (Helmreich & Spence, 1978). That is, a preference for challenges (mastery need) and for working hard was positively related to actual career success, but interpersonal competitiveness, of wanting to outdo others, was not positively related to actual career success. The distinction between striving for career achievement thus needs to be separated from a competitive, hostile, and impatient disposition.

As a result of these and other findings, researchers have come to focus on selected aspects of the Type A pattern as leading to disease. The focus in recent years has been on hostility and anger (Siegman, 1994b; Thomas, 1993), which is similar to the "irritability" variable described by Spence et al. (1987, 1988). However, the "impatience" variable described by Spence and her colleagues has been relatively neglected in recent years, with far less emphasis placed on time urgency (impatience) than on hostility and anger in the Type A pattern. Although time urgency was considered important in the original description of the Type A personality, this component has not been studied extensively and thus still requires better understanding. People who are impatient and place themselves unnecessarily under time pressure may make themselves vulnerable to incomplete information processing for available cues, and if this occurs, it could perpetuate preconceptions of distrust and hostility.

Time pressure can alter information processing. Heaton and Kruglanski (1991) found a significant primacy by time pressure interaction for judgments about another individual. When college students were given information about a fictitious job candidate, those under time pressure of 30 seconds to make a judgment used more of the first set of information whereas persons under no time constraints used more later information. If externally imposed time pressure can alter the way information is processed, self-imposed time pressure could do the same. Although contemporary studies on Type A patterns do not focus on the role of impatience and time urgency, that variable deserves greater scrutiny in the constellation of factors involving anger, hostility, and disease.

People who increase their arousal when they confront novel or unexpected stimuli were identified on a Trait Arousability Scale (Mehrabian, 1995). Scores on that scale correlate with incidence of illness as well as with increase in diastolic blood pressure when the person is angry in a confronted situation. Blood pressure reactivity, especially diastolic blood pressure, has been linked to anger expression in many studies (Siegman, 1994a), and high hostility is linked with high proneness to anger. Thus, from a broad range of investigations, the relationship between anger, hostility, and heightened cardiovascular arousal has been well established.

One can lessen heart increase by feedback and reward for lower heart rate. This was found (Larkin, Manuck, & Kasprowicz, 1989) with college students who were engaged in a competitive game. Although feedback and reward for lowered heart rate lessened heart rate increase while the subjects engaged in the game, it is not known whether this approach has long-term effects. More information is needed on how to lessen heart rate increase for Type A individuals in real-life competitive situations.

Anger can change hormone activity in addition to cardiovascular reactivity. In men, anger can relate to increased production of testosterone (a male sex hormone). Men with high testosterone levels tend to show more anger, angry men create more testosterone, and testosterone seems to increase risk of CHD (Siegman, 1994a). More study is needed to yield a better understanding of this three-way relationship between anger, testosterone, and CHD. The *expression* of anger more than its *experience* plays a significant role in processes leading to CHD. Whereas blood pressure reactivity has been linked with anger expression, heart rate (rather than blood pressure) reactivity was found to occur for subjects who repressed rather than expressed feelings of anger (Siegman, 1994a). The separate factors of anger expression versus anger experience were studied in relation to CHD only after the early research on Type A personality. Evidence now exists that anger *expression* relates to cardiovascular disease, but anger *experience* relates more to immune-related diseases (Siegman & Smith, 1994).

Overall, when anger is maladaptively expressed, repressed, inhibited, or denied, the risks increase significantly for many illnesses. People who score high on hostility scales tend to score high on anger scales, to drink more heavily, to smoke more, and to express anger in more volatile ways. All these factors have been identified as leading to more illness and disease. Gender differences have been found consistently, with men receiving higher ratings than women in hostility, anger expression, cardiovascular reactivity in stressful situations, and risk for CHD (Stoney & Engebretson, 1994). Age and race also have significant effects. Personality factors, social learning, hormonal factors, and cultural variations all play significant roles in anger experience, anger expression, hostility, and proneness to CHD. For interpersonal effectiveness and for disease prevention, positive anger management is exceedingly helpful.

Stress and low self-esteem are the two factors most likely to lead to frequent experiences of anger and to ineffective anger management. How one appraises the actions of self and others fits life patterns and life goals, which means some individuals are more likely than others to appraise external events as threats to self-esteem and hence to experience anger. Moreover, once anger has been experienced, the lower the person's self-respect, the less likely is the anger expression to be effective. Programs based on building self-respect, building respect *for* others, and disengaging from conflict so that one communicates expectation of respect *from* others (Messer, 1996) have been helpful for im-

proving anger management at work and at home. Messer, Coronado-Bogdaniak, and Dillon (1993) base their approach on Adlerian principles and have helped a wide range of men and women learn effective anger management techniques. Although the relationship between anger and disease has been found to be different for men and women in many studies, a number of training programs have helped both men and women with far-reaching social as well as medical benefits.

Support groups can lessen stress and help raise self-esteem. They have also been used effectively for positive anger management (Yahne & Long, 1988). Cognitive modification methods have been useful to minimize the hostile beliefs that trigger anger, and groups of patients with cardiovascular illness have been successfully helped to change their Type A patterns (Friedman et al., 1986). Behavior modification, psychoanalytic therapeutic treatment, cognitive psychotherapy, and Adlerian approaches all have been used with varying degrees of success to help individuals deal with hostility and with their experience and expression of anger.

SUMMARY

Many factors influence success and failure on a task and many attributions are possible to explain a person's success or failure. Humans make attributions about many aspects of their lives, in part for understanding and in part for helping them develop effective coping strategies.

Weiner initially proposed two attribution dimensions for explaining success and failure in achievement tasks, and he based his proposals on the work of Heider. The two dimensions were internal versus external and unstable versus stable explanations. Later he added the third dimension of controllability. This dimension was relevant to whether emotions like anger were evoked. Uncontrollable negative events would evoke less censure or anger than controllable ones.

Questions remain whether attributions about others' achievement are similar or different from attributions about one's own achievement. Spence and Helmreich found that high needs for mastery over tasks and for hard work were related to career success, but interpersonal competitiveness was not. Persons who in addition to having a high motivation for mastery and hard work also were high on competitiveness did *not* have high career success. This suggests that the kinds of attributions one makes about others' and about one's own success in achievement situations is related to competitiveness, with competitiveness diminishing one's actual success.

Seligman studied attributions in terms of long-term dispositions called "explanatory style." That style involved the internal-external and stable-unstable dimensions of Weiner, but instead of controllability the third dimension was global-specific. A pessimistic style of internal, stable, and global explanations for bad events was found to relate to poorer grades in college than a style of external, unstable, and specific explanations for bad events.

Besides the universal specific facial muscle activity associated with anger (found by Ekman and his colleagues) many other facial and body movements occur, and these are closely related to social learning. People in different cultures learn when to be angry, how to show anger, and what the rules are about anger experience and anger expression. Contrary to Ekman's biopsychological evolutionary perspective, Averill proposed a social psychological evolutionary perspective that identifies cultural variations concerning the emotion of anger.

Similar to the appraisal theory of Lazarus, Dreikurs emphasized that anger occurs in the context of personal-social meaning. The activation of a power goal regarding "who is boss?" leads to the emotion of anger. This contrasts to a goal of attention, which leads to irritation but not anger.

Anger leads to autonomic nervous system activity and skin temperature changes which are different from those evoked by fear. Neurochemical and physiological studies have shown anger to be similar to as well as different from other emotions.

Solomon proposed that anger does not have an opponent process. His theoretical perspective concerns noncognitive processes. Other psychologists have examined related questions, such as whether "venting anger" leads to dissipation of anger. Another question is whether cognitive restructuring permits dissolving anger. If venting anger strengthens an opponent process, this in time should bring release, but research has tended to show the reverse effect. Anger venting often leads to more, not less, anger. Cognitive restructuring and relaxation training appear to be most effective in diminishing anger. Indirect support is thus found for Solomon's proposal that anger does not have an opponent process.

Berkowitz examined what kinds of situations give rise to anger. He posited a cognitive-neoassociationistic theory, which states that any unpleasant occurrence can lead to anger. Any negative event or state sets off automatic reactions of rudimentary fear and rudimentary anger. The former is escape associated with the fear and the latter is aggression associated. Frustration can lead to anger, and belief about the source of the frustration only partly affects the anger. Even when attributions involve uncontrollability, anger is still evident when frustration occurs, according to this theory.

Anger can be measured as a state and as a trait. Anger suppression and anger shown by attacking or blaming are not as healthy (in terms of anxiety and illness) as discussing one's anger. The latter is more likely to help in problem solving and in improving the circumstances that evoked the anger.

Hostility involves beliefs (like suspicion), emotion (like contempt or anger), and behavior (like uncooperativeness). Various measures of hostility have been used, especially in relationship to risk for illness. Persons with Type A personality were compared with those with Type B personality, following the work of cardiologists Friedman and Rosenman who found Type A individuals more prone to cardiovascular illness than Type B individuals. Type A individuals were found to be more hostile than Type B individuals, and they were more impatient and irritable than Type B persons.

Anger expression is different from anger experience, and the two have different risk factors for different kinds of disease. Hostile persons tend to score high on anger scales and to express anger in more volatile ways than persons who are less hostile. Anger management programs and support groups have helped individuals to reduce anger and hostility and thereby also to lessen their risk for disease.

CHAPTER 12

Aggression, Power, and Mastery

We need to distinguish between aggression, which is behavior, and anger, which is an emotion. Aggression can occur without anger and anger can occur without aggression. Both are closely tied to motivation. When a person is angry, the anger reflects a goal and provides energy for action, and aggression is the behavioral expression of motivated, directed energy. The motivation for anger need not be the same as for aggression, although in many cases it is the same.

Aggression may be used to assert dominance in a competitive or power relationship, and it may be used defensively to deter attack by another. Aggression also may occur as an act of revenge to counteract previous experiences of hurt. Aggression may reflect a temporary motivational state or it may reflect an action program that is an expression of a long-term motivational disposition. Aggression occurs in nonhuman animals and in humans. In humans aggression can have far-reaching consequences, as in spousal or partner abuse (Magdol et al., 1997) and abusive family relationships (Emery & Laumann-Billings, 1998). An important distinction also is made for humans between mastery and aggression.

WHAT IS MEANT BY AGGRESSION?

Two characteristics of aggression are important. One is that aggression refers to a class of negative *behaviors* in which one individual attacks or threatens another, or inflicts injury or harm. The other refers to the *motivation* associated with aggression, which is usually described in terms of intention,

such as intending to assert dominance, to defend oneself or one's young, or to harm another. Some writers insist that aggression should be described only in behavioral terms, without including the motivational component of *intention* (Loeber & Hay, 1997), on the basis that intention cannot be observed and that many persons who behave aggressively deny their intent to harm. However, congruent with the emphasis in the present book, most psychologists conceptualize aggression in motivational terms (to name just a few, Berkowitz, 1993; R. J. Blanchard, Hori, Tom, & Blanchard, 1988; Ferguson, 1982; O'Neal, 1991).

The Motivational Aspects of Aggression

Some writers (e.g., Geen, 1990) distinguish between "affective aggression," which involves some type of emotion relevant to the aggression, and "instrumental aggression," in which the person does not specifically seek to inflict harm and the aggressive action is primarily a means to some other goal. Psychologists tend to agree that in affective aggression the behavior is negative (hurting or instilling fear) and that the goal is negative (to defeat, demean, or harm another). Aggression has also been studied in the context of *defense*. In defense, the motivation may be fear and the goal pain avoidance rather than primarily an intent to harm another. Many controversies exist in the literature, regarding whether fear-induced aggression should be viewed in the same way as offensive attack with intent to harm another.

Defensive aggression in some species involves

posturing but not inflicting hurt or harm. Although offensive attack involves negative behavior, in many animal species the aggression by an attacker against other members of the species does not necessarily inflict serious hurt or wounds (see Figure 12.1). Human aggression, in contrast, has been found to involve many negative actions that inflict serious harm.

Complex motivations are involved in aggression. Aggressive behavior may be motivated by pain or other forms of extreme arousal, or by pleasure seeking. Some aggressive acts reflect a mixture of offense and defense. Studies also have found that aggressive actions can be pleasurable. From studies of rats living in colonies and burrows, D. C. Blanchard and R. J. Blanchard (1984) observed that animals with a previous history of victory in combat appear to gain pleasure from the combat and seem to seek out interactions that permit display of offensive aggression. Studies with humans have provided considerable evidence that aggressive behavior for some individuals and in some circumstances can become pleasurable (Berkowitz, 1993). A very different type of motivation for aggression may in-

FIGURE 12.1
Rival fight between marine iguanas. Above: two males fighting by butting their heads together; below: the loser (right) lies flat in a submissive posture before the victor.

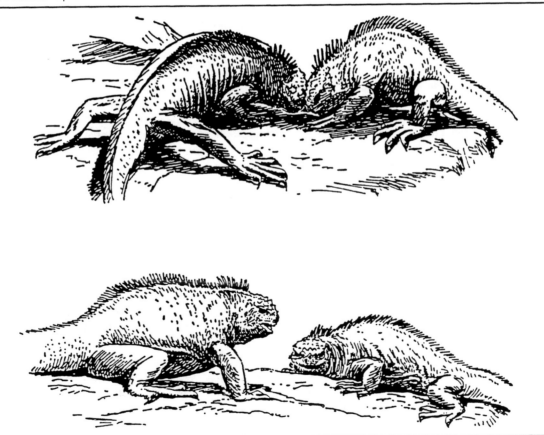

Source: From photographs by the author, Eibl-Eibesfeldt, 1972, p. 67.

volve a positive intention, like a mother animal protecting its young.

The Frustration-Aggression Hypothesis

The previous chapter described the theory of Berkowitz (1990, 1993) and supportive studies in which frustration led to anger. A much older formulation concerned the relationships between frustration and aggression. An influential 1939 book was reprinted in 1961 by Dollard, Doob, Miller, Mowrer, and Sears (1961). Its fundamental premises were taken from Freudian theory, and the relationship between frustration and aggression was stated as follows: "the occurrence of aggressive behavior always presupposes the existence of frustration" and furthermore, "the existence of frustration always leads to some form of aggression" (Dollard et al., 1961, p. 1). Many studies tested this set of statements. Although the frustration-aggression hypothesis is not accepted as valid today, in earlier days it stimulated a large body of research. Today the evidence is that frustration can lead to many forms of behavior and not only to aggression, and aggression has many sources besides the existence of frustration.

Berkowitz (1990) related frustration and anger and he proposed that this anger could, but need not, lead to aggression. He indicated that once people became cognizant of their anger, they could contemplate various ways of responding, and the more aware they were of their emotion, the less likely it was that they would behave aggressively. Persons who were not aware of their anger would be more likely to react to the frustration with aggression. Thus, a two-step process was proposed by Berkowitz (1990), in which frustration can lead to anger and, depending on the person, this can then lead to aggression. This two-step formulation differs radically from the frustration-aggression hypothesis described above.

Dollard et al. (1961, p. 7) defined frustration as involving (a) a clear sequence of acts and (b) the prevention of that sequence from continuing to its end of goal satisfaction or attainment. Generally, psychologists conceptualize frustration more broadly, considering that frustration occurs only when goal attainment is thwarted or blocked. Dollard et al., (1961), basing their ideas on drive theory, stated that

it does not matter what the source of interference is to prevent full occurrence of the behavioral sequence. Contemporary researchers are likely to focus on attributions regarding the nature of the goal interference or blocking, with attributions playing a large role in determining a person's emotional and behavioral reactions to frustration. Mere thwarting or blocking of goal attainment has been found in many studies not to lead to aggression, and attributions mute anger, as shown by Berkowitz (1990). Many studies show that circumstances ordinarily considered to lead to frustration do not necessarily do so (Berkowitz, 1993).

Depending on the source of the frustration, nonhuman animals as well as humans show a variety of reactions when a clear and predicted behavioral sequence is prevented from leading to goal satisfaction. For example, if subordinate rats are prevented from obtaining food in a set location because a dominant male interferes with the food-obtaining sequence, the food seeker behaves differently than when the interference is by an even more subordinate animal. Aggressive behavior is replaced by fleeing in the former case but not in the latter. Various behaviors by animals and humans have been observed in response to frustration, including regression, fleeing, and overcoming the frustration by problem solving and adoption of new behavioral strategies.

A different approach was taken by Amsel (1962). He emphasized nonreward occurrence for previously rewarded behavior and called it "frustrative nonreward." He considered frustration to be an unlearned (primary) aversive motivational state, resulting from reduced or eliminated reward when previously a set of behaviors was followed by the reward. His studies showed that if sometimes reward occurs and sometimes not, response persistence occurs as a reaction to frustration. Current work of Amsel (1990) concerns the effect of nonreward frustration on attention in nonhuman animals and human children. His concern is not with aggression as a reaction to frustration but with what processes heighten persistence and attention in normal animals and children and diminish persistence and attention under various conditions of pathology or drugs.

Not all psychologists agree with Amsel (1990)

that cessation of previously provided rewards necessarily leads to a motivational state of frustration. Moreover, most psychologists consider frustration far more broadly than the narrow meanings given by Dollard et al. (1961) and by Amsel (1990). Frustration can be defined in terms of a procedure imposed on an animal or human, that is, thwarting or preventing the subject from attaining a goal or blocking the subject from obaining an anticipated pleasure. However, this procedure need not create frustration as an internal aroused state. In humans, attributions about the source of the thwarting are important determinants for whether the person subjectively feels frustrated when a goal is blocked. If the nonreward or the failure to attain a goal is appraised as due to unavoidable or reasonable sources, reactions other than a subjective feeling of frustration can occur, and aggressive behavior is not likely.

When nonreward does lead to aggression, is it similar to the aggression induced by painful or other aversive circumstances? Studies of brain areas involved in aggression have addressed that question. Other issues are also pertinent in considering aggression. The discussion of anger focused on humans, because anger is not readily studied in nonhuman animals. However, a large literature exists on animal aggression, which is the next topic to be considered.

AGGRESSION IN ANIMALS

Is There an Aggression Drive?

Ethologists are zoologists who seek to understand how animals behave in their natural environments. Some ethologists have argued that there is an aggression drive, or a need to be aggressive (Eibl-Eibesfeldt, 1972; Lorenz, 1966). They believe not only that aggression is instinctive, but that when animals are deprived of the opportunity to aggress there is increased likelihood the animals will show aggressive behavior. They cite data that presumably reveal an innate need to aggress, and they extrapolate from observations of dogs, wolves, and apes to conclude that there is also an aggression drive for humans. That extrapolation has gone so far as to lead to the proposition that war, as an expression of such an aggression drive, is inevitable. Strong counters

have been written to this view (e.g., Groebel & Hinde, 1989). Many psychologists have questioned the inevitability of war based on an aggression instinct. They have further questioned the view that there is an aggression drive which, independent of suitable circumstances, makes mammals (including humans) inevitably act aggressively.

Certain groups and individuals advocate practices based on the belief that there is an innate need for aggression. Some communities set aside opportunities for sanctioned aggression, on the premise that "young people need to release pent up aggressive urges." This reflects cultural biases and practices but not a scientifically valid fact. Attempts to document that animals as well as humans have a need for aggression, and that this builds up by deprivation of aggression, have not been effective. Young animals do need to be active for muscle growth and many forms of sensory-motor learning, and as part of social learning young mammals of many species tussle and "roughhouse" in mock aggressive play, but such activity characteristically differs in behavior and intention from acts of aggression. Instead of emphasizing an aggressive drive, most psychologists focus on the role of species characteristics, learning, neurobiological processes, and situational factors. Species differ in terms of their peacefulness or aggressiveness. Individuals within a species also have unique learning experiences, and they may have unique neurobiological processes that interact with their learning background. It is known that some situations are far more likely than others to lead to aggressive behavior. With humans, socialization and neurobiological and developmental processes all interact with situational variables to increase or decrease aggression and violent behavior (American Psychological Society, 1997).

Conspecific Aggression

The term *conspecific* refers to animals of the same species, and conspecific aggression refers to aggressive behavior between animals of the same species. Although interspecies aggression also occurs, "aggression" usually refers to harmful actions against a member of one's own species. The term *agonistic* (Scott, 1958) has also been used to describe this type of aggression, in contrast to the term *predatory,* used for interspecies aggression.

Moyer (1976) reviewed many studies of animal aggression. These were mostly laboratory studies rather than observations made in naturalistic settings. Moyer proposed seven categories: predatory, intermale, fear-induced, irritable, maternal, instrumental, and sex-related. These categories differ in their characteristic patterns of behavior, the types of situations that tend to elicit them, and their neural and endocrine bases. Predatory aggression refers to attack on natural prey, or more generally, attack on members of another species. Instrumental aggression is the type that is not generated by emotion or motivation or the goal of intending harm, but rather is learned like any other behavior according to training and reinforcement of specific behaviors. In humans, instrumental aggression might be the action of shooting or bombing in response to orders by a commander. The seven categories initially were useful but later were found to be too limiting. When agonistic interactions of nonhuman animals were observed in naturalistic settings, Moyer's scheme was found to be inadequate. Later schemes, focusing on functional categories, emphasized the diversity of behavior patterns and their regulatory mechanisms across species (e.g., Archer, 1988). That is, different species may achieve similar functional ends by means of activation of different mechanisms.

Like anger, aggression is primarily social. The antecedent and the target for aggressive behavior ordinarily occur in the context of social interaction, although in some circumstances aggressive acts will be directed toward inanimate objects, such as when a nonhuman animal is in pain or is given other negative stimulation (Azrin, Hutchinson, & Hake, 1967; Azrin, Hutchinson, & Sallery, 1964; Azrin, Rubin, & Hutchinson, 1968). If an animal is given painful shock it will bite objects of wood, rubber, or metal when no other animal is present. However, when the animal receives painful stimulation and a conspecific is present, the other animal becomes the target of attack.

Nonsocial aggression is not usual but it may be artificially created for research purposes. For example, undomesticated as well as domesticated rats

will bite a leather glove when it is the apparent source for painful stimulation, but in natural settings aggression is ordinarily part of social interaction. D. C. Blanchard and R. J. Blanchard (1984; R. J. Blanchard et al., 1988) have documented that when animals live in a colony, the aggressive behavior of an attacking animal is finely matched with that of the defending animal. How the attacker behaves fits with how the defending animal behaves, and the defender varies his behavior in terms of the way the attacking animal behaves.

The Blanchards used "ethoexperimental" observations of aggression that were similar to their method for studying fear (D. C. Blanchard & Blanchard, 1987; R. J. Blanchard, Blanchard, & Hori, 1989). This method uses observation of naturally occurring behavior, which is the perspective of ethologists, and in addition, the researchers introduce into the animal colony systematic manipulation of experimental variables. The colony provides data that reveal natural behavioral patterns, like the establishment of dominance hierarchies. The Blanchards found with rat colonies that one male tends to initiate most of the fights, and subordinate males respond defensively (running away or rearing up to face the attacker without making a counterattacking motion). In this way, the "alpha" animal assumes dominance. This same animal is likely to be the one to attack an intruder rat placed into the colony. The Blanchards found that offensive attack was very different from defensive attack, and each type of aggressive behavior follows a typical set of patterns for a species. Certain types of situations are likely to lead to aggressive acts, and stereotypical behaviors are shown by members of the species.

Aggressive male behavior is characteristic for establishing dominance in a social hierarchy (D. C. Blanchard & Blanchard, 1990). Intermale aggressive behavior differs from mixed-sex or interfemale aggressive behavior in the kinds of behavior patterns typically shown and in the types of circumstances that elicit the behavior. Overall, males within a species show much more aggressive activity than do females within a species. Exceptions are found, like the golden hamster in which females are more aggressive than males (Moyer, 1976). In rat colonies studied by the Blanchards (1984, 1990), the dominant or alpha male shows the most frequent attacks on territorial intruders and is likely to be the most successful in fending off competitors for mating with an estrous female. This has been observed in many mammalian species in addition to rats, including baboon troops (DeVore, 1965) and Richardson's ground squirrels (Pellis, MacDonald, & Michener, 1996).

Response stereotyped aggression has been studied in many species. For example, Richardson's ground squirrels were observed during mating season in a free-living environment (Pellis et al., 1996). The lateral display (see Figure 12.2) was observed, and biting was recorded during agonistic encounters. Bites were far more frequent on the upper back than on any other part of the body. During chases, the attacking animal moved past the rump and bit the shoulders or upper back. Most of the agonistic encounters were between two males, although some male-female encounters were observed, if a male approached a female not yet in estrus or the female was already pregnant.

Monkeys have more varied ways than rodents for showing aggression, and threatening facial expressions are a potent form. Exline's study (1972) of rhesus macaques revealed that a "hard" menacing look occurs as an early stage of threat display in response to eye contact with other monkeys or humans. Like humans, monkeys may seek to avoid eye contact. If they select a more aggressive reaction, they will show an "anger threat" facial display, and when more aggressive, a leaping attack. Analysis of monkeys' responses showed that if facing a downcast glance, monkeys are likely to respond nonaggressively, but if facing a challenging glance, threat and attack are very likely. This is part of dominance patterning. As suggested by Exline (1972, p. 196), "maintenance of eye engagement (the mutual glance) serves as a dominance challenge to the rhesus macaque whether the contender is another rhesus" or a human or a member of another primate genus. Likewise, another's gaze aversion inhibits the monkey's threat display. Monkeys living in caged environments show response characteristics similar to those found in monkeys living in their natural environment.

Species characteristics can be studied by com-

FIGURE 12.2

Schematic representation shows a dorsal view of a Richardson's ground squirrel in three forms of lateral movement which involve pivoting around a vertical axis. The pivot point of each is represented by an X, and the dotted image of the squirrel represents the position following the lateral movement. The three pivot points are the pelvis (A), the shoulders (B), and the mid-body (C).

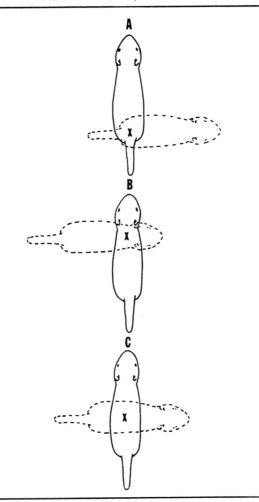

Source: From Pellis, MacDonald, & Michener, 1996, p. 125.

paring feral (wild) and domesticated animals. For example, feral and domesticated rats are alike in that alpha attacks on intruders occur to the back and not to the abdomen, and offensive and defensive attacks are very distinct behavioral patterns. However, differences also exist between feral and labo-ratory-raised rats, in part due to breeding and in part due to conditions in which the animals were raised. Such differences are evident especially with regard to defensive attack behaviors (R. J. Blanchard & Blanchard, 1987). For example, when an anes-thetized conspecific was brought by hand to an an-imal, feral rats (but not laboratory-raised rats) screamed and jumped at the animal.

Situational Variables

A situation that typically engenders or modifies ag-gressive behavior is that of an intruder entering another's territory. Another type of situation that provokes aggressive behavior is competition for mating. Situations requiring protective action can also engender or modify aggressive behavior. Ma-ternal activity may be stimulated more by some than other situations. Situational variables play a powerful role in all aggressive actions, including defensive attack.

Mice show defensive patterns that are similar to but not the same as those of rats (R. J. Blanchard et al., 1995). Mice, cats, pigs, and mountain sheep all show differences in attack behavior patterns that are offensive as distinct from defensive. The immediate situation determines whether the behavior is offen-sive or defensive. For example, when animals are regrouped, with the more dominant males removed, formerly subordinate males that had shown little of-fensive attack become far more aggressive, and previously dominant males in interaction with more dominant males become far less aggressive. Such regrouping effects have been found with many species. Greater alcohol consumption by subordi-nates, in natural as well as regrouping rat colonies, reflects stress experienced by subordinates, and in one regrouping study (R. J. Blanchard, Flores, Magee, Weiss, & Blanchard, 1992), higher volun-tary alcohol consumption was found in the post-grouping subordinates.

Response stereotyping occurs, with characteris-tic ways of responding for offensive and for defen-sive attack, and these stereotypical patterns are closely tied to characteristic elicitors or situations. Dawkins (1989, pp. 79–80) described how the fa-

mous ethologist Tinbergen moved two male stick-leback fish back and forth, each in a test tube. When the fish were moved toward the region where one stickleback had built its nest in a large fish tank, that fish took an attacking posture and the other took a retreat posture, and when the fish in the test tubes were moved toward the other nest area, the animals reversed their movements within the test tube. Ac-cording to the situation into which they were placed, behavior changed from offense to defense.

Animals respond to high incentive situations dif-ferently than to low incentive situations. For exam-ple, rats are more likely to fight over high-quality than over ordinary rat food (D. C. Blanchard & Blanchard, 1984). D. C. Blanchard and R. J. Blan-chard (1984) found that different types of behaviors occur if an animal is threatened in a familiar as op-posed to a novel situation, and the prior learning history of an animal modifies both the offensive and defensive types of behaviors shown. Fear appears to be the motivational variable mediating defensive attack, and anger-associated motivation underlies offensive aggressive actions. Anger and offensive attack apparently can be rewarding. In a colony, victorious animals and alpha animals were found to seek offensive attack behaviors.

Social situations affect the frequency of fighting. How docile or aggressive the conspecifics are influ-ences the behavior of the alpha animal. When alpha rats interacted with aggressive compared with more submissive subordinates, the agonistic behavior of the alpha rats was far more frequent and intense (R. J. Blanchard et al., 1988). Likewise, the number of males seeking access to an estrous female will determine the number of biting attacks in agonistic encounters involving competition for mating. When male Richardson's ground squirrels patrolled and sought to defend areas containing estrous fe-males, many more male-male agonistic encounters were recorded than male-female or female-female encounters during the key mating hours of late af-ternoon or early evening (Pellis et al., 1996).

The social circumstances in which aggressive behavior occurs also alter the effects of brain stim-ulation and lesions. Stimulation of specific brain areas in the absence of provocation from conspe-cific can produce aggressive behavior, but the social status of the animal being stimulated has been found to determine the quality and quantity of the aggressive behavioral displays (Delgado & Mir, 1969). Lesions in the hippocampus were found to affect rats' attack behavior differently when the rat was paired with a conspecific than when it was alone (R. J. Blanchard, Blanchard, & Fial, 1970).

Maternal aggressive behavior occurs when an animal protects its young. Studies of whether maternal attack behavior resembles the territorial behavior of male alpha animals has shown some similarities. Female rats with young have been found to use the lateral attack sequence of alpha male rats, but they also use a jump-bite attack, as a broadly defensive maneuver, which is not shown by alpha male rats. In a study of female rats with pups (Lucion & de Almeida, 1996), one group was first exposed to a real (and docile) cat and another group was exposed to a toy stuffed cat. The researchers found important differences between the groups in the maternal rats' attack behavior to a subsequent conspecific male intruder placed into the cage. Those who first encountered the real cat before confronting the male intruder reacted to the intruder with more defensive jump-attacks and less offensive boxing, lateral attacks, and biting.

Female compared with male aggressive behavior differs according to the species of the animals. In rats, females consistently have been found to be less aggressive and to show more defensive behavior than males, but in hamsters and especially in the spotted hyenas, females show more aggression than do males (Monaghan & Glickman, 1993). Observation of mountain gorillas (Watts, 1994) revealed that female-female fighting can occur in competition for access to males, and observations of the woolly spider monkey in Brazil (Strier, 1990) showed that the females have equal domination with males, neither males nor females showing obvious dominance hierarchies.

Play fighting behaviors are shown by various species, and animals display different types of play fighting at different ages. Although male and female adults tend to show different patterns of non-play attack behavior (R. J. Blanchard & Blanchard, 1989), for various species, prior to puberty the two sexes show similar play fighting. At the age of pu-berty males and females differ in their play fighting (Smith, Field, Forgie, & Pellis, 1996). The social situation also affects the pattern of play in adult animals. When adult subordinate male rats interact they show more adult-like defense behavior with one another, but when they interact with a dominant animal they show more juvenile forms of defensive behavior (Pellis, Pellis, & McKenna, 1993). Thus, whether in offensive attack, defensive attack, or play fighting, situational factors, especially social factors, strongly influence the kinds of behavior shown by members of a given species.

Interspecies Aggressive Behavior

Animals show aggression not only to members of their own species but also to members of other species. Rhesus macaques show threatening facial expressions to humans who engage the monkeys in eye contact, and feral rats will bite a gloved human hand in defensive attack. Such interspecies aggression is different from predatory killing for food. A lion killing an antelope concerns the motivation of hunger, not the behaviors and goals of aggression.

In the laboratory, one type of interspecies aggression that has been studied is that of mouse killing by rats. The percentage of rats that spontaneously kill mice has ranged from about 70% in wild (feral) Norway rats (Karli, 1956) to 4% in domestic rats (Galef, 1970). Interspecies aggression can occur for goals that are similar to conspecific aggression, like competition for a common food supply. To test whether interspecies attacks might be related to competition for food, investigators have examined if food deprivation affects mouse killing in domestic rats. Milner (1974) tested three groups of albino rats after different conditions of food availability. One group had a period of food deprivation, one group was allowed a period of free access to food after being food deprived, and a control group had no deprivation and had continued free access to food. Out of a total number of possible kills, the food-deprived group showed nearly 49% kills, the control group had 16%, and the group allowed free access to food following food deprivation had close to 4% mouse killing.

Successful prior competitive intraspe-

riences did not relate to mouse killing in one study (Baenninger & Baenninger, 1970). This suggests different factors are involved in interspecies aggression compared with conspecific aggression. One important factor is social familiarity. Animals normally have far more prior social and emotional experiences with members of their own than with members of other species. Familiarity and interspecies social experiences can mitigate the effect of food deprivation on interspecies aggression. If a rat is first exposed to a mouse, this can lessen the incidence of mouse killing. Even for a hungry rat, prior exposure to a mouse may inhibit its killing reaction due to the social experience. Milner (1974) concluded that in some studies no increased mouse killing occurred under conditions of food deprivation because there was prior exposure to the mouse. Interspecies social experiences alter the way animals interact. For example, some studies (Hall & Latané, 1974; Walton & Latané, 1973) found that even though rats prefer the company of other rats in comparison with interspecies contact, rats do seek social contact with other rodents like hamsters and gerbils. Moreover, if animals are raised together from early infancy and have strong social bonding akin to imprinting, natural enemies like cats and rats can live peaceably with one another (Kuo, 1938, 1960).

Familiarity can also be a factor in defensive attack. For example, when a colony of rats was observed in a burrow living arrangement (R. J. Blanchard et al., 1989) the rats showed markedly altered behavior after a cat was placed in a location above the burrow. Their movements and eating patterns were very much altered as part of a defensive pattern, and if they were close to the cat, the dominant male would show defensive attack behavior. However, if a nonmoving cat was present for a long period of time, some of the rats actually showed some approach to the cat. It was as if the rats began to question whether the cat was indeed "a predator/danger after a long period of nonmovement" (R. J. Blanchard et al., 1989, p. 134). This approach behavior appeared to be part of risk assessment. If another animal or foreign object was familiar and found not to be dangerous, the less likely was it to be the target of defensive attack. R. J. Blanchard

and colleagues (1989) identified risk assessment as a category of defensive behavior that plays an important role in situations involving aggression, both in conspecific and interspecies encounters.

BRAIN AREAS AND HORMONES

Brain Areas

Studies to identify which brain areas have a role in aggressive behaviors have followed the general pattern of research reviewed in studies seeking to find brain systems for hunger and satiation as well as for reward. The chapters on hunger and on reward described studies dealing with either stimulation or lesions of specific areas of the brain. In the same way, brain areas for aggressive behavior or its inhibition have been examined from the time of the 1930s. A good review of the history of this research is found in Renfrew (1997).

Key names worth noting will credit the early researchers who made important contributions. Papez (1937) identified the limbic system in the brain as important for emotion. Hess (1957) found that stimulation of specific areas of the hypothalamus in cats led to aggressive behavior. MacLean and Delgado (1953) showed that stimulation of the amygdala and hippocampus in cats and monkeys produced attack behavior. Flynn (1973; Wasman & Flynn, 1962), in electrical stimulation studies with cats, found that different areas of the hypothalamus led to different types of attack behavior toward rats, one type being affective (more like conspecific anger-induced attack) and one type being nonaffective and more closely resembling predatory behavior, such as stalking a prey.

Two kinds of brain areas were found to lead to attack behavior, especially to biting attack, in several animal species. One area was related to an aversive process, such as the experiencing of pain. When animals are presented with painful stimulation, like electric shock to the body, they bite inanimate objects like wood or rubber. When specific brain areas are stimulated, animals bite objects in the same way. Brain areas identified with this type of aversively motivated attack behavior are said to involve an Onset Aggression System (Renfrew,

1997), in contrast to other brain areas thought to involve an Offset Aggression System. Brain stimulation of the ON areas led to biting attack, whereas *offset* of brain stimulation of the OFF areas led to biting attack. The offset areas seemed to be the same as the "reward areas" that deal with pleasure, and this suggests that cessation of pleasure led to the biting attack. This is reminiscent of the frustration-aggression hypothesis, with cessation of reward leading to frustration and to attack. However, far more needs to be known before one can conclude that this type of study supports the frustration-aggression hypothesis.

Relatively less is known about the OFF system than about the ON system with regard to aggression. It is not clear to what extent removal of reward or pleasure, either through brain area stimulation offset or through behavioral nonrewarding, leads to aggression. Behavioral nonrewarding is more likely to lead to aggression in animals than in humans, and some evidence exists that offset of stimulation of pleasure areas leads to aggression in animals. Very little is known about the effect of removal of rewarding brain stimulation with humans. Moyer (1976, p. 109) reported the case of a patient who seemed addictively to require brain stimulation that led to relaxation, and without the stimulation the patient showed extreme aggressiveness. Beyond such rare data, little is known about brain stimulation offset and aggression in humans.

From studies with nonhuman animals certain ON areas have been identified. Specific areas in the amygdala, hippocampus, and septum have been found to lead to aggression when stimulated and to lead to docility when lesioned. The best documented brain area in which lesions lead to reduced aggressiveness is the amygdala. However, amygdala lesioning leads not only to less aggressive behavior but also to other changes, especially to impaired interpretation of information (Kalat, 1992). Removal of the temporal lobe in rhesus monkeys by Klüver and Bucy (1939) led to very tame and far less fearful animals, with a pattern of behavior known as the Klüver-Bucy syndrome. The critical area of lesion that led to the tameness was the amygdala. Various brain areas thought to be involved in aggression are depicted in Figure 12.3.

Hormones

In many animal species aggression appears to be related to the sex of the individual, so it is reasonable to ask if sex-related hormones play a role in aggression for nonhuman animals and for humans. Androgens are a class of male hormones, of which the major hormone, testosterone, is produced in the testes. Female hormones, estrogen and progesterone, are produced by the ovaries. Both male and female hormones have been studied in relation to aggression. In most species, the pattern of male aggressive behavior differs from the pattern of female aggression. Testosterone levels increase significantly during puberty, when aggressive behavior in males also increases significantly in many species. Although a naive guess might lead one to think that males fight because they have testosterone, and that the more testosterone they have the more they fight, this is not a valid formulation. As noted in Chapter 11, the relationship between testosterone and anger is far from simple, and the relationship between testosterone and aggression is even more complex. Most studies of adult nonhuman animals have shown that the amount of aggression or dominance does not reflect the overall level of testosterone. For example, in one study (Pellis, Pellis, & Kolb, 1992) some of the male rats soon after birth received testosterone injections and then were observed for play fighting in a later juvenile period and in adulthood. The initiation of playful attacks during the juvenile period was significantly greater for the experimental compared with control animals, but nonplayful attack in adulthood was unrelated to the neonatal testosterone treatment.

Researchers have measured base levels of testosterone, but it is important to note that levels of testosterone do not remain stable over time. They follow a circadian rhythm, and their levels vary according to many types of social interactions. During a fight the testosterone level goes up, and afterward it stays up for the victor and drops for the loser. Winning seems to be a big factor in raising testosterone levels. A review of salivary testosterone measures revealed that "testosterone affects behavior, but the outcome of behavior also affects testosterone levels" (Dabbs, 1993, p. 117). Testosterone levels rise and fall with success and failure in social

FIGURE 12.3
Schematic drawing of brain areas involved in emotions (anger, fear) and aggression.

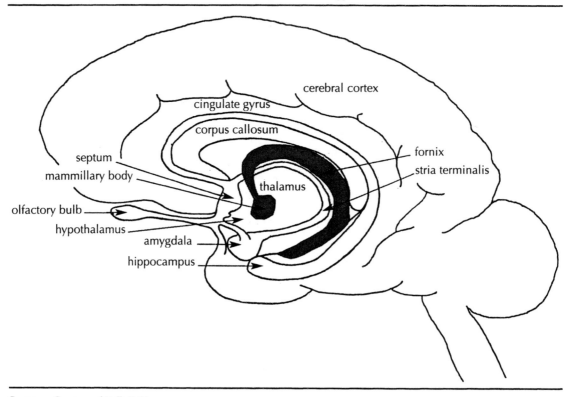

Source: Courtesy of B. E. F. Wee.

encounters. When rhesus monkeys won fights their serum testosterone level rose, and it dropped when they lost. When humans played varsity tennis, salivary testosterone increased when team members won a match and decreased when they lost. Before a match, testosterone was higher than on control days, as if the anticipation of competition heightened the testosterone levels. In chess matches, testosterone levels dropped for losing players and remained high or increased for winning players. The more astounding the win, the greater the effect. Vicarious winning also was found to change testosterone levels. College basketball fans were sampled over a number of weeks with respect to various matches of their college team, and testosterone levels dropped after losing games but remained or increased after winning games. Analogous to the

competitive wining and losing encounters, real or anticipated sexual activity in nonhuman animals and in humans was found to increase testosterone levels, and it did so for women as well as men (Dabbs, 1993).

Berkowitz (1993) reviewed studies on the relationship between testosterone and other male sex hormones and aggression. He drew an important distinction between the effect of prenatal or immediately postnatal testosterone levels, which have an organizing effect on the developing central nervous system, and testosterone levels in later life. Male sex hormones in utero in some instances were found to affect later aggressive behavior in girls as well as boys, presumably due to the organizing effect of prenatal male sex hormones.

Many studies have shown testosterone-related

organizational effects (Monaghan & Glickman, 1993). Castration of male mice up to the first few days after birth significantly decreases their testosterone levels and decreases their later aggressive behavior. When castration occurs in older animals their male-male aggression is decreased, but if they receive testosterone injections, the castrated animals show normal aggression. Testosterone injections do not lead to normal male aggression in mice if the castration occurs soon after birth. This is because neonatal castration alters brain organization, which is not reversed with later testosterone injection. If female mice have their ovaries removed up to about 1 month after birth and are then given testosterone daily, their later aggressiveness is very much increased compared with that of intact female mice. *Organizational* processes are thus evident when gonads are removed soon after birth, and *activational* processes are evident when gonads are removed and testosterone treatment is given in adulthood (Monaghan & Glickman, 1993).

Two additional types of animal studies demonstrate organizational processes, of fetal androgen levels affecting aggressive behavior after birth and into adulthood. One type of study with mice concerns the placement of the fetuses within the uterus. The other type of study involves spotted hyenas. In the study of mice, female fetuses located next to males are more aggressive in later life than female fetuses located in utero next to other females. Palanza, Parmigiani, and Vom Saal (1995) found that the female fetuses located next to males were exposed to the males' androgen, and although such exposed female fetuses did not differ in adulthood from other females in how they behaved toward their litter of pups, they did show more agonistic behavior toward intruders of both sexes. The study of spotted hyenas provides further evidence about an androgen-aggression relationship. The female spotted hyenas are larger, tend to be more dominant, and in certain types of interchanges they show more aggression than do the males (Glickman et al., 1992). Fetal androgens and estrogens have been implicated as leading to the masculinization of the spotted hyenas in their outward appearance (hyperdeveloped external genitalia that resemble a male penis) and in their aggressiveness and social dominance.

Some effects of sex hormones in adult animals are related to olfactory cues. Sex hormones change pheromones, and urine seems to provide the critical odor cues that alter aggression. Moyer (1976) described studies that showed that the odor either inhibits or triggers aggression in conspecifics. If castrated male mice have urine from an intact male mouse put on their fur, they receive far more aggressive acts than control castrates with plain water rubbed on their fur, and they receive hardly any aggressive acts if the urine is from a female mouse. Even intact stranger male mice show reduced aggression between them if one of the animals is rubbed with urine from an adult female mouse.

That hormones are only a part of the total picture is evident from studies involving social processes. For example, Monaghan and Glickman (1993) described studies of male dusky-footed woodrats, that when castrated fought as much as intact males when tested in a neutral area but when tested in social and natural house-defending environments were not as vigorous as intact males. In rhesus monkeys, androgen given to pregnant females alters the aggressive behavior of their female offsprings when tested in situations lacking normal social groupings, but does not do so within normal group life. Other studies show that when male rhesus monkeys are placed together into new groups, their testosterone levels prior to group formation do not correlate with their later dominance rank. However, after the ranks are made stable, alpha male testosterone levels rise very sharply, especially soon after the animal becomes the alpha male. No significant correlation was found between dominance rank and testosterone levels in long-term stable (normally formed) male groups, which suggests that social patterns lead to testosterone changes and not that initial testosterone levels lead to specific social and dominance patterns.

Studies with humans have shown mixed results, but overall, when confounding variables have been controlled or counteracted, testosterone levels and aggressiveness have not been found to be significantly related. One interesting study sought to evaluate the relationship in a laboratory setting (Berman, Gladue, & Taylor, 1993). College men volunteers provided saliva for measurement of testosterone levels before and after a competitive task. Reaction time was used to determine if the subject or his presumed "opponent" (in fact a computer) was the first to provide shock to the other. Aggression was defined by the magnitude of shock that the subject selected for the "opponent." The level of pretask testosterone was significantly related to aggression, with high testosterone subjects giving higher shock levels. This would suggest a direct link between the sex hormone and aggressive behavior. However, over trial blocks the aggression levels increased, with significantly and consistently higher shock settings given over trial blocks, and the testosterone levels decreased. Thus, an inverse relationship appeared over time between testosterone level and aggression. This study illustrated that for humans as for nonhuman animals, aggression and male sex hormone levels in adulthood are complexly and inconsistently related.

In addition to sex hormones, levels of serotonin and measures of certain serotonin metabolites have been thought to be related to aggression. A chemical compound called tryptophan is a precursor to serotonin, and some foods, like corn, are low in tryptophan. At one time it was thought that a significant relationship may exist between tryptophan depletion and aggression in humans, but neither carbohydrates (also thought to bear on aggression) nor tryptophan in the diet are clearly related to aggression in humans (Spring, Chiodo, & Bowen, 1987). Other data, including measures of a specific serotonin metabolite (5-HIAA, or 5-hydroxy-indole-acetic acid), have been studied. Some studies have found a relationship between aggression and serotonin turnover (Kalat, 1992, p. 479). Low turnover was related to aggression and high turnover was related to inhibition of aggression. Subordinates in a rat colony were found to have a high level of the serotonin metabolite 5-HIAA, and testosterone-induced dominance was found to be reversed by certain kinds of serotonergic agonists (Bonson & Winter, 1992). Serotonin is thought to inhibit impulsive behavior, and data from various animal studies suggest a relationship exists between low levels of serotonin and impulsive acts of aggression.

The relationship between hormones and aggres-

sion is complex. Some evidence exists that specific hormones in adult animals and humans are correlated with aggressive behavior, but one cannot make a conclusion about causality from such correlational relationships. Social experiences shape behaviors and modify hormonal activity, and because hormonal levels are modified by social experiences, cause and effect are not easily determined.

For a number of reasons, and because hormones like testosterone and serotonin have been found to relate to aggression, some researchers are exploring the role of genetic factors in individual differences in aggression. Complex relationships have been found between hormonal levels and situational factors, and genetic variables may contribute to these relationships. Study of animals living in groups and studies of regrouping (like those of R. J. Blanchard et al., 1992) provide important information about how early learning experiences, hormonal and genetic variations, and differences in a given situation can interact to heighten or diminish aggressive behavior of individual animals within the group. Far more studies are needed to show how early experiences and social situations affect the relationship between hormones and aggressive behavior in humans, especially in human adults.

SELF-INTEREST VERSUS COLLECTIVE INTEREST: COMPETITION AND HUMAN AGGRESSION

Self-Interest Versus Collective Interest

Humans show aggressive behavior in a wide range of circumstances and in a large variety of ways. Some ways are very subtle. If a person deprives another of a fair share of resources, this may be expressed by, "I was only looking out for myself, not trying to deprive you of your share!" The question arises, does "looking out for number one" fall into the category of "harm doing" and thus aggression? Controversy exists whether competition in the form of striving to be superior to others is subtly aggressive. Looking out for one's own interest is considered by many to represent individualism and not aggression. Do competition and individualism involve different kinds of motivation, and does one but not the other involve aggression?

Researchers have studied competitive sports to arrive at possible answers to the difference between individualism and competition and how they relate to aggression. For example, in some sports, like figure skating, one can try to perform at the highest possible achievement to win first place, with the motivation of maximizing one's own position but not being motivated to demean or harm a competitor. In team sports, in contrast, maximizing one's own position may undermine team achievement, so that individualism directly harms the performance of the team as a whole. Thus, one way of assessing to what extent individualism involves aggression is to examine the social context in which the individualistic aims occur. If the individualistic actions hurt group action, harm doing is evident. Not all circumstances are easily analyzed into group versus individual welfare, however, and so considerable debate exists about individualism and aggression in terms of the motivation of intent to harm others.

The way competitiveness and individualism affect aggression is complex. Looking out for one's own individualistic interests can have the same effect as competitively outdoing others, and this may be experienced by one's opponent as aggression. Actions that intentionally disregard the dignity or value or needs of the other person in a transaction, regardless of the verbalized intent, involve aggression. An alternative approach involves the aim of protecting collective interest. In protecting collective interest one protects the interests of the self as well as of the members of the group. One can strive for high achievement in oneself as well as in others, or one can place oneself in opposition to others. The motivation and actions are different in these two circumstances.

Human aggression can occur for similar reasons that nonhuman animals show aggression, that is, to dominate, to defend, to offset pain, or to retaliate against inflicted pain. Not all theorists agree with the biological reductionistic interpretation of human aggression given by E. O. Wilson (1979), but instead take a strong social learning emphasis or a more contemporary evolutionary perspective

(Buss, 1999). The later view focuses on evolutionary forces that shape how species adapt to specific circumstances. The manifestation and intent of human aggression show that aggressive behavior is far more varied and far more complex than shown by nonhuman animals, and human aggression has relatively few preset patterns. Human aggression can involve behaviors that are also shown by nonhuman animals, but for some behaviors there is no parallel. Similarities can be seen in that humans like animals will fight and bite. Biting as aggression can be seen in small children who seek to get their own way or as a method of defensive attack. However, humans use verbal or physical weapons unlike the way aggression occurs in nonhuman animals.

Many human groups as well as individuals within groups show the intent to be superior to others. Having a large house, a glamorous spouse, the fastest car, the most attractive clothes often reflect a striving to be superior. For norm-defying adolescents, having the lowest grades, using substance-abuse drugs, and going in untidy clothes to school also can reflect behaviors that demean others (like parents and teachers) and that reflect superiority strivings. Aggression need not reflect brutish efforts to win or to conquer.

Psychologists have developed forms and questionnaires that measure aggression, and they reveal human aggression to be varied and complex. The Buss and Perry (1992) aggression questionnaire, for example, yielded four factors: physical aggression, verbal aggression, anger, and hostility. The hostility factor in that questionnaire combined the resentment and suspicion scales of the earlier Buss and Durkee (1957) hostility inventory. Human aggression in symbolic form is often unrelated to territory or food or mating, and forms of demeaning others can occur in an almost unlimited variety of competitive situations. Competition offers a study of aggression, although more violent forms of aggressive behavior occur in countless other circumstances.

Sports and Games

One of the ways humans in many societies channel aggressive behavior is through sport. At one level, sport is defined as fun and as exercise, but most sports involve a competitive win-loss set of outcomes, and some form of attack behavior often takes place with the aim of turning the competition into a win rather than a loss for the aggressor. Parents and other adults influence children's values concerning sport at an early age (Roberts, Treasure, & Hall, 1994). Values that favor task mastery lead to positive and prosocial behaviors (Treasure & Roberts, 1994), whereas values concerning self-elevation and ego rewards are more likely to lead to negative and aggressive behaviors. Terms like *one upmanship* or *besting* someone have been used to describe the competitive spirit that is likely to lead to actions that demean or thwart others.

Many professionals in recreation and social services urge the adoption of *cooperative games* or win-win games and sports, in which all participants play for the joy of the game (Harris, 1976; Lentz & Cornelius, 1950; Orlick, 1978; Schneider, 1976; Sobel, 1983). The aim is to share activities and pleasure, not to defeat an opponent. To the extent that cooperative games and sports are geared toward mastery and challenge, all participants experience a sense of achievement and a type of "win." Such games and sports minimize combat and aggression, maximize prosocial concern for the welfare of others, and minimize the negative emotional consequences of lowered self-confidence and "feeling defeated." Just as competitive games and sports have tended to teach the desirability of winning at the expense of others, cooperative games and sports teach the value of cooperation and of sharing positive outcomes. Even though teamwork and sharing within a cooperative framework are desirable, modern social living in industrialized nations has emphasized competitive rather than cooperative approaches to sports and games.

Psychologists and other scientists have studied "gamesmanship" in the laboratory by means of a Prisoner's Dilemma Game (PDG). This is a widely used approach to test hypotheses in *game theory,* which deals with theoretical formulations about the way people make choices in games of strategy. Researchers study the strategies people use when having to make choices that lead to outcomes (rewards or gains versus punishments or losses). Many recreational games, especially those using dice or cards, involve a mixture of strategy and luck (the roll of the dice or the draw of the cards), but in the PDG only the choices of the players determine the outcome for each "move" or trial. Figure 12.4 illustrates the way gains and losses can occur when the two players in a PDG make either a cooperative or a competitive choice on a given trial.

Many writers use the term *noncooperative* rather than the term *competitive* for PDG choices that are not cooperative. In discussing allocation of resources (Knight & Chao, 1991) as well as the PDG (Komorita & Parks, 1995), various writers distinguish between "competitive" and "individualistic" choices. The latter focuses on maximizing self-gain and the former focuses on besting another. However, the present discussion uses the term *competition* to highlight the fact that in the PDG a noncooperative choice serves both self-interest and superiority over the other and does not serve collective interest. Whereas in a zero-sum game the players have opposing interests (the more one player wins the less the other player can win), the PDG is a mixed-motive game, with the players having a conflict between the motivation to cooperate and the motivation to compete.

There are several types of mixed-motive games, of which the PDG is the best known. The usual payoff matrix for costs and benefits is one in which collective gains would *not* maximize one's own personal gains. When players make choices that are in

FIGURE 12.4
Prisoner's Dilemma game.

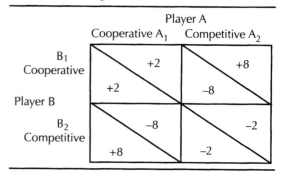

Source: Patterned after Ferguson, 1982, p. 349, Fig. 11.1.

their best collective interest, these choices do not maximize personal individual gains (Rapoport, 1970). In the example in Figure 12.4, players A and B have available a cooperative and a competitive strategy. The payoffs to the left of the diagonal lines are for player B and to the right of the diagonal lines are for player A. If both players make cooperative choices (cell A_1B_1) they collectively get the most total gains, but individually they do not gain as much as they would if they had split choices. If A selects the cooperative choice and B selected the cooperative choice, B would gain only 2 points, but if B made the competitive choice (A_1B_2), B would receive 8 points (and A would lose 8 points). Note that a strategy to maximize collective gains brings collective gains *only* if both players follow that strategy. As soon as the other player makes a competitive choice, the player making the cooperative choice gets a heavy penalty. This poses a dilemma. If both players consistently made the competitive choice (A_2B_2) they would lose a lot of points.

In some mixed-motive games players may have verbal or physical interchange, but in many investigations players are permitted only choice behavior without other forms of interchange. Thus, mixed-motive games are likely to show subtle aggression (sometimes called "defection") which does not involve aggression in the usual sense of verbal or physical combat. However, noncooperation leading to the defeat of another person in favor of self-elevation fits the characteristics of "intent to harm or demean or defeat" which are ordinarily considered aggression.

Thibaut and Kelley (1959) used the concept of the PDG for describing dominance patterns in real-life interactions. They called one pattern "mutual fate control," and it resembled a PDG with a payoff matrix similar to that of Figure 12.4. In this circumstance, called an *exchange* situation, the interacting persons might elect to help each other by selecting the A_1B_1 choices. They also can elect to harm each other. Another pattern, called "mutual behavior control," is like a PDG with a payoff matrix that gives gains or rewards to both persons for A_1B_1 *and* A_2B_2 choices (and gives losses or punishments to both persons for A_2B_1 and A_1B_2 choices, as described by Kelley, 1997, p. 144).

The mutual behavior control circumstance is referred to as a *coordination* situation. In this pattern the possible gains for the collective good come from two combinations in the payoff matrix, in contrast to only one combination of choices in the mutual fate control. In exchange situations a promise-threat interaction is likely, with compliance to a command being rewarded and noncompliance being punished. Coordination situations lend themselves to initiative-taking interactions, with the person taking the initiative depending on the other to follow the example. Kelley (1997) considered it important to separate the two kinds of dominance patterns, the first being more concerned with pursuit of self-interest and the second more concerned with pursuit of common interests. Communication patterns differ when interacting parties have a conflict of interest compared with commonality of interests.

Several players in N-person games (called social dilemmas) have been studied to show processes in coalition formation, trust, and cooperation (Messick & Librand, 1995; Orbell, Dawes, Schwartz-Shea, 1994). How much cooperation or competition is shown is influenced by many variables. In the PDG the gains and losses of the payoff matrix have a large influence (Antonides, 1994). Payoffs and losses can be biased to lead to more cooperation or to more competition. Enzle, Hansen, & Lowe (1975) found that payoff matrices significantly affected amount of cooperative versus competitive choices in the PDG, and Deutsch and Kraus (1962) in a game similar to the PDG showed clearly that the greatest losses of money occurred when both players had punitive capabilities. Without punitive capabilities, the interacting persons cooperated and both gained money. Being able to punish an opponent appears to increase competitive and aggressive behavior, even when verbal interaction and negotiation are possible (Raven & Kruglanski, 1970). Threats (and promises) are clearly ways of controlling another's actions. Threats can be used as acts of aggression, to intimidate another, and these need not involve physical harm. Limiting another's options, removing rewards, coercion into doing unwanted behaviors, and demeaning another's status can be considered aggression insofar as they lead to the recipient's experience of discomfort and stress.

Interactions in games, even those presumed to involve fun and not actual monetary profit, often provide instances of such aggression.

The PDG is used to simulate business decision making. Players without exchange of real money can nevertheless reveal pregame stereotypes and attitudes. In one PDG study (Ferguson & Schmitt, 1988), men and women college students played a simulated business game that involved bogus corporate profits and losses. Information about the game was provided on a computer screen and responses were made on a computer keyboard. The subjects were told their "partner" was in another room. Half the subjects played against "John Morrison" and the other half against "Jane Morrison," and they received "responses" from their presumed partner over 30 trials. Both partner and subject were to make a response concurrently, and as soon as the subject made his or her choice the response of the partner, along with information about accumulated profits and losses, was shown on the screen. In fact, the partner's responses were preprogrammed to be overall nonbiasing 50% cooperative responses (the computer gave the same sequence of responses to all the subjects), regardless of what strategy the subject chose. A maximum possible profit for the subject and a maximum possible loss for the partner would have occurred if 0% of the choices were cooperative. In other words, gainful self-interest and punitive loss for the "other" was assured with a 100% competitive strategy across all trials.

As seen in Figure 12.5, when the subjects began the trials, between 40% and 50% of their choices were cooperative, regardless of the sex of the partner. However, by the last set of trials, far fewer cooperative responses were given to the "man partner" than to the "woman partner" by both the men and women subjects. Subjects' gender was not a significant factor, but that of the partner was significant, and it became so increasingly over trials. Thus, although the partner gave the same responses to all subjects, depending on which gender the subjects believed their partner to be, over identical experiences their responses diverged rather than converged. From the subjects' behavior one can infer that different rules exist for how much self-interest

FIGURE 12.5
Prisoner's Dilemma mean percent of cooperative responses as a function of sex of subject, sex of "partner," and trial blocks.

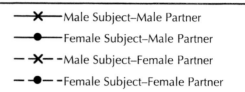
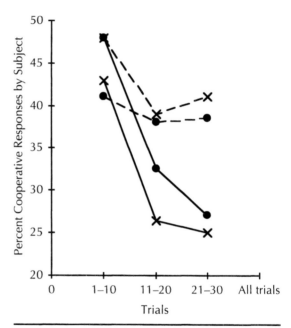

Source: From Ferguson & Schmitt, 1988.

compared with common interest is to be shown to men versus women. The stereotype that one can (or should) be more competitive with men than with women was evident in these PDG choices.

Culture

Cultures vary in how much they foster competition and aggression. For example, Montague (1978) reported that Tahitian and Inuit societies teach nonaggression and have nonviolent and gentle societies.

The characteristics of highly aggressive and even violent societies and highly peaceful and nonviolent societies are markedly different. Robarchek and Robarchek (1992) compared the aggressive Ecuadorian Amazon Waorani people and the peaceful Malaysian rainforest aboriginal Semai people. These two peoples have different world views, self-images, social relations, and social control patterns. Individualism is key in the warlike Waorani and emphasis on group cohesion and mutual support is key in the Semai. After missionaries offered a peaceful alternative to the incessant retaliatory killings of the Waorani, the Waorani soon rejected their strong aggressive approaches, relieved to live more peacably. Robarchek and Robarchek (1992) attribute the initial aggression to the cultural meanings the Waorani gave to the events in their lives. With new cultural beliefs and new methods of dealing with interpersonal conflicts their warlike behaviors also changed.

Kohn (1986) distinguished between *structural* and *intentional* competition. Structural competition is imposed by the situation. One example of a structural factor is the payoff matrix in situations like the PDG, which influences how much or how little competitiveness is likely to occur. Intentional competition refers to a given person's competitiveness, and this can be manifest in situations with little or no structural competition. For example, a person coming to a party can competitively focus on his or her superior skills or charms even when others at the party are not competitively concerned. Kohn (1986) further distinguished between *intergroup* and *intragroup* competition. As described by Robarchek and Robarchek (1992), the extreme aggressiveness of the Waorani was evident in both their intergroup and intragroup behavior. Both outsiders and persons within the group were met with extreme violence, even sometimes for minimal infractions. Other cultures have strong intragroup cohesion with marked concern for the common interest, but there is strong intergroup competition and fierce aggressive attack on outsiders.

In comparing many cultures and countries, Kohn (1986) found that the United States appears to be the most competitive. Real-life situations and laboratory studies support that conclusion, although controversy exists whether competition or individualism is the key variable. Parks and Vu (1994), using the concept of individualism rather than competition to describe the American culture, compared Americans' dilemma game playing (social dilemmas and PDG) with that of South Vietnamese, whose culture is collectivist. These researchers found that cooperative choices declined far more for the American than the South Vietnamese subjects in the PDG. Kohn (1986) considered that children in American schools are trained far more to be competitive than cooperative. In spite of this, when children have an opportunity for cooperative training and cooperative games, they strongly prefer these to the competitive approach, and achievement in school can occur without competitive training. High achieving children are not necessarily also high in competitiveness. This supports the data of Spence and Helmreich (1983) already cited, that very high achieving adults were not found to be very high in competitive striving.

Kohn (1986) provided a wide range of studies to counter the sociobiology view (E. O. Wilson, 1979) that aggression and competition are intrinsic to human nature. He cited studies that show that competitiveness is not universal and that competitiveness is not necessarily in the best interest of the individual. Moreover, competitiveness is often not in the best interest of the community or group. Kohn (1986) indicated that the most effective way to change individual *intentional* competition is to change the culture and its practices, that is, to change *structural* competition.

The conceptualization of Kohn (1986) concurs with Adlerian writing (Adler, 1930, 1933/1964; Dreikurs, 1992; Dreikurs & Grey, 1992; Dreikurs, Grunwald, & Pepper, 1998). Dreikurs (1971/1992) described how a vertical competitive belief in superiority versus inferiority is damaging to all members of the society. It leads to anxiety, defensiveness, unnecessary demeaning of others, and continuous self-doubt. To retrain individuals and communities for minimizing competition, new values need to replace old values, and new methods of interpersonal relationships need to be implemented. The values and beliefs held by individuals and the culture will increase or decrease cooperation compared with competition. Since the 1920s, Adlerians urged that training for cooperation and minimizing of competition benefits the individual and the society as a whole (Ferguson, 1958, 1989, 1989/91, 1995, 1996). The Adlerian approach emphasizes both the individual and the group. An either-or approach is not beneficial: A primary emphasis on the individual's gains is damaging to the group and this eventually comes to hurt the individual; a primary emphasis on the group's gains neglects the needs of each individual, and this eventually comes to hurt the group. To be effective, actions must be geared to help the interest and welfare of both the individual and the group. Many specific Adlerian techniques have been developed for increasing cooperation, to the benefit of the individual, the family, the school, the work place, and the community.

HUMAN AGGRESSION: POWER, AROUSAL, AND LEARNING

Human aggression is often direct and hurtful. Violent behavior, as an extreme form of aggression, occurs in homes and on the streets. Family violence appears to be on the increase (American Psychological Society, 1997). Children and spouses are physically and verbally abused. Defenseless persons, including the elderly, are targets of aggression in many countries. Rules of conduct and the norms of a community differ, so that some groups accept or even condone aggression much more than do others. Psychologists have assessed the situational factors that tend to lead to aggression and the reasons people use aggression when nominally it is not sanctioned. The stated belief in American society is that exchanges in interpersonal relationships should be peaceful, yet aggressive behavior is shown frequently and in ways that are not sanctioned. A full treatment of this topic is beyond the scope of the present book, but some issues are considered here.

Power

In autocratic societies, people in power use coercion to enforce obedience. Aggression by the person in power, but not by the subordinate, is sanctioned. In democratic societies, negotiation rather than coercion and aggression tends to be advocated. The relationship between power and aggression has interested historians, politicians, and economists as well as psychologists.

Milgram's Studies of Obedience. Milgram (1963, 1965), in a series of experiments, showed that many persons will perform painfully aggressive actions as acts of obedience when a person with power of status and authority commands such actions. An experimenter with authoritarian demeanor instructed subjects to be "teachers" and to give electric shock to a "learner" whenever that person made a mistake in his learning. Unbeknownst to the subjects, the learner was the experimenter's confederate and never received any shock. In the initial experiments, the learner was in another room from the subject and only voice contact was available. In later experiments, visual contact was also available. Because the subjects believed they were actually giving shocks, of concern to the researcher was the question of how much painful shock a subject was willing to deliver to a stranger who never attacked or harmed the subject, simply on the basis of obedience to a powerful authority.

Subjects were to start at the first shock level of presumably 15 volts, and from then on to increase the punishment for mistakes. Increasingly strident promptings from the experimenter occurred (e.g., "It is absolutely essential that you continue") if the subject hesitated to give higher voltages of shock. The findings dismayed a great many people (laypersons, the media, and psychologists alike). In one study 65% of the subjects gave the maximum shock level, even though that went beyond the point where the learner had screamed in pain and subsequently was silent due to undisclosed misery. As Miller, Collins, and Brief (1995, p. 5) pointed out, "the power of the situation" led to obedience of such an extreme form. Some persons disobeyed the authority on the basis of humanitarian concerns for the learner, but a very large number of subjects gave shock levels that would have inflicted a lot of pain had the shock been real. A researcher (Elms, 1995, p. 25) who helped conduct the initial experiments stated "We were gratified when any subject resisted authority. . . . As more and more subjects obeyed every command, we felt at first dismayed" and then increasingly distressed. Milgram was attempting to understand the phenomenon of obedience, but had not anticipated how much harm doing would result from obedience.

The nature of the situation was crucial. When the "learner" was in the same room as the subject, obedience (of maximum shock level given) decreased. Empathy for the learner nullified some of the obedience to the authority. Also, when the experimenter was not in the room but gave instructions by phone, the obedience sharply decreased. The studies reviewed by Milgram (1974) are of interest because two processes occurred: One was aggressive behavior, of the attacks on the learner, and the other was obedience to authority in a power-oriented situation. Because there was no clear evidence of intent to harm the learner and because different procedures used by Milgram showed that obedience was the main factor, different interpretations regarding the findings of Milgram are possible. Miller and colleagues (1995, p. 6) argued that aggression was not involved, only obedience was. However, attack on the learner did occur. For many subjects the emotion was contrary to the attack behavior (many subjects had strong negative emotional reactions when giving such high shock levels), but the attack in fact was knowingly made (not accidental). The attack behavior thus tends to fit what was described by Moyer (1976) as *instrumental aggression*. As the studies of Milgram showed, such attack behavior was clearly a function of power in the situation.

French and Raven: Bases of Power. Various theories about power have been advanced by psychologists, and one of the best known is that of French and Raven (1959). Aggression played a role in only one of their categories of power. For these authors, power means influencing others. The theory cited five different bases of power, with informational influence not called a power basis but being a sixth basis of influence (Raven, 1993).

In the original (French & Raven, 1959) formulation the five bases of power were: *reward* power,

coercive power, *legitimate* power, *referent* power, and *expert* power. In his description many years after the initial formulation, Raven (1993) included *informational influence*, of persuading others to a course of action based on providing relevant information. The power to reward is clearly a way to influence others, and on its own it does not involve aggression or intent to harm. In contrast, coercive power is based on the punitiveness of the more powerful person, and this often can involve aggression by the more powerful person. Legitimate power rests upon values and internalized standards that allow the less powerful to accept the legitimacy of being influenced by the more powerful. Referent power is based on a desire to identify with a more powerful person because of that person's status or attractiveness. Expert power is based on the more powerful person having greater knowledge than the less powerful, who accepts the influence by the expert.

Further work by Raven (1993) showed that the more confident influencers used more informational power bases, while less confident influencers relied on other bases, like legitimate or coercive power. Cross-cultural differences were also evident in terms of ways that children sought to influence each other. Coercive power was likely to be used by children in Italy and Argentina, whereas children in Japan were likely to use referent power. In developing the "bases of power" postulations beyond the original formulation, Raven (1992; Gold & Raven, 1992) added that bases of power can lead to inverse consequences, such as a subordinate doing the opposite of what the influencer intended. This depends on the subordinate's assessment of the influencer's motivation. If the subordinate assesses that the more powerful person is exerting influence primarily for his or her own interest or gain, resistance is likely, and if coercive power is used, a spiral of negative interactions is likely.

Analysis of political figures' actions (Raven, 1990), such as Churchill influencing Franklin Roosevelt, showed that effective influencing avoided use of coercive power, which could have led to noncompliance. A survey of women executives (Oyster, 1992), selected from the National Association of Female Executives, showed that former bosses of these women used different types of power bases, with significant differences between best and worst bosses. Those judged as best bosses most often used *referent power,* and worst bosses were reported as using *coercive* and *legitimate* power most often.

The work by Raven on power did not deal extensively with aggression, but the applications are evident. Autocratic control as coercive power is used frequently by political dictators, strict teachers, and autocratic parents. If this is interpreted by the subordinate as not in the best interest of the subordinate, resistance is likely. Moreover, the fact of using coercive power rather than informational power alters attributions of both the subordinate and the person in power. In real life and even in a laboratory study this occurs in complex ways. In one laboratory study (O'Neal, Kipnis, & Craig, 1994), different influence methods were randomly allocated to different persons, and the influencer's appraisal of the target person's reactions to the influence (in terms of "dominance") was found to vary as a function of the mode of influence. That is, subjects using informational methods of influence judged their target persons to be significantly less dominant than subjects using more coercive power approaches. When one uses coercive power, even if that is not one's personal choice, one is more likely to attribute resistance to others and thus to appraise them as more dominant than when one seeks to influence others informationally.

When in real life the autocratic use of coercive power leads to resistance by the subordinate and to the powerful person describing the subordinate as being not submissive (that is, having "dominance"), the person in power is likely to use more punitive action. Thus a cycle of aggression and counteraggression is likely to occur. With animals as well as humans, research has shown that the induction of pain can lead to aggressive responses. As a defensive attack against pain or humiliation, children and adults are likely to use counteraggression against coercion by the more powerful. Children who were hit or beaten by adults often have been found to retaliate by counteraggression in some way. Moreover, once coercion and aggression have been used

by the powerful, this suggests to the less powerful that rules of conduct include aggression, and that aggression may be sanctioned. Belief in use of aggression as a mode of influence becomes established when subordinates observe aggression in the actions of powerful others.

Power and Male Gender Role. Considerable controversy exists whether men are more aggressive than women. Researchers have sought to identify under what circumstances there is more aggression by men and under what other conditions there is minimal gender difference in aggression (Bettencourt & Miller, 1996; Knight, Fabes, and Higgins, 1996).

Men in many countries follow a belief system that in popular culture is called "macho." Early in the 20th century Adler described the negative impact of the presumed powerfulness and superiority of men (versus women). Using the term *masculine protest* (Adler, 1910/1978, 1933/1964; Bottome, 1939, pp. 194–199; Keenleyside, 1937), he noted that society's pressures for men to be superior and powerful induced stress and malaise in both men and women, with women resistant to a subordinate role and men under stress from the pressure to live up to the mythical masculine ideal. He pointed out that this pressure for male power and superiority led to dysfunction in the individual and in a marriage relationship, and that it was a potential source of stress in all relationships between men and women. Testing men subjects, Eisler and Blalock (1991) developed a measure that is congruent with Adler's postulation. With their measure of masculine gender role stress (MGRS) they found five factors relating to such stress. The stress-inducing masculine beliefs included reliance on aggression and power as ways of coping. Their data provide support for Adler's concepts. Rigidly held gender role beliefs regarding masculinity led to dysfunction and vulnerability to health problems in men.

One of the dysfunctional manifestations associated with macho beliefs is high alcohol consumption. A study of over 4,000 male military veterans (Windle, 1994) showed that men who followed more of the masculine active behavioral patterns tended to have higher testosterone levels, alcohol consumption, and aggression. The data could be interpreted to mean that higher testosterone levels led to the higher aggression, but from a correlational perspective and from other known facts, it is as likely that these men's macho beliefs led to increased aggressive "acting out," testosterone levels, and alcohol consumption.

Alcohol and Aggression.   As described in an earlier chapter, alcohol consumption is found to be related to the need for power (McClelland, 1973) and to aggressive behavior (S. P. Taylor, 1993; S. P. Taylor & Chermack, 1993). Bailey and Taylor (1991) showed that intoxicated individuals with fairly high aggressive dispositions responded more aggressively to provocation than did intoxicated individuals with low tendencies for aggression. Pharmacological effects have been identified to relate alcohol ingestion with aggression (Chermack & Taylor, 1995). Inhibitions are loosened with alcohol consumption. Additional variables have also been identified to account for the increase of aggressive behavior with alcohol ingestion. Although in general alcohol ingestion increases aggressive behavior, not all individuals behave aggressively when intoxicated. The amount of frustration that individuals experience, and people's belief that alcohol increases aggression (Ito, Miller, & Pollock, 1996; Murphy & O'Farrell, 1996), have been found to increase aggressiveness under intoxication.

Laplace, Chermack, and Taylor (1994) studied in the laboratory whether people who have a tendency to use aggressive behavior as a method for solving interpersonal conflicts are likely to decrease their usual socialized inhibitions under alcohol consumption. Three groups of 20 men college student volunteers were selected on the basis of their self-reported patterns of low, moderate, and high alcohol consumption. Half the subjects in each group received a high, and half a low, dose of alcohol (relative to body weight). Neither group knew what amount they consumed. Subjects received the experimental task after a 25-minute wait, to allow the peak blood alcohol concentration to be reached. Before the start of the experiment they had been in-

formed that in one of the tasks they would receive mild electric shock.

The experimental procedure involved each subject's receiving shocks to his wrist to determine his unpleasantness threshold, and he was told his "opponent" was receiving the same procedure. (There was no actual opponent.) The task was to be a reaction time competition containing 10 shock intensities, with 10 corresponding to the subject's unpleasantness threshold. If the subject was faster than the opponent the subject would select a level of shock from 1 to 10 to *give* the opponent, and the subject would *receive* shock set by the opponent if the latter were faster than the subject. For each trial the subjects had visual information about the level of shock the opponent set. A total of 21 trials with increasing provocation (higher shock levels) was preprogrammed. On half the trials the subject "lost" and received shock. Thorough debriefing occurred at the end of the study. Aggression was measured by the magnitude of shock the subjects selected during the trials for the opponent.

The results showed that preexperimental alcohol patterns and experimental dosage had a significant interaction effect on the mean shock levels subjects selected to give the "opponent." Within the low-experience group, those given the low-dosage experimental alcohol consumption set the lowest mean shock levels of all subject groups across trials, but those given the high-dosage set the highest mean shock levels. This showed that the effect of alcohol dosage increased aggression the most for those men whose prior alcohol consumption history was a low amount of drinking. In addition to this interaction, the experimental alcohol dosage had a significant main effect on amount of aggression, as shown by shock levels given to the opponent. For example, for all three groups overall, on the initial trials the high-dose subjects set a mean shock level of 5.5 compared with 4.2 for the low-dose subjects. The fact that confrontation raised aggression was seen by the fact that at the end of the 21 trials, all three groups gave significantly higher shock levels than at the start of the trials. The study revealed a number of important findings about the role of prior drinking experience in the way that alcohol affects aggression, and it confirmed the fact that increased quantity of alcohol consumed leads to increase in aggressive behavior.

Arousal and Learning

Aggression can be expressed instrumentally, without affect, and it can be expressed with incongruous affect, as in the Milgram studies, in which many subjects experienced self-blaming emotions and intense distress regarding the extreme attacks they were inflicting. Aggression can be expressed with emotions of anger, rage, disgust, or even joy. For some individuals under special circumstances, the joy of excitement can be the affect involved in aggression. Seeking arousal sometimes can instigate aggression.

Some individuals behave aggressively in line with a thrill-seeking motivation. Aggression raises testosterone level and various physiological indicators of arousal, like blood pressure and heart rate. Increasingly, newspapers and magazines report hideous aggressive actions in urban as well as rural areas that appear to be motivated by seeking of excitement and thrills. Evidence on this point is still sparse. A thrill-seeking personality type (Type T personality) has been described by Farley (see, for example, Morehouse, Farley, & Youngquist, 1990) and others (Nelson, 1992). Some evidence exists that the combination of impulsivity and thrill seeking leads to aggressive behavior (Pfefferbaum & Wood, 1994). To what extent such aggression-based thrill seeking is learned and to what extent an individual is disposed physiologically to this type of behavior is still not clear.

As evident in the Milgram type of obedience study, a person can attack others without being provoked or attacked by another. In the Milgram studies the emotion was not anger nor was the emotion congruent with the attack behavior. Depending on the motivation of the subject, the goal was to oblige or placate the authority rather than to harm the person being shocked. However, other types of studies, in which the target also had not provoked or attacked the person, found aggression was accompanied by a congruent affect and a goal of harm-doing. The best known area of research on this topic

deals with the effects of media violence. Some controversy remains about the findings of this area of research, but overall, it is established that people behave more aggressively after viewing videos or movies containing highly aggressive visual content. Many explanations for this effect have been offered, and they include reference to "expectancy-value-cognitions" (Betsch & Dickenberger, 1993), arousal (S. L. Taylor, O'Neal, Langley, & Butcher, 1991), and learning processes of various kinds, such as modeling (Bandura, 1965; O'Neal, Macdonald, Cloninger, & Levine, 1979), priming (Bushman & Geen, 1990), and norm acquisition (Liebert & Sprafkin, 1988). Although for some persons observing aggression can lead to disgust, aversion, and activation of help giving, observing aggression can also arouse an individual and activate learned aggression reactions and cognitions. Observing aggression on videos or movies can also communicate expectations and teach beliefs about norms of appropriate behavior.

Effects of Media Aggression.   Examples of aggression, especially violent assault, in movies or videos can have serious consequences in terms of increasing aggressive behavior of viewers and altering viewers' beliefs regarding aggression as a means of solving interpersonal problems. Berkowitz (1993) reviewed many studies and their findings with respect to the role of media aggression and subsequent aggressive behaviors. The effect of media aggression has been found in the behavior of both children and adults. Some effects are transitory, such as effects from physiological arousal induced in the viewer and from priming due to aggressive content triggering aggressive associations. Some effects are cumulative, because large-scale beliefs about norms of the culture are likely to be developed by the viewing of aggressive content. The more that peers and authorities appear to sanction aggressive behavior, the more likely are individuals to use aggressive action for a wide range of interpersonal conflicts.

In the original study on modeling (Bandura, Ross, & Ross, 1963), children watched a person in a room physically and aggressively attack a large inflated clown doll ("bobo doll"). Then they were frustrated (told they could not play with some promised desirable toys) and put back in the room in which they had seen the clown doll attacked. Children who had observed the aggressive model showed what appeared to be more aggressive actions toward the doll (imitation) than did children who had not previously observed the adult model. However, the data with the bobo doll may not have been as convincing as at first thought for illustrating the effect of modeling on aggression. Smith (1988), on viewing films from the bobo doll experiment, suggested that the children's punching reflected play fighting and not aggression.

Geen and Thomas (1986) indicated that imitation of specifically performed behavior observed on film or television can explain a number of aggressive actions due to the role of modeling. Observing aggression toward a target has been shown in many studies to increase one's aggressive behavior toward an innocent, nonprovoking target. The effect of pornographic violence on subsequent aggression may relate to later rape (Malamuth, 1984), and viewing pornographic violence was found in a laboratory study to increase generalized aggressive responses to women. Giving electric shocks supposedly as punishment for another person's task performance was used as a measure of aggression. Donnerstein (1980) had control subjects watch a short videotape containing bland content and another group watch an intimate heterosexual scene, whereas a third group watched a movie containing violent rape. The erotic nonviolent sex viewing did not lead to more aggression compared with the content viewed by the control group, but viewing of the rape scene did lead to more aggression, and it elicited more aggression to a woman than a man target.

The extent to which the culture generally condones aggression appears to play a major role. Sanctioned aggression heightens the effects of viewed aggression on later aggressive behavior. Many variables influence the role of media violence on aggression. In adults, whether subjects consume alcohol before viewing videotapes plays a role (Sayette, Wilson, & Elias, 1993), and in children the history of their television violence viewing plays a role (Viemero & Paajanen, 1992). Children who had

seen much TV violence had more aggressive fantasies, and fantasy was positively correlated with real-life aggressive behavior as measured by judgments of peers and by self-ratings of aggressiveness.

Childhood Experiences. Many studies have shown that children who are rejected show the consequence of the rejection in poorer social competence and impaired information-processing skills (Moore, Hughes, & Robinson, 1992). Children who have experienced early physical abuse are likely to have altered patterns of behavior and processing of social information. They are more likely to behave aggressively and to misattribute social cues (Crick, 1995; Dodge, Pettit, Bates, & Valente, 1995; Quigle, Garber, Panak, & Dodge, 1993). Parents who aggress against their children with physical abuse also have disturbance in social information processing (Milner, 1993). Children who experience parental aggression thus directly learn aggressive behavior by example, and they are likely to learn cognitive strategies and ways of interpreting social information that bias them toward using aggressive actions. Not only social information processing but also the kinds of attributions adults give have been found to be related to aggressive responding against provocation (Kogut, Langley, & O'Neal, 1992; S. L. Taylor et al., 1991).

In general, a person is *less likely* to resort to ineffective or inappropriate aggressive action (a) the more diverse information-processing methods the person has for interpreting social cues, (b) the more varied response strategies the person has for dealing with provocation, and (c) the more the individual has been rewarded in the past for nonaggressive methods of coping. Individuals can be trained, even in adulthood, to decrease their aggressive actions (Lau & Pihl, 1996). However, when children are rejected or frequently are the target of coercion, they may become submissive or withdrawn *or* they can become aggressive. If they have a history of being rewarded for aggression as a mode of reaction, they may come to use that mode even when it is inappropriate or ineffective.

Children learn at an early age to be aggressive. As very young children, when first learning to scream or hit or bite, they receive adult reactions that either reward or admonish aggression and nonaggression. By age 3 or 4, children have clearly learned response patterns and modes of interpreting events around them, although these change with further learning. Studies of children aged 4 to 7 years reveal developmental patterns and changes in aggressive behaviors. In one study (Hartup, 1974) 102 children were observed over a 10-week period. The older children initiated more hostile acts and made more verbal or physical attacks on another child for the purpose of protection of self-esteem. In contrast, the younger children displayed significantly more impersonal goal-oriented acts aimed at retrieving an object, territory, or privilege. Per unit of time, the younger children displayed more overall aggressive acts than did the older children. In interpersonal aggression, older children less often resorted to hitting and more often used insults or verbal attack on another's self-esteem than did the younger children. Threats to self-esteem as well as blocking an action or goal led to acts of aggression, but all the children used verbal rather than physical attacks to defend against derogation.

Developmental and longitudinal studies have shown that aggressive behavior at the age of 8 is likely to predict aggressive behavior in adulthood (Hamalainen & Pulkkinen, 1995; Pulkkinen & Pitkanen, 1993), and to do so for girls as well as boys. From early school years onward, emotional and behavioral patterns have been observed to be fairly stable (Pulkkinen, 1996a, 1996b). Individual differences in aggressiveness have been noted by various writers. Some interpret these differences as due to psychobiological factors, although most psychologists recognize that early family experiences shape personality, including patterns of aggressiveness. From all that is known about the effects of family constellation and parent-child patterns of interactions, it is clear that family patterns lead to relatively stable personality indicators of all kinds, including aggressiveness.

Ways of coping with stress, frustration, and achievement of goals are a function of cognitive, motivational, and emotional learning. Controversy exists concerning causal factors and how individual differences should be interpreted. That is, some psychologists give less credit to early *family influ-*

ences and believe that *psychobiological* variables (involving neurochemical and physiological processes) shape apperceptions and appraisals as well as ways of behaving and coping. Others believe that the later childhood and adult physiological differences that are correlated with aggressiveness result from learning in early childhood (before age 7), and that the learning involves many kinds of appraising and behaving. From that perspective, aggressiveness results from early learning, and the correlated physiological reactions are the result rather than the cause of the aggressiveness.

MACHIAVELLIANISM, MASTERY, AND ASSERTIVENESS

Machiavellianism

A variable that is related to aggression but also different from it is *Machiavellianism*. The term is taken from political history, based on Machiavelli who advocated ruthless pursuit of power in his book *The Prince*. On the basis of Machiavelli's destructive approach to other people for the attainment of self-serving goals, Christie and Geis (1970) developed a Machiavellian scale. High Machs, who score high on the scale and use manipulation for self-serving goals, are successful in getting what they want, and they readily violate moral principles in the process. Although high Mach persons are self-reliant they do not score very high on a test for nAch. They use manipulation rather than seek successful attainment of high standards of excellence. High Mach persons, compared with low Machs, are more likely to manipulate people by means of emotional control and nonverbal communication (Barth, 1974; Exline, Thibaut, Hickey, & Gumpert, 1970), and power is a means to an end.

For the high Mach person, other people are perceived as objects or pawns to be used and manipulated. High Machs do not consistently have real-world success (Wilson, Near, & Miller, 1996) and their approach may be highly maladaptive (McHoskey, 1995) in specific circumstances. High Mach persons use mastery over others (using others as pawns), and for them the term *mastery* is likely to describe conquest or dominance over others.

Some individuals with Machiavellian tendencies consider mastery to include conquest of others as well as mastery over tasks, thus associating mastery with aggressiveness. In one study of college students (Driscoll & Yankeelov, 1995), persons prone to be aggressive indicated that they experienced a feeling of mastery when involved in aggression. Some people enjoy competition because of the thrill of defeating others, and mastery of the game becomes confused with power and aggression. However, in modern psychological use the term *mastery* is used to refer to tasks rather than people.

Mastery

The distinction between being a master over others and mastering a task is an important one. Being master over others reflects power and Machiavellianism. In many situations that is not likely to aid in mastery over a task. Confusion between task mastery and aggression may arise because a person associates passivity in tasks with submissiveness in interpersonal relationships. If a person seeks to avoid such passivity (submissiveness) by resorting to an active approach, this can become mistakenly linked to interpersonal aggression. Rehabilitation to avoid such confusions is possible. Roberts and Treasure (1992) point out in describing sports for children that sports that focus on *mastery motivation* are more adaptive for achievement than are those that focus on competitive defeating of opponents.

A competitive attitude can undermine task satisfaction and task mastery. A study by Deci (Deci, Betley, Kahle, Abrams, & Porac, 1981) showed a different effect on intrinsic motivation from a competition versus a task mastery orientation. The researchers had college students solve interesting puzzles in the presence of another student. Half the subjects were told to compete and solve the puzzles faster than the other person, and half were told to work quickly and finish in the allotted time (task mastery). Upon completion of the experimental task, intrinsic motivation was measured in terms of how long the subjects worked on similar puzzles when alone in the room. As expected, intrinsic motivation was lower for subjects who were competing, because trying to win focuses a person on ex-

trinsic rewards rather than on intrinsic aspects of the task.

In the process of socialization, children are taught to learn mastery over tasks. They themselves and/or their parents may focus on an active perspective, and in the process children may confuse mastery with aggression. Preschool children's fantasy was examined in one study, and gender differences concerning mastery and aggression were found already by the ages of 3 to 5 (Libby & Aries, 1989). Boys revealed more aggressive fantasy figures in their stories, with aggressive activity involved in their attempts to master situations. In that study, girls were found to tend to describe caretaking fantasy figures.

Cultural factors play a role in whether gender differences of this type occur. Socioeconomic and family-dynamic factors play a role in whether preschool children are taught the distinction between mastery over tasks and aggressive styles in relating to people. During their development they learn to sort out for themselves how to interact actively with their environment. Pressures by family and teachers to master tasks may appear to the child to conflict with requirements by society not to be aggressive toward other people. For many children, learning to master tasks and not to be aggressive to other persons poses a formidable challenge. Unfortunately, for many children the reverse takes place (Hinshaw, 1992): they learn to be aggressive to others but do not learn effectively to master tasks, especially academic tasks.

Assertiveness

Just as psychologists distinguish mastery over tasks from mastery over persons, so also do they distinguish *assertiveness* from aggression. Aggression, either in subtle or direct ways, aims to demean or harm another, whereas assertiveness aims to put one's own needs or wishes forward and not to harm another. The aim for assertiveness is to attain one's own goal or safeguard one's own rights without harming or belittling another person. The child who insists that she or he gets a turn with a toy and is also willing to have another child get a turn is being assertive, not aggressive. An example of assertiveness is the customer who clearly points out that a suit for purchase is not as advertised and that she or he expects to get what was advertised, but the customer does not berate or demean the sales clerk or behave in any way harmful or attacking. In contrast, if the customer in protecting her or his rights, also attacked or demeaned the store personnel, the action would be called aggression. When one protects one's rights or needs while concurrently assuring that the other person is not demeaned, the action is assertive.

During the 1970s, to counteract a gender bias that women would be labeled "aggressive" and be rejected if they asserted their rights, many counseling programs were established to provide "assertiveness training." Assertiveness refers to protecting the rights or needs of an individual while also assuring the rights or needs of the other person. In one's peer relations as well as in commercial dealings, assertiveness is likely to be more positive and effective than submission or self-denial, and the benefit extends to all parties in the transaction. Researchers addressed some of these issues. For example, in one study (Sharp, 1995) students aged 13 to 16 years were given a questionnaire regarding coping strategies and bullying that they had experienced. Many reported strong negative reactions to being bullied. Coping strategies went from passive walking away to assertively standing up for themselves but not using physical aggression to aggressive actions like fighting.

Teaching children effective ways of dealing with peers involves showing them alternatives to submission other than the use of aggression. If aggression is to be avoided, young children need to have alternative skills. In one study (Wall & Holden, 1994), inner-city preschool children were observed for frequency of aggressive, assertive, and submissive behavior in play interaction with their mothers. Boys were found to be significantly more assertive but not more aggressive or submissive than girls. A problem—that not everyone dissociates assertive from aggressive behavior—was identified in a different study (Hegland & Rix, 1990). Researchers observed and teachers rated 5- to 7-year-old children. The researchers' observations showed that assertive behaviors correlated with instrumental ag-

gression and with positive social behavior, but assertiveness did not correlate with hostile aggression. In contrast, the teachers' ratings of assertiveness did correlate with ratings of hostile aggression. The teachers' ratings did not dissociate hostile aggression and assertiveness, whereas the researchers' observations did.

In a study with undergraduate business students, researchers (Slama & Celuch, 1995) sought to measure self-presentation style, which is the way one presents oneself to others. Students with an "acquisitive self-presentation style" revealed more assertive consumer behavior in their answers to a consumer behavior questionnaire than did students with a "protective self-presentation style." Assertiveness in business activities thus was shown to be part of a broader social pattern. In a study of college students and community residents (Hobfoll, Dunahoo, Ben-Porath, & Monnier, 1994), gender differences were found. Men reported more aggressive action, and women reported more assertive action, in professional and interpersonal situations. Training can explain such differences. Both in the larger society and within the culture of the family, one learns in which situation to be assertive and in which to be aggressive, and gender roles may shape that training.

School, socioeconomic factors, and various experiences throughout childhood and adolescence shape the way children cope with stress and challenges. Small children, especially boys, are likely to be trained at an early age to be assertive. With increasing exposure to competitive and aggressive actions by others, by the time they are adults, men are more likely to make use of aggressive coping strategies and women are more likely to use prosocial assertive strategies. The complexity of experiences people have by the time they reach adulthood will inevitably shape their styles of self-presentation and coping.

The importance of competition was seen in the Deci et al. (1981) study, which found that competition can diminish intrinsic motivation in a task. Later research by Deci (Reeve & Deci, 1996) showed that if the focus is on self-competence and not on a controlling necessity to win, and the person who is winning interprets the winning as favorable information about self-competence, then competition can increase intrinsic motivation. This type of finding applies to issues of assertiveness and aggression. Depending on the kinds of feedback individuals receive in interpersonal situations, they may come to adopt assertive *or* aggressive strategies, according to whether the feedback diminishes or enhances their self-competence valuations. If girls and women learn that their competence is more valued when they are assertive rather than aggressive, and boys and men learn that their competence is more valued when they are aggressive rather than assertive, gender differences in adults' aggressive and assertive behaviors are likely to occur. A society burdened with aggression can find alternative values and methods of training boys and girls and can replace acts of aggression with use of assertiveness and constructive acts of cooperation.

SUMMARY

Aggression is behavior, motivated by the intent to harm another in some way, to assert dominance, or to defend oneself or one's young by attack on another. Aggression can occur without anger, and anger can occur without aggression.

The frustration-aggression hypothesis was proposed in the 1960s. It stated that frustration always leads to some form of aggression and that when aggressive behavior occurs it is due to frustration. Contemporary researchers found that frustration can lead to anger but that does not necessarily lead to aggression, and many kinds of aggression occur without being evoked by frustration. Amsel found that under some circumstances frustrative nonreward, of previously rewarded behavior not leading to consistent further reward, leads to persistence rather than to aggression.

Whereas at one time ethologists (animal behaviorists) suggested that animals and humans have an innate aggression drive, a more contemporary evolutionary perspective examines how species functionally adapt to specific situations. Species differences exist, and aggressive behavior varies with specific situations, with developmental experiences and social learning, and in humans, with larger cultural variables.

Aggression with members of one's own species (conspecifics) has been called agonistic aggression. Various types of aggression have been identified, including intermale, fear induced, irritable, maternal, instrumental, and sex related. Interspecies aggression is called predatory.

Aggression is social, and social variables strongly influence aggression when animals and humans live in groups. Species have characteristic behaviors for aggression, and these may be different for domesticated compared with feral (wild) members of the species.

Territorial behavior patterns have been studied in detail in some species. The Blanchards have documented many types of aggressive behaviors in their ethoexperimental studies of rats living in groups. Female and male aggressive behaviors differ within a species and between species. Interspecies aggression has been studied with "mouse killing" in rats. Interspecies aggression can be minimized by prior familiarity between target and attacker.

Brain areas related to aggression (the amygdala, hippocampus, and septum) have been identified. Specific hormones, like testosterone and serotonin, have also been linked with aggression. Because testosterone level rises according to a wide range of situations, evidence suggests that in many cases testosterone level rises due to, rather than leads to, competition and aggressive behavior. Dominance level of the alpha male in group living seems to lead to, rather than result from, higher testosterone level.

Individualism has been contrasted with competitiveness by some researchers. When striving to protect one's own self-interest leads to harming others, such aggression can be as injurious as aggression from competitiveness. Sports and games can be played so as to maximize aggression or in ways that lead to cooperation. Mixed-motive games have been used to study cooperation and competition. Payoff matrixes can increase or decrease the amount of cooperation shown by players. People's built-in biases also can affect how much cooperation is shown to men and women opponents.

Culture increases or decreases competition and aggression. Children's values and attitudes toward competition and aggression are learned through many experiences, including family, school, and sports.

Milgram's studies of obedience showed that harming another person may be done when an authority directs such action. Persons in power can create situations that heighten aggression and they can themselves use aggression for domination. French and Raven described different types of power. Many types did not involve aggression but one did, coercive power, which uses punishment for obedience or submission.

In many societies men are rewarded for aggression and show more aggression than do women. Situational factors also determine to what extent there are gender differences in aggression. The relationship between alcohol and aggression has been studied especially in men, and data show that alcohol often does, but need not, increase aggressive behavior.

Some persons show aggressive behavior as part of seeking excitement. Increased arousal, by viewing certain types of films or videotapes, can lead to heightened aggressiveness. The effects of television and film violence are complex. To the extent that they model or sanction violence, and not merely prime aggressive reactions and thoughts, they can have long-term debilitating effects.

Children learn what aggression means from many persons. They learn rules as well as behaviors of aggression. Attributions, self-concept, and cultural beliefs shape children's and adults' use of aggression (and shape refraining from such use).

Machiavellianism, the use of destructive behaviors toward others for one's own self-interest, can be measured and is different from task mastery. Persons who are high Machs have not attained special real-world success, although they do use others as pawns for their own gains.

Mastery over tasks is likely to lead to higher achievement than mastery over other people (power). Task mastery is different from aggression, but for small children there may be confusion about this. Children can be taught the distinction.

Assertiveness refers to protecting one's rights but not demeaning or harming others in the process. Assertiveness differs from aggression. However, some observers may mistakenly judge a given behavior as aggressive when in fact it is assertive. Young children can be taught the distinction between assertiveness and aggression, and they can learn that assertiveness is preferable over aggression, both for themselves and for others.

CHAPTER **13**

Fear and Anxiety

As noted in the last chapter, aggressive behavior can occur as part of defensive protection of self or one's young. When others attack us, we may be afraid yet seek to protect ourselves by aggressive means, such as counterattacks. Fear can lead to aggression and to many other types of behavior. The present chapter deals with situations that give rise to fear and to anxiety. It is concerned with what effects fear and anxiety have on a wide range of behavioral, emotional, and cognitive variables.

GENERAL CONSIDERATIONS

At different times in the history of psychology fear and anxiety were considered to be emotions *or* motivations. In the more behavioristic period up to the 1970s, they were investigated as motivational states (Ferguson, 1982), whereas in contemporary work they are more often considered to be emotions. In either case fear and anxiety have been studied as states and as traits. Fearfulness as a disposition refers to a trait, like timidity, and fear is also a short-term state. Some contemporary writers focus on fear as an innate response to a specific stimulus that has evolutionary significance as a sign of danger, and others consider how fear is learned by means of Pavlovian (classical) conditioning.

Human fear also can be considered in much broader terms. For example, Averill (1991) distinguished between the *occurrence* and *disposition* of fear, with the occurrence a relatively brief fright reaction and the disposition lasting anywhere from hours to weeks. Defensive actions are involved in both, but longer-term defensive maneuvers charac-

terize the disposition of fear. Averill (1991) considered the longer-term fear as the counterpart to hope. Different theorists emphasize different facets of fear and anxiety. Some are concerned with the physiology and neurochemistry, some focus on how fear and anxiety are learned, and some focus on innate and evolutionary factors. Some writers focus on the impact of fear and anxiety on various types of behaviors, and others are concerned with individual differences in anxiety. All agree that hurtful and/or punishing events are related to the intervening variables of fear and anxiety.

Some theorists propose that fear is focused on a specific stimulus or event, whereas anxiety is more diffuse (nonspecific). Others distinguish between fear of physical danger, in contrast to anxiety, which concerns self-esteem or self-value. Many psychologists consider specific concrete events to be involved in fear, whereas uncertain and more abstract (symbolic) processes are involved in anxiety (Lazarus, 1991). Anxieties of all kinds have been identified in humans, including test-taking anxiety in achievement-related circumstances. Interest in the topic of fear and anxiety has come from many sources. Anxiety, in particular, has been given prominence in theories of psychopathology. Freud (1926) emphasized anxiety in his study of personality functioning and problems of neurosis. Many theorists considered anxiety to be a malaise of humans in modern times, due to pressures of a technological age and the conflicts within and between people. Anxiety was the cornerstone of neurosis in the theories of many clinical psychologists, social anthropologists, and psychiatrists, who, like Horney (1937), noted that modern humans live in an age of anxiety and in a neurotic time.

Fear and anxiety associated with pathological difficulties, like phobias and anxiety neurosis, go beyond the scope of the present chapter. The present chapter focuses on research devoted to understanding the basic processes of fear and anxiety within normal functioning. Because of ethical considerations, much of the research on fear has been conducted with nonhuman animals rather than with human beings, but many studies of anxiety have been conducted with human subjects.

EARLY EXPERIMENTAL WORK

In the early 1900s, Pavlov (1928, 1941) did work on experimental neurosis, in which he showed that dogs trained to make fine discriminations can be confronted with such difficult discriminations that they develop intense negative emotional reactions and show signs of extreme distress and anxiety. Subsequent researchers studied classical conditioning of fear, like the work described previously, in which Watson and Rayner (1920) trained the infant Albert to fear a white rat. Later, operant conditioning studies under the leadership of Skinner (1938, 1953) added knowledge about the effects of aversive stimuli (Estes & Skinner, 1941). In the 1940s and 1950s, Hullian drive theorists conceptualized fear and anxiety as learned motivations. Miller (1948) proposed that fear is a motivation. Motivation leads to learning of new behaviors, and fear leads to learning of many new responses. Investigations with animals by Miller (1948) and Mowrer (1940, 1950) were followed by studies on human anxiety by Taylor (1951, 1953) and Spence (1964; Spence & Taylor, 1951).

Escape and Avoidance Conditioning Studies of Fear and Anxiety

Escape conditioning is a form of instrumental or operant conditioning that involves an aversive stimulus that can be terminated by a response the investigator designates. A typical experiment would involve placing a rat in a Skinner box, turning on a shock, and stopping the shock after the an-

imal presses a bar. The time (latency) between shock onset and bar pressing is quite long at first, because the animal makes the "correct" response only by chance. After several occasions the animal learns the response, and the latency of responding becomes very short. The animal has learned the designated escape behavior. The shock cannot be prevented but it can be escaped very rapidly. In a shuttle box the escape occurs literally, with the animal escaping (running) from a shocked to a non-shocked compartment.

Negative Reinforcement and Punishment. Skinner (1953) used the term *negative reinforcement* when behavior leads to the cessation of an aversive stimulus. It is a type of reinforcement because it follows the behavior to be learned. It brings a "relatively" positive outcome (by stopping the aversive event), and like positive reinforcement, it leads to the acquisition and strengthening of responses. This differs from a *punishment,* which is the term used when a noxious stimulus is given after a specific response, and the response subsequently decreases. Punishment refers to the *presentation* of an aversive event following a designated behavior, whereas negative reinforcement refers to the *cessation* of an aversive event following the designated behavior. In punishment, an aversive event occurs *after* the designated behavior, whereas in negative reinforcement, the aversive event occurs *before* the behavior. Figure 13.1 illustrates the difference.

In real-life circumstances the use of aversive control tends to involve both punishment and negative reinforcement. An example is a wife who does not speak to her husband the next morning (punishes him) for "going out with the guys" the previous night instead of going with her to a movie, and she then continues "the silent treatment" (negative reinforcement) until he apologizes and the next night goes with her to a movie. Problems occur with using aversive control, however, in that the "silent treatment" may in time lead to resentment and retaliation, which can prove to be more distressing than the original problem behavior.

Escape and Avoidance Conditioning. Avoidance conditioning differs from escape conditioning in

FIGURE 13.1
Comparison of negative reinforcement and punishment.

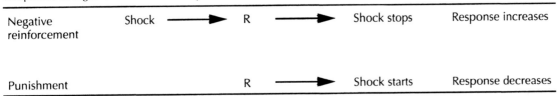

Negative reinforcement	Shock ⟶ R ⟶ Shock stops	Response increases
Punishment	R ⟶ Shock starts	Response decreases

that prevention of the aversive event is possible. Various kinds of avoidance conditioning procedures have been used. One is a nondiscriminative type of avoidance conditioning, named after the person who first reported use of the method, the *Sidman* (1953) avoidance conditioning procedure. In this, the animal makes the appropriate response and thereby postpones the aversive stimulus, like shock, for a specified period. If the animal fails to respond in a designated interval, the aversive stimulus occurs. For example, if the animal fails to respond in 10 seconds since the last shock, then shock is received, but if the animal makes the response, shock can be avoided. Rate of responding is the dependent variable in this type of procedure. Another procedure, called *passive* avoidance conditioning, has already been discussed. The animal learns to withhold responses (Mowrer, 1960). If an animal is shocked when it steps onto a grid floor in a compartmentalized box, in time the animal stops going onto the grid and does not even approach that side. How long the animal refrains from making the response is the dependent variable in this type of procedure. A third type is called *active* avoidance conditioning. In this procedure a discriminative cue, like a light, comes on and remains on long enough for an instrumental response to be made, prior to onset of the aversive event. In time the animal learns to associate the cue and the aversive stimulus. Latency of response, following the cue, is the dependent variable in this procedure.

Active avoidance studies have been used frequently in studies of anxiety. Typically, a two-compartment shuttle box is used. The animal is in one compartment in which a cue (like a light) precedes the aversive stimulus (like shock). Early in the

training the animal does not associate light and shock, but manifests escape learning by running from the shocked compartment to the other compartment. In a two-way shuttle box, the light and shock occur in the alternate compartments, so that what was the safe (nonshocked) side becomes the shocked side. During the course of learning, the escape occurs with decreasing time after shock onset, and periodically the animal leaves the shocked side after light onset and before shock onset. When that happens, the animal does not *escape* the shock but *avoids* it. With repeated trials, the animal typically shows no escape behavior, only avoidance behavior. As soon as light appears, the animal runs to the other side. In this way, the animal can shuttle back and forth for a long time and never receive shock.

Unlike escape learning, in which curtailment of shock (by escape) provides a negative reinforcer for the response, in avoidance there is no obvious negative reinforcement because the animal does not receive shock. One explanation of how reinforcement may occur is that the light is feared, and because fear is a negative condition, escape from the feared stimulus provides the negative reinforcement. Mowrer (1951) posited a two-factor theory, one factor relating to the escape behavior and the other to learning fear as a secondary motivation. Although he did not use these exact terms, his main points were that learning of the escape response occurs due to reinforcement, which involves operant or instrumental conditioning, and *learning of fear occurs through classical conditioning,* due to the contiguity and association of shock and light. The light (initially a neutral stimulus) becomes a CS by being paired with the pain of shock as the US. The light becomes feared, and fear is a learned (secondary) motivation. These two factors were used as a model for learning anxiety. Whereas a specific stimulus (like light) is feared, the more diffuse context of the shuttle box leads to a less focused anxiety. The connection between anxiety and avoidance conditioning in the shuttle box was demonstrated by Solomon and Wynne (1954).

Contemporary researchers differ from this approach. Fear conditioning tends to be studied with other types of apparatus than shuttle boxes or Skinner boxes. Place preference is studied, with foot shock given in one chamber and no shock given in the other chamber. Also, the negative emotion conditioned to the context of the chamber in which shock occurred is called fear in contemporary studies, not anxiety (Anagnostaras, Maren, & Fanselow, 1995; Fanselow, 1994; Young, Bohenek, & Fanselow, 1995). For example, in one chamber a tone can be given immediately before footshock, or footshock can be given without a tone. Rats will learn to fear the tone and they will also learn to fear the chamber. Instead of bar presses, behavior of freezing when given the tone or placed in the chamber indicates the conditioned fear. Research has shown that different brain areas are involved in fear to the tone compared with fear to the environmental context of the chamber (Young et al., 1995). Thus, what earlier researchers in animal studies called anxiety is more likely called fear in contemporary studies, but the *distinction* between *fear to a specific stimulus* and the negative emotion to the more *nonspecific context* is still found to be important. Whereas earlier researchers used two terms, fear and anxiety, contemporary researchers call them both fear but recognize that two types exist, with different brain systems involved in the two negative emotions.

Punishment, Fear, and Anxiety

Use of aversive events for controlling and altering behavior has a very long history, and punishment is still used widely today. Punishment occurs in the treatment of humans as well as nonhuman animals (pets and work animals). Aside from the suffering caused by punishment and other forms of aversive control, these methods tend not to be effective in

changing behavior. Skinner (1953) and others (Dreikurs & Grey, 1992) have shown that aversive means of control lead to a wide range of effects, some of which may be far more destructive and unwanted than the original behavior to be altered. Skinner's admonishments are worth noting:

> Punishment does not actually eliminate behavior from a repertoire, and its temporary achievement is obtained at tremendous cost in reducing the over-all efficiency and happiness of the group. (1953, p. 190)

Animal studies have focused on what conditions elicit fear and how fear affects behavior, and they show that punishment decreases responding. When shock and tone are paired repeatedly, the tone elicits fear. The tone can then be used as *conditioned punishment* and used as a learned (secondary) punisher in the same way that a tone paired with food can be used as a conditioned (secondary) reward. A rat in a Skinner box can be operantly conditioned with a positive reinforcer by receiving food after bar pressing, and this can be followed by conditioned punishment training with tone and shock in another chamber. If upon being returned to the Skinner box the animal receives both food and tone after bar pressing, the bar press responding markedly decreases, presumably because the response is punished (Mowrer & Aiken, 1954).

In a different procedure, *conditioned emotional response* or CER training (Estes & Skinner, 1941) the neutral stimulus and shock are given in the same apparatus as the bar press conditioning. In this procedure the animal learns the bar pressing with food reinforcement, then tone is paired with shock independently (noncontingently) of bar pressing, and later the bar press response is followed by both tone and food. As with the conditioned punishment procedure, the operantly conditioned response is markedly decreased. This type of response suppression has been studied extensively with rats and other animals, and the suppression of responding is assumed to be due to fear (McAllister & McAllister, 1971).

A different approach tested dogs in a two-way shuttle box (Solomon, Kamin, & Wynne, 1953). The animals received a buzzer in one compartment and 1 second later a gate between the two compartments was raised. This allowed the dog to jump over a barrier separating the two compartments. If during the 10 seconds of the warning buzzer the dog did not jump, intense shock was given through the grid floor on which the dog stood. Escape was possible by jumping to the other, shock-free, side. Every 3 minutes a new trial began, with buzzer and shock on alternating sides. Soon the animals learned not only to escape but to avoid the shock. This avoidance response persisted for a very long time, even though no shock occurred. Typically, shuttle-box avoidance conditioning is very resistant to extinction. The animal does not have the experience that in extinction shock will not occur, because in fact the animal does not remain in the compartment long enough to learn that shock will not occur. As reported by Solomon et al. (1953), as many as 490 trials were given during which the animal would jump across the barrier in less than 1.5 seconds and thus not receive shock. Solomon and Wynne (1954) noted that there were no obvious signs of emotional upset when the animal jumped within short latencies. However, if the animal happened to have a long response latency, clear signs of anxiety were evident, and very short latencies were given on subsequent trials. The anxiety reaction occurred after the animal had jumped. The researchers noted that the emotion was not to a specific stimulus and thus fear, but was diffuse and thus anxiety.

Learned Helplessness and Flooding

The early shuttle-box avoidance studies of Solomon and his colleagues and students were followed by a variation in procedure, which led to unexpected and dramatic effects. The procedure involved strapping the experimental animal into a harness and giving it intense and unsignaled shock that lasted several seconds and from which the animal could not escape. After a number of such shocks, the animal was put into the two-way shuttle box the next day. Unexpectedly, it showed very poor escape conditioning compared with control animals also strapped into a harness but not given shock. Control animals learned the usual escape and avoidance conditioning but the experimental animals made very few instrumental responses to

the shock in spite of strong emotional distress. The experimental animals seemed resigned and "to take" the shock. Overmier and Seligman (1967) and Seligman and Maier (1967) showed that giving dogs intense inescapable shock, which was independent of and not controlled by any of the dog's behavior, led 24 hours later to seriously impaired two-way shuttle-box escape learning. When the procedure of giving uncontrollable shocks was repeated over many sessions and not merely during one session, the effect of the *learned helplessness* extended over many days (Seligman & Groves, 1970).

The animal appeared to learn a kind of defensive passivity. When escape involved an active instrumental response, the prior uncontrollable shock impaired active response learning like bar pressing to terminate shock (Dinsmoor & Campbell, 1956). However, if the animal had only to flee shock, by running to a safe box in which it never received shock, prior uncontrollable shock did not impair fleeing but even facilitated it (DeToledo & Black, 1967). Controlled studies with humans were sparse, but the phenomenon of learned helplessness was demonstrated with rats and goldfish as well as dogs, and the early literature was well reviewed by Seligman, Maier, and Solomon (1971). The explanation favored by the early researchers was in terms of expectancy. That is, in the normal course of escape conditioning an animal learns that its behavior leads to shock cessation. Maier, Seligman, and Solomon (1969) suggested that the incentive for active instrumental responding is greatly reduced when initially the animal learns to expect that its behavior has no effect on the shock. Thus, even though in the later situation the animal has control over the aversive events, the animal fails to learn effective responding and acts helplessly. The findings of learned helplessness from animal studies were later used to explain depression in humans, with the depressed person also assumed to experience the emotions and beliefs of learned helplessness (Seligman, 1975).

The "learned helplessness" of animals first given inescapable and uncontrollable shock is the opposite of the persistent responding shown by animals with successful avoidance conditioning. In both cases the response pattern is not congruent with the objective task characteristics. In the case of the passive learned helplessness, active and effective responding for pain cessation and prevention is not made. In the case of successful avoidance conditioning, the response fails to extinguish, and responding seems inappropriate when there is no longer any shock. With learned helplessness the animal would be more effective by responding; with extinction of active avoidance the animal would be more effective by nonresponding. Both types of reactions have been used as models for human psychopathology. Persons with pathological anxieties and phobias are presumed to continue a learned avoidance behavior that realistically should have been extinguished, and persons who are depressed are presumed to have learned helplessness. In the language used by some clinical psychologists, both patterns represent failed "reality testing."

The procedure of *flooding,* or response prevention, differs from the above procedures. It was developed to provide a means for successful extinction of a learned avoidance response. Most researchers assumed that difficulty in extinction occurs because the animal continues to be fearful or anxious about an event (like shock) which won't happen. To enable the animal to find out that the noxious event won't occur, flooding is done by leaving the animal in the environment long enough to extinguish the fear or anxiety. When the animal is in the environment and shock does not occur, this presumably breaks the CS-US association, the US (shock) not occurring in the presence of the CS (chamber). Once fear is extinguished, the escape or avoidance response is also more readily extinguished.

Flooding was found to hasten extinction of avoidance responding (Baum, 1970). For example, a rat would be placed in a box with a grid floor that provided shock. A retractable ledge served as a safety platform during avoidance conditioning but would be removed during flooding. *During avoidance conditioning,* shock would be given if the rat failed to jump onto the ledge within 10 seconds. After a period, the platform was briefly retracted to put the animal again on the grid floor and this would start a new trial. After avoidance responding was well established, *flooding* was given (Siegeltuch &

Baum, 1971). No shock occurred during flooding. By being in the box for some time (anywhere from 5 to 30 minutes) without being able to make the learned response, associations previously learned become extinguished. After flooding, the animal typically is removed briefly from the box and the ledge again is presented in order to test for extinction (to assess if the previously learned escape or avoidance response still occurs).

Extinction would be complete when the rat no longer jumps to the ledge and remains on the non-shocked grid for some time, like 5 consecutive minutes. An analogous type of treatment for removing excessive anxiety or fear in humans is called *implosive therapy* (Stampfl & Levis, 1968). Like flooding, it involves exposing the person to the fearful stimulus and letting the person learn that no traumatic event follows the stimulus. Successful treatment of phobias has been reported with this technique (Watson & Marks, 1971). Contemporary researchers have not actively investigated flooding or implosive therapy, but studies on extinction of conditioned aversions and conditioned fear have shown that both contextual changes and forgetting can lead to recovery of fears and responses that had become extinguished (Bouton, 1993, 1994; Rosas & Bouton, 1997), so it is not firmly known how long the effects of flooding remain or whether the conditioned fears do return.

CONTEMPORARY RESEARCH IN FEAR LEARNING

Psychobiological Findings

Researchers extended the kinds of studies described above to obtain a greater understanding of the details of psychobiological and behavioral processes involved in fear, anxiety, and learned helplessness.

Conditioning and the Search for Brain Areas Involved in Fear. Over a 30-year period, Gray (1991) sought to identify the crucial neuroanatomical and neurophysiological systems responding to and responsible for fear and anxiety. By assessing avoidance conditioning studies with strains of rats specifically bred to be either high or low in fearful emotionality, and by comparing effects of drugs as well as effects of lesions in different brain areas, Gray proposed that septal and hippocampus areas were involved in fear and anxiety. He compared the results of passive avoidance conditioning studies with those of active avoidance conditioning. This led to his postulating that passive avoidance involves a system directed only to learned punishment and fear, whereas active avoidance involves a different system that is based on learned reward and hope, because in active avoidance learning the animal (or person) learns that safety exists.

Drugs that tend to impair passive avoidance conditioning do not impair active avoidance learning, presumably because different systems are involved. Gray (1991) concluded from the effects of drugs that reduce anxiety (anxiolytic drugs) that response suppression reflects the action of fear and anxiety but active avoidance does not. He reviewed studies of rats bred to be high in fearful emotionality, called the Maudsley reactive rats. They show high passive avoidance and high response suppression, whereas the Maudsley nonreactive rats, who are low in fearful emotionality, show more active avoidance. Frustrative nonreward has similar effects to fear, in that passive avoidance responding increases when animals experience frustrative nonreward. He also cited data to suggest that fear and anxiety increase attention to novel cues. Some of the hypotheses of Gray (1991) have found support and others have not. For example, data from habituation studies are mixed in providing support for his hypothesis regarding the way anxiety increases attentiveness to novel stimuli. If high anxiety increases attentiveness, then high anxiety (compared with low anxiety) individuals should habituate more slowly to novel stimuli.

Data from a study by Ferguson (1987) may help shed light on Gray's formulation. College students, half high and half low in trait anxiety, were individually given a noxiously loud (90-db) 1,000-Hz tone through earphones. Each tone lasted 2 seconds and occurred on the average every minute until a criterion of three consecutive low-amplitude electrodermal responses (trials) was reached. The high anxiety subjects reached the first nonresponse (low-amplitude) trial significantly sooner than did the low anx-

iety subjects. This is counter to Gray's hypothesis about high anxiety individuals being more attentive to novel stimuli. However, the tone was noxiously loud, so a defensive mode of information processing can be expected for the high anxiety subjects. More than defensive processing occurred, however. Support for Gray's hypothesis, that anxiety leads to greater attentiveness, was found in the way that the high and low anxiety subjects differed after they initially tuned out the tone. Once the low anxiety subjects tuned out the stimulus and had low electrodermal responses, they reached the criterion of three consecutive nonresponse trials quickly. In contrast, the high anxiety subjects periodically kept responding to the tone, and thus they reached the strict criterion of consecutive nonresponding at nearly the same number of trials as did the low anxiety subjects. The fact that the high but not the low anxiety subjects kept responding to the tone long after their initial nonresponse is in support of Gray's formulation that high anxiety individuals keep attending to novel stimuli.

Various researchers provided evidence regarding the brain areas crucial for fear and anxiety, and the findings tend only partially to support Gray's (1991) postulation that the important areas are septal and hippocampal. Other researchers focused on the amygdala as the brain area crucial for emotion (LeDoux, 1986, 1989, 1991; Rolls, 1990) and especially crucial for fear (LeDoux, 1995). LeDoux (1995) reviewed many studies of conditioning and concluded that overwhelmingly the evidence points to the amygdala as the important brain area. It is assumed by various researchers that the amygdala is involved in preverbal, possibly preconscious, primitive information processing. The amygdala may be involved in procedural learning of emotions that are not verbalized (Kentridge & Aggleton, 1990), and it may allow emotional processing to be fast but not to involve strong or detailed representation (LeDoux, 1991).

Ongoing research is exploring the possible brain areas involved in fear and anxiety by using the conditioning procedures of the earlier experimenters. For example, Wilson, Brooks, and Bouton (1995) on the basis of their studies suggested that the hippocampus system is important in the formation of context-US associations (but not in other types of learning about the context), so that fear learned to context in passive avoidance may be mediated by the hippocampus. Anagnostaras and colleagues (1995) also found contextual fear conditioning to be dependent on the hippocampal system. Maren, Aharonov, Stote, and Fanselow, (1996) additionally found the amygdala to be necessary for learning and expressing fear conditioning to contextual cues. Thus, support has been found for the views of both Gray and LeDoux, and research continues to assess how different aspects of fear learning are mediated by various brain systems.

Human and Nonhuman Fear, Anxiety, and Neurotransmitters. The early researchers studied human and nonhuman animal fear and anxiety with a focus on how these emotions and motivations are *learned.* They sought to identify what kinds of situations and what kinds of experiences lead a human or nonhuman animal to learn to be afraid or anxious. Little consideration was given to the evolutionary significance of these emotions. In contrast, many contemporary researchers focus on *evolutionary* factors, and for some researchers this means emphasizing innate rather than learned aspects of fear and anxiety. In science as in everyday life, "the pendulum" of emphases often swings from one to another perspective. Animals do learn, and animals also have innate fears to certain stimuli and they have species-specific defense reactions (Bolles, 1970). Psychobiologically oriented animal researchers tend to focus on the evolutionary survival value of emotions (LeDoux, 1995; Kentridge & Aggleton, 1990). Within this approach, fear is considered to sensitize the animal to specific types of stimuli and to activate specific defensive responses. Other researchers more broadly direct their efforts to understanding how learning, social experiences, and innate characteristics combine. For example, depending on the circumstances, rats show freezing (immobilization), flight, or defensive attack when fear is aroused (Blanchard, Hori, Rodgers, Hendrie, & Blanchard, 1989), and some researchers seek to identify the underlying processes that lead to behavioral variations.

Some researchers assessed how the intensity of

a noxious stimulus leads to different kinds of fear responses. For example, a moderately strong footshock given immediately after placing rats in a chamber leads to freezing, defecation, and conditioned analgesia (of a learned lowering of pain sensitivity), but a strong immediate shock leads to a transient unconditioned response of analgesia (Fanselow, Landeira-Fernandez, DeCola, & Kim, 1994). Strength of fear or of threat seems to play a role in which types of innate species-specific defense responses occur in rats (Fanselow, DeCola, De Oca, & Landeira-Fernandez, 1995). Such findings cannot be translated readily to human reactions, and each species of nonhuman animals has its own patterns of defensive responses. However, humans, like nonhuman animals, have rapid reactions to fear-arousing stimuli. Due to sympathetic nervous system activity, humans as well as nonhuman animals show the "fight or flight" syndrome. Contemporary researchers seek to understand what neurochemicals are involved in human fear and anxiety, in part because such understanding helps in the development of antianxiety (anxiolytic) drugs.

Epinephrine and norepinephrine have been studied with regard to human anxiety. The literature suggests that it is not resting level of epinephrine but rather the rise in level as a reaction to stressful events that differ between high and low anxiety individuals. Studies in this field take into account different types of stressors and different methods of coping with stress (Netter, 1991). Although amount of pain and amount of cognitive stress determine the strength of affective and neurochemical reactions, Netter (1991) found that both high and low anxiety subjects reacted more strongly to the pain condition used in her study than to a stressful cognitive task. Additionally, the high anxiety individuals responded with a larger epinephrine increase to anxiety-inducing stress (pain and cognitive stress) than did the low anxiety individuals. Effort spent on coping with stress was found to be related to norepinephrine levels (Netter, 1991), lower levels being associated with less effective coping.

The anxiety induction of course examinations raises norepinephrine levels in college students. McClelland, Ross, and Patel (1985) measured salivary norepinephrine levels during relaxation, immediately after a mid-term examination, and 105 minutes after the exam. After the examination the levels were significantly higher than during relaxation. Persons high in the need for power, compared with those high in the need for affiliation, had significantly higher levels of norepinephrine. One cannot be certain that the need for power was a more effective coping strategy with respect to the course examination, but indirectly the data of that study support the findings of Netter (1991), that styles of coping are sensitive to norepinephrine levels.

Learned Helplessness.   What has been found with human norepinephrine levels has also been found in animal studies with learned helplessness. Exposure to inescapable, but not to escapable, shock lowers norepinephrine levels (Maier, 1991; Peterson, Maier, & Seligman, 1993). Also, when norepinephrine is lowered by chemically induced methods, escape learning is impaired when there are irrelevant cues (Peterson et al., 1993) in the same way as found when animals are first inescapably shocked (learned helplessness) and later given escape training.

Maier (1991) proposed that inescapable shock appears to alter what the animal later attends to. This was also the conclusion of Overmier (Dess & Overmier, 1989; Overmier & Wielkiewicz, 1983), who used conditioning studies in which some animals received shock (US) unrelated to a tone (CS). Overmier (Dess & Overmier, 1989; Overmier & Wielkiewicz, 1983) found that such noncontingent CS-US presentations led to impaired conditioning later. He explained this as due to "learned irrelevance" and likened his findings that such learning impairs later conditioning to the phenomenon of learned helplessness. Further studies of learned irrelevance (Linden, Savage, & Overmier, 1997) show it can occur with pigeon's key peck responses and appetitive conditioning and not only with dogs and aversive conditioning. Differences exist between learned helplessness and learned irrelevance, in that the former involves both a motivational and associative deficit and the latter involves only an associative deficit. It may be that the associative deficit found for learned irrelevance also explains the associative deficit found in learned helplessness, but learned irrelevance is not likely to explain

all aspects (especially the motivational aspects) of learned helplessness.

Maier (1991) refuted the early explanation that learned helplessness was due to expectancy in a different way than that of learned irrelevance. Maier accounted for the learned helplessness behavior in terms of altered attention. He proposed that the animal first given inescapable shocks appears to be biased toward external rather than internal cues. The animal shows impaired escape learning subsequent to inescapable shock because the animal attends to irrelevant stimuli. The impairment in learning is not due to faulty expectancy or to passivity (decreased motor activity), as was initially thought in the early work on learned helplessness, but is due to inappropriate attention. A number of neurochemical processes have been identified as modulating the behavioral effects (Peterson, et al., 1993).

Associative as well as motivational processes are involved in learned helplessness. In addition to attention being altered, as described by Maier (1991), other processes are altered by inescapable shock. Long-term potentiation (LTP) in the hippocampus (a measure of neural plasticity that is important in associative memory formation) was found to be severely impaired for rats given inescapable shock in comparison with those given escapable shock (Shors, Seib, Levine, & Thompson, 1989). The decreased neural plasticity induced by inescapable shock would mean that animals given inescapable shock are likely to be impaired in forming new learning. The researchers also suggested that in part the decreased LTP of animals given inescapable shock could have been due to the inescapable shock lowering arousal. A direct test of the role of arousal and of increased activity due to motivation was given in an investigation that compared water-deprived and nondeprived rats (Stromberg, Bersh, Whitehouse, Neuman, & Mongeluzzi, 1997). Inescapable shock led to a significant decrease in later escapable shuttle-box performance in the nondeprived animals, but water-deprived animals had minimal loss, being similar in later escape performance to control animals not given inescapable shock. The additional water deprivation mitigated the learned helplessness effect from prior inescapable shock, presumably by inducing arousal and activity that matched those of the control subjects. Thus, inescapable shock compared with escapable shock lowers both the neural plasticity involved in associative learning and motivated (aroused) activity.

Human Conditioning Studies

Conditioning procedures were used in treatment for human anxiety and phobias in the 1950s and 1960s. Some therapists used flooding and implosive therapy, already described, which involved presenting to the individual the often traumatic full-blown fear-arousing stimuli or events. An alternative method was used by Wolpe (1958, 1963), called "systematic desensitization." In this method an anxiety or fear hierarchy was established, consisting of a progression of related items from least feared to most feared. Extinction and counterconditioning procedures usually began with the least feared items until eventually the most feared items could be readily tolerated.

Fear of Snakes and Other Fears. One of the most active researchers using Wolpe's method was Peter Lang, who between the 1960s and 1990s conducted many conditioning and desensitization studies. In early work, Lang therapeutically altered fear of snakes (Lang & Lazovik, 1963; Lang, Melamed, & Hart, 1970). Subjects were volunteer undergraduate women who indicated on a pretest questionnaire that they had a strong snake fear. In the laboratory, they received a snake avoidance test, in which the subject would be asked to approach as closely as possible to a live and harmless boa constrictor enclosed in a glass cage. Fear was measured by how close the subject came to the snake and by self-rating of fear by the subject on a 10-point scale. Various therapeutic methods were utilized, including an automated desensitization device (Lang et al., 1970). Relaxation methods were used as part of the therapeutic methods, and physiological measures were recorded. Characteristically, heart rate rose in tandem with verbalized fear ratings. As also occurs with fear or pain in nonhuman animals (Gardner & Malmo, 1969), heart rate in humans increases dramatically as a function of fear.

In addition to studying fear of snakes, Lang studied fear of public speaking and fear of spiders (Lang et al., 1970). He found fear of specific animals, like snakes and spiders, to show a different physiological and behavioral pattern than a social fear like that of public speaking. An important difference is the visual imaging of the feared event or stimulus. Fears of specific animals yield more vivid images than do social fears.

Continuing to explore fear within a conditioning perspective, Lang (1995; Bradley & Lang, 1993; Lang & Bradley, 1990) obtained a number of reliable findings and developed a broad set of hypotheses regarding not only fear but also positive emotions. He focused on appetitive versus aversive processes and showed that different imagery is involved in the two systems. Reviewing many studies, he concluded that unpleasant images potentiate startle reflexes (increase their strength and probability), but pleasant images inhibit the startle reflex. For example, if a loud sound is presented unexpectedly, humans will reflexively blink. If the startle is tested during an activity containing fear stimuli, like recalling sentences with fear content (Vrana & Lang, 1990), or the person is experiencing a fear emotion, the blink is larger and heart rate is faster than if the startle is tested when the person processes neutral content or is in a relaxed state. In one study (Bradley & Lang, 1993) subjects viewed pleasant, unpleasant, and neutral pictures and they were tested for habituation of the startle reflex under each type of picture condition. He found the startle reflex to be more sensitive to the type of picture than were physiological patterns of heart rate and skin conductance. He proposed that the affect-startle effect is not determined by general arousal or simple attention (Lang & Bradley, 1990) but reflects the dual nature of the affect-motivational system (of aversive versus appetitive processes).

Can Fear Learning Occur Without Awareness? Related to the work of Lang, Öhman (1996) explored whether fearful responding can occur without conscious processing of the fear-evoking stimuli. He postulated that certain stimuli are more likely than others to be feared because of an evolutionary determined preparedness. Thus, some stimuli are more easily learned to be feared than others. Other researchers had found this. Although fear of snakes in rhesus monkeys need not be innate (Mineka, 1992), observing fear in a conspecific leads to rapid learning of snake fear in originally nonfearful animals. Different stimuli are far less readily learned to arouse fear.

Öhman and colleagues (Esteves, Parra, Dimberg, & Öhman, 1994) found that angry faces could be used to lead to electrodermal fear-relevant conditioning but happy faces could not. Using an "uncomfortable" but not painful shock as the US, the researchers presented photographic slides of happy, angry, or emotionally neutral faces to college student volunteers. Conditioning and extinction trials were given. In one of the experiments, some subjects received the angry face as the target CS and some received the happy face as the target CS during conditioning. To prevent the subjects from consciously recognizing the stimuli, the stimuli were masked by superimposing a neutral face on the briefly presented target face. (The mask occurred either 30 msec or 500 msec after the onset of the target.) During the conditioning phase, each subject was shown both the happy and the angry face pictures, but only one (called CS+) was paired with shock. During the extinction trials no shock was given and subjects again were shown both types of pictures, but this time without a mask and for a longer duration of 2 seconds. Because of the brief and masked earlier presentations, the subjects were not able to state which pictures had been paired with shock.

To test if fear conditioning had taken place, skin conductance responses were measured during extinction trials, when no shock was given. If during extinction trials the subjects gave a higher skin conductance response to the target stimulus (CS+) than to the nontarget stimulus (CS–, which had not been paired with shock), fear conditioning can be said to have occurred.

As seen in Figure 13.2, skin conductance responses during extinction were overall the largest for subjects who had the angry faces (the angry CS+) paired with shock during conditioning. Additionally, a significant difference in responding to CS+ versus CS– occurred only for the subjects who

FIGURE 13.2

Mean magnitude (square root transformed) skin conductance responses (SCRs) to angry and happy faces for the six groups in the extinction phase of Experiment 2. Half of the groups had 30-ms stimulus onset asynchrony (SOA) and the other half had a 500-ms SOA. Within each SOA, one group was conditioned to an angry face (angry CS+) and another to a happy face (happy CS+), and the third group was a sensitization control group.

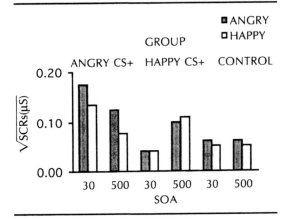

Source: From Esteves, Parra, Dimberg, & Öhman, 1994.

had the angry CS+. Thus, only the angry face gave fear conditioning. For the subjects receiving the happy face CS+ and for the control group, skin conductance responses were essentially the same for the happy as for the angry faces during the extinction trials. The investigators had predicted this, because they had theorized that due to evolutionary preparedness, angry faces would be the easier stimuli to learn to fear. That the angry faces are more readily learned as feared stimuli was found in other studies as well (Öhman, 1996).

Preparedness, or the ease of establishing certain types of conditioning, was described in earlier chapters on taste aversion and bait shyness studies (Garcia & Rusiniak, 1979), and it is a concept that has been well documented in animal studies. The question is whether this works in humans the same way as in nonhuman animals. That angry faces can be more easily feared is evident from the above study, but the explanation of why this occurs is open to dispute. Do the conditioning data of Esteves et al. (1994) demonstrate an evolutionary preparedness? Critics would argue for alternative ex-

292

planations. Human adults have had years of experience with human faces, and it is possible that a *learning history* has occurred in which angry but not happy faces consistently were accompanied by punishments or other aversive circumstances. Such variables need to be assessed to rule out prior learning in favor of evolutionary preparedness. For example, do very young infants show this difference in conditionability between stimuli? Do cultures with rare facial expressions of anger also show this difference between angry and happy faces?

A useful investigation to address these issues (Campos, Bertenthal, & Kermoian, 1992) assessed whether fear of heights in human infants is innate, in the sense of a maturational unfolding that occurs in all members of the species. Evolutionary adaptiveness has been advanced to account for this fear. However, as Campos et al. (1992) found, locomotor experience is the critical variable to lead to such a fear. For example, an orthopedically handicapped infant was tested longitudinally and did not show this fear as long as he had no locomotor experience. Moreover, regardless of the age when the infant begins to crawl, duration of locomotor experience, not age, predicted the avoidance of heights. More research is needed to clarify the extent to which prior learning, not evolutionary factors, play a role in human fear learning.

Regardless of whether the study by Esteves and colleagues (1994) illustrated evolutionary preparedness, the data did show that a person can learn emotionally relevant physiological responses without awareness. Learning without awareness has been suggested for a long time by various theorists and psychotherapists. Emotions as well as beliefs can be learned and acted on without a person being aware of the processes (Brewin, 1989, 1996). Increasingly, studies within cognitive psychology have shown that information processing can take place without awareness. One can take note of fleeting images without awareness that one has done so, and later they can influence behavior in certain ways.

Unaware learning to associate aversive stimuli (like shock) with previously nonfeared stimuli (pictures of faces) can be considered an example of unaware information processing. Some would question whether the physiological responses in the

Esteves et al. (1994) study signify emotion. For example, cognitive emotion theorists would argue that emotion consists of more than skin conductance reactivity, and that without further elaboration (like appraisal), what is learned is not fear as an emotion but merely selective physiological responding. To understand the effects of such conditioning, it would be important to know how long such learning lasts, to what extent the learning alters future emotional experiences, and whether cognitive appraisals in later emotional encounters will make the unconscious learning relevant or irrelevant.

Social Variables Involved in Fear Learning

Although human learning of fear can occur by means of Pavlovian conditioning of a CS with a US, much of human fear learning occurs through more complex and more cognitive processes. Fear can be learned in the kinds of ways already discussed for anger. Modeling is an important way for children to learn fear. When children observe emotional responses in adults who are significant in their lives, they come to adopt such emotions for themselves. Children's stories provide information about what is dangerous, and the incessant tales of harm and danger in newspapers and on television serve a similar function for adults. Verbal information and graphic depiction of dangers serve as bases for fear development. Real-life fear development occurs in many ways. In one study, children (ages 9 to 12) and their parents were given fear surveys and trait anxiety tests (Muris & Steerneman, 1996). The researchers found that the children's fearfulness was related to that of their mother and was due to modeling. Moreover, trait anxiety in the children was associated with trait anxiety of both the mother and the father.

Parental modeling and reinforcements will vary according to the type of fear the parent has. If the mother is afraid of thunder and lightning, she is likely to take the children indoors or possibly even to take them to bed with her whenever a storm occurs. Parents who fear persons of another race or ethnic group are likely to teach that fear by countless admonishments and examples. By many actions, people convey fear and anxiety and train it in others. Equally, by many actions people convey that safe events exist and fear is inappropriate. Teaching children effective coping skills can train them *not* to fear events that could be dangerous but are safe when dealt with appropriately.

The way others respond to a person's fear expression affects fear experiences. If parents give attention to the fearful child without teaching ways of coping with fear, they may inadvertently teach the child to become increasingly fearful. Fear that is reinforced by special attention can be learned instrumentally. In social living, fear is part of interpersonal experiences. Parents respond to emotional expressions of their children from the time infants are at an early age (Huebner & Izard, 1988). Children also show emotions of varying kinds in their relationships with peers. A study of social conflict in children from the third through the sixth grade revealed that different types of provoking situations led to different kinds of distress (Crick, 1995), and disturbance in relationships was found to be particularly distressing to girls. In school, many kinds of fears exist, and fear of losing friends or of being disliked can be powerful emotions.

Counseling with parents has shown that how parents respond to fear in their children has significant effects on the type of fears the child has, the intensity of the fears, and the way the child copes with fears (Dreikurs & Soltz 1992). Many fears are in reaction to real dangers, such as crime, AIDS, and traffic accidents. Preventive coping methods along with self-efficacy and a belief in internal locus of control can help reduce such fears. How one copes after a fear experience is also important. For example, in adults, talking about one's emotional reaction concerning a fearful and distressing event after it occurs can lower a person's later fear and distress upon experiencing the event a second time (Mendolia & Kleck, 1993).

Fear in humans is enormously complex. It is learned in a wide variety of ways, and appraisal and coping play a crucial role in many aspects of human fear experiences. Studies with nonhuman animals and humans have assessed how fear is learned and later modified or replaced. Social experiences are the major source of fear in humans, and social experiences also provide occasions of fear for animals. Dominance versus submission is related to aggression versus fear in animals and it can also be evident in humans. Dominant animals in a colony are more aggressive and domination can lead to aggression in humans; subordinate animals show fearful behavior, and subordinate status in humans can lead to fear and fearfulness. Dominance versus submission shapes aggression and fear in parent-child and spousal relationships. Violence in married and dating partners produces ongoing fear as well as cycles of offense and defense aggression (Koss et al., 1994).

In humans, cognitive restructuring can alter appraisals and thus alleviate fears. Therapeutic programs have been developed for treatment of many kinds of fears, including certain types of intense fears, like panic attacks (Craske & Barlow, 1993). Fear can be incapacitating, but fear and anxiety can also have valuable protective and defensive value. Learning to attend to signals of danger or pain or harm can help prevent the occurrence of the dangerous negative event. *Appropriate* fear and anxiety can help keep individuals safe from aversive events. Humans and nonhuman animals can learn fear by means of classical (Pavlovian) conditioning, and fear can be a motivation for learning a wide range of behaviors by means of escape and avoidance conditioning. Species differ in terms of which stimuli are more readily fear arousing and they differ in what behavior is displayed when fear is activated. Evolutionary factors have been identified in animal fears, some stimuli being more readily feared than others by members of a given species, and evolutionary factors may play a role in human fears. Human fear can be protective by helping individuals avoid dangers, and effective coping skills can be learned that forestall dangers and also prevent the debilitating effects of fear.

ANXIETY, INDIVIDUAL DIFFERENCES, COGNITION, AND COPING

With their capacity for abstract representations, humans are able to fear events that are not immediately tangible, and they can fear events in terms of a wide time span. We can fear events that will occur in 6 months, and due to creative and complex cog-

nitions, we can imagine dangers both real and fictitious. Humans can fear events that are misconstrued
and they can have anxieties that hinder rather than
help them attain desired goals.

An earlier chapter discussed fear of failure in relationship to achievement motivation. Human fears
are often not directed toward specific stimuli in the
way that animal fears are, and for humans the distinction between fear and anxiety can be blurred.
This was evident in the way "fear of failure" was
conceptualized and measured in terms of trait anxiety (Atkinson & Littwin, 1960). Human fear can
range from being extremely specific to being relatively intangible. At times human fear may blend
with and be indistinguishable from anxiety. Nevertheless, many writers distinguish between fear and
anxiety. Barlow (Antony, Brown, & Barlow, 1992)
considered fear as a cohesive emotion that is accompanied by an intense desire to escape a situation; fear is a reaction to immediate danger. In contrast, anxiety is loosely structured and serves to
prepare the individual to deal with possible future
threats. Anxiety involves vigilance and shifting attention toward presumed unpredictable and uncontrollable events. For Barlow, fear and anxiety are
stored in memory and activated by various cues.
Lazarus (1991) also distinguished anxiety from fear
but in a way that differs from that of Barlow.
Lazarus considered fear in terms of tangible events,
whereas anxiety always concerns threat to one's
sense of self or ego identity ("existential threat").
Both Lazarus and Barlow agree, however, that anxiety does not pertain to tangible events in the way
fear does. Many psychologists agree that anxiety in
humans tends to relate to central and personal concerns. The literature on fear includes animal studies, but studies of anxiety have focused primarily
on human rather than on animal motivation and
emotion. Anxiety has social significance, like the
anxiety many persons have about the impression
they make on others (Geen, 1991). Many other issues also bear on the study of anxiety.

State and Trait Anxiety

The state versus trait distinction is important in research on anxiety. Individuals can be anxious in a

given situation and then within a short time the anxiety can be diminished, and this transience can
occur with state anxiety and not only fear. The uncertainty of outcomes and of consequences gives
the state a diffuseness that is different from the
specificity of fear. Suppose an instructor in a course
has just graded an examination, and before handing
back the tests the instructor informs the class that
all the grades of the examination will be read aloud,
with each student identified by name. This is likely
to create anxiety in many students. No specific danger is known, and only a general uncertainty of consequences exists ("will my grade be bad?" or "I will
be sure to be embarrassed, regardless if my grade is
high or low!"), so that the motivational state is not
one of fear but of anxiety. If the instructor then
looks at the perturbed expressions of the students
and says "I've changed my mind, I'll just pass out
the tests as usual," for many students the anxiety
state will diminish significantly. For some, the anxiety about the outcome (high or low grade) may still
remain, but anxiety triggered by the uncertain consequences of public disclosure will be gone.

Trait anxiety refers to a long-term disposition to
be anxious. State anxiety refers to anxiety at a given
time. State anxiety is usually manifested by autonomic nervous system reactivity. Various endocrine
changes occur, muscles may become tight, thoughts
may be fast and not follow a logical progression,
worries may focus attention on a narrow topic, and
the person may show a variety of behaviors reflecting suboptimum functioning. High versus low *trait*
anxiety may not bring significant differences on
some response measures even though differences
occur as a function of high versus low *state* anxiety.
For example, in one study (Grillon & Ameli, 1993)
subjects were tested for the startle reflex. The researchers presented a loud sound and observed eye
blinks. There was no difference in fear-potentiated
startle as a function of high and low trait anxiety,
but there was a difference according to whether the
subjects had high versus low state anxiety.

Various tests have been devised to measure both
state and trait anxiety. An early well-known paper-
and-pencil test, the Taylor Manifest Anxiety Scale
(MAS), sought to measure anxiety as a means of activating generalized drive (Taylor, 1953). Other

tests sought to measure test-taking anxiety (Alpert & Haber, 1960; Mandler & Sarason, 1952). Tests that measure both state and trait anxiety are the IPAT scale by Cattell (1957, 1966) and the widely used Spielberger (1983; Spielberger, Gorsuch, & Lushene, 1970) State-Trait Anxiety Inventory (STAI). In the state scale subjects rate themselves for reactions at the moment, and in the trait scale they rate themselves for their usual reaction in anxiety-producing situations. Individual scores are compared with group norms and then converted to percentile scores. Correlations between trait and state anxiety scores for groups of subjects typically vary between low and high positive.

Persons who score high on the trait scale in specific circumstances may score low on the state scale, for example if they are in a calm situation or feel relaxed and confident. Likewise, persons who score low on the trait scale in some circumstances may score high on the state scale, for example if they are in a very pressured situation or feel demeaned and personally vulnerable. After performing well on a task persons with high trait anxiety may show relatively low state anxiety, and after performing poorly on a task persons with low trait anxiety may show relatively higher state anxiety (Ferguson, 1983).

What Is Trait Anxiety? Many studies have explored trait anxiety, its effect on behavior, and how one therapeutically can help persons with high trait anxiety (Zinbarg, Barlow, Brown, & Hertz, 1992). The literature on this topic is too vast to cover in the present book, but some pertinent issues are considered. Good reviews are given by M. W. Eysenck (1987b, 1997). Many studies have shown how trait anxiety affects goals, emotions, coping strategies, physiological responding, and many other aspects of cognition and behavior.

Trait anxiety is considered an *individual differences* variable. Long-term differences exist between people in their tendency to become anxious. People who are high in trait anxiety need not all become anxious about the same events nor manifest their anxiety in the same way. Various theorists have proposed alternative models of what is meant by trait anxiety, but in general, there is agreement that trait

anxiety is multidimensional (see, for example, Endler, Edwards, Vitelli, & Parker, 1989). Various dimensions are represented by trait anxiety, one being anxiety about physical pain or danger. Several dimensions of anxiety pertain to interpersonal processes, such as anxiety about how one is socially evaluated by others. Because highly anxious individuals tend to be sensitive to threatening stimuli or events (Mineka & Sutton, 1992), anxiety has been considered by many to be similar to the concept of repression-sensitization proposed by Byrne (1964). That is, sensitizers, like highly anxious persons, are sensitive to threatening stimuli or events, whereas repressors avoid such stimuli or events. Repressors tend to rate themselves as low on trait and state anxiety scales, but their physiological arousal is high. In this as well as other ways repressors differ from genuinely low anxiety individuals.

Trait Anxiety, Neuroticism, and Introversion. As described in an earlier chapter, H. J. Eysenck (1967) proposed a model of personality with two independent dimensions, one being neuroticism and the other introversion-extraversion. Many studies confirmed that there is a relationship between trait anxiety and being emotionally labile, as measured by scores on a scale of neuroticism. Some researchers have suggested that trait anxiety is also related to introversion. For example, Gray (1991, pp. 349–351) suggested that extraverts are less sensitive to punishment than are introverts and thus are not likely to develop fear. Gray also suggested that introverts have a tendency to pessimism, and that introverts are sensitizers who perform better with threatening stimuli than with neutral ones. Various factor analytic studies have found that extraverts are high in impulsivity and sociability, and Gray proposed that due to their impulsivity, extraverts are sensitive to stimuli depicting rewards. According to Gray, persons high in trait anxiety are likely to be high on neuroticism and introversion and to be highly sensitive to stimuli depicting punishment. In line with this formulation, individuals with high trait anxiety should show better conditioning than those with low trait anxiety when a noxious stimulus is used for the US. Data from research by Spence (1964) on eye blink conditioning, with an aversive puff of air as the US, provided support for the proposals of Gray (1991). The high anxiety subjects did show better conditioning.

Spence (1964) did not test the formulation of Gray, and instead considered his conditioning data as showing support for Hullian generalized drive theory. According to Spence, persons with high anxiety have higher generalized drive than those with low anxiety. Drive theorists predicted one set of effects for a noncompetitional task like classical conditioning (J. A. Taylor, 1951), in which only a single response is learned, and other effects for a task that had many responses, with interference for learning. In a task with high response interference, according to drive theory (Spence, Farber, & Mc-Fann, 1956), high drive subjects should do worse than low drive subjects. This is because under high drive, more than under low drive, there is a differential increase in response strength of all competing responses. Thus, for drive theorists, anxiety should facilitate conditioning but not multiple response learning in which many interfering responses occur. Gray and Spence would agree on what the effects of anxiety should be on classical conditioning, but they would disagree on how anxiety would affect performance on complex, multiple-response tasks. For Gray, aversive conditions should facilitate performance for high trait anxiety (that is, introverted) individuals, regardless of task characteristics.

Data other than conditioning did support Gray's formulation. McCord and Wakefield (1981) studied children in a classroom. Teachers were rated according to whether they tended to use praise as reward or blame as punishment. The children had been given personality testing. Those who were more introverted tended to improve the most with punishment, whereas those who were more extraverted tended to improve the most with rewards. Gray interpreted these findings on the basis of biological factors, based on hypothesized differences in predisposition and in brain activity between introverts and extraverts. Although these data suggest support for Gray's formulation, alternative *learning* explanations for the difference in reactions to punishment and reward between introverts and extraverts can also apply.

Biological variables like the ones suggested by Gray (1991) may not be as valid an explanation for long-term individual differences as are alternative explanations. Knowledge of child-rearing practices needs to be obtained. It is well known that different ways of raising children lead to their adopting different strategies and methods of coping. Many variables need to be investigated to permit fuller understanding of how high versus low trait anxiety or introversion and extraversion are associated with physiological, attitudinal, and behavioral differences. Davidson (1995; Sutton & Davidson, 1997) has found consistently that the left prefrontal cortex is a substrate of positive emotions and approach behavior and the right prefrontal cortex is a substrate of negative emotions and avoidance (withdrawal or inhibition). As already discussed in a previous chapter, significantly different electrical activity is recorded from these brain regions, depending on whether the person is in an approach or inhibition state (Sutton & Davidson, 1997). Individuals with high trait anxiety might thus show different prefrontal cortex electrical activity than would self-confident and optimistic individuals. What is important to consider is that an eletrophysiological correlate does not indicate constitutional or biological determinism, of individuals being preprogrammed to be high or low in anxiety. Depending on the kinds of learning experiences an individual had from early childhood, different electrophysiological activity can be expected during a given momentary state. Differences in physiological activity do not signify what the causal factors are that led to the individual differences.

How children are socialized is likely to affect whether they tend to be anxious. A simple learning explanation might be that children who are given more punishment could become more introverted, especially if impulsive and sociable behavior is punished. Higgins and colleagues (Higgins, Roney, Crowe, & Hymes, 1994) in their study of adults' self-regulation had an approach different from that of Gray or Spence. Individuals may be guided by "ideal" self-guides or by "ought" self-guides. From that perspective, the McCord and Wakefield (1981) findings could represent different ways the children were trained, with anxious introverted children trained to pay attention to duty and what "ought" to be done, and low anxious extraverted children trained to pay attention to what "ideally" should be done. Such training could explain the defensive "avoid punishment" strategy of the anxious introverted children and the "approach reward" strategy of the low anxious extraverted children. Regardless of what explanations best fit the McCord and Wakefield (1981) findings, interest has been shown by a number of researchers for identifying whether persons with high trait anxiety are selectively sensitive to punishing events.

Cognition and Coping

Cognitive Tasks and Anxiety. M. W. Eysenck (1987b, 1991; Derakshan & Eysenck, 1997), as well as many others studying cognitive task performance, found that individuals with high trait anxiety are selectively sensitive to threatening and punitive content. Data from many studies suggest that trait rather than state anxiety is the key factor in this sensitivity (Williams, Mathews & MacLeod, 1996), but contrary evidence also exists that it is a state rather than trait anxiety that affects this sensitivity (Green, Rogers & Hedderley, 1996) in nonclinical populations.

To examine this sensitizing phenomenon, researchers have used a method that is based on a well-known task developed by Stroop (1935). In the original Stroop test, subjects are shown words in colored lettering and asked to name that color. What makes the task unexpectedly difficult is that the semantic content of the word is a different color from that of the lettering, and subjects tend to name the semantic meaning rather than the surface color. For example, if the word content is "blue" and the lettering for that word is red, subjects to name the lettering are likely to err and describe the lettering as blue. The time taken to name the semantic color content is significantly shorter than that needed to name the color of the lettering. This occurs in part because of the vast experience adults have had in reading semantic content and ignoring the color in which the word is written. A modified Stroop task, known as the emotional Stroop task, takes advantage of the fact that the more the subject pays attention to and processes the semantic word content, the

longer will it take the subject to name the color of the letters. Thus, how long it takes for subjects to give the color name for different kinds of words has been used to study the effects of word content.

The emotional Stroop test has been used in studies evaluating patient groups (with clinical depression, phobia, or anxiety) and it has been used with college students differing in high versus low anxiety. Threat-related words were compared sometimes with neutral and positively valenced words and sometimes just with neutral words. Color naming of threat-related words was found to take longer than naming of neutral words for clinically anxious persons (Mathews & MacLeod, 1985) and for nonclinical subjects with high trait anxiety (Richards & Millwood, 1989). However, it has also been found that both types of anxious subjects show impaired color naming of affectively positive material (Mogg & Marden, 1990). This suggests the possibility that the crucial variable is how relevant the words are to immediate concerns of the subjects, rather than whether the words contain threatening content. Support for this was found in a study by Green et al. (1996). These researchers found that state but not trait anxiety led to selective threat sensitivity. In their study, college students in the experimental group watched a 10-minute negative mood-induction film about a nuclear explosion and those in the control group saw no film but sat in a separated area for 10 minutes. No positive mood manipulation was used because previously the researchers had found no color-naming effects from positive mood induction. At the start of the study all subjects completed the Spielberger et al. (1970) state and trait tests and did color naming of neutral, negative, and positive words. Following the experimental manipulation (film or no film), the color-naming task was presented again after one of three delay conditions: 0, 5, or 15 minutes. Red, green, purple, blue, and yellow lettering was used. After the second color naming, the subjects filled out another state anxiety form.

Complex results were found. The delay conditions interacted with the main experimental variable (film or no film). The experimental subjects named the threat-related words more slowly than the neutral words but this was found only in the 0- and 5-

minute groups. It was evident that the mood-induction effect wore off by the time of the 15-minute delay, because the significant increase in state anxiety for the experimental subjects was found only for the 0- and 5-minute groups. No significant state anxiety increase between first and second testing occurred for the control subjects. Importantly, the control subjects did *not* show slowed color naming for the threat-related versus neutral words. Positive words were named more slowly by both experimental and control groups under the 0-minute delay condition. In this study trait anxiety did not have a significant effect on color naming. Studies using other types of tasks did find significant characteristics in cognitive processing for high trait individuals, especially in contrast to persons considered to be repressors (Derakshan & Eysenck, 1997). Other studies have shown coping strategies that differ between high and low trait anxiety subjects. One way for high trait anxiety subjects to overcome the interference of threatening words is to speed up their overall color-naming latencies (Williams et al., 1996). Thus, even on neutral words the high trait anxiety subjects in some studies gave faster color naming than did the low trait anxiety subjects.

In the Green et al. (1996) study, the affective pull of positive and negative words was shown, but only the pull for negative words was strongly related to anxiety. The positive words were slowed comparably for the control and the experimental groups, and slowing occurred only for the 0-minute delay condition. Whatever attention was demanded by the positive words was fleeting and not related to anxiety. The Green et al. study highlights the need to consider effects of both trait and state anxiety in carefully controlled studies. Evidence that nonconscious processes can be involved in differential responding to words on the emotional Stroop task was found by MacLeod and Hagan (1992), who gave words like "disease" subliminally. Women were tested before a gynecological examination and the degrees of anxiety and depression experienced by the women who later received a diagnosis of pathology was predicted by their color naming of the situationally threatening words 2 months earlier.

Data are needed to show not only how low trait anxiety subjects perform on cognitive tasks when they are under high state anxiety but also how high trait anxiety subjects perform when they are in a low state anxiety. Under low state anxiety they might perform in a way that is similar to low trait anxiety subjects. Persons with high trait anxiety are likely to perform differently than low trait anxiety subjects in situations in which they feel threatened (have high state anxiety), but the question remains of how they perform when they are not anxious and don't feel threatened. Data reviewed by Williams and colleagues (1996) show that with nonclinical subjects (like college students), the relatedness of words to current concern, both for positive and negative words, is the key factor that leads to interference (slower color naming) on the emotional Stroop task. However, whether high trait anxiety subjects perform like low trait anxiety subjects in low state anxiety circumstances is still to be determined.

It is possible that high trait anxiety persons maintain high state anxiety because of a habitual sensitivity to threatening stimuli. Such sensitivity would ensure that one is very often exposed to threat and thereby must remain in a high state of anxiety. It may be that such sensitivity has a protective function. Would a person with a less defensive mode of meeting environmental inputs have a stronger discomfort if and when painful or threatening events do occur? A large literature unrelated to anxiety shows that signaled compared with unsignaled shock is preferred, and predictable shock or pain overall is preferred to one that is unpredictable (Ferguson, 1982). This occurs in part because preparatory pain-inhibiting maneuvers can be made. If the highly anxious person has a bias to expect aversive events, then "being prepared" for threatening or punishing events may mitigate the aversiveness.

An important distinction needs to be made between cognitive processes that are *self-generated* and those that occur as part of task demands. Many studies have shown that high versus low trait anxiety persons differ in their self-generated cognitions. For example, persons with high trait anxiety worry more than do those with low trait anxiety, and this occurs even when state anxiety is comparable (M. W. Eysenck, 1984). The kinds of events they remember, the internal scripts they recite to themselves, and many of their coping strategies are different. Unresolved questions still remain to what extent they differ in information processing of new material that does not have personal significance.

Anxiety, Self-Esteem, and Coping. Individuals who have experienced anxiety know not only that it is an unpleasant experience but that in many ways it can be debilitating. Anxiety can be related to stress-induced illness (Peterson et al., 1993) and to lower immune system activity (Cohen & Herbert, 1996), and it is associated with lowered productive energy (Thayer, 1989). Although in noncompetitional tasks like eye blink conditioning anxiety has been found to be facilitating (Spence, 1964), in complex tasks with interfering responses and varied attentional demands, anxiety characteristically reduces processing efficiency (M. W. Eysenck, 1987a, see Table 12.1 and p. 357). Memory, attentional control, and retrieval efficiency tend to suffer when an individual is anxious. State and trait anxiety have wide-ranging consequences, many of which have a spiral effect. That is, high trait anxiety people are more pessimistic and more prone to take note of threatening information than are persons with low anxiety (M. W. Eysenck, 1991). In turn, if people expect negative events (pessimism) and then find them (selective attention to threatening or negative inputs), that process will fortify and even enhance the anxiety. Covington (1992) reviewed many studies of anxiety in achievement situations and found that measures of *worry* were the best predictor of academic performance decrease. Worry misdirects attention from the task to task-irrelevant considerations, and during test taking the anxious student shows various forms of retrieval deficit, of not remembering prior learned material. Anxiety also was found to lead to poor study habits, with resulting deficit in skill of learning the necessary material. A fear of failure for many students becomes an emotional preoccupation, and this leads to coping strategies that increase rather than decrease the likelihood of failure in achievement tasks.

Anxious individuals have a low sense of well-being. Emmons and Diener (1985) asked college students to keep a daily mood report for many days. The subjects also completed a life satisfaction scale

and several personality tests. Anxiety was found to relate significantly to an overall negative affect score, and for one sample of students anxiety was inversely related to life satisfaction. In studies of personal strivings, in which subjects state what they try to do in their daily life, Emmons (1989) found that anxious persons show significant ambivalence, that is, unhappiness when they had successfully accomplished (consummated) their strivings.

As Folkman and Lazarus (1990) pointed out, a key factor in coping effectiveness is the appropriateness of the strategy with the actual circumstances. Problem-focused coping is most effective when the person has control of the outcome and can bring about the desired outcome. When a person has no control over a situation or over the outcome of events, emotion-focused coping, which is geared to reduce the amount of distress, is more effective. If anxious individuals are ambivalent when they do achieve what they have striven to attain, as described by Emmons (1989), ineffective coping is clearly indicated. Bringing task achievements in line with aspirations (Covington, 1992), and emotional satisfaction with strivings (Emmons, 1989) are ways to reduce anxiety. Data on coping strategies and on anxiety in achievement situations showed that persons with low anxiety do bring task achievements in line with aspirations and they do have congruent emotional satisfaction with their strivings, whereas highly anxious persons have not been effective in these ways.

Moos (1992a) developed a coping responses inventory that identified positive (effective) and negative (ineffective) ways of coping with stressful situations. Both adolescents and adults showed a range of styles of dealing with stressful events (Moos, 1992b). Problem solving and positive reappraisal methods were used as coping by individuals who reported good interpersonal relationships with friends and family. A spiraling effect was evident. People are not only influenced by stressors, but they can cause stressors to occur by ineffective coping. Intervention strategies need to take both aspects into account.

It is clear from a wide range of studies that trait and state anxiety have significant effects on many aspects of people's lives. Researchers have shown that cognitive processes differ between persons with high versus low trait anxiety and that they differ for individuals when they experience high versus low state anxiety. Pessimistic versus optimistic explanatory styles (Peterson et al., 1993) are in part based on, and in turn perpetuate, low or high self-confidence. Expanding a person's sense of self-worth (Covington, 1992) helps the anxious person to be more confident, to adopt more effective coping methods, and thereby to reverse an ineffective cycle. Social support systems play a crucial role in this process (Moos, 1992b). Cognitive and social variables play major roles in human fear and anxiety and in the ways individuals can reduce inappropriate fear and anxiety. Models based on animal fear and anxiety are useful and instructive. However, many additional variables need to be considered in order to understand and remediate human fear and anxiety.

SUMMARY

At different times in the history of psychology, fear and anxiety have been studied as emotions and as motivations. Contemporary studies identify the two variables as emotions. Most theorists consider fear to relate to tangible and immediate events of threat or harm, and anxiety to relate to less specific events. Anxiety more than fear is linked to threats concerned with self-esteem.

Escape and avoidance conditioning are two kinds of instrumental conditioning in which responses lead to cessation or prevention of a noxious stimulus. Negative reinforcement refers to the offset of a noxious stimulus after a response occurs. Punishment refers to the onset of a noxious stimulus after a response occurs.

Learned helplessness describes the fact that after animals are given intense inescapable shock, when later given escapable shock their escape conditioning is decreased compared with control animals never given inescapable shock. Various explanations have been given for why the inescapable shock leads to learned helplessness. Associative as well as motivational and attentional processes seem to be altered by the inescapable shocks.

Flooding involves restraining an animal in a previously shocked chamber in which instrumental responding had occurred and was subsequently prevented. The procedure is presumed to extinguish fear as well as the learned escape or avoidance response. Data on extinction show that contextual changes and forgetting make extinction of learned fear unlikely. Alternative methods are available for modifying or replacing fear.

The amygdala and hippocampus are brain systems involved in fear. Different brain areas seem to be involved in the conditioning of fear to specific stimuli than to contextual stimuli. Levels of the neurotransmitters epinephrine and norepinephrine are raised with anxiety.

Fear can be learned in humans by Pavlovian conditioning, and such learning can occur without awareness. Adult fear learning is far more likely to involve cognitive processes, and cognitive reorientation is successful in modifying fear in humans.

Anxiety is studied as a trait and as a state. A person with high trait anxiety may experience moments of low state anxiety, and a person with low trait anxiety may have high state anxiety at times. Persons with high trait anxiety tend to be sensitive to threatening stimuli. Persons with high trait anxiety are more readily conditioned with an aversive stimulus like a puff of air to the eye, but it is not firmly established what other ways distinguish the learning and cognitive processes of high compared with low trait anxiety individuals. The emotional Stroop test has been used to study how individuals respond to threatening compared with affectively neutral words.

Anxious persons tend to generate interfering thoughts. They often have ineffective coping strategies that interfere in their performance on tasks. Various kinds of rehabilitative methods have been used effectively with persons suffering from anxiety and also with persons suffering from the intense fear of panic disorder.

CHAPTER 14

Sex, Gender, and Love

Nonhuman animals and humans interact with members of their species in many ways. Aggression and fear, described in the previous chapters, involve negative emotions and processes of antagonism or harm. However, members of a species also approach each other in positive ways. In the human community, cooperation, empathy, and mutual support provide the means for individuals and the community to thrive. When individuals experience love and friendship, they have deeply satisfying positive emotions. A person's health and energies are heightened with long-term positive emotions and approach motivations compared with negative emotions and avoidance motivations (Ader & Cohen, 1993; S. Cohen & Herbert, 1996). Positive emotions, approach motivation, and mutual support for working toward shared or compatible goals enable group members to merge skills, strengths, and energies for productive achievements and creative enjoyments. Cooperation makes emotional demands on people, but many satisfactions come from prosocial ways of interacting with others. When persons strive to maximize positive outcomes for themselves and for others and to form relationships based on equality (a prosocial value orientation), their patterns of interaction are more satisfying and their attachments are more secure than are individualistic and competitive modes of interaction (Van Lange, Otten, De Bruin, & Joireman, 1997).

Love has many dimensions, and human affections are of many kinds. Sexual motivation also helps nonhuman animals and humans to approach members of their species. For many species, sexual motivation is a "primary drive" in the sense of being biologically driven. In contrast to other primary drives like hunger and thirst, sexual motivation does not lead to survival of the individual but, instead, ensures survival of the species. In lower animals sexual motivation is largely shaped by a limited range of biological determinants and triggered by highly specific stimuli. In higher mammals, and especially in humans, sexual motivation is broadly varied and largely a function of individual learning experiences and social contexts. Considerable debate exists whether humans select sexual partners and mates according to evolutionary principles, but all researchers agree that human sexual arousal, sexual behavior, and the targets of these arousals and behaviors vary widely for individuals and across cultures.

Sex differences in neurochemistry, physiology, and behavior are found in vertebrates and in many invertebrate species. Human behaviors, cognitions, emotions, and motivations also have been found to relate to sex differences that are largely a function of culture and social learning. For this reason, the term *gender* is used, to denote cultural effects and social learning rather than sex as a biological variable. Gender affects many aspects of human life. Considerable controversy exists about what differences do exist as a function of gender and about how to interpret gender differences (Baumeister & Sommer, 1997; Cross & Madson, 1997; Martin & Ruble, 1997).

HORMONAL EFFECTS, SEXUAL DIMORPHISM, AND SEXUAL MOTIVATION

Gonadal Steroid Hormones

The gonads (testes and ovaries) produce steroid hormones. The effects of these are wide ranging. Prenatally they affect the development of the central nervous system (CNS) and they determine the peripheral genital and reproductive organ development pertinent to a male or female. In puberty they are responsible for further body changes and certain types of related behavioral changes. Their role differs for various species.

The testes produce *androgens,* of which *testosterone* has the widest effects on sexual motivation. The adrenal gland also produces androgens. Ovaries produce *estrogens,* the notable one being *estradiol,* and *progestins,* the notable one being *progesterone* (involved in pregnancy). In many mammalian species, both estrogen and progesterone have been linked to sexual receptivity in females. Because testosterone is a precursor to estrogen, the ovaries also make testosterone. Also, estrogen is a metabolite of testosterone, which leads to the testes secreting small amounts of estrogens. In mammals, both sexes make both classes of hormone, but these occur in different proportions. The gonadal steroid hormones can regulate gene expression and in this way they exert major influences on the development and differentiation of cells (Becker & Breedlove, 1992).

Genetic sex (whether the individual has XX or Y chromosomes) determines gonadal sex (whether there are ovaries or testes) due to a gene on the Y chromosome. This gene is responsible for the development of the testes. During early embryonic development, the undifferentiated gonad has the potential to become either an ovary or a testis. If the gene on the Y chromosome is present, the gonad will develop into a testis. If the gene is absent (as in the normal XX female), the gonad develops into an ovary. The hormones secreted by the testes determine many changes; without these hormones, the internal reproductive structures, external genitalia, gonads, and brain development follow a female pattern.

Ovulation in females after onset of puberty is governed by the pituitary. Postpubertal ovulation can be altered in rats prenatally or shortly after birth by surgical graft of testicular tissue in females, and by castration and surgically implanted ovaries in males. Such prenatal or neonatal alteration permits postpubertal male rats to support ovulation and postpubertal female rats not to support ovulation. Thus, prenatally and for a brief period postnatally, gonadal hormones have been found in rats to control the way the pituitary functions in terms of male or female characteristics (Breedlove, 1992).

Sexual Dimorphism. Sexual dimorphism refers to an organ or physical feature having a different appearance for the two sexes. Sexually dimorphic features include manes in lions, deer antlers, and bright coloration of male birds. Sexual dimorphism also has been demonstrated for parts of the brain in birds and mammals. Differences exist between rats and primates with regard to which centers of the brain are sexually dimorphic. Evidence of sexual dimorphism exists in the human brain, but how that is related to possible behavioral differences between men and women is still very much an open question. There is evidence that brain weight differs at birth between the sexes, and the differences are more pronounced in adulthood, due in part to different body size and weight in men versus women. In adults, more lateralization (specialized functioning in left and right brain hemispheres) appears to occur in men compared with women, but this may be due in part to different life experiences for men compared with women. Also, certain hypothalamic centers were found to be sexually dimorphic (Breedlove, 1994). Studies of adults does not readily permit one to know if life experiences lead to the differences in brain structure or if the sexual dimorphism is due to the impact of male and female hormones prenatally on brain development.

To assess such questions, information about newborns is needed. One study (Sakai, Baker, Jacklin, & Shulman, 1995) tested newborn monozygotic (identical) and dizygotic (fraternal) twins by analysis of their umbilical cord blood. All twin pairs were of the same sex. Differences in hormone levels were found within a twin pair, pointing to the importance of intrauterine environmental factors. Also, progesterone and testosterone levels were significantly higher for the boys than the girls but zygosity was not a significant factor. Intrauterine environment as well as genetic factors play a role in levels of neonatal sex hormones. Enormous complexity exists in the way genes, sex hormones, prenatal environment, and life experiences shape brain and behavior, and especially postnatal environmental factors have far-reaching influences on these interactions.

Sexual Behavior. In nonhuman animals, sexual behavior normally refers to all interactive behaviors between a female and a male of a species, which lead up to and include behavior that will lead to reproduction. In mammals, that involves copulatory behavior, with ejaculation by the male and potential fertilization of the female. Fishes and amphibians have a variety of sexual behaviors, including courtship. Reproduction occurs in most cases by the male depositing sperms on the eggs that the female has laid. Because sexual behavior leading to reproduction ordinarily occurs only within a species, each species has developed unique patterns. Birds have characteristic song patterns or plumage displays. Some invertebrates are hermaphrodites, which means they have both male and female reproductive organs and can reproduce as either sex. Nonsexual behavior can occur, in which the hermaphrodites have self-fertilization, and sexual behavior can occur also in hermaphrodites, when reproduction involves interaction between two individuals (Breedlove, 1992). Many variations in sexual behavior occur for different species (Crews, 1992).

In rats, the female is receptive to the male when she is in estrus (time of ovulation). If the male approaches her at other times during her ovarian cycle, she will fend him off and not show receptivity. She shows receptivity by arching her back in a characteristic fashion, called *lordosis*, which facilitates the male's mounting her and achieving penile intromission. Receptivity is closely tied to the levels of estrogen and progesterone in the female rat, and amount of sexual behavior in the male rat is partly related to his level of testosterone. For animals living in a colony, social factors play a large role in the male rat's sexual behavior, in terms of the dominance of the male.

In normal male rats and mice, testosterone that is present at birth has an *organizing* effect by acting on the nervous system. Castration (removal of the testes, the primary source of testosterone) soon after birth abolishes normal male sexual behavior. That is, the brain and other parts of the nervous system are altered (demasculinized) by the lack of the male hormone shortly after birth. Castration in the adult is likely to diminish sexual behavior, but this reflects the *activating* effect of the male hormone. Hormone replacement, in some cases even after a long delay following castration, can reinstate copulatory behavior to precastration levels, as was found in one study with a specific strain of mice (Wee, Weaver, & Clemens, 1988). Other species, like dogs, cats, and rhesus monkeys, have been reported to copulate for some years after castration in adulthood, but sexual behavior in rats and mice is more dependent upon gonadal hormones (reviewed in Meisel & Sachs, 1994). Nevertheless, strain differences in the retention of sexual behavior after castration have been found. For example, 30% of the males of one strain (B6D2F1 genotype) of mice continued to ejaculate many weeks after castration, even though gonadal hormone levels were reduced to a level comparable to that of other strains of mice that lost copulatory behavior (Clemens et al., 1988).

Neurochemicals other than gonadal hormones also affect sexual behavior. In female rats, chemicals that enhance cholinergic neurotransmission facilitate the occurrence of lordosis behavior, and scopolamine, a cholinergic antagonist, inhibits lordosis in naturally cycling female rats and in females that have had their ovaries removed and been given hormone replacement (Dohanich, 1995). Scopolamine also inhibits other components of female sexual behavior, including solicitation of the male by the female, pacing of sexual contacts with a stimulus male (Dohanich et al., 1993), and male preference. Regarding male preference, female rats given scopolamine avoided a compartment containing a sexually intact male rat and preferred a compartment containing a castrated male rat (Wee, Francis, Lee, Lee, & Dohanich, 1995). The control group rats, given saline injections, showed the opposite preference. In addition to acetylcholine, several other neurochemicals, including dopamine, norepinephrine, and serotonin, have been found to affect female rats' sexual receptivity (Carter, 1992b).

Gonadal hormones play a different role in rats and mice than in many other species, including primates. The estrous cycle determines receptivity in female rats and in many nonprimate species, and it has an apparent effect on the timing of male baboon sexual approach behavior (DeVore, 1965). In humans, copulation occurs at any time, even for some women during menstruation. Human adult sexual behavior is not controlled by levels of sex hormones in either men or women except in extreme hormonal deficiencies. Even in these cases, like in castration, sexual activity has been found to continue rather than to cease (Carter, 1992a, p. 132). Moreover, sexual behavior need not occur in human adults even with adequate levels of sex hormones. Sexual behavior does not seem to be determined by estrogen levels, but estrogen levels may affect sexual motivation in women, with highest sexual arousal at specific times in the menstrual cycle.

Although the hypothalamus and amygdala are known to be crucial areas of the brain for mediation of sexual behavior and sexual motivation, variations in crucial brain areas exist across many species (Baum, 1992). The complexity of sexual behavior and sexual motivation makes localizing of brain areas far more difficult than localizing crucial brain areas for hunger and satiety, for example. Moreover, as seen in the chapters on hunger, even in hunger and satiety there is uncertainty about which brain areas are important. Sexual behavior is determined in some species by highly specific stimuli and in other species by complex social variables. Neurochemicals affect sexual behavior differently in many species, and specific brain areas are not yet fully understood in their relationship to sexual behavior and sexual motivation.

Social Animals: Prairie Voles and Spotted Hyenas

In mammalian species, female preference tends to determine the sexual activity of the copulating pair. In animals like rats, the female rat's preference is controlled by the ovarian cycle. In other animals, a variety of processes occur that lead to the female's choice of sexual behavior in terms of when it should occur and with which male. Animals with strong and clear-cut social patterns, like prairie voles and spotted hyenas, provide important insights for clarifying the role of social dynamics in sexual behavior.

Using field and laboratory observations of prairie voles, Getz and Carter (1996) found that the first estrus in a virgin female is stimulated by a specific pheromone in a male's urine, acquired by the female sniffing the genitals of the male. She does not sniff the genitals of familiar males, only an unfamiliar male. During autumn and winter, prairie voles are highly communal, and litter mates and other close relatives may live together for an extended period. Thus, a nonfamiliar male aids in preventing excessive inbreeding. Within two days of sniffing the pheromone, she achieves estrus and mates. After giving birth, she again achieves estrus and mates. If she lives within an extended family, another pheromone is produced, this time by the reproductively active female. It serves to suppress reproductive activity of young females, so that male genital sniffing won't as easily activate the virgin female.

If an unfamiliar male is present, the sexually active female won't mate with her brothers or her father. But if an unfamiliar male is not present, the females do sometimes mate with family members. Of importance in showing the significance of *social motivation* in the sexual behavior of these animals is the finding that if the female's mother is present, the daughter won't mate with her father. Males living in family groups do not become sexually active unless they interact with unfamiliar animals. In spite of the large number of animals that a female can encounter in a large community, mating is largely monogamous. This is accomplished for the most part by the male. One way he does so is by rejecting unfamiliar virgin females from sniffing his genital area. Another is to exclude unfamiliar males from his area. Getz and Carter (1996) hypothesized that the special mating system of prairie voles and their social organization evolved as a means of adapting to low-food habitats. In low-food habitats, offspring would survive better staying home, and males would not wander. The social organization involves not only extended family members living together harmoniously, but also the males contributing actively to nest building, grooming the young, and rearing the offspring. With predators like snakes a constant danger, their cooperative communal living and safeguarding sexual patterns help the small prairie voles survive.

A different pattern of social and sexual behaviors is evident in the spotted hyenas. The females are bigger and heavier than the males and maternal rank is the key to many behaviors. Females in the wild dominate males and males react subordinately. Females have a hypertrophied clitoris that is fully erectile and looks like a male penis. Mating and birth occur through the urogenital canal, which is the length of the clitoris. The masculinization of the external genitalia is closely related to the female's high levels of androgens (Glickman, Frank, Davidson, Smith, & Siiteri, 1987). In the wild, the females remain in the group of their birth (natal clan) for life and the males join other clans when they are adults. Females and males acquire their mother's rank. Until they leave their clan, sons of high-ranking females are dominant to females whose rank is lower than that of the sons' mother (Zabel, Glickman, Frank, Woodmansee, & Keppel, 1992). Spotted hyenas display a considerable amount of coalition formation, in which two or more animals aggress together against one or more targets. Dominant females tend not to be targets.

All females in a clan can breed, but daughters of high-ranking females are likely to have higher reproductive success. Male and female offspring of high-ranking mothers also have an advantage during feeding. Although low-ranking females rarely aggress against high-ranking females, one instance was observed in the research colony in which a high-ranking female attacked an offspring of a low-ranking female. The low-ranking mother then attacked the high-ranking animal, with maternal defense overriding hierarchical patterns (Zabel et al., 1992).

In the research colony, when females played in same-sex groups they were observed to play more frequently and vigorously than males in same-sex groups (Glickman et al., 1992; Pedersen, Glickman, Frank, & Beach, 1990), which reverses the pattern

found in many species. In humans, rough-and-tumble play has been reported to be more evident in boys than in girls, and this difference has been linked by some to possible brain sexual dimorphism due to prenatal androgen levels. Because the spotted hyena females have unusually high androgen levels, their rough-and-tumble play need not be due to brain differences but could be due instead to their presently high androgen levels. Whether the play difference between the sexes is a function of brain differences or not, indirect support for an androgen-roughhousing relationship is provided by the play behavior of these animals in same-sex play. Far more important is the role of *social* grouping. The role of androgen in the play of the spotted hyenas was found to depend on their social context. When the males and females played in same-sex groups they differed in their play, but when males and females played together, no sex differences were evident.

In the wild and in the research colony after puberty, females are more dominant than males and the high-ranking offspring are dominant (Jenks, Weldele, Frank, & Glickman, 1995). In the wild, the only known time when males will form a coalition and attack a female is when she is close to estrus (Frank, Glickman, & Zabel, 1989). In estrus she is receptive to males. Before they leave for another clan, males in the wild will make sexual overtures to females in the natal clan. However, females do not accept the sexual approach and instead mate with immigrant males that join the clan (Smale & Holekamp, 1993).

The spotted hyenas and their social life provide a glimpse into unusual relationships among environmental factors, hormones, and various facets of behavior. The fact that the males in the wild have to travel away from their natal den appears to play a large role in their low dominance, because in the research colony, which they do not leave, different dominance patterns than in the wild are shown. Thus, environmental factors (leaving or staying) and social experiences (the male taking low rank when finding a new clan) play a major role in the types of dominance-submission shown by the female and male spotted hyenas. Additionally, androgen hormones can play a significant role in the females' aggressiveness. This may be due to a direct effect or because the prenatal androgens add size and weight to the female. In the wild, females and males have an uneasy truce, and sexual behavior appears to be partly determined by the female's estrus, when she appears to forego her dominance to males.

Human Studies

Human sexual motivation and sexual behavior are functions of many factors. Overwhelming data from clinical observation and scientific studies reveal that early childhood experiences have an enormous impact on the kinds and number of sexual partners a person chooses in adulthood, the frequency of sexual experiences, and the attitudes and beliefs a person has about sexual behavior. In addition to childhood, the culture during adulthood has enormous effects. In different times in history, various types of sexual practices were considered normal as well as ideal, and in contemporary society, fears of contagious disease have a significant impact on sexual practices. Fear of AIDS has had a profound impact on the sexual behavior of many persons (for example, see Weinberg, Williams, & Pryor, 1994). The beliefs of one's family and community, independent of the larger culture, also shape sexual beliefs and practices.

Reproductive Behavior. Sexual behavior has many characteristics, one being that it is instrumental behavior. In many respects, sexual behavior is learned similarly to the way other instrumental behavior is learned. An individual can increase sexual behavior because of the consequent rewards, or an individual can decrease sexual behavior because it leads to pain or danger. Sexual behavior can be used for many purposes. It occurs to procreate young and continue the family or clan. However, in humans that has been changing with alterations in society and culture. For example, artificial insemination without sexual intercourse has been used increasingly for reproduction, sometimes for reasons of fertility problems in the couple and, more recently, because women want a child but not a relationship with the biological father.

Tragically, reproductive behavior has also been used not to continue a lineage but to destroy it and to destroy the identity of a group. Reproductive behavior as a violent and not a sexual behavior has been used ghoulishly to exterminate the ethnic genetic character of a group of people. This happened in the 1990s, in the region once known as Yugoslavia. Military orders led soldiers of one ethnic group to rape women of another ethnic group, for the avowed purpose of "ethnic cleansing," so that the offspring are no longer a true representation of the mother's ethnic group. Such actions not only use sexual intercourse in the violent act of rape, but they also use reproductive behavior for destruction.

Evolutionary-oriented conceptualizations have been offered to explain human mate selection in terms of reproductive behavior (Buss, 1989, 1996; Symons, 1979). Psychologists favoring an evolutionary psychological approach do not emphasize individual choices or individual learning and life experiences. They focus, instead, on presumed universal characteristics that over evolutionary time have benefited the species. Buss (1989, p. 1) posited that preferential mating patterns arise because "powerful reproductive consequences" result from mating preferences. He collected demographic data from 37 cultures. He concluded that male mate preferences in most of these cultures showed men to value characteristics that signal high reproductive capacity, defined by the fact that for men but not women, physical attractiveness in the partner and a young age were highly valued (Buss, 1989, p. 12). He interpreted men's preferred choice of young women as mates (just under 25 years old) to signify the woman's *fertility* value.

Many psychologists account for the data in other ways than in terms of fertility value and reproductive capacity. For example, men may prefer a woman of a young age because a young woman has less worldly experience (and is more likely to be naive and innocent) than an older woman, which means the younger one can be more readily influenced. Furthermore, a young woman is stronger than an older woman and thus can provide more physical labor. Many interpretations of the data are possible, and a life experience and social learning explanation is in closer agreement with the way individual human beings actually select their mates.

Researchers investigating mate selection in mammals, birds, and fish have found strong learning factors based on *individual* experiences to influence mate selection. In describing mate selection in nonhuman animals, for example, Domjan (1992) wrote:

> Given the importance of reproductive behavior, one might predict that it would not be left open to the vagaries of individual experience. Nevertheless, learning experiences have been shown to influence various aspects of reproductive behavior in a range of species . . . learning influences on the stimulus control of sexual behavior seem especially relevant to the analysis of mate choice. p. 48

Social and developmental explanations of individuals' mating preferences are based on data different from the data gathered by evolutionary theorists (Buss, 1989). For any specific individual, mating preference is shaped by motivational and personality variables and not usually by concern over a woman's maximal reproductive capacity. According to evolutionary theory (Buss, 1996), women prefer to marry men who are good economic providers because these men can ensure future success for their offspring. However, many women and men choose not to have offspring, and many contemporary women choose to have offspring without husbands, so *individual* choices of whom to marry are not necessarily related to such evolutionary variables. People are likely to marry those who are similar to close members of their own family, and personal needs, goals, and satisfactions are likely to shape mate preference and mate selection (Dreikurs, 1999). Researchers also have found variables such as interpersonal attachment styles, which offer mutual support and secure relationships (Kobak & Hazan, 1991), to be significant in mate selection. Reproduction is important for the species, but many personality and cultural factors affect a specific person's choice of whom to select for a mate.

Other Aspects of Human Sexual Behavior. A distinction is made in contemporary society between consensual sexual behavior and the use of sexual acts for coercion and aggression. Violent sexual ac-

tions such as rape (sexual intercourse perpetrated on a nonconsenting person) are acts of aggression (see Sorenson & White, 1992). Laws as well as research on rape have defined rape as assault and violence, not as sexual behavior, whether it is perpetrated against a woman or a man. In recent years, increasing research has been devoted to this social problem and to its effect on the victims, their family, and the larger community.

Other than procreation, sexual behavior is instrumental in bringing enjoyment and pleasure. When sexual behavior is shared between two people, it can serve to bring bonding and closeness to the couple. The diversity of motivations leading to sexual behavior is enormous. Sexual motivation in the sense of sexual arousal is distinct from reproductive motivation.

Sexual behavior can occur for pleasure and it can occur for gaining power and wealth. For a given person, sexual behavior may serve the purpose of retaliation against another person. Sexual behavior also can be used for self-enhancement of status (in some adolescent groups as well as with some older persons, the more sexual partners one has the more status one gains). The reasons people give for sexual behavior may not fully reflect their motivation, because self-awareness of motivation often is inexact. Sexual behavior and sexual motivation vary widely, and so do stimuli that lead to sexual arousal.

Stimuli that lead to sexual arousal, called erotic stimuli, vary with the culture and with individuals. Masters and Johnson (1966, 1970) described a wide range of ways that lead to heightening of sexual arousal. The senses of touch and vision provide much of human erotic stimulation, but stimuli of all kinds can serve arousal functions for human sexual behavior. Countless books have been written regarding the large variety of human sexual behavior, sexual motivation, and stimuli providing human sexual arousal (Allgeier & McCormick, 1983; Docter, 1988; Kinsey, Pomeroy, & Martin, 1948; Kinsey, Pomeroy, Martin, & Gebhard, 1953; Langevin, 1985; Money & Ehrhardt, 1972; Weinberg, et al., 1994; Williams, 1983). Only a brief discussion of this vast topic is possible in the present chapter.

Sexual arousal has been distinguished from sexual arousability (Whalen, 1966). Sexual arousal refers to sexual excitement at a given moment, whereas sexual arousability refers to the time taken to reach maximum sexual arousal (orgasm). Physiological measures like heart rate, skin conductance, and muscle tension have all been used by researchers to measure sexual arousal, especially when subjects are viewing or listening to erotic material. In addition, penile erection and vaginal lubrication have been used to study sexual arousal. The four phases of sexual arousal identified by Masters and Johnson (1966) are excitement, plateau, orgasm, and resolution. Cognitive variables strongly influence both arousal and arousability. Learning and cognition can heighten sexual pleasure (Masters & Johnson, 1975) as well as inhibit it. Many subtle as well as major worries and concerns can significantly affect sexual arousal and arousability (Abramson, 1994).

Stable emotional dispositions and values have been found to shape attitudes toward sexual behaviors. In particular, permissiveness (Leak & Gardner, 1990) or indiscriminant (Simpson & Gangestad, 1991) sexual behavior is closely linked to social attitudes concerning involvement and caring. An avoidant attachment style, of withdrawing from close relationships, was identified to lead to indiscriminant sexuality (Simpson & Gangestad, 1991). Leak and Gardner (1990) studied sexual attitudes in relationship to Adler's theory and the concept of *social interest,* which refers to a social commitment of belonging and contributing to the welfare of others. College students were given two measures of social interest and a sexual attitude test. Four subscales of the Hendrick, Hendrick, Slapion-Foote, and Foote (1985) sexual attitude scale were given, which measured attitudes toward sexual permissiveness, responsibility, communion, and instrumentality. Social interest showed a significant negative correlation with the sexual permissiveness scale. That is, the subjects who did not feel a sense of belonging to others and did not seek to contribute to others' welfare had the higher acceptance of casual sex with many partners and without commitment. Sexual communion as an attitude toward sexual behavior had a significant positive correlation with one of the social interest scales. Sexual instrumentality, seeking sexual activity for one's own pleasure, was neg-

atively correlated with social interest but not significantly. The data reveal how attitudes toward sexual behavior are closely related to larger issues of social concern and attachment.

The age of first intercourse is a function of many variables, an important one being the larger culture and its permissions or prohibitions. For example, the overall mean age of reported first intercourse in an Australian study (Dunne et al., 1997) was just over 20 years of age. This is considerably older than the mean age generally identified for Americans. The American and Australian cultures differ in a number of characteristics, with the American culture being far more sexually permissive. Australia has undergone a large cultural transition in the past decades, and this was reflected in the significant difference in the mean age of reported first intercourse for the younger (27 to 40 years) versus the older subjects (41 to 70 years). For the younger subjects the mean age of first intercourse was 18.94 years and for the older subjects it was 21.10 years. Thus, within the Australian sample and between Australians and Americans, cultural variables can explain differences in age of when individuals have their first sexual intercourse.

The study used men and women twins, monozygotic as well as dizygotic, and this enabled the researchers to look for genetic as well as environmental factors. The researchers found evidence for genetic determinants, but they were different for men than for women and different for the younger than for the older sample of subjects. Age of gaining gonadal hormonal maturity in adolescence may be one of the contributing genetic factors. Other variables clearly are involved, in view of the fact that variation in the role of genetic factors occurred according to the age and the sex of the subjects.

How social learning experiences versus gonadal hormones and brain sexual dimorphism affect human sexual behavior has been of interest to researchers. Clinical data have been helpful in this regard. For example, in one area of the Dominican Republic individuals with XY chromosomes were found who were born with ambiguously identified external genitalia and raised as females (Breedlove, 1992). At puberty these persons developed masculine build and male external genitalia, and they took on a masculine way of life, including girlfriends. The example of these individuals has been interpreted to mean that the fetal testosterone masculinized their brains and thus social influence from the way they were raised had no effect. However, as Breedlove (1992) suggested, the villagers may have treated these persons differently because they knew of this type of condition, so social factors cannot be ruled out.

A different type of clinical evidence was reported by Money (1961) who studied hermaphrodites (persons with both male and female sex characteristics). Although controversy exists regarding some of these data, the study reported that those hermaphrodites who were raised as boys later responded erotically to girls in the same way as did other men in the culture, and those raised as girls responded erotically to men. Overall, social learning and family patterns influence people's sexual behavior. The issue of what factors give rise to sexual orientation is quite complex and has received considerable attention in the 1990s. Research, based on autopsies, has reported that specific brain areas are different for homosexual than for heterosexual men (see the review by Breedlove, 1994). Clinical data have shown that family dynamics and early childhood experiences can shape sexual orientation. Life experiences are known to alter neural structures, which leaves open the question whether brain differences found in autopsies of homosexual compared with heterosexual men are a *cause* or a *result* of sexual orientation and sexual behavior.

GENDER

The Importance of Gender

For many years psychologists have taken note of differences between men and women in a variety of behaviors, motivations, and cognitions. Most, but not all, researchers realized that cultural variables were crucial in their effect on men and women. The term *gender* takes into account cultural influences. This term has come to be used instead of the word "sex," which tends to be used only when biological gonadal variables are considered.

Gender affects the way humans act and interact. In every human society, cultural definitions of gender and gender roles exist for men and women. Individuals' biological strengths and weaknesses were probably noted early within human groups, and depending on the group, these biological differences became more, or less, important in the life and functioning of that society. Men are taller and tend to be physically stronger than women, and women bear children. Societies differ in regard to how much they assign gender roles according to these biological differences. In societies in which production of offspring is considered important, women's reproductive functions are likely to influence the way the female gender role is defined. If reproductive functions are less important in the life of the society, and the kind of work people do requires talents other than muscular strength, biological differences may come to be minimized in defining gender roles.

In contemporary computer age societies that rely on information-processing skills, and in which small families with few children are desired, the physical strength of men and the child-bearing ability in women become more irrelevant. As men increasingly have choices that include being "house husbands," definitions of gender roles are also likely to change. In a technological and information-processing age the way gender influences motivations and behaviors of individuals inevitably will differ from that of previous generations.

Democratization also brings enormous changes in the ways society treats biological categories like those of age and sex. Children in many countries are given increasing rights for health and education. Egalitarian sharing of power and responsibilities for work and home is increasing between women and men. In some societies, a very large difference exists in the way power and responsibility are divided between adults and children and between women and men, and in other societies the differences are minimal. When power and responsibility are divided very unevenly between men and women, gender roles (ways of behaving in accord with gender) and gender schemas (ways of thinking in accord with gender) are likely to differ markedly for men versus women. When the division is egalitarian, gender roles and gender schemas are likely to differ far less. Democratization in human relationships has tended to reduce differences in gender roles and gender schemas. Democratization has led to men and women increasingly performing comparable work and attaining increasingly comparable esteem and status within the culture. Use of gender-related categories remain (Skitka & Maslach, 1996), but how gender roles and gender schemas are defined is changing.

Because gender affects emotions, motivations, and cognitions, the topic is important. A very large literature has developed on the topic of gender, and only some of that can be presented in this chapter.

Gender Identity, Gender Schema, and Gender Differences

What Is Gender Identity? Considerable debate has arisen about the way gender identity develops and how it is defined and measured. There is general consensus that *gender identity* refers to self definition, of "I am a girl" and "I am a woman," or "I am a boy" and "I am a man," and with it, a "basic psychological sense of belongingness" (Spence, 1993, p. 625) to one's own sex. Not all researchers agree with Spence (1993), however, when she states that most people in very early childhood develop a firm sense of gender identity corresponding to their biological sex, and that this remains a core part of their self-concept or self-image.

Spence (1985, p. 80) described gender identity as a "primitive, unarticulated concept of self" developed by the age of 2 1/2 and thus formed at "an essentially preverbal state of development and maintained at an unverbalized level." This sense of self as belonging to a gender permeates other awarenesses that develop at later ages. She suggested that a person adopts roles and tasks that may only loosely fit gender stereotypes, and ordinarily gender identity is not altered. How much one's later behavior fits gender stereotypes will be shaped by cultural factors rather than by gender identity. Spence (1985) suggested that the vast majority of people believe themselves as having a given gender ("masculine" or "maleness" for men and "feminine" or "femaleness" for women) without evalua-

tive labels (like strong, weak, dominant, submissive, good, bad) and even without regard to sexual orientation. The way Spence described stability of gender identity in the face of changes in behaviors over a lifetime fits with the way core aspects of self-concept are usually considered.

Ehrhardt (1985) reviewed the history of the terms *gender* and *gender identity* and their introduction into the fields of psychology and medicine. Reviewing studies of individuals who had abnormal prenatal hormones for a variety of medical reasons, Ehrhardt drew the conclusion that factors like rough-and-tumble outdoor play (which tends to be more prevalent among boys than girls) and nurturing parenting behavior (such as shown in children's doll play, and which tends to be more prevalent among girls than among boys), may be influenced by prenatal as well as postnatal hormones. To what extent hormones play a major role in these behaviors is not fully established, but clearly both types of behaviors are shaped by the way the family and the larger community permit or inhibit such activities.

For most psychologists, gender identity is a psychological and social variable. Gender identity is based on a person's recognition of his or her biological sex and it is largely independent of the actions of hormones or brain sexual dimorphism. Theorists differ in their conceptualization of what is meant by gender identity, however. Not all agree with Spence (1993) that it is formed in early childhood and remains relatively primitive and unchanged in the life of the individual.

Some considered gender identity to be made up of different attributes and attitudes. Others formulated gender identity as developing in stages over a number of years rather than as a global, primitive, early self-image (see Frable, 1997 for a review). The stages include (1) correctly identifying oneself and others (labeling), (2) understanding that the identity continues over time (stability), and (3) understanding that neither one's wish to change nor experiences of altered cultural cues will change one's identity (constancy). Some theorists argue that gender identity is part of one's fundamental self-concept and relates to issues of self-esteem, whereas others conceptualize gender identity as quite specific and shaped by one's immediate environment and context. Most theorists consider gender identity to be shaped largely by the child's early emotional and social learning. Many consider various attributes or sets of roles to be complexly associated with one another and in this way to make the composite gender identity.

Measuring Gender Identity. Two well-known tests have been used widely to measure gender identity, although over time some researchers have come to question to what extent these tests do measure this identity. The two tests contain items that at the time reflected society's gender stereotypes (of what society at that time considered to characterize men and women). The stereotypes were that men are active and achievement oriented, and women are more concerned with expressing emotions and with nurturing. Terms used for these dichotomies, such as *instrumental* versus *expressive,* and *agentic* versus *communal,* represented masculine and feminine stereotypes.

The PAQ (Personal Attributes Questionnaire) was designed to measure gender identity. The test was developed and refined by Spence and Helmreich (1978). It consists of items describing socially desirable instrumental (I) traits and socially desirable expressive (E) traits. Persons taking the test were given pairs of descriptors, like "very passive" and "very active." Respondents were asked to identify, with a mark on a 5-point scale, where they fit between these opposites. When men and women took the test, within each sex the I and the E items were found to be independent of each other (uncorrelated).

Another test, designed to measure "sex typing," is called the BSRI (Bem Sex-Role Inventory) developed by Bem (1974). The items belong to either a masculinity (M) or a femininity (F) scale. Many of the items were instrumental (M) or expressive (F) desirable traits. The respondents were given personal descriptors, like "self-reliance," and had to mark on a scale from 1 to 7 how true the descriptor was for the person. The BSRI typed both men and women according to their M and F scale scores. *Androgynous* persons were those who scored high on both scales, and *undifferentiated* persons were

those who scored low on both scales. Sex-typed men scored high on the M and low on the F scale, and sex-typed women scored high on the F and low on the M scale.

In the original test development, the researchers indicated that sex typing and androgyny could be measured by the PAQ. Later, Spence (1993) reconsidered this. Originally, Spence and Helmreich (1978) considered the PAQ to measure gender identity, but later considerations led Spence (1985, 1993) to propose that gender identity is much broader than the kinds of characteristics measured by the PAQ. She concluded that the PAQ measures the desirable instrumental and expressive traits people believe they have, but these traits only partially provide the characteristics that people attribute to themselves. Moreover, these traits only partially represent their maleness or femaleness (gender identity). In contrast, Bem (1985) considered the BSRI to measure gender schema and sex typing, with androgynous and undifferentiated persons non-sex-typed or "gender aschematic."

Gender Schema. Schemas are perspectives and cognitions with which people organize perceptions and by which they interpret events in the internal and external environment. Gender schemas are thus gender-developed and gender-relevant perspectives and cognitions. Bem (1985) pointed out that sex typing shapes gender schemas, and she defined schema as (Bem, 1985, p. 187) "a cognitive structure, a network of associations that organizes and guides an individual's perception. A schema functions as an anticipatory structure, a readiness to search for and assimilate incoming information in schema-relevant terms."

Children identify with the parent of the same sex, and children learn by observation as well as reinforcements what behaviors are expected of girls and boys and women and men. Bem (1985) proposed a *gender schema theory,* which specifies that gender-schematic processing shapes sex typing. Children learn the way society defines gender, and thus which attributes should become part of their own self-concept. Children are motivated to regulate their behavior to conform to these cultural definitions of gender (maleness and femaleness). Sex-typed individuals are those who organize their self-concept and behavior on the basis of gender. These organizing cognitions are not conscious. People who are not sex typed, however, evaluate new information on the basis of a variety of dimensions or criteria, whereas people who are sex typed evaluate that same information on the basis of its gender relevance. For example, "Do I want to learn to ski?" becomes processed in a gender-schematic way when the question is assessed on the basis of, "Is it a manly or a womanly thing to do?" and it is processed aschematically when the person uses other assessment criteria ("Will I get hurt? Is it hard to learn? Can I afford it?").

Bem (1985) cited data to show that sex-typed individuals process gender-relevant information differently than do non-sex-typed persons. Sex-typed persons recall more gender-relevant versus other items, and they respond faster to gender-relevant than to other items. She suggested that gender schema serve as a filter for processing a specific type of information, that of gender. This works in the same way that other schema serve as organizing principles for processing other types of information. In the 1970s Bem advocated androgyny, because the androgynous person has the best characteristics of both men and women. Later (Bem, 1985, 1993) she reconsidered that view. Because androgyny means a person (man or woman) has the desirable qualities of both genders, the criteria for processing information and directing one's behavior remain gender linked. Having the desirable qualities of both genders does not mean one is free of the biasing effects of gender.

In her later theorizing, Bem suggested that the assumption of having a femininity or a masculinity "within" a person, as if that were an internal reality, is erroneous. Gender itself is a cognitive construct, not something within a person. Culture prescribes what are appropriate and inappropriate male versus female beliefs and actions. Prescriptions and approbation are given according to whether one is a man or a woman, and thus gender itself is a cultural construction. To be androgynous does not remove the gender construct. It merely means that one has accepted both male and female gender as part of one's self-concept. Bem considered that the more effec-

tive approach is for society to be as gender aschematic as possible and for people not to use gender as a filter for processing information and guiding action.

Research has found support for gender-schema theory. For example, Park and Hahn (1988) asked subjects to respond to hypothetical characters (Michael or Linda) in a story, by saying a trait did or did not describe that person. Reaction time was measured. Non-sex-typed subjects did not differ significantly from each other (androgynous versus undifferentiated) in their reaction times for judgments, but feminine sex-typed persons were significantly faster than masculine sex-typed persons in responding to the female character. The cultural gender schema described by Bem (1985) were evident in the fact that subjects responded significantly faster to masculine descriptors (like aggressiveness) for the male character and faster to feminine descriptors for the female character. Moreover, they responded "yes" (the descriptor fits) to a significantly larger number of masculine items for the male character and a greater number of feminine items for the female character. To the extent that "gender" of the character affected people's response patterns, the study supported the proposal by Bem that gender schema function as cultural filters. The variable of sex-typing proved to be less robust in that study.

Many studies have found support for the fact that gender schema bias perception, cognitions, and behavior. Less clear-cut support has been found for sex-typing effects. However, indirect evidence, with related constructs like "traditional beliefs," has shown that variables similar to sex-typing can affect a wide range of behaviors. For example, data show that although individuals following the traditional gender roles are attracted to and marry one another, their marriage may be prone to more stress and eventual dissolution (Ickes, 1993). As expected, however, other factors besides traditional beliefs play a role in marriage and its stability (Peplau, Hill, & Rubin, 1993).

Gender beliefs in young men aged 15 to 18 were found to have potential health hazards, insofar as those with traditional gender beliefs were less likely to use condoms during intercourse and more likely to view pregnancy as an affirmation of their masculinity (Pleck, Sonenstein, & Ku, 1993). Such beliefs have impact on teen pregnancy and spreading of AIDS. What is clear from the literature on gender beliefs and sex-typing is that beliefs about masculinity and femininity have a profound impact on sexual behavior and on intimate relationships. Additional variables also play significant roles in how individuals cope with complexities of marriage and intimate relationships.

Men as well as women have experienced limitations in terms of gender schema, and both genders have witnessed significant changes in the culture. Some of these changes have brought new opportunities and some have brought new interpersonal problems. Gender schema are shaped in childhood, but with cultural transformations and new gender schema, the schema from childhood need to be changed. Many persons, both men and women, have difficulties with these changes and with the pressure of adapting to the culture of adulthood. After the "women's movement" developed in the 1960s and 1970s, a "men's movement" and a growing "men's issues" literature has developed, which reflect men's search for new gender schema that are more adaptive in the 1990s and beyond (Abbott, 1987; Brod, 1987; Thompson, 1994; Weiss, 1990).

Gender Differences. Men and women have many similarities. More differences occur *within* than *between* gender groups. Nevertheless, some between-group effects have been found regarding ways that people judge their own adequacy and ways they react to specific social, cognitive, and motivational circumstances. Many characteristics have been identified that purportedly show important differences between men and women, but these vary with countries and with time, and there is considerable disagreement about the specific ways men and women differ (Baumeister & Sommer, 1997; Cross, & Madson, 1997). It is not clear to what extent differences represent culture compared with biologically linked differences.

Reference has been made already to the rough-and-tumble outdoor play of boys versus girls, and to the hypothesis that androgen levels account for the difference. Data on how parents play with their

infants are still far too sparse to counter an androgen explanation. However, if it is the case that fathers and mothers play differently with their female and male children from the time the child is a few weeks old, the amount of rough-housing play a child experiences when small could account for the way the child plays outdoors when older.

The way people interact with one another is shaped by culture, and the effects are pervasive (Wade, 1993). Cultural factors were identified in an earlier chapter in reference to girls' and women's eating disturbances and their anxiety about weight. Studies have shown that girls and women rely on physical appearance for their overall self-evaluation more than do boys and men (Jackson, Hodge, & Ingram, 1994), but that pattern is changing, in that boys and men also are increasingly relying this way on their self-evaluation. Gender differences can strain work relationships (Studd, 1996). Events and cues are often interpreted differently by men and women who work together. Motivations are tied to evaluations of events and cues and they can lead to various types of sexual harassment (Deaux, 1995; Fiske & Glick, 1995).

Many studies have found differences between boys and girls and men and women in *cognitive abilities*. Most of the studies have not sampled across a wide range of cultures. The data tend to come from cultures with formal schooling, which build in gender biases, so it is hard to interpret the findings. Boys have been reported to be better in mathematics and in spatial and perceptual motor skills, whereas girls have been reported as better in verbal skills (Halpern, 1992). Comparisons are not commonly available between countries that value verbal skills in men and countries that value verbal skills in women. The same holds for spatial and perceptual motor skills. In some cultures, men are valued for their intellect, and values in the upper socioeconomic classes demean physical labor and perceptual motor skills for men. In other cultures, men are expected to know "how to fix things." Data on abilities of boys and girls and men and women from such widely different cultures would be very helpful in providing a clearer understanding of gender differences in cognitive abilities.

Studies that have assessed both gender and culture tend to find cultural differences to be far greater than gender differences in motivations and attitudes. These differences in turn can affect performance on ability tests. A study done in Israel with Jewish and Arab 9th-grade students (Birenbaum & Kraemer, 1995) illustrates the value of cross-cultural comparisons. The investigators assessed causal attributions for success and failure in mathematics and language examinations. Ethnicity had a larger effect than did gender. Arab students gave more success attributions and less failure attributions than did Jewish students on math as well as language examinations.

Within very broad limits, girls tend to have better verbal skills and boys to have better spatial skills (Halpern, 1992), but these differences are not the same at different ages. Variations within each gender group are very large (Caplan, Crawford, Hyde, & Richardson, 1997). Child-rearing patterns for the comparison groups usually are not reported, nor are data provided on how much time per day the children devote to various activities. Thus, it is hard to interpret the findings. For example, if boys are encouraged to engage more in outdoor rough-and-tumble play, the more quiescent girls could be more exposed to books and television (which involve verbal content). Moreover, large motor activity outdoors is likely to help children gain spatial and perceptual motor skills. If one engages in outdoor rough-and-tumble play and one wants to avoid constant bruises and fractures, it soon is evident that one needs to attend to space and to the consequences that arise from perceptual motor activity.

Cultural changes occur within a society, and these may bring associated changes in gender-related skills and self-concepts. For example, in a recent study (Jackson et al., 1994) girls and women were found to have higher academic self-concepts than boys and men, and academic self-concept was a slightly better predictor of overall self-evaluation for the girls and women. These findings contrasted with earlier data, which found either no difference between genders or higher academic self-concepts for boys and men. Without understanding the cultural and child-rearing patterns of a sample, explanations of gender differences are hard to assess.

In a variety of cognitive tasks, data show that boys and men use the two cerebral hemispheres differently than do girls and women. Data are reported that males are more lateralized than females (Breedlove, 1994; Halpern, 1992) in infancy and in later years, with males using one or the other hemisphere for a given task whereas females are more likely to use both hemispheres. However, inconsistent results have been obtained on this variable, and research is ongoing whether prenatal gonadal hormones have an influence. Like so many issues involving brain and behavior, it is hard to know if lateralization in the brains of women and men is different as part of prenatal hormonal organizing effects or whether different modes of thinking linked to gender schemas alter later hemispheric functioning.

Although males have been found to show better mathematical and spatial ability than females, the differences in means are often small. Moreover, gender differences in cognition are typically absent in young children, the differences increase with age up through adulthood, and over years of research the differences have not remained the same (Richardson, 1997). Clearly, culture and life experiences play a critical role in reported cognitive differences between males and females. Eccles (1985) studied 300 students over 2 years and found a number of attitudinal variables to be important. Although boys and girls scored comparably on math achievement, girls did not choose math classes as often as boys did and they did not value math classes as important for themselves, whereas boys did. The belief of both boys and girls was that mathematics is important for boys but not for girls. Other studies showed that parents tend to hold the same beliefs. A few studies sought to identify the role of culture, and they have shown possible experiential factors as an explanation of gender differences in spatial abilities. Reviewing some cross-cultural studies, Halpern (1992) reported data on Eskimos and New Zealand tribal groups that revealed cultural variables to have an influence on spatial abilities.

Comparison of mean differences in performance between males and females does not provide all the evidence regarding gender differences. One issue concerns the variance, or spread of scores within a group. Addressing this problem, Hedges and Nowell (1995) used samples involving thousands of children and youths, and found that the variability in cognitive task performance is considerably greater among males than females. As a result, among exceptionally high performing individuals a disproportionate number will be males, but among exceptionally low performing individuals a disproportionate number also will be males. Adding up all the findings, it is not surprising that Stein and Bailey (1973) some years ago found that children as early as sixth grade considered mechanical and spatial skills to be masculine and social and verbal skills to be feminine. The question remains, whether the children's gender schemas *resulted* from or *caused* gender differences in spatial and verbal abilities.

Fear of Success.   A different type of gender difference was identified by Horner (1972). She proposed that women with high achievement strivings have conflict about these strivings because they fear bad consequences from success in achievement. Horner called it a motive to avoid success due to a fear of success. In hundreds of later studies, fear of success was abbreviated as FOS. Horner asked subjects to give stories, following the model developed by McClelland (1955, 1961) for the projective test measurement of nAch. Her materials were not pictures but verbal descriptions of social situations, like a character (Anne) being at the top of her medical school class. Men subjects received male names and social situations, and women subjects received female names and social situations. Horner found that achievement motivation themes were prevalent in men subjects, and themes for the motive to avoid success were prevalent in women subjects. Women tended to downgrade successful female characters but men approved of successful male characters.

Many later studies sought to replicate this finding. Spence (1974) gave descriptions in which the successful medical student was either a single male, a single female, or a married female. She found women subjects to be positive to all three characters and men subjects to be positive to the married female and the single male. The FOS motive was not evident the way Horner had predicted. Horner had suggested that the more capable the woman was

and the more achievement she had actually attained, the more she would have the motive aroused to avoid success. FOS was not always studied from that perspective. Initially there was support for FOS, and in some studies it was found in men as well as women. By the late 1980s inconsistent and contradictory results led to proposals to modify the original FOS formulation (Piedmont, 1988). Some researchers (Mednick, 1989) indicated that the fear of success was no longer accepted as a reliable scientific construct. To explain lack of high achievement in women compared with men on the basis of FOS did not seem viable, because many variables contributed to whether capable women attained high achievement. Sex role socialization was likely to be one significant factor.

The original work of McClelland (1961), based on studies with boys, showed that training at home was crucial for the development of a high achievement motivation, with training for independence a key. An important study with African-American preschool children and their mothers (Carr & Mednick, 1988) added the factor of sex role socialization to the formulation of McClelland. Carr and Mednick (1988) found that the effect of sex-role socialization on high achievement motivation interacted with socioeconomic class, and that overall, traditional sex role socialization for boys and nontraditional sex role training for girls led to higher achievement motivation for the children.

Several reasons were given to explain why FOS was not found in the stories of women of the 1980s and 1990s as Horner found in her research in the 1960s. Some researchers question whether FOS ever occurred. Piedmont (1995) explained that FOS was closely related to such variables as anxiety, conscientiousness, neuroticism, and fear of failure. He suggested that a different motivational formulation concerning FOS was needed. Other suggestions are that FOS was a valid phenomenon in the 1960s, but by the late 1980s many cultural changes occurred that could have led to motivational changes. Medical schools enrolled a very high percentage of women, and what might have appeared as an unusual and anxiety-provoking situation (the woman medical student) in the 1960s became almost commonplace two decades later. The consensus is that fear of *success* in women as originally conceptualized is probably no longer a reliable occurrence, but that fear of *failure* remains and is in part a reflection of continuing cultural forces.

Researchers in general have indicated that many women, regardless of race or ethnic background, still lack confidence in task attainment compared with men (Carr, Thomas, & Mednick, 1985). Moreover, in the work force, women still do not advance as much as do men, and salaries are lower in general for women (Phillips & Imhoff, 1997). Thus, aspects of cultural change seem to have brought about some changes in women's motivation, but lack of other cultural changes have meant that some kinds of motivations remain. To the extent that some countries continue to exert inhibitions on women's high achievement, it is possible that FOS remains in those countries. In some countries women are largely forbidden to gain an advanced education, and it is possible that in those cultures any women who attain achievement success would also fear negative consequences. Thus, FOS may occur for capable women in countries that continue to give women strong negative consequences for successful achievement.

LOVE

There are many kinds of love. In this chapter only a limited consideration of love is possible, and the focus is on only some kinds of love.

Parent-Child Love

The human infant depends for life maintenance upon care from other individuals. Adler (1927/1959, 1930) related the capacity for humans to develop bonding and social interest (feeling of belonging and contributing to others' welfare) to the fact that the human infant is born small and helpless and relies on others for survival. The earliest social learning, of affection and belonging, grows in infancy.

Bonds of belonging begin with the earliest close relationships. Research is slowly revealing aspects of this bonding. For example, in newborns and 2-week old infants, ingestion of sucrose solution had a calming effect, but by 4 weeks of age and older, visual contact was needed to maintain the calm stage (Blass, 1992). Without eye contact with a caretaker the infant was found to cry within a short time following the sucrose ingestion. Bonding may involve a parent or any other individual who takes on a parental role, regardless if the person is the child's biological parent.

At one time, and still in many communities, the initial bonding has been strongest between mother and child. As fathers take on increasingly nurturing roles, that pattern is changing. Following the child's initial attachments come an increasingly wider set of interactions that lead to loving relationships. With increased maturity of the child, bonds of *asexual* love develop between friends. In adolescence and adulthood, *sexual* love occurs between partners. The way parents treat their offspring in a large measure sets the patterns for love and attachment developed in later years. The social, cognitive, and emotional experiences of childhood set a prototype of ways of relating to intimate others. Total family patterns form models for later relationships. Because families are also parts of larger social, cognitive, and emotional networks, how the communal group relates to the young has an important effect on parent-child relationships and on the relationships the young have after leaving the confines of parents.

The Work of Harlow. Early research that was revolutionary at the time was the work of Harlow (1958) on infant attachment to a "mother." He studied rhesus monkeys. Some were separated from their biological mothers and given substitute, or surrogate, mothers. The infants became attached with deep affection to inanimate "mothers" made of cloth, but they failed to make such attachment to surrogates made of wire. Once the affection was developed, the infant was lonely and unhappy when removed from the cloth surrogate, and the monkey was relaxed and contented when the surrogate was present. The strong bond that ties infant monkeys and infant humans to their parent or parent substitute provides deep emotional satisfactions that extend beyond reduction of hunger, fear, and pain. The higher primates are social animals, for whom the need for bonding is as basic as hunger. Harlow (1971) described the bonding as due to a need for "contact comfort." In the early part of a rhesus monkey's life, the cloth surrogate seemed to provide that contact comfort.

Harlow did what other researchers do also, which is to measure the strength of the attachment of the infant to its mother or surrogate in terms of how much distress the infant shows when separated from the loved one. Whereas Harlow explained a human or monkey infant's love for its mother as due to a need for contact comfort, others had different explanations. Field (1996, p. 557) suggested that the distress experienced by a human infant's separation from its mother or other exclusive intimate caregiver occurs because that person provides "stimulation and arousal modulation" and because others ordinarily are "not as familiar with the child's individual needs for stimulation and arousal modulation." Some of the bonding between child and others very likely is due to such a process. However, Field's explanation assigns too passive a role to the infant. It conceptualizes the infant's attachment and distress in terms of the mother's efforts, and in terms of events external to the infant. Harlow's work focused on the directional aspects of *internal* motivation. The position advanced by Field and others who emphasize the mother's reinforcement, stimulation, and arousal modulation implies a passive infant instead of one that actively reaches out emotionally in the relationship.

An explanation that relies solely on caregiver behavior cannot apply to Harlow's monkeys, who gave active love to the nonmoving and inanimate cloth surrogate. The inanimate surrogate was not able to provide reinforcements or to give active stimulation and arousal modulation. The surrogate was there for the infant to act upon. The cloth surrogate was not as effective as a real mother nor could the surrogate provide healthy emotional growth for a long time. By 6 months of age the rhesus monkey required much more than the surrogate for normal emotional development. By that age, an active role from a living monkey, to provide interaction, was essential. For example, peers had a strong positive impact on infant monkeys. The Harlow studies highlighted the fact that a complete theory of attachment must acknowledge internal processes within primate infants. It is not enough to conjecture what the external environment provides.

The position taken here, and by others who em-phasize the *transactional nature of motivation and emotion,* is that the need to love is an approach motivation that is primary in human infants (and probably also in monkey infants). Regardless of how much or little the "mother" stimulates and modulates, the infant has an inner need to *give* love to another who represents warmth and safety. In a social species, it is very likely that infants have a *need to give love.* Contact with a caregiver who provides comfort and safety is essential in early infancy. The more attuned the caregiver is to the infant, the more the love and attachment grow. Rather than causing or creating love, external sources enable the love of an active, giving infant to flourish and grow. Clearly, the more the caregiver provides stimulation, comfort, arousal modulation, and many other important aspects of social life, the stronger the transactional bonding will be.

Imprinting.   Although many birds are social, their attachment behavior is more stereotyped and occurs in more rigid and fixed action sequences than the types of behaviors studied by Harlow. Geese and ducks, for example, show *imprinting* (Hess, 1959). If they follow a moving target at a certain time in their life, called "critical period," they develop a life attachment to that object or to one just like it. A young duck would normally follow its mother, and thus become imprinted on members of its own species. If it follows a human or inanimate object some time between 18 and 26 hours after hatching, normal social and sexual attachment to its own species will not occur. The type of imprinting that takes place in a very narrow span of time is very different from the slowly evolving and complex bonding and attachment that monkeys and humans have for their caregivers. Bonding in primates is in many ways different from imprinting, and it is important to draw that distinction. Social-emotional bonding in primates and other highly social species is complex, occurs over a long time span, and typically involves many relationships by the time of adulthood.

The Work of Ainsworth.   Ainsworth (1982) studied mother-infant attachment for many years. She used a "strange situation" in which a mother and her toddler were in an unfamiliar environment containing toys. The researcher observed their actions over four kinds of prearranged conditions. The conditions might vary, but always involved four distinct characteristics: the mother was present with the child, the mother left the room, a stranger was alone with the child, and the mother returned. Typical reactions occurred under the four conditions. When the mother was present, following some initial adjustment to the new surroundings, the child felt relaxed and played with the toys. After the mother left, the child showed a lot of distress and no longer played with the toys. An unfamiliar person tried to comfort the child, but the distress was not eased. Only when the mother returned did the child's distress ease, and more clinging was evident than before the mother's departure. Children varied in their reactions, but the above patterns were typical for many children. The attachment studies of Ainsworth related to and supported the formulations of Bowlby (1979).

The reactions found in the research settings allowed Ainsworth and others to identify three types of attachment patterns (Ainsworth, Blehar, Waters, & Wall, 1978). A secure pattern is one in which the parent (or whoever is the significant caregiver) is responsive to the signals of the child and gives assurance of safety to the child, and in this pattern the child is relaxed and permits physical closeness. In a secure relationship, when the child is in new surroundings the child explores them in a relaxed way when the parent is present. A second pattern, called anxious/ambivalent, is one in which the parent responds inconsistently to the child's signals, and in new surroundings the child does not appear reassured or comforted in the presence of the parent. The child does not explore the way the child in a secure relationship does. A third pattern, called avoidant, is one in which the parent rebuffs or rejects the child, and in new surroundings the child does not seem to seek the parent. Although variations may be observed, many researchers have found the description of these three patterns to be helpful in understanding the interactions between caregivers and children. Although the work of Ainsworth provided valuable insights, her research and conceptual focus did not extend sufficiently to include attachment between child and father or siblings, and other close relationships (Field, 1996).

Other Considerations. Human contact provides many signals from which the child gains social, emotional, and cognitive learning. Much of the learning with caregiving adults is at a nonverbal level. Emotions of comfort and distress are basic for the young child. From the relationships formed in the early months and years, children learn to extend their love and develop wider emotional associations. Questions have been raised whether the child should be protected from distress. The literature has shown that humans need mild stresses in childhood, especially when these lead to effective coping strategies. They need such learning to be emotionally stable and courageous in later years. Studies with rats have found that handling them or providing other mild stressors in their infancy (Denenberg, 1964; Nunez & Ferre, 1995) helps them to be less anxious in later life. Human and monkey children, also, have better adjustment when mild stressors occur that are part of normal give-and-take learning. The requirement for normal give-and-take learning was found in the research of Harlow (1971). If the infant had only a cloth surrogate mother and no monkey interactions, serious emotional consequences occurred after some months. The monkey had no stressors, but what the monkey needed was interaction, not an absence of stressors. Up to 6 months of age, if the monkey with a cloth surrogate had peers for interaction, deprivation effects were reversible. Without other monkeys to teach social skills, emotional development and later social relationships were seriously impaired.

The early childhood attachment studies of Ainsworth (1982) led to other researchers' conceptualizations regarding people's later attachments in crucial love relationships (Shaver & Hazan, 1993). Attachment styles that were developed in early childhood appear to carry into later loving relationships. The relationships between all members in the immediate family are of great importance in the way the individual develops (Ferguson, 1995). Sibling relationships are especially powerful in shaping adult personality (Ferguson, 1958). It would be valuable to have a description of attachment styles between all dyads and all combinations of relationships in the immediate family. Moreover, with divorce, remarriage, and blended families, many more variables have an impact on a child's attachment to significant persons.

Increasingly, fathers are raising children, either as house husbands or as single parents. The kinds of loving relationships fathers have with their children are often similar to those mothers have with their children, but possible differences exist, and they warrant further study. One study compared divorced fathers and divorced mothers who were raising their children themselves (O. Cohen, 1995). The study focused on the felt well-being of the parent rather than on the loving relationship between children and parent. The data bear on that relationship, however, because a single parent with a felt well-being is likely to be more openly loving. The findings were that the parent's sense of well-being was increased by an androgynous concept of the parent's sex role and a coping style that was problem oriented. As a group, fathers compared with mothers did not differ in felt well-being, although fathers received less social support. That lack of social support has also been noted in other reports for house-husband fathers, who tend not to be as included in social conversations with other parents when they take their children to a park or other outings.

Cultural variables are important in terms of fathers' roles. As more fathers become significant caregivers in the lives of their children, new factors will emerge regarding the emotional, social, cognitive, and motivational processes involved in the loving parent-child relationship. For example, when two-parent families who shared parenting equally were compared with traditional two-parent families (Fagot & Leinbach, 1995), the parents with a sharing style treated their sons and daughters similarly. Their children had less clear cognitions regarding gender compared with children in the traditional families.

At times in the past, fathers tended not to play as important a role in the life of the child as did mothers, but it is likely that in coming years fathers will do so. Over the past two decades a slow change has occurred in this regard. One study illustrates the role of fathers when current college students were growing up (Haigler, Day, & Marshall, 1995). College student men and women reported on attachment to their parents, measured by an attachment self-report test. Overall, the subjects reported greater attachment to their mother than their father. Men and women, overall, were comparable in their attachment to parents, but other variables were significant. Attachment to parents was greater for persons sex-typed on the Bem sex-role inventory (BSRI) as feminine or androgynous (versus masculine or undifferentiated). Also, women reported higher attachment to peers than did men.

How parents relate with each other teaches children emotional and social coping skills and norms of human relationships that touch many aspects of the child's later relationships with others. Parental loving styles become models for later peer loving styles, and, unfortunately, parental physical abuse (father to mother or mother to father) also becomes a predictor of such abuse in later peer relationships. Violence in the parental relationship was found to lead to a greater amount of violent behavior in both same-sex and opposite-sex peer relationships of college-age young adults (Cantrell, MacIntyre, Sharkey, & Thompson, 1995). Many patterns in parents' style of marital interaction affect the growing child's and late adolescent's peer relationships.

Peer Relationships and Friendship

The importance of peers is documented in all child psychology and developmental psychology textbooks. Specific studies of friendship and its relationship to peer adjustment are still relatively rare, however, with notable exceptions (Parker & Asher, 1993). Although focusing on the importance of the mother-child rather than peer relationships in the early years, Freud (1964) identified the period from ages 6 to 12 as the time for same-sex friendships, when sexual urges are dormant (latent). Adler (1930) differed from Freud in many ways, one being Adler's emphasis on sibling relationships as crucial for personality development (Ferguson, 1958). Whereas peer relationships in adolescence have been given prominence by many theorists, less attention has been paid to the importance of peer friendships in preadolescence.

Harlow's work with rhesus monkeys (Harlow, 1971) showed that if a monkey had only a relationship with its mother and no peer relationships, in early childhood this would provide positive emotional well-being, but in later childhood it would be less and less positive. Eventually, a mothered monkey without peers showed impaired social skills and disturbed emotional well-being. In contrast, if a monkey had only peer relationships and no mother, in early childhood this would be socially and emotionally impairing, but after the first year of life the monkey would show normal social and emotional maturity. The early life without an adult leads to clumsy and immature behavior and relationships, but these become replaced by appropriate behavior and normal social relationships. Peers provide many opportunities that are not available in any other type of relationship, for monkey or human children.

Peers living together show physiological concordance. Observations of menstrual cycles of women in dormitories showed a tendency toward cycling synchronicity, and in a wide range of settings, adults living together have shown congruent physiological rhythms. Infant monkeys also showed this pattern. Reite and Capitanio (1985) obtained physiological measures for two pigtail monkeys reared together, who had a strong attachment bond, and these were compared with measures of two mother-reared monkeys who were not familiar with each other. The heart rates of the bonded peers were correlated when they were together and the correlation decreased when they were separated. Heart rates of the other monkeys were not correlated. Amount of delta sleep was correlated for the bonded peers but not for the other monkeys. This kind of rhythm entrainment is possibly a sensitive measure of peers' emotional and motivational bonding.

Friendships among very young children can be deep and enduring, and with increasing age, peers partially replace parents in the scope of sharing and attachment (Shaver & Hazan, 1993). An illustrative investigation (Jones & Costin, 1995) studied friendships in boys and girls in 6th, 8th, and 10th grades by means of self-report measures. The results showed differences between the grades and between boys and girls. However, regardless of gender, the more the individual was expressive (versus being instrumental), the more positive was the quality of the person's friendships. Overall,

girls were more communal (versus agentic) than boys, and girls revealed a more positive satisfaction in their friendships.

A different approach to the study of peer relationships was that of Sternberg (1987), who reviewed many formulations that compared liking and loving. Various theorists have acknowledged the depth of emotion in friendships, such as being someone's best friend. In his own theory, which he called the "triangular theory of love," Sternberg included liking of the kind that close friends share. He considered liking to involve *intimacy* but not to involve *long-term commitment* (Sternberg, 1987, p. 340). Intimacy and long-term commitment are two components of the triangle. One can challenge his point that liking in friendship lacks long-term commitment in contemporary times. People may have several marriages, but they are likely to retain one or more "best friends" throughout a lifetime, and they do so by commitment rather than chance. The third component of the triangular theory, *passion,* is absent in the love of a friend, and this distinguishes the liking between friends and sexual love.

Developmental psychologists have studied how peer relationships differ over childhood years. The size of the closely interacting group increases from age 2 to adulthood, and the gender composition of friendship groups tends to be different at various ages. Preschool children form smaller groups than do older children. Although variations occur in terms of the community and neighborhood, same-sex friendships tend to be dominant between ages 4 and 15. Friendship patterns in a class have been documented through sociometric analysis (Ferguson, 1957), which identifies the isolates and popular children as well as cliques within a large group.

Bonding in human peer relationships, from sibships to friendships, from very young to very old, has been given less attention than other love relationships in modern psychology. Far more attention has been given to sexual relationships, both in theory and research. The importance of peer relationships in several nonhuman species has received research focus, with social relationships studied in dogs, hyenas, elephants, and nonhuman primates. However, human peer relationships are far more varied and complex than those of other species, and increased empirical investigations regarding bonding in human peer relationships are needed to show how such relationships develop and change. Bonding and love in human peer relationships, between friends and siblings, play a very important role in people's lives.

Romantic Love and Adult Love Relationships

Sternberg: Triangular Theory and Love as Story. As already mentioned, Sternberg (1986, 1987, 1988, 1995) developed a triangular theory of love in which the three components are intimacy, passion, and commitment. Different kinds of love have different combinations of these components. For instance, romantic love comprises of intimacy and passion, empty love involves only commitment, and consummate love has all three components. Sternberg (Beall & Sternberg, 1995) considered the functions of love to be important. Cultural factors play a role in how love is experienced and how it changes over time. Intimacy connects lovers to one another, and passion draws them together with sexual consummation. Commitment is a goal orientation to remain with a partner. In that sense, Sternberg identifies love as multidimensional, including behavior, cognition, emotion, and motivation. Love is an active process that involves selective appraisal and continuing evaluation. Partners help to build love, and family and community foster love between the partners. As cultures permit marriage to be less formal and to serve less of an economic function, love becomes the means of bringing partners together and keeping them together. Each culture defines love, and two partners in sharing the culture also share some of that meaning. However, each relationship has unique, idiosyncratic aspects. Individuals and couples regulate their thoughts, feelings, and actions in their love according to a story format.

Sternberg (1994, 1995) conceptualized love as a story, with characters and a type of script. The story is about the relationship and it concerns each partner's role. Each partner brings a theme, and each brings a story with a plot. Relationships are best when both partners have compatible kinds of stories. Stories are creations, and how the relationship evolves is also created by the partners. A person is not a victim but a participant in a relationship. Some stories can be fantasy. Although Sternberg did not give that example, many persons have a fantasy story of Cinderella and the prince.

In a large table of categories of stories, Sternberg (1994, Table 1) described different kinds of stories and how these are manifested. For example, in a story that "love is gardening" the pertinent belief focuses on the nurturing of the relationship and the belief that without nurturing, the relationship will die. The roles of the partners involve one as gardener and the other as the garden. The benefit is that the partner is cared for and the relationship is tended. A possible disadvantage is a lack of spontaneity in the relationship. According to this formulation, the potential for success of such a relationship is very good.

Compared with a gardening story, a police story is likely to lead to a poor outcome for the relationship. The beliefs in a police story focus on keeping tabs on the partner, wanting to know everything the partner does. The roles are likely to have one person as the police officer and the partner as a suspect. This may bring the benefit of having an interest in the partner's life, but it may also bring the disadvantage of the partner feeling confined. These kinds of stories are people's constructions and they set a direction for what the individuals want in the relationship. The story indicates what a person believes is important. When both partners' stories are compatible, the relationship is likely to last and bring satisfaction. If one person changes and prefers another story, this may jeopardize the relationship.

This story approach of Sternberg (1994) describes a person's mode of thought and indicates the complementary roles taken by the partners in the relationship. Certain relationships have much more chance of mutual satisfactions than others, and certain stories are more likely to bring "a happy ending" than other stories. According to Sternberg, love relationships do not involve attributes. People do not select a partner on the basis of traits or attributes but according to (Sternberg, 1994, p. 7) "who presents us with the love story we like best." These stories are at a preconscious level and not formulated rationally. Each story represents an ideal, and the amount of positive emotion felt in the relationship is a function of the match a person believes to exist between actual events and an ideal story. The ideals are generated within a culture, and probably would not be created in another culture, but they are also unique for each individual. Within each culture, many stories are possible.

Attachment Style. On the basis of the work of Ainsworth (1982; Ainsworth et al., 1978), several researchers have examined love and love relationships in terms of attachment style (Feeney & Noller, 1992; Kobak, & Hazan 1991). Individuals may have a history of relationships involving a *secure* attachment style, in which the individuals are sensitive and responsive to each other. Others have an *avoidant* style, in which closeness is avoided. Still others have an *anxious/ambivalent* style, in which closeness and avoidance are mixed. This approach with adult attachments was first reported by Hazan and Shaver (1987). The researchers predicted that adult love would be similar to the love an infant has for a parent or parent substitute. Love involves seeking and maintaining close physical proximity, relying on the other person's availability, and seeking the person for comfort. The researchers also postulated that adult attachment styles would be related to styles the persons recalled from childhood. The researchers surveyed adults across a broad age range with a self-report measure that assessed the three attachment styles Ainsworth had observed with infants.

The items on the attachment questionnaire required subjects to indicate on a scale from 1 to 7 whether the subject disagreed or agreed with the item. An example of an item is, "I find it relatively easy to get close to others and am comfortable depending on them. I don't often worry about being abandoned or about someone getting too close to me." The researchers found that persons of all three attachment styles had some common experiences associated with romantic love, but differences between the styles were evident. Persons with primarily avoidant attachment in relationships had fears of intimacy and reported low incidence of positive relationship experiences. The person with an anxious/ambivalent attachment style tended to have

high and low emotional swings and a likelihood of jealousy. Persons with a secure attachment style had relationships of trust and closeness and they lacked fear of intimacy. Adult love relationship styles were closely related to the kinds of relationships the persons had with parents in childhood.

These findings have been replicated with subjects in different countries and cultures (Shaver & Hazan, 1993). The three attachment styles did not differ according to gender. No gender differences were found in the distribution of attachment styles within subject samples. In various studies, a majority of persons revealed a secure style, and the other two styles were each shown by about a fifth of the people. The various studies also revealed that persons with certain attachment styles were not likely to form romantic relationships. For instance, a relationship between two persons with an avoidant attachment style was very unlikely. The fact that adult love relationships continued experiences from childhood had positive as well as negative consequences. For example, adults in love relationships with abusive partners were likely to have been physically and emotionally abused by a parent in childhood. Data on this come from researchers using the theoretical perspective of attachment style (Shaver & Hazan, 1993) and from others. For example, Reuterman and Burcky (1989) studied high school students in their dating patterns. The researchers found that among those who were in a dating relationship that involved physical abuse, a significant number also had a parent who had physically abused them at home during childhood.

Many explanations can be offered for core styles of love relationships continuing from childhood into adult love relationships. An emotional learning explanation provides some answers. Learning to relate certain kinds of interpersonal experiences with early love relationships will later transfer to new love relationships. As example, one woman in a clinical setting remarked that her father hit her frequently when she was a child and that she was his favorite. She had come to believe that love means hitting someone, and if a person did not do so, the person did not love her. There are many other explanations regarding aspects of social and emotional learning that bear on personality dynamics, relationships, and motivation. Love relationships involve deep emotions and goals as well as core self-concepts, and often they are learned without the person's awareness.

Change in love relationships is possible through new learning. Sternberg (1994) suggested that partners' stories can be examined and altered to become more congruent when the relationship falters. Also, partners can learn to modify their ideal story to permit it to come closer to reality and what is truly possible. In a similar vein, when couples learn that their attachment styles need to be modified, with help and insight they often can do so. Feeney and Noller (1992) studied attachment style for college students whose romantic relationships dissolved. Those with an avoidant attachment style were the most likely to dissolve their relationships. Thus, when individuals want to learn alternative patterns in their love relationships, a change in attachment style may be required.

Other Approaches. An evolutionary biological perspective differs from a focus on individuals, and considers species characteristics. For example, Buss (1987) wrote on "love acts" and suggested that fidelity, commitment, and intimacy serve species survival functions, with the emphasis being reproductive success. Women will select mates who provide economic resources and men will select mates who show reproductive capability, and these are characteristics needed by the species. Jealousy is a manifestation of mate guarding, and serves an evolutionary value. Jealousy by the man guards the reproductive resource provided by the woman. Love acts function in order to promote reproduction, in that "both males and females have been selected to maximize gene replication" (Buss, 1987, p. 102). For gene replication (Buss, 1987), evolutionary theory posits that jealous guarding by males leads to reproduction.

The evolutionary perspective shares in common with other theories of love an emphasis on fidelity, commitment, and intimacy, but is incongruent with other theories of love by its emphasis on the value of jealousy and economic resources. At the level of the *individual,* rather than at the level of evolutionary concerns with reproductively oriented species

survival, much evidence has shown that jealousy has *harmful* consequences for individuals' love relationship. In the story approach of Sternberg (1994), jealousy plays a less healthy function than do other interacting styles, and in the formulation of Shaver (Shaver & Hazen, 1993), the most effective bonding is in the secure attachment style, which is based on trust and not on jealousy.

Researchers from various perspectives found that attitudes play significant roles in love relationships between adults. Reference was made already to the study by Leak and Gardner (1990) concerning the way the Adlerian construct of social interest related to sexual behavior. In that same study, the researchers also found social interest to relate to the "love styles" proposed by Hendrick and Hendrick (1986). The styles are given the names of Eros, Ludus, Storge, Pragma, Mania, and Agape. Eros refers to romantic, passionate love with strong emotional attachment and commitment. Storge is love based on respect, affection, permanence, and friendship, whereas Agape is unselfish and unconditional humanitarian love. These are prosocial styles that would be expected to relate positively to social interest. The other two love styles are not prosocial but instead are primarily self-serving. Ludus refers to love that avoids involvement and deep feelings, is manipulative, and views relationships in terms of a contest to be won. Mania refers to a possessive adolescent love style that is more like infatuation and reflects insecurity. Leak and Gardner (1990) found that the Storge love style was correlated significantly and positively with social interest, in support of the Adlerian prediction. That is, those subjects who reported on the love scale that their most recent love relationship was based on respect, affection, and friendship (Storge love style) also had high social interest. The Ludic love style was correlated significantly and negatively with social interest, also in support of the prediction. That is, subjects who in their most recent love relationship avoided involvement and had a manipulative approach had the lowest social interest.

The issue of realism was considered in Sternberg's (1994) love story formulation, and many theories of love focus on that aspect. The secure attachment style discussed by Shaver and Hazan

(1993), for example, involves realism about others and oneself. Goals for oneself and others are realistic, and others are trusted and trust is also directed to oneself. Studies of dating persons have consistently found that individuals with realistic expectations find their dating relationships far more satisfying than individuals with unrealistic expectations. Sullivan and Schwebel (1995) tested college students in dating relationships and gave them several self-report instruments. A dyadic adjustment scale that assessed relationship adjustment and a relationship satisfaction scale was used. The data showed that persons with more realistic expectations (measured by another scale) had significantly better adjustment, and they had higher satisfaction in their dating relationship, than did persons with more unrealistic expectations. For couples who seek counseling to improve their love relationship, one important change may be to set more realistic expectations for the relationship.

The characteristics described by Leak and Gardner (1990), and by the attachment style researchers, help couples develop long-term relationships that provide great value to the individuals. Attachment research (Van Lange et al., 1997) and Adlerian theory point out that jealousy and competitive or individualistic emphases are counterproductive to relationships and dysfunctional for individuals. Love that serves the couple and the community requires prosocial qualities and characteristics. The predisposition to help (Rubin, 1970), to trust, to nurture, support, and provide empathy are the characteristics that help develop stable and nurturing love relationships. Adler used the following words in describing love within marriage, but his words describe deep love of any kind. For Adler, love meant (Adler, 1929/1969, p. 113) "to see with the eyes, hear with the ears, and feel with the heart of another." Social, cognitive, emotional, and motivational theories of love concur with that description.

SUMMARY

Positive approach emotions and motivations bind humans together. Love has a powerful bonding role in social life. Many kinds of love exist, and some are discussed in the chapter. Sex as a biological variable is distinguished from gender as a sociocultural and cognitive variable.

Gonadal hormones are androgens, with testosterone important as a male sex hormone, and estrogens (estradiol and progestin) for female hormones. Sexual dimorphism (an organ or feature which differs for the two sexes) is evident in many characteristics, including parts of the brain in birds and mammals. Testosterone present at birth in male animals is said to have an organizing effect on the brain. This differs from the activating effect of sex hormones, which concerns the display of sexual behavior.

Social animals like the prairie vole and spotted hyena show different male and female behaviors than do other kinds of animals. The social dynamics in groups of nonhuman animals and in humans have strong effects on their sexual as well as peer behaviors. Whereas human boys have been generally observed to play more vigorously than human girls, in same-sex prepubertal play the spotted hyena females play more vigorously than the males. The importance of social grouping is evident by the fact that when spotted hyenas play in mixed-sex groups there is no difference between male and female playing. High levels of androgen in spotted hyena females have been associated with a variety of complex social behaviors. Females are dominant over males, and rank of mothers affects behaviors and privileges of their offspring.

Sexual behavior can occur for motivations other than to gain pleasure or for bonding. Sexual behavior can be used as acts of aggression and for gaining power. Sexual arousal is different from sexual arousability. Cognitive, social, and motivational variables can affect both arousal and arousability.

Gender identity refers to a person's sense of belonging as being a girl or a boy, a woman or a man. Spence considered gender identity to be a part of one's self-concept. Gender identity is different from gender stereotypes, which refer to beliefs held in society about male and female characteristics. Terms like *instrumental* versus *expressive,* and *agentic* versus *communal,* were used to express masculine and feminine stereotypes. Sex-typing was measured by one test, with androgynous and undifferentiated persons not having high male or high female sex-typing.

Gender schemas are gender-relevant cognitions. Children learn what behaviors are expected of boys and girls, and children think in terms of gender-related cognitions as part of their daily living. Gender schemas bias perception, cognition, and behavior. Bem advocated that society should move away from gender schemas as biasing people's information processing and actions.

Controversy exists to what extent men and women differ in cognitive skills and in various other characteristics. Controversy also exists to what extent various differences are due to culture as distinct from hormone-related brain characteristics.

A motivational disposition called "fear of success" was believed to occur in women striving for achievement. Although the topic was once studied extensively, evidence in support of it has been weak or lacking. Because some persons may fear being successful, such a motivation may occur at an individual level, but in studies of American women it has not been found to be a characteristic, as was thought at one time.

Love occurs in many kinds of relationships. Parent–child relationships foster love and attachment. Data from studies of rhesus monkeys have shown that loving attachment is not a passive process, in that the infant is not the passive recipient of maternal action. Love involves transaction. Contact comfort and security have been identified as important for love and attachment in infancy. How parents interact with their children, and how they interact with each other, has long-term effects on how children later form relationships with peers and mates.

Peer and sibling relationships are very important for development. Siblings have an impact on personality development, and peer relationships are the basis for many kinds of important social, emotional, and motivational learning.

Romantic love has been studied from many perspectives. How people relate to each other and what they expect from relationships has been studied in terms of attachment styles and stories. Realistic expectations and trust have been identified as important for stable and satisfying love relationships. Persons with a secure attachment style for relationships are also likely to be prosocial in their concerns for the welfare of self and others.

References

Abbott, F. (Ed.). (1987). *New men, new minds: Breaking male tradition—how today's men are changing the traditional roles of masculinity.* Freedom, CA: The Crossing Press.

Abramson, L. Y., Seligman, M. E. P., & Teasdale, J. D. (1978). Learned helplessness in humans: Critique and reformulation. *Journal of Abnormal Psychology, 87,* 49–74.

Abramson, Z. (1994). Sexuality, sex therapy, and Adlerian theory. *Individual Psychology: The Journal of Adlerian Theory, Research, and Practice, 50,* 110–118.

Achermann, P., & Borbely, A. A. (1990). Simulation of human sleep: Ultradian dynamics of electroencephalographic slow-wave activity. *Journal of Biological Rhythms, 5,* 141–157.

Ader, R., & Cohen, N. (1993). Psychoneuroimmunology: Conditioning and stress. *Annual Review of Psychology, 44,* 53–85.

Adler, A. (1910/1978). Masculine protest and a critique of Freud. In H. L. Ansbacher & R. R. Ansbacher (Eds.), *Cooperation between the sexes.* New York: Anchor Books. Pp. 32–74.

Adler, A. (1927/1959). *Understanding human nature.* Greenwich, CT: Fawcet.

Adler, A. (1927/1971). *Practice and theory of Individual Psychology.* New York: Humanitas Press.

Adler, A. (1928). Feeling and emotions from the standpoint of Individual Psychology. In M. L. Reymert (Ed.), *The Wittenberg Symposium.* Worcester, MA: Clark University Press.

Adler, A. (1929/1969). *The science of living.* New York: Anchor Books.

Adler, A. (1930). *The education of children.* New York: Greenburg.

Adler, A. (1932). *What life should mean to you.* London: Allen & Unwin.

Adler, A. (1933/1964). *Social interest: A challenge to mankind.* New York: Capricorn.

Adler, K. A. (1961). Depression in the light of Individual Psychology. *Journal of Individual Psychology, 17,* 56–67.

Ainsworth, M. D. S. (1982). Attachment: Retrospect and prospect. In C. M. Parkes & J. Sevenson-Hinde (Eds.), *The place of attachment in human behavior.* New York: Basic Books. Pp. 3–30.

Ainsworth, M. D. S., Blehar, M. C., Waters, E., & Wall, S. (1978). *Patterns of attachment: Assessed in the strange situation and at home.* Hillsdale, NJ: Erlbaum.

Allgeier, E. R., & McCormick, N. B. (Eds.). (1983). *Changing boundaries: Gender roles and sexual behavior.* Palo Alto, CA: Mayfield.

Alpert, R., & Haber, R. N. (1960). Anxiety in academic achievement situations. *Journal of Abnormal and Social Psychology, 61,* 207–215.

Amabile, T. M., & Hennessey, B. A. (1992). The motivation for creativity in children. In A. K. Boggiano & T. S. Pittman (Eds.), *Achievement and motivation: A social-developmental perspective.* New York: Cambridge University Press. Pp. 54–74.

American Psychological Society (1997). Reducing violence: A research agenda. *Human Capital Initiative, Report 5* (October), 4–24.

Amsel, A. (1962). Frustrative nonreward in partial reinforcement and discrimination learning: Some recent history and a theoretical extension. *Psychological Review, 69,* 306–328.

Amsel, A. (1990). Arousal, suppression, and persistence: Frustration theory, attention, and its disorders. *Cognition and Emotion, 4,* 239–268.

Anagnostaras, S. G., Maren, S., & Fanselow, M. S. (1995). Scopolamine selectively disrupts the acquisition of contextual fear conditioning in rats. *Neurobiology of Learning and Memory, 64,* 191–194.

Anderson, D. E., & Brady, J. V. (1971). Preavoidance blood pressure elevations accompanied by heart rate decreases in the dog. *Science, 172,* 595–597.

Anderson, J. R. (1985). *Cognitive psychology and its implications.* New York: W. H. Freeman.

Anderson, J. R., & Bower, G. H. (1973). *Human associative memory.* Washington, DC: Winston.

Anderson, K. J. (1990). Arousal and the inverted-U hypothesis: A critique of Neiss's "Reconceptualizing arousal." *Psychological Bulletin, 107,* 96–100.

Antonides, G. (1994). Mental accounting in a sequential Prisoner's Dilemma game. *Journal of Economic Psychology, 15,* 351–374.

Antony, M. M., Brown, T. A., & Barlow, D. H. (1992). Current perspectives on panic and panic disorder. *Current Directions in Psychological Science, 1,* 79–82.

Arankowsky, S. G., Stone, W. S., & Gold, P. E. (1992). Enhancement of REM sleep with auditory stimulation in young and old rats. *Brain Research, 589,* 353–357.

Archer, J. (1988). *The behavioral biology of agression.* Cambridge, UK: Cambridge University Press.

Arendt, J. (1995). *Melatonin and the mammalian pineal gland.* London: Chapman & Hall.

Arendt, J. (1997). Safety of melatonin in long-term use? *Journal of Biological Rhythms, 12,* 673–681.

Arendt, J., Skene, D. J., Middleton, B., Lockley, S. W., & Deacon, S. (1997). Efficacy of melatonin treatment in jet lag, shift work, and blindness. *Journal of Biological Rhythms, 12,* 604–617.

Aschoff, J. (1979a). Circadian rhythms: Influences of internal and external factors on the period measured in constant conditions. *Zeitschrift fuer Tierpsychologie, 49,* 225–249.

Aschoff, J. (1979b). Circadian rhythms: General features and endocrinological aspects. In D. Krieger (Ed.), *Endocrine rhythms.* New York: Raven Press. Pp. 1–61.

Aschoff, J. (1981). *Handbook of behavioral neurobiology, Vol 4: Biological Rhythms.* New York: Plenum Press.

Aschoff, J., & Pohl, H. (1978). Phase relations between a circadian rhythm and its zeitgeber within the range of entrainment. *Naturwissenschaften, 65,* 80–84.

Aschoff, J., & Wever, R. (1976). Human circadian rhythms: A multioscillatory system. *Federation Proceedings, 35,* 2326–2332.

Aschoff, J., & Wever, R. (1981). The circadian system of man. In J. Aschoff (Ed.), *Handbook of behavioral neurobiology, Vol 4: Biological rhythms.* New York: Plenum Press. Pp. 311–331.

Astington, J. W., & Gopnik, A. (1990). Developing understanding of desire and intention. In A. Whiten (Ed.), *Mindreading: The evolution, development and stimulation of second order representations.* Oxford: Blackwell. Pp. 30–56.

Aston-Jones, G., Rajkowski, J., Kubiak, P., & Alexinsky, T. (1994). Locus coeruleus neurons in monkey are selectively activated by attended cues in a vigilance task. *Journal of Neuroscience, 14,* 4467–4480.

Atkinson, J. W. (1957). Motivational determinants of risk-taking behavior. *Psychological Review, 54,* 359–372.

Atkinson, J. W. (Ed.). (1958). *Motives in fantasy, action, and society.* Princeton, NJ: Van Nostrand.

Atkinson, J. W. (1964). *An introduction to motivation.* Princeton, NJ: Van Nostrand.

Atkinson, J. W. (1983). *Personality, motivation, and action: Selected papers.* New York: Praeger.

Atkinson, J. W., & Birch, D. (1970). *The dynamics of action.* New York: Wiley.

Atkinson, J. W., & Birch, D. (1978). *An introduction to motivation* Rev. ed. New York: Van Nostrand Reinhold.

Atkinson, J. W., & Littwin, G. H. (1960). Achievement motive and test anxiety conceived as motive to approach success and motive to avoid failure. *Journal of Abnormal and Social Psychology, 60,* 52–63.

Atkinson, J. W., & O'Connor, P. A. (1966). Neglected factors in studies of achievement-oriented performance: Social approval as an incentive and performance decrement. In J. W. Atkinson & N. T. Feather (Eds.), *A theory of achievement motivation.* New York: Wiley. Pp. 299–325.

Austin, J. T., & Vancouver, J. B. (1966). Goal constructs in psychology: Structure, process, and content. *Psychological Review, 120,* 338–375.

Averill, J. R. (1969). Autonomic response patterns during sadness and mirth. *Psychophysiology, 5,* 399–414.

Averill, J. R. (1982). *Anger and aggression: An essay on emotion.* New York: Springer-Verlag.

Averill, J. R. (1991). Intellectual emotions. In C. D. Spielberger, I. G. Sarason, Z. Kulcsar, & G. L. Van Heck (Eds.), *Stress and emotion: Anxiety, anger, and curiosity.* Vol. 14. New York: Hemisphere. Pp. 3–16.

Averill, J. R. (1994). In the eyes of the beholder. In P. Ekman & R. J. Davidson (Eds.), *The nature of emotion.* New York: Oxford University Press. Pp. 7–14.

Ax, A. (1953). The physiological differentiation between fear and anger in humans. *Psychosomatic Medicine, 15,* 433–442.

Azrin, N. H., & Lindsley, O. R. (1956). The reinforcement of cooperation between children. *Journal of Abnormal and Social Psychology, 52,* 100–102.

Azrin, N. H., Hutchinson, R. R., & Sallery, R. D. (1964). Pain aggression toward inanimate objects. *Journal of the Experimental Analysis of Behavior, 7,* 223–228.

Azrin, N. H., Hutchinson, R., & Hake, D. F. (1967). Attack, avoidance, and escape reactions to aversive shock. *Journal of the Experimental Analysis of Behavior, 10,* 131–148.

Azrin, N. H., Rubin, H. B., & Hutchinson, R. R. (1968). Biting attack by rats in response to aversive shock. *Journal of the Experimental Analysis of Behavior, 11,* 633–639.

Babkoff, H. Caspy T., & Mikulincer, M. (1991). Subjective sleepiness ratings: The effects of sleep deprivation, circadian rhythmicity, and cognitive performance. *Sleep, 14,* 534–539.

Bachmann, T. (1991). Microgenesis in visual information processing; Some experimental results. In R. E. Hanlon (Ed.), *Cognitive microgenesis: A neuropsychological perspective.* New York: Springer Verlag. Pp. 240–261.

Baell, W. K., & Wertheim, E. H. (1992). Predictors of outcome in the treatment of bulimia nervosa. *British Journal of Clinical Psychology, 31,* 330–332.

Baenninger, L. P., & Baenninger, R. (1970). Spontaneous fighting and mouse-killing by rats. *Psychonomic Science, 19,* 161.

Bailey, D. S., & Taylor, S. P. (1991). Effects of alcohol and aggressive disposition on human physical aggression. *Journal of Research in Personality, 25,* 334–342.

Baldeweg, T., Ullsperger, P., Pietrowsky, R., Feham, H. L., & Born, J. (1993). Event-related brain potential correlates of self-reported hunger and satiety. *Psychophysiology, 30,* 23–29.

Balleine, B., & Dickinson, A. (1994). Role of cholecystokinin in the motivational control of instrumental action in rats. *Behavioral Neuroscience, 108,* 590–605.

Balleine, B., Davies, A., & Dickinson, A. (1995). Cholecystokinin attenuates incentive learning in rats. *Behavioral Neuroscience, 109,* 312–319.

Bandura, A. (1965). Influence of models' reinforcement contingencies on the acquisition of imitative responses. *Journal of Personality and Social Psychology, 1,* 589–595.

Bandura, A. (1977). Self-efficacy: Toward a unifying theory of behavioral change. *Psychological Review, 84,* 191–215.

Bandura, A. (1982). Self-efficacy mechanism in human agency. *American Psychologist, 37,* 122–147.

Bandura, A. (1986). *Social foundations of thought and action: A social cognitive theory.* Englewood Cliffs, NJ: Prentice-Hall.

Bandura, A. (1989). Human agency in social cognitive theory. *American Psychologist, 44,* 1175–1184.

Bandura, A. (1991). Self-regulation of motivation through anticipatory and self-reactive mechanisms. In R. Dienstbier (Ed.), *Nebraska symposium on motivation, 1990.* Vol. 38. Lincoln: University of Nebraska Press. Pp. 69–164.

Bandura, A. (1997). *Self-efficacy: The exercise of control.* New York: W. H. Freeman.

Bandura, A., & Jourden, F. J. (1991). Self-regulatory mechanisms governing the impact of social comparison on complex decision making. *Journal of Personality and Social Psychology, 60,* 941–951.

Bandura, A., Ross, D., & Ross, S. A. (1963). Imitation of film-mediated aggressive models. *Journal of Abnormal and Social Psychology, 66,* 3–11.

Bare, J. K. (1959). Hunger, deprivation, and the day-night cycle. *Journal of Comparative and Physiological Psychology, 52,* 129–131.

Barefoot, J. C., & Lipkus, I. M. (1994). The assessment of anger and hostility. In A. W. Siegman & T. W. Smith (Eds.), *Anger, hostility, and the heart.* Hillsdale, NJ: Erlbaum. Pp. 43–66.

Barinaga, M. (1995). "Obese" protein slims mice. *Science, 269,* 475–476.

Barlow, D. H. (Ed.). (1993). *Clinical handbook of psychological disorders: A step-by-step treatment manual.* 2nd ed. New York: Guilford Press.

Barth, R. (1974). Developmental and personality assessment of high Mach female adults. Unpublished master's thesis, Southern Illinois University at Edwardsville.

Bartoshuk, L. M. (1989). The functions of taste and olfaction. In L. H. Schneider, S. J. Cooper, & K. A. Halmi (Eds.), *The psychology of human eating disorders: Preclinical and clinical perspectives.* Vol. 575. *Annals of the New York Academy of Sciences.* New York: New York Academy of Sciences. Pp. 353–361.

Bates, F. C., & Horvath, T. (1971). Discrimination learning with rhythmic and non-rhythmic background music. *Perceptual and Motor Skills, 33,* 1123–1126.

Baum, A., & Grunberg, N. (1995). Measurement of stress hormones. In S. Cohen, R. C. Kessler, & L. U. Gordon (Eds.), *Measuring stress: A guide for health and social scientists.* New York: Oxford University Press. Pp. 175–192.

Baum, M. (1970). Extinction of avoidance responding through response prevention (flooding). *Psychological Bulletin, 74,* 276–284.

Baum, M. J. (1992). Neuroendocrinology of sexual behavior in the male. In J. B. Becker, S. M. Breedlove, & D. Crews (Eds.), *Behavioral endocrinology.* Cambridge, MA: MIT Press. Pp. 97–130.

Baumeister, A., Hawkins, W. F., & Cromwell, R. L.

(1964). Need states and activity level. *Psychological Bulletin, 61,* 438–453.

Baumeister, R. F., & Showers, C. J. (1986). A review of paradoxical performance effects: Choking under pressure in sports and mental tests. *European Journal of Social Psychology, 37,* 1251–1281.

Baumeister, R. F., & Sommer, K. L. (1997). What do men want? Gender differences and two spheres of belongingness: Comment on Cross and Madson (1997). *Psychological Bulletin, 122,* 38–44.

Baumeister, R. F., Hutton, D. G., & Cairns, K. J. (1990). Negative effects of praise on skilled performance. *Basic and Applied Social Psychology, 11,* 131–148.

Bayton, J. A., & Whyte, E. C. (1950). Personality dynamics during success-failure sequences. *Journal of Abnormal and Social Psychology, 45,* 583–591.

Beall, A. E., & Sternberg, R. J. (1995). The social construction of love. *Journal of Social and Personal Relationships, 12,* 417–438.

Beck, A. T. (1963). Thinking and depression: I. Idiosyncratic content and cognitive distortions. *Archives of General Psychiatry, 9,* 324–333.

Beck, A. T. (1983). Cognitive therapy of depression: New perspectives. In P. J. Clayton & J. E. Barrett (Eds.), *Treatment of depression: Old controversies and new approaches.* New York: Raven Press. Pp. 265–290.

Beck, A. T., & Greenberg, R. L. (1996). Brief cognitive therapies. In J. E. Groves (Ed.), *Essential papers on short-term dynamic therapy.* New York: New York University Press. Pp. 230–247.

Beck, A. T., & Young, J. E. (1985). Depression. In D. H. Barlow (Ed.), *Clinical handbook of psychological disorders: A step-by-step treatment manual.* New York: Guilford Press. Pp. 206–244.

Beck, A. T., Ward, C. H., Mendelsohn, M., Mock, J. E., & Erbaujh, J. K. (1961). An inventory for measuring depression. *Archives of General Psychiatry, 4,* 561–571.

Beck, M., & Galef, B. G., Jr. (1989). Social influences on the selection of a protein-sufficient diet by Norway rats (*Ratus norvegicus*). *Journal of Comparative Psychology, 103,* 132–139.

Becker, J. B., & Breedlove, S. M. (1992). Introduction to behavioral endocrinology. In J. B. Becker, S. M. Breedlove, & D. Crews (Eds.), *Behavioral endocrinology.* Cambridge, MA: MIT Press. Pp. 3–37.

Belinger, C. (1994). Effect of cholecystokinin on gastric motility in humans. In J. R. Reeve, Jr., V. Eysslelein, T. E. Solomon, & V. l. W. Go (Eds.), *Cholecystokinin.* Vol. 713. *Annals of the New York Academy of Sciences.* New York: New York Academy of Sciences. Pp. 219–225.

Bem, S. L. (1974). The measurement of psychological androgyny. *Journal of Consulting and Clinical Psychology, 42,* 155–162.

Bem, S. L. (1985). Androgyny and gender schema theory: A conceptual and empirical integration. In T. B. Sonderegger (Ed.), *Nebraska Symposium on Motivation, 1984.* Vol. 32. Lincoln: University of Nebraska Press. Pp. 179–226.

Bem, S. L. (1993). *The lenses of gender: Transforming the debate on sexual inequality.* New Haven, CT: Yale University Press.

Berk, M. L., & Finkelstein, J. A. (1981). An autoradiographic determination of the efferent projections of the suprachiasmatic nucleus of the hypothalamus. *Brain Research, 226,* 1–13.

Berkowitz, L. (1990). On the formation and regulation of anger and aggression: A cognitive-neoassociationistic analysis. *American Psychologist, 45,* 494–503.

Berkowitz, L. (1990.) On the formation and regulation of anger and aggression: A cognitive-neoassociationistic analysis. *American Psychologist, 45,* 494–503.

Berkowitz, L. (1993). *Aggression: Its causes, consequences, and control.* New York: McGraw-Hill.

Berman, M., Gladue, B., & Taylor, S. (1993). The effects of hormones, Type A behavior pattern, and provocation on aggression in men. *Motivation and Emotion, 17,* 125–138.

Berndt, R. M., & Berndt, C. H. (1952). *The first Australians.* Sydney: Ure Smith.

Bernstein, I. L. (1968). Learned taste aversion in children receiving chemotherapy. *Science, 200,* 1302.

Berridge, K. C., Venier, I. L., & Robinson, T. E. (1989). Taste reactivity analysis of 6-hydroxydopamine-induced aphagia: Implications for arousal and anhedonia hypotheses of dopamine function. *Behavioral Neuroscience, 103,* 36–45.

Betsch, T., & Dickenberger, D. (1993). Why do aggressive movies make people aggressive? An attempt to explain short-term effects of the depiction of violence on the observer. *Aggressive Behavior, 19,* 137–149.

Bettencourt, B. A., & Miller, N. (1996). Gender differences in aggression as a function of provocation: A meta-analysis. *Psychological Bulletin, 119,* 422–447.

Bills, R. E. (1953). A comparison of scores in the Index of Adjustment with behavior in level of aspiration tests. *Journal of Consulting Psychology, 17,* 206–213.

Birch, L. L., & Fisher, J. A. (1996). The role of experience in the development of children's eating behavior. In E. D. Capaldi (Ed.), *Why we eat what we eat: The psychology of eating.* Washington, DC: American Psychological Association. Pp. 113–141.

Birenbaum, M., & Kraemer, R. (1995). Gender and ethnic-group differences in causal attributions for success and failure in mathematics and language examinations. *Journal of Cross Cultural Psychology, 26,* 342–359.

Black, R. W. (1965). On the combination of drive and incentive motivation. *Psychological Review, 72,* 310–317.

Blanchard, D. C., & Blanchard, R. J. (1984). Affect and aggression: An animal model applied to human behavior. In R. J. Blanchard & D. C. Blanchard, (Eds.), *Advances in the study of aggression, Vol. I.* Orlando, FL: Academic Press. Pp. 1–62.

Blanchard, D. C., & Blanchard, R. J. (1990). Behavioral correlates of chronic dominance-subordination relationships of male rats in a seminatural situation. *Neuroscience & Behavioral Reviews, 14,* 455–462.

Blanchard, D. C., Hori, K., Rodgers, R. J., Hendrie, C. A., & Blanchard, R. J. (1989). Attenuation of defensive threat and attack in wild rats (*Rattus rattus*) by benzodiazepines. *Psychopharmacology, 97,* 392–401.

Blanchard, R. J., & Blanchard, D. C. (1987). An ethoexperimental approach to the study of fear. *The Psychological Record, 37,* 305–316.

Blanchard, R. J., & Blanchard, D. C. (1989). Antipredator defensive behaviors in a visible burrow system. *Journal of Comparative Psychology, 103,* 70–82.

Blanchard, R. J., Blanchard, D. C., & Fial, R. A. (1970). Hippocampal lesions in rats and their effect on activity, avoidance, and aggression. *Journal of Comparative and Physiological Psychology, 71,* 92–102.

Blanchard, R. J., Blanchard, D. C., & Hori, K. (1989). An ethoexperimental approach to the study of defense. In R. J. Blanchard, P. F. Brain, D. C. Blanchard, & S. Parmigiani (Eds.), *Ethoexperimental approaches to the study of behavior.* Boston: Kluwer Academic Publishers. Pp. 114–136.

Blanchard, R. J., Flores, T., Magee, L., Weiss, S., & Blanchard, D. C. (1992). Pregrouping aggression and defense scores influences alcohol consumption for dominant and subordinate rats in visible burrow systems. *Aggressive Behavior, 18,* 459–467.

Blanchard, R. J., Hori, K., Tom, P., & Blanchard, D. C. (1988). Social dominance and individual aggressiveness. *Aggressive Behavior, 14,* 195–203.

Blanchard, R. J., Parmigiani, S., Bjornson, C., Masuda, C., Weiss, S. M., & Blanchard, D. C. (1995). Antipredator behavior of Swiss-Webster mice in a visible burrow system. *Aggressive Behavior, 21,* 123–136.

Blankenship, V. (1987). A computer-based measure of resultant achievement motivation. *Journal of Personality and Social Psychology, 53,* 361–372.

Blass, E. M. (1992). The ontogeny of motivation: Opioid bases of energy conservation and lasting affective change in rat and human infants. *Current Directions in Psychological Science, 1,* 116–120.

Blass, E. M., Shide, D. J., & Weller, A. (1989). Stress-reducing effects of ingesting milk, sugars, and fats: A developmental perspective. In L. H. Schneider, S. J. Cooper, & K. A. Halmi (Eds.), *The psychology of human eating disorders: Preclinical and clinical perspectives.* Vol. 575. *Annals of the New York Academy of Sciences.* New York: New York Academy of Sciences. Pp. 292–305.

Block, S., Lemeignan, M., & Aguilera, N. (1991). Specific respiratory patterns distinguish among human basic emotions. *International Journal of Psychophysiology, 11,* 141–154.

Boivin, D. B., & Czeisler, C. A. (1998). Resetting of circadian melatonin and cortisol rhythms in humans by ordinary room light. *Neuroreport, 9,* 779–782.

Bolles, R. C. (1965). Readiness to eat: Effects of age, sex, and weight loss. *Journal of Comparative and Physiological Psychology, 60,* 88–92.

Bolles, R. C. (1967). *Theory of motivation.* New York: Harper & Row.

Bolles, R. C. (1970). Species-specific defense reactions and avoidance learning. *Psychological Review, 77,* 32–48.

Bolles, R. C. (1975). *Theory of motivation.* New York: Harper & Row.

Bonson, J. R., & Winter, J. C. (1992). Reversal of testosterone-induced dominance by the serotonergic agonist quipazine. *Pharmacology, Biochemistry and Behavior, 42,* 809–813.

Booth, D. A. (1989). Mood and nutrient-conditioned appetites: Cultural and physiological bases for eating disorders. In L. H. Schneider, S. J. Cooper, & K. A. Halmi (Eds.), *The psychology of human eating disorders: Preclinical and clinical perspectives.* Vol. 575. *Annals of the New York Academy of Sciences,* New York: New York Academy of Sciences, Pp. 122–135.

Borbely, A. A. (1982). A two process model of sleep regulation. *Human Neurobiology, 1,* 195–204.

Borbely, A. A. (1994). Sleep homeostasis and models of sleep regulation. In M. H. Kryger, T. Roth, & W. C. Dement (Eds.), *Principles and practice of sleep medicine.* Philadelphia: W. B. Saunders. Pp. 309–320.

Bottome, P. (1939). *Alfred Adler: Apostle of freedom.* London: Faber and Faber.

Boulos, Z., Campbell, S. S., Lewy, A. J., Terman, M., Dijk, D. J., & Eastman, C. I. (1995). Light treatment for sleep disorders: Consensus report. VII. Jet lag. *Journal of Biological Rhythms, 10,* 167–176.

Bouton, M. E. (1993). Context, time, and memory retrieval in the interference paradigms of Pavlovian learning. *Psychological Bulletin, 114,* 80–99.

Bouton, M. E. (1994). Conditioning, remembering, and

forgetting. *Journal of Experimental Psychology: Animal Behavior Processes, 20,* 219–231.

Bower, G. H. (1981). Mood and memory. *American Psychologist, 36,* 129–148.

Bower, G. H. (1983). Affect and cognition. *Philosophical Transactions of the Royal Society of London, Series B, 302,* 387–403.

Bower, G. H. (1992). How might emotions affect learning? In S.-A. Christianson (Ed.), *The handbook of emotion and memory.* Hillsdale, NJ: Erlbaum. Pp. 3–31.

Bower, G. H. (1994). Some relations between emotions and memory. In P. Ekman & R. J. Davidson (Eds.), *The nature of emotion: Fundamental questions.* New York: Oxford University Press. Pp. 303–305.

Bower, G. H., & Mayer, J. D. (1985). Failure to replicate mood-dependent retrieval. *Bulletin of the Psychonomic Society, 23,* 39–42.

Bower, G. H., Gilligan, S. C., & Monteiro, K. P. (1981). Selectivity of learning caused by affective states. *Journal of Experimental Psychology: General, 110,* 451–473.

Bower, G. H., Monteiro, K. P., & Gilligan, S. G. (1978). Emotional mood as a context for learning and recall. *Journal of Verbal Learning and Verbal Behavior, 17,* 573–587.

Bowlby, J. (1979). *The making and breaking of affectional bonds.* London: Tavistock Publications.

Bradley, M. M., & Lang, P. J. (1993). Emotion, novelty, and the startle reflex: Habituation in humans. *Behavioral Neuroscience, 107,* 970–980.

Brazier, M. M. (1996). Effects of present and former deprivation on consummatory contrast. *The Psychological Record, 46,* 187–200.

Breedlove, S. M. (1992). Sexual differentiation of the brain and behavior. In J. B. Becker, S. M. Breedlove, & D. Crews (Eds.), *Behavioral endocrinology.* Cambridge, MA: MIT Press. Pp. 39–68

Breedlove, S. M. (1994). Sexual differentiation of the human nervous system. *Annual Review of Psychology, 45,* 389–418.

Brehm, J. W., & Self, E. A. (1989). The intensity of motivation. *Annual Review of Psychology, 40,* 109–131.

Brehm, J. W., & Self, E. A. (1989). The intensity of motivation. In M. R. Rosenzweig & L. W. Porter (Eds.), *Annual review of psychology.* Vol. 40. Palo Alto, CA: Annual Reviews, Inc. Pp. 109–131.

Brewin, C. R. (1989). Cognitive change processes in psychotherapy. *Psychological Review, 96,* 379–394.

Brewin, C. R. (1996). Theoretical foundations of cognitive-behavior therapy for anxiety and depression. *Annual Review of Psychology, 47,* 33–57.

Broadbent, D. E., & Gregory, M. (1967). Perception of emotionally toned words. *Nature, 216,* 581–584.

Broadhurst, P. L. (1957). Emotionality and the Yerkes-Dodson Law. *Journal of Experimental Psychology, 54,* 345–352.

Brod, H. (Ed.). (1987). *The making of masculinities: The new men's studies.* Boston: Unwin Hyman.

Bronson, F. H., Heideman, P. D., & Kerbeshian, M. C. (1991). Lability of fat stores in peripubertal wild house mice. *Journal of Comparative Physiology B, 161,* 15–18.

Brosschot, J. F., Gebhardt, W. A., & Godaert, G. L. R. (1994). Internal, powerful others and chance locus of control: Relationships with personality, coping, stress, and health. *Personality and Individual Differences, 16,* 839–852.

Brown, J. L. (1956). The effect of drive on learning with secondary reinforcement. *Journal of Comparative and Physiological Psychology, 49,* 254–260.

Brown, P. J., & Konner, M. (1987). An anthropological perspective on obesity. In R. J. Wurtman & J. J. Wurtman (Eds.), *Human obesity.* Vol. 499. *Annals of the New York Academy of Sciences.* New York: New York Academy of Sciences. Pp. 29–46.

Brown, T. A., O'Leary, T. A., & Barlow, D. H. (1993). Generated anxiety disorder. In D. H. Barlow (Ed.), *Clinical handbook of psychological disorders: A step-by-step treatment manual.* 2nd ed. New York: Guilford Press. Pp. 137–188.

Brownell, K. D., & O'Neil, P. M. (1993). Obesity. In D. H. Barlow (Ed.), *Clinical handbook of psychological disorders: A step-by-step treatment manual* 2nd ed. New York: Guilford Press. Pp. 318–361.

Buck, R. (1985). Prime theory: An integrated view of motivation and emotion. *Psychological Review, 92,* 389–413.

Buckner, D. N., & McGrath, J. J. (Eds.). (1963). *Vigilance: A symposium.* New York: McGraw-Hill.

Burger, J. M. (1985). Desire for control and achievement-related behaviors. *Journal of Personality and Social Psychology, 48,* 1520–1533.

Burns, D. D. (1989). *The feeling good handbook: Using the new mood therapy in everyday life.* New York: William Morrow.

Bushman, B. J., & Geen, R. G. (1990). Role of cognitive-emotional mediators and individual differences in the effects of media violence on aggression. *Journal of Personality and Social Psychology, 58,* 156–163.

Buss, A. H., & Durkee, A. (1957). An inventory for assessing different kinds of hostility. *Journal of Consulting Psychology, 42,* 155–162.

Buss, A. H., & Perry, M. (1992). The aggression questionnaire. *Journal of Personality and Social Psychology, 63,* 452–459.

Buss, D. (1999). *Evolutionary psychology.* Needham Heights, MA: Allyn & Bacon.

Buss, D. M. (1987). Love acts: The evolutionary biology of love. In R. J. Sternberg & M. L. Barnes (Eds.), *The psychology of love.* New Haven, CT: Yale University Press.

Buss, D. M. (1989). Sex differences in human mate preferences: Evolutionary hypotheses tested in 37 cultures. *Behavioral and Brain Sciences, 12,* 1–49.

Buss, D. M. (1996). Sexual conflict: Evolutionary insights into feminism and the "battle of the sexes." In D. M. Buss & N. M. Malamuth (Eds.), *Sex power, conflict: Evolutionary and feminist perspectives.* New York: Oxford University Press. Pp. 296–318.

Byrne, D. (1964). Repression-sensitization as a dimension of personality. In B. A. Maher (Ed.), *Progress in experimental personality research.* Vol. I. New York: Academic Press. Pp. 169–220.

Cacciopo, J. T., & Berntson, G. G. (1992). Social psychological contributions to the decade of the brain. *American Psychologist, 47,* 1019–1028.

Cagnacci, A., Krauchi, K., Wirz-Justice, A., & Volpe, A. (1997). Homeostatic versus circadian effects of melatonin on core body temperature in humans. *Journal of Biological Rhythms, 12,* 509–517.

Campbell, B. A., & Sheffield, F. D. (1953). Relation of random activity to food deprivation. *Journal of Comparative and Physiological Psychology, 46,* 320–322.

Campbell, S. S., & Murphy, P. J. (1998). Extraocular circadian phototransduction in humans. *Science, 279,* 396–399.

Campfield, L. A., & Smith, F. J. (1990). Systemic factors in the control of food intake: Evidence for patterns as signals. In E. M. Stricker (Ed.), *Neurobiology of food and fluid intake. Handbook of behavioral neurobiology.* Vol. 10. New York: Plenum Press. Pp. 183–206.

Campfield, L. A., Smith, F. J., Guisez, Y., Devos, R., & Burn, P. (1995). Recombinant mouse OB protein: Evidence for a peripheral signal linking adiposity and central neural networks. *Science, 269,* 546–549.

Campos, J. J., Bertenthal, B. I., & Kermoian, R. (1992). Early experience and emotional development: The emergence of wariness of heights. *Psychological Science, 3,* 61–64.

Candland, D. K., & Nagy, Z. M. (1969). The open field: Some comparative data. In E. Tobach (Ed.), *Experimental approaches to the study of emotional behavior.*

Annals of the New York Academy of Sciences, 159, 831–851.

Cannon, W. B. (1929). *Bodily changes in pain, hunger, fear and rage.* 2nd ed. New York: Appleton.

Cannon, W. B. (1932). *The wisdom of the body.* New York: W. W. Norton.

Cannon, W. B., & Washburn, A. L. (1912). An explanation of hunger. *American Journal of Physiology, 29,* 441–454.

Cantor, N. (1990). From thought to behavior: "Having" and "doing" in the study of personality and cognition. *American Psychologist, 45,* 735–750.

Cantor, N., & Fleeson, W. (1994). Social intelligence and intelligent goal pursuit: A cognitive slice of motivation. In W. D. Spaulding (Ed.), *Nebraska Symposium on Motivation.* Vol. 41. Lincoln: University of Nebraska Press, Pp. 125–179.

Cantrell, P. J., MacIntyre, D. I., Sharkey, K. J., & Thompson, V. (1995). Violence in the marital dyad as a predictor of violence in the peer relationships of older adolescents/young adults. *Violence and Victims, 10,* 35–40.

Cantril, H., & Hunt, W. A. (1932). Emotional effects produced by the injection of adrenalin. *American Journal of Psychology, 44,* 300–307.

Capaldi, E. D. (1996). Introduction. In E. D. Capaldi (Ed.), *Why we eat what we eat: The psychology of eating.* Washington, DC: American Psychological Association. Pp. 3–9.

Capaldi, E. D., Owens, J., & Palmer, K. A. (1994). Effects of food deprivation on learning and expression of flavor preferences conditioned by saccharin or sucrose. *Animal Learning and Behavior, 22,* 173–180.

Caplan, P. J., Crawford, M., Hyde, J. S., & Richardson, T. E. (Eds.). (1997). *Gender differences in human cognition.* New York: Oxford University Press.

Card, J. P., & Moore, R. Y. (1989). Organization of lateral geniculate-hypothalamic connections in the rat. *Journal of Comparative Neurology, 284,* 135–147.

Carlson, N. R. (1998). *Physiology of behavior.* 6th Edition. Needham Heights, MA: Allyn & Bacon.

Carr, P. G., & Mednick, M. T. (1988). Sex role socialization and the development of achievement motivation in Black preschool children. *Sex Roles, 18,* 169–180.

Carr, P. G., Thomas, C. G., & Mednick, M. T. (1985). Evaluation of sex-typed tasks by Black men and somen. *Sex Roles, 13,* 311–316.

Carrier, J., Monk, T. H., Buysse, D. J., & Kupfer, D. J. (1997). Sleep and morningness-eveningness in the "middle" years of life (20–59). *Journal of Sleep Research, 6,* 230–237.

Carter, C. S. (1992a). Hormonal influences on human sexual behavior. In J. B. Becker, S. M. Breedlove, & D. Crews (Eds.), *Behavioral endocrinology*. Cambridge, MA: MIT Press. Pp. 131–142.

Carter, C. S. (1992b). Neuroendocrinology of sexual behavior in the female. In J. B. Becker, S. M. Breedlove, & D. Crews (Eds.), *Behavioral endocrinology*. Cambridge, MA: MIT Press. Pp. 71–95.

Carton, J. S., & Nowicki, S. (1994). Antecedents of individual differences in locus of control of reinforcement: A critical review. *Genetic, Social, and General Psychology Mongoraphs, 120,* 31–81.

Cattell, R. B. (1957). *Handbook for the I.P.A.T. Anxiety Scale.* Champaign, IL: Institute for Personality and Ability Testing.

Cattell, R. B. (1966). *Handbook of multivariate experimental psychology.* Skokie, IL: Rand McNally.

Cattell, R. B., Eber, H. W., & Tatsuoka, M. M. (1970). *Handbook for the Sixteen Personality Factor questionnaire (16 PF).* Champaign, IL: Institute for Personality and Ability Testing.

Cervone, D., Jiwani, N., & Wood, R. (1991). Goal setting and the differential influence of self-regulatory processes on complex decision-making performance. *Journal of Personality and Social Psychology, 61,* 257–266.

Chapman, D. W., & Volkman, J. (1939). A social determinant of the level of aspiration. *Journal of Abnormal and Social Psychology, 38,* 225–238.

Chermack, S. T., & Taylor, S. P. (1995). Alcohol and human physical aggression: Pharmacological versus expectancy effects. *Journal of Studies on Alcohol, 56,* 449–456.

Christianson, S.-A., & Loftus, E. F. (1987). Memory for traumatic events. *Applied Cognitive Psychology, 1,* 225–239.

Christie, R., & Geis, F. (Eds.). (1970). *Studies in Machiavellianism.* New York: Academic Press.

Clark, L. A., Watson, D., & Leeka, J. (1989). Diurnal variation in the positive affects. *Motivation and Emotion, 13,* 205–234.

Clark, M. S., Milberg, S., & Ross, J. (1983). Arousal cues arousal-related material in memory: Implications for understanding effects of mood on memory. *Journal of Verbal Learning and Verbal Behavior, 22,* 633–649.

Clemens, L. G., Wee, B. E. F., Weaver, D. R., Roy, E. J., Goldman, B. D., & Rakerd, B. (1988). Retention of masculine sexual behavior following castration in male B6D2F1 mice. *Physiology & Behavior, 42,* 69–76.

Cofer, C. N., & Appley, M. H. (1964). *Motivation: Theory and research.* New York: Wiley.

Cohen, L. D. (1954). Level-of-aspiration behavior and feelings of adequacy and self-acceptance. *Journal of Abnormal and Social Psychology, 49,* 84–86.

Cohen, O. (1995). Divorced fathers raise their children by themselves. *Journal of Divorce and Remarriage, 23,* 55–73.

Cohen, R. A., & Albers, H. E. (1991). Disruption of human circadian and cognitive regulation following a discrete hypothlamic lesion: A case study. *Neurology, 41,* 726–729.

Cohen, S., & Herbert, T. B. (1996) Health psychology: Psychological factors and physical disease from the perspective of human psychoneuroimmunology. *Annual Review of Psychology, 47,* 113–142.

Coleman, L. M., Jussim, L., & Isaac, J. L. (1991). Black students' reactions to feedback conveyed by White and Black teachers. *Journal of Applied Social Psychology, 21,* 460–481.

Collier, G., & Levitsky, D. (1967). Defense of water balance in rats: Behavioral and physiological responses to depletion. *Journal of Comparative and Physiological Psychology, 64,* 59–67.

Collier, G., Hirsch, E., & Hamlin, P. H. (1972). The ecological determinants of reinforcement in the rat. *Physiology and Behavior, 9,* 705–716.

Collins, A. M. & Loftus, E. F. (1975). A spreading activation theory of semantic processing. *Psychological Review, 82,* 407–428.

Collins, A. M., & Quillian, M. R. (1969) Retrieval time from semantic memory. *Journal of Verbal Learning and Verbal Behavior, 8,* 240–247.

Collins, B. (1974). Four separate components of the Rotter I-E scale: Belief in a difficult world, a just world, a predictable world and a politically responsive world. *Journal of Personality and Social Psychology, 41,* 471–492.

Colombo, G., Agabio, R., Lobina, C., Reali, R., Zocchi, A., Fadda, F., & Gessa, G. L. (1995). Sardinian alcohol-preferring rats: A genetic animal model of anxiety. *Physiology and Behavior, 57,* 1181–1185.

Condry, J., & Stokker, L. G. (1992). Overview of special issue on intrinsic motivation. *Motivation and Emotion, 16,* 157–164.

Cook, W. W., & Medley, D. M. (1954). Proposed hostility and pharasaic-virtue scales for the MMPI. *Journal of Applied Psychology, 38,* 414–418.

Corban, C. M., & Gournard, B. R. (1976). Types of music, schedules of background stimulation and visual vigilance performance. *Perceptual and Motor Skills, 42,* 662.

Corbett, W. W., & Keesey, R. E. (1982). Energy balance of rats with lateral hypothalamic lesions. *American Journal of Physiology, 242,* E273–279.

Coren, S. (1988). Prediction of insomnia from arousability predisposition scores: Scale development and cross-validation. *Behavior Research and Therapy, 26,* 415–420.

Coren, S. (1990). The arousal predisposition scale: Normative data. *Bulletin of the Psychonomic Society, 28,* 551–552.

Coren, S., & Aks, D. J. (1991). Prediction of task-related arousal under conditions of environmental distraction. *Journal of Applied Social Psychology, 21,* 189–197.

Courts, F. A. (1942). The influence of practice on the dynamogenic effect of muscular tension. *Journal of Experimental Psychology, 30,* 504–511.

Covington, M. V. (1992). *Making the grade: A self-worth perspective on motivation and school reform.* New York: Cambridge University Press.

Covington, M., & Omelich, C. (1979). Are causal attributions causal? A path analysis of the cognitive model of achievement motivation. *Journal of Personality and Social Psychology, 37,* 1487–1504.

Covington, M. V., & Omelich, C. L. (1991). Need achievement revisited: Verification of Atkinson's original 2 × 2 model. In C. D. Spielberger, I. G. Sarason, Z. Kulcsar, & G. L. Van Heck (Eds.), *Stress and emotion: Anxiety, anger, and curiosity.* Vol. 14. New York: Hemisphere. Pp. 85–105.

Craig, K. D. (1968). Physiological arousal as a function of imagined, vicarious, and direct stress experiences. *Journal of Abnormal Psychology, 73,* 513–520.

Craik, F. I. M., & Tulving, E. (1975). Depth of processing and the retention of words in episodic memory. *Journal of Experimental Psychology: General, 104,* 268–294.

Craske, M. G., & Barlow, D. H. (1993). Panic disorder and agoraphobia. In D. H. Barlow (Ed.), *Clinical handbook of psychological disorders: A step-by-step treatment manual.* 2nd ed. New York: Guilford Press. Pp. 1–47.

Crespi, L. P. (1942). Quantitative variation of incentive and performance in the white rat. *American Journal of Psychology, 55,* 467–517.

Crews, D. (1992). Diversity of hormone-behavior relations in reproductive behavior. In J. B. Becker, S. M. Breedlove, & D. Crews (Eds.), *Behavioral endocrinology.* Cambridge, MA: MIT Press. Pp. 143–186.

Crick, N. R. (1995). Relational aggression: The role of intent attributions, feelings of distress, and provocation type. *Development and Psychopathology, 7,* 313–322.

Cross, H. R., Halcomb, C. G., & Matter, W. W. (1967). Imprinting or exposure learning in rats given early auditory stimuli. *Psychonomic Science, 7,* 233–234.

Cross, S. E., & Madson, L. (1997). Models of the self:

Self-construals and gender. *Psychological Bulletin, 122,* 5–37.

Czeisler, C. A. (1995). The effect of light on the human circadian pacemaker. In D. J. Derek & K. Ackrill (Eds.), *Circadian clocks and their adjustment.* (Ciba Foundation Symposium, 183). Chichester: Wiley. Pp. 254–302.

Czeisler, C. A., Johnson, M. P., Duffy, J. F., Brown, E. N., Ronda, J. M., & Kronauer, R. E. (1990). Exposure to bright light and darkness to treat physiologic maladaptation to night work. *New England Journal of Medicine, 322,* 1253–1259.

Czeisler, C. A., Kronauer, R. E., Allan, J. S., Duffy, J. F., Jewett, M. E., Brown, E. N., & Ronda, J. M. (1989). Bright light induction of strong (Type 0) resetting of the human circadian pacemaker. *Science, 244,* 1328–1333.

Czeisler, C. A., Moore-Ede, M. C., & Coleman, R. M. (1982). Rotating shift work schedules that disrupt sleep are improved by applying circadian principles. *Science, 217,* 460–463.

Daan, S., & Pittendrigh, C. S. (1976). A functional analysis of circadian pacemakers in nocturnal rodents. II. Variability of phase response curves. *Journal of Comparative Physiology A, 106,* 253–266.

Daan, S., Beersma, D. G. M., & Borbely, A. (1984). Timing of human sleep: Recovery process gated by a circadian pacemaker. *American Journal of Physiology, 246,* R161–R178.

Dabbs, J. M., Jr. (1993). Salivary testosterone measurements in behavioral studies. In D. Malamud & L. A. Tabak (Eds.), *Saliva as a diagnostic fluid. Annals of the New York Academy of Sciences, 694,* 177–183.

Dachowski, L., & Flaherty, C. F. (Eds.). (1991). *Current topics in animal learning: Brain, emotion, and cognition.* Hillsdale, NJ: Erlbaum.

Dallett, K. M. (1962). The transfer surface re-examined. *Journal of Verbal Learning and Verbal Behavior, 1,* 91–94.

Danziger, K. (1997). *Naming the mind: How psychology found its language.* Thousand Oaks, CA: Sage.

Darley, J. M., Glucksberg, S., & Kinchla, R. A. (1986). *Psychology.* 3rd ed. Englewood Cliffs, NJ: Prentice-Hall.

Darwin, C. (1972/1965). *The expression of emotion in man and animals.* London: John Murray.

Davidson, J., Ekman, P., Saron, D., Senulis, A., & Friesen, W. V. (1990). Approach-withdrawal and cerebral asymmetry: Emotional expression and brain physiology. *Journal of Personality and Social Psychology, 58,* 330–341.

Davidson, R. J. (1984). Affect, cognition, and hemispheric specialization. In C. E. Izard, J. Kagan, & R. B. Zajonc (Eds.), *Emotions, cognition, and behavior.* New York: Cambridge University Press. Pp. 320–365.

Davidson, R. J. (1992). Emotion and affective style: Hemispheric substrates. *Psychological Science, 3,* 39–43.

Davidson, R. J. (1993). Cerebral asymmetry and emotion: Conceptual and methodological conundrums. *Cognition and Emotion, 7,* 115–138.

Davidson, R. J. (1994). Asymmetric brain function, affective style, and psychopathology: The role of early experience and plasticity. *Development and Psychopathology, 6,* 741–758.

Davidson, R. J. (1995). Cerebral asymmetry, emotion and affective style. In R. J. Davidson & K. Hugdahl (Eds.), *Brain asymmetry.* Cambridge, MA: MIT Press. Pp. 361–387.

Davidson, R. J., & Fox, N. A. (1982). Asymmetrical brain activity discriminates between positive versus negative affective stimuli in human infants. *Science, 218,* 1235–1237.

Davidson, R. J., & Fox, N. A. (1989). Frontal brain asymmetry predicts infants' response to maternal separation. *Journal of Abnormal Psychology, 98,* 127–131.

Davidson, R. J., & Tomarken, A. J. (1989). Laterality and emotion: An electrophysiological approach. In F. Boller & J. Grafman (Eds.), *Handbook of neuropsychology.* Vol. 3. Amsterdam: Elsevier. Pp. 419–441.

Davidson, R. J., Schwartz, G. E., Saron, C., Bennett, J., & Goleman, D. J. (1979). Frontal versus parietal EEG asymmetry during positive and negative affect. *Psychophysiology, 16,* 202–203.

Dawkins, R. (1989). *The selfish gene.* 2nd ed. New York: Oxford University Press.

Dawson, G., Klinger, L. G., Panagiotides, H., Hill, D., & Spieker, S. (1992). Frontal lobe activity and affective behavior of infants of mothers with depressive symptoms. *Child Development, 63,* 725–737.

de Castro, J. M. (1987). Circadian rhythms of the spontaneous meal pattern, macronutrient intake, and mood of humans. *Physiology & Behavior, 40,* 437–446.

de Castro, J. M. (1988). Physiological, environmental, and subjective determinants of food intake in humans: A meal pattern analysis. *Physiology & Behavior, 44,* 651–659.

de Castro, J. M. (1991). Bout pattern analysis of ad libitum fluid intake. In D. J. Ramsay & D. Booth (Eds.), *Thirst: Physiological and psychological aspects.* New York: Springer Verlag. Pp. 345–353.

de Castro, J. M., & Elmore, D. K. (1988). Subjective hunger relationships with meal patterns in the spontaneous

feeding behavior of humans: Evidence for a causal connection. *Physiology & Behavior, 43,* 159–168.

De Giorgio, R., Stanghellini, V., Maccarini, M. R., Morselli-Labate, A. M., Barbara, G., Franzoso, L., Rovati, L. C., Corinaldesi, R., Barbara, L., & Go, V. L. W. (1994). Effects of dietary fat on postprandial gastrointestinal motility are inhibited by a cholecystokinin Type A receptor antagonist. In J. R. Reeve, Jr., V. Eysselein, T. E. Solomon, & V. 1. W. Go (Eds.), *Cholecystokinin.* Vol. 713. *Annals of the New York Academy of Sciences.* New York: New York Academy of Sciences. Pp. 226–231.

Deaux, K. (1995). How basic can you be? The evolution of research on gender stereotypes. *Journal of Social Issues, 51,* 11–20.

DeCharms, R. (1968). *Personal causation: The internal affective determinants of behavior.* New York: Academic Press.

Deci, E. L. (1971). The effects of externally mediated rewards on intrinsic motivation. *Journal of Personality and Social Psychology, 18,* 105–115.

Deci, E. L. (1972). Intrinsic motivation, extrinsic reinforcement, and inequity. *Journal of Personality and Social Psychology, 22,* 113–120.

Deci, E. L. (1975). *Intrinsic motivation.* New York: Plenum Press.

Deci, E. L. (1980). *The psychology of self-determination.* Lexington, MA: D.C. Heath (Lexington Books).

Deci, E. L., & Ryan, R. M. (1991). A motivational approach to self: Integration in personality. In R. A. Dienstbier (Ed.), *Nebraska symposium on motivation, 1990.* Vol. 38. Lincoln: University of Nebraska Press. Pp. 237–288.

Deci, E. L., Betley, G., Kahle, J., Abrams, L., & Porac, J. (1981). When trying to win: Competition and intrinsic motivation. *Personality and Social Psychology Bulletin, 7,* 79–83.

Deci, E. L., Eghrari, H., Patrick, B. C., & Leone, D. R. (1994). Facilitating internalization: The self-determination theory perspective. *Journal of Personality, 62,* 119–142.

Deffenbacher, J. L. (1988). Cognitive-relaxation and social skills treatments of anger: A year later. *Journal of Counseling Psychology, 35,* 234–236.

Deffenbacher, J. L. (1992). Trait anger: Theory, findings, and implications. In C. D. Spielberger & J. N. Butcher (Eds.), *Advances in personality assessment.* Vol. 9. Hillsdale, NJ: Erlbaum. Pp. 177–201.

Delgado, J. M. R., & Mir, D. (1969). Fragmental organization of emotional behavior in the monkey brain. *Annals of the New York Academy of Sciences, 159,* 731–751.

Denenberg, V. H. (1964). Critical periods, stimulus input and emotional reactivity: A theory of infantile stimulation. *Psychological Review, 71,* 335–351.

Derakshan, N., & Eysenck, M. W. (1997). Interpretive biases for one's own behavior and physiology in high-trait-anxious individuals and repressors. *Journal of Personality and Social Psychology, 73,* 816–825.

Derryberry, D. (1989). Effects of goal-related motivational states on the orienting of spatial attention. *Acta Psychologica, 72,* 199–220.

Derryberry, D. (1993). Attentional consequences of outcome-related motivational states: Congruent, incongruent, and focusing effects. *Motivation and Emotion, 17,* 65–89.

Dess, N. K. (1997). Ingestion after stress: Evidence for a regulatory shift in food-rewarded operant performance. *Learning and Motivation, 28,* 342–356.

Dess, N. K., & Overmier, J. B. (1989). General learned irrelevance: Proactive effects on Pavlovian conditioning in dogs. *Learning and Motivation, 20,* 1–14.

DeToledo, L., & Black, A. H. (1967). Effects of preshock on subsequent avoidance conditioning. *Journal of Comparative and Physiological Psychology, 63,* 493–499.

Deutsch, J. A. (1990). Food intake: Gastric factors. In E. M. Stricker (Ed.), *Neurobiology of food and fluid intake. Handbook of behavioral neurobiology. Vol. 10.* New York: Plenum Press. Pp. 151–182.

Deutsch, M., & Kraus, R. M. (1962). Studies of interpersonal bargaining. *Journal of Conflict Resolution, 6,* 52–76.

DeVore, I. (1965). Male dominance and mating behavior in baboons. In F. A. Beach (Ed.), *Sex and behavior.* New York: Wiley.

Dickinson, A., & Balleine, B. (1990). Motivational control of instrumental performance following a shift from thirst to hunger. *The Quarterly Journal of Experimental Psychology, 42B,* 413–431.

Dickinson, A., & Balleine, B. (1994). Motivational control of goal-directed action. *Animal Learning and Behavior, 22,* 1–18.

Dickinson, A., & Balleine, B. (1995). Motivational control of instrumental action. *Current Directions in Psychological Science, 4,* 162–167.

Dickinson, A., & Dawson, G. R. (1989). Incentive learning and the motivational control of instrumental performance. *The Quarterly Journal of Experimental Psychology, 41B,* 99–112.

Diener, E., & Emmons, R. A. (1984). The independence of positive and negative affect. *Journal of Personality and Social Psychology, 47,* 1105–1117.

Diener, E., Larsen, R. J., Levine, S., & Emmons, R. A. (1985). Intensity and frequency: Dimensions underlying positive and negative affect. *Journal of Personality and Social Psychology, 48,* 1253–1265.

Diener, E., Smith, H., & Fujita, F. (1995). The personality structure of affect. *Journal of Personality and Social Psychology, 69,* 130–141.

Dijk, D. J., & Czeisler, C. A. (1995). Contribution of the circadian pacemaker and the sleep homeostat to sleep propensity, sleep structure, electroencephalographic slow waves, and sleep spindle activity in humans. *Journal of Neuroscience, 15,* 3526–3538.

Dill, J. C., & Anderson, C. A. (1995). Effects of frustration justification on hostile aggression. *Aggressive Behavior, 21,* 359–369.

Dinkmeyer, D., & Dreikurs, R. (1963). *Encouraging children to learn: The encouragement process.* Englewood Cliffs, NJ: Prentice-Hall.

Dinsmoor, J. A., & Campbell, S. L. (1956). Escape-from-shock training following exposure to inescapable shock. *Psychological Reports, 2,* 43–49.

Docter, R. F. (1988). *Transvestites and transsexuals: Toward a theory of cross-gender behavior.* New York: Plenum Press.

Dodge, K. A., Pettit, G. S., Bates, J. E., & Valente, E. (1995). Social information-processing patterns partially mediate the effect of early physical abuse on later conduct problems. *Journal of Abnormal Psychology, 104,* 632–643.

Dodson, J. D. (1915). The relation of strength of stimulus to rapidity of habit-formation in the kitten. *Journal of Animal Behavior, 5,* 330–336.

Dohanich, G. D. (1995). Cholinergic regulation of female sexual behavior. In P. E. Micevych & R. P. Hammer (Eds.), *Neurobiological effects of sex steroid hormones.* New York: Cambridge University Press. Pp. 184–206.

Dohanich, G. D., Ross, S. M., Francis, T. J., Fader, A. J., Wee, B. E. F., Brazier, M. M., & Menard, C. S. (1993). The effects of a muscarinic antagonist on various components of female sexual behavior. *Behavioral Neuroscience, 107,* 818–826.

Dollard, J., Doob, L. W., Miller, N. E., Mowrer, O. H., & Sears, R. R. (1961). *Frustration and aggression.* New Haven, CT: Yale University Press.

Dominowski, R. L., & Ekstrand, B. R. (1967). Direct and associative priming in anagram solving. *Journal of Experimental Psychology, 74,* 84–86.

Domjan, M. (1992). Adult learning and mate choice: Possibilities and experimental evidence. *American Zoologist, 32,* 48–61.

Domjan, M. (1998). *The principles of learning and behavior.* 4th ed. Pacific Grove, CA: Brooks/Cole.

Donnerstein, E. (1980). Aggressive erotica and violence against women. *Journal of Personality and Social Psychology, 39,* 269–277.

Dougherty, D. M., & Cherek, D. R. (1994). Effects of social context, reinforcer probability, and reinforcer magnitude on humans' choices to compete or not to compete. *Journal of the Experimental Analysis of Behavior, 62,* 133–148.

Douvan, E. (1956). Social class and success strivings. *Journal of Abnormal and Social Psychology, 52,* 219–223.

Dreikurs, R. (1946/1990). *The challenge of marriage.* New York: New American Library.

Dreikurs, R. (1947). The four goals of children's misbehavior. *Nervous Child, 6,* 3–11.

Dreikurs, R. (1948/1990). *The challenge of parenthood.* New York: New American Library.

Dreikurs, R. (1950/1992). *Fundamentals of Adlerian psychology.* Chicago: Adler School of Professional Psychology.

Dreikurs, R. (1960). *Group psychotherapy and group approaches: Collected papers.* Chicago: Adler School of Professional Psychology.

Dreikurs, R. (1967a). Guilt feelings as an excuse. In R. Dreikurs (Ed.), *Psychodynamics, psychotherapy, and counseling.* Chicago: Adler School of Professional Psychology. Pp. 229–239.

Dreikurs, R. (1967b). The function of emotions. In R. Dreikurs (Ed.), *Psychodynamics, psychotherapy, and counseling.* Chicago: Adler School of Professional Psychology. Pp. 205–217.

Dreikurs, R. (1969). Social interest: The basis of normalcy. *Counseling Psychologist, 1,* 45–48.

Dreikurs, R. (1971/1992). *Social equality: The challenge of today.* Chicago: Adler School of Professional Psychology.

Dreikurs, R. (1972). Family counseling: A demonstration. *Journal of Individual Psychology, 28,* 202–222.

Dreikurs, R. (1982). The function of emotions. In R. Dreikurs (Ed.), *Psychodynamics, psychotherapy, and counseling.* Chicago: Adler School of Professional Psychology.

Dreikurs, R. (1992). *The challenge of parenthood.* New York: Penguin.

Dreikurs, R. (1999). *The challenge of marriage.* Philadelphia: Taylor & Francis.

Dreikurs, R., & Cassel, P. (1990). *Discipline without tears.* New York: Dutton-Penguin.

Dreikurs, R., & Grey, L. (1992). *Logical consequences: A new approach to discipline.* New York: Penguin.

Dreikurs, R., & Mosak, H. H. (1966). The tasks of life. I.

Adler's three tasks. *Individual Psychologist, 4,* 18–22.

Dreikurs, R., & Soltz, V. (1992). *Children: The challenge.* New York: Penguin.

Dreikurs, R., Grunwald, B. B., & Pepper, F. C. (1998). *Maintaining sanity in the classroom: Classroom management techniques.* 2nd ed. Washington, DC: Taylor & Francis.

Drewnowski, A. (1991). Obesity and eating disorders: Cognitive aspects of food preference and food aversion. *Bulletin of the Psychonomic Society, 29,* 261–264.

Drewnowski, A. (1996). The behavioral phenotype in human obesity. In E. D. Capaldi (Ed.), *Why we eat what we eat: The psychology of eating.* Washington, DC: American Psychological Association. Pp. 291–308.

Driscoll, J. M., & Yankeelov, P. A. (1995). Feelings of mastery in high aggression-history aggressors. *Journal of Social Behavior and Personality, 10,* 693–706.

Duffy, E. (1932). The measurement of muscular tension as a technique for the study of emotional tendencies. *American Journal of Psychology, 44,* 146–162.

Duffy, E. (1934). Emotion: An example of the need for reorientation in psychology. *Psychological Review, 41,* 184–198.

Duffy, E. (1941). An explanation of "emotional" phenomena without the use of the concept "emotion." *Journal of General Psychology, 25,* 283–293.

Duffy, E. (1951). The concept of energy mobilization. *Psychological Review, 58,* 30–40.

Duffy, E. (1957). The psychological significance of the concept of "arousal" or "activation." *Psychological Review, 64,* 265–275.

Duffy, E. (1962). *Activation and behavior.* New York: Wiley.

Duffy, V. B., & Bartoshuk, L. M. (1996). Sensory factors in feeding. In E. D. Capaldi (Ed.), *Why we eat what we eat: The psychology of eating.* Washington, DC: American Psychological Association. Pp. 145–170.

Dunne, M. P., Martin, N. G., Statham, D. J., Slutske, W. S., Dinwiddie, S. H., Bucholz, K. K., Madden, P. A. F., & Heath, A. C. (1997). Genetic and environmental contributions to variance in age at first sexual intercourse. *Psychological Science, 8,* 211–216.

Dunning, D., Leuenberger, A., & Sherman, D. A. (1995). A new look at motivated inference: Are self-serving theories of success a product of motivational forces? *Journal of Personality and Social Psychology, 69,* 58–68.

Dweck, C. S. (1991). Self-theories and goals: Their role in motivation, personality, and development. In R. A.

Dienstbier (Ed.), *Nebraska symposium on motivation, 1990.* Vol. 38. Lincoln: University of Nebraska Press. Pp. 199–235.

Dweck, C. S. (1992). The study of goals in psychology. *Psychological Science, 3,* 165–167.

Eason, R. G., & Dudley, L. M. (1970). Physiological and behavioral indicants of activation. *Psychophysiology, 7,* 223–232.

Easterbrook, J. A. (1959). The effect of emotion on cue utilization and the organization of behavior. *Psychological Review, 66,* 183–201.

Eastman, C. I. (1990). Natural summer and winter sunlight exposure patterns in seasonal affective disorder. *Physiology and Behavior, 48,* 611–616.

Eastman, C. I., Hoese, E. K., Youngstedt, S. D., & Liu, L. (1995). Phase-shifting human circadian rhythms with exercise during the night shift. *Physiology and Behavior, 58,* 1287–1291.

Eccles (Parsons), J. (1983). Expectancies, values, and academic behavior. In J. T. Spence (Ed.), *Achievement and achievement motivation.* San Fracisco: W. H. Freeman. Pp. 75–146.

Eccles, J. (1985). Sex differences in achievement patterns. In T. B. Sonderegger (Ed.), *Nebraska Symposium on Motivation, 1984.* Vol. 32. Lincoln: University of Nebraska Press. Pp. 97–132.

Eccles, J. S. (1984). Sex differences in achievement patterns. In T. Sonderegger (Ed.), *Nebraska symposium on motivation.* Vol. 32. Lincoln: University of Nebraska Press. Pp. 97–132.

Eccles, J. S. (1993). School and family effects on the ontogeny of children's interests, self-perceptions, and activity choices. In J. E. Jacobs (Ed.), *Nebraska Symposium on Motivation 1992.* Vol. 40. Lincoln: University of Nebraska Press. Pp. 145–208.

Eccles, J. S., & Wigfield, A. (1995). In the mind of the actor: The structure of adolescents' achievement task values and expectancy-related beliefs. *Personality and Social Psychology Bulletin, 21,* 215–225.

Edgar, D. M., Dement, C., & Fuller, C. A. (1993). Effect of SCN lesions on sleep in squirrel monkeys: Evidence for opponent processes in sleep-wake regulation. *Journal of Neuroscience, 13,* 1065–1079.

Ehrenfreund, D. (1971). Effect of drive on successive magnitude shift in rats. *Journal of Comparative and Physiological Psychology, 72,* 418–423.

Ehrhardt, A. A. (1985). Gender differences: A biosocial perspective. In T. B. Sonderegger (Ed.), *Nebraska Symposium on Motivation, 1984.* Vol. 32. Lincoln: University of Nebraska Press. Pp. 37–57.

Eibl-Eibesfeldt, I. (1972). *Love and hate: The natural history of behavior patterns.* New York: Holt, Hinehart, and Winston.

Eisler, R. M., & Blalock, J. A. (1991). Masculine gender role stress. Implications for the assessment of men. *Clinical Psychology Review, 11,* 45–60.

Ekman, P. (1972) Universals and cultural differences in facial expressions of emotion. In J. K. Cole (Ed.), *Nebraska symposium on motivation, 1971.* Vol. 19. Lincoln: University of Nebraska Press. Pp. 207–283.

Ekman, P. (1984). Expression and the nature of emotion. In K. S. Scherer & P. Ekman (Eds.), *Approaches to emotion.* Hillsdale, NJ: Erlbaum.

Ekman, P. (1989). The argument and evidence about universals in facial expressions of emotion. In H. Wagner & A. Manstead (Eds.), *Handbook of social psychophysiology.* New York: Wiley. Pp. 143–163.

Ekman, P. (1992a). An argument for basic emotions. *Cognition and Emotion, 6,* 169–200.

Ekman, P. (1992b). Are there basic emotions? *Psychological Review, 99,* 550–553.

Ekman, P. (1992c). Facial expressions of emotion: An old controversy and new findings. *Philosophical Transactions of the Royal Society of London, Series B, 335,* 63–69.

Ekman, P. (1992d). Facial expressions of emotion: New findings, new questions. *Psychological Science, 3,* 34–38.

Ekman, P. (1993). Facial expression and emotion. *American Psychologist, 48,* 384–392.

Ekman, P. (1994a). All emotions are basic. In P. Ekman & R. J. Davidson (Eds.), *The nature of emotion: Fundamental questions.* New York: Oxford University Press. Pp. 15–19.

Ekman, P. (1994b). Strong evidence for universals in facial expressions: A reply to Russell's mistaken critique. *Psychological Bulletin, 115,* 268–287.

Ekman, P., & Friesen, W. V. (1982). Felt, false, and miserable smiles. *Journal of Nonverbal Behavior, 6,* 238–252.

Ekman, P., Davidson, R. J., & Friesen, W. V. (1990). The Duchenne smile: Emotional expression and brain physiology II. *Journal of Personality and Social Psychology, 58,* 342–353.

Ekman, P., Friesen, W. V., & Ancoli, S. (1980). Facial signs of emotional experience. *Journal of Personality and Social Psychology, 39,* 1125–1134.

Ekman, P., Friesen, W. V., & Ellsworth, P. (1972). *Emotion in the human face.* New York: Pergamon Press.

Ekman, P., Levenson, R. W., & Friesen, W. V. (1983). Autonomic nervous system activity distinguishes among emotions. *Science, 221,* 1208–1210.

Elliott, E. S., & Dweck, C. S. (1988). Goals: An approach to motivation and achievement. *Journal of Personality and Social Psychology, 54,* 5–12.

Ellis, A., & Dryden, W. (1997). *The practice of rational emotive behavior therapy.* 2nd ed. New York: Springer.

Ellis, H. C., & Ashbrook, P. W. (1988). Resource allocation model of the effects of depressed mood states on memory. In K. Fiedler & J. Forgas (Eds.), *Affect, cognition and social behavior: New evidence and integrative attempts.* Zurich: C. J. Hogrefe. Pp. 25–43.

Ellis, H. C., & Hunt, R. R. (1989). *Fundamentals of human learning and cognition.* 4th ed. Dubuque, IA: Wm. C. Brown.

Ellis, H. C., Ottaway, S. A., Varner, L. J., Becker, A. S., & Moore, B. A. (1997). Emotion, motivation, and text comprehension: The detection of contradiction in passages. *Journal of Experimental Psychology: General, 126,* 131–146.

Ellis, H. C., Thomas, R. L., & Rodriguez, I. A. (1984). Emotional mood states and memory: Elaborative encoding, semantic processing, and cognitive effort. *Journal of Experimental Psychology: Learning, Memory, and Cognition, 10,* 470–482.

Ellison, G. D., & Potthoff, A. D. (1983). Social models of drinking behavior in animals: The importance of individual differences. In M. Glanater (Ed.), *Recent developments in alcoholism.* Vol. 2. New York: Plenum Press. Pp. 17–36.

Elms, A. C. (1995). Obedience in retrospect. *Journal of Social Issues, 51,* 21–31.

Emery, R. E., & Laumann-Billings, L. L. (1998). An overview of the nature, causes, and consequences of abusive family relationships. *American Psychologist, 53,* 121–135.

Emmons, R. A. (1989). The personal striving approach to personality. In L. A. Pervin (Ed.), *Goal concepts in personality and social psychology.* Hillsdale, NJ: Erlbaum. Pp. 87–126.

Emmons, R. A., & Diener, E. (1985). Personality correlates of subjective well-being. *Personality and Social Psychology Bulletin, 11,* 89–97.

Emmons, R. A., & Diener, E. (1986). A goal-affect analysis of everyday situational choices. *Journal of Research in Personality, 20,* 309–326.

Emmons, R. A., & King, L. A. (1989). Personal striving differentiation and affective reactivity. *Journal of Personality and Social Psychology, 56,* 478–484.

Endler, N. S., Edwards, J. M., Vitelli, R., & Parker, J. D. A. (1989). Assessment of state and trait anxiety: Endler Multidimensional Anxiety Scales. *Anxiety Research, 2,* 1–14.

Engel, B. T. (1959). Some physiological correlates of hunger and pain. *Journal of Experimental Psychology, 57,* 389–396.

Enright, T. E. (1981). Methodology. In J. Aschoff (Ed.). *Handbook of behavioral neurobiology, Vol 4: Biological rhythms.* New York: Plenum Press. Pp. 11–19.

Enzle, M. E., Hansen, R. D., & Lowe, C. A. (1975). Causal attribution in the mixed-motive game: Effects of facilitory and inhibitory environmental forces. *Journal of Personality and Social Psychology, 31,* 50–54.

Epstein, A. N. (1960). Reciprocal changes in feeding behavior produced by intrahypothalamic chemical injections. *American Journal of Physiology, 199,* 969–974.

Epstein, A. N. (1990). Prospectus: Thirst and salt appetite. In E. M. Stricker (Ed.), *Neurobiology of food and fluid intake. Handbook of behavioral neurobiology. Vol. 10.* New York: Plenum Press. Pp. 489–512.

Epstein, L. H., & Wing, R. R. (1987). Behavioral treatment of childhood obesity. *Psychological Bulletin, 101,* 331–342.

Ervin, G. N. (1994). Cholecystokinin and satiety: A time line. In J. R. Reeve, Jr., V. Eysslelein, T. E. Solomon, & V. 1. W. Go (Eds.), *Cholecystokinin. Vol. 713. Annals of the New York Academy of Sciences.* New York: New York Academy of Sciences. Pp. 232–235.

Erwin, R. J., & Ferguson, E. D. (1979). The effect of food and water deprivation and satiation on recognition. *American Journal of Psychology, 92,* 611–626.

Eskin, A. (1979). Identification and physiology of circadian pacemakers. *Federation Proceedings, 38,* 2570–2572.

Estes, W. K., & Skinner, B. F. (1941). Some quantitative properties of anxiety. *Journal of Experimental Psychology, 29,* 390–400.

Esteves, F., Parra, C., Dimberg, U., & Ohman, A. (1994). Nonconscious associative learning: Pavlovian conditioning of skin conductance responses to masked fear-relevant facial stimuli. *Psychophysiology, 31,* 375–385.

Evans, K. R., & Vaccarino, F. J. (1990). Amphetamine- and morphine-induced feeding: Evidence for involvement of reward mechanisms. *Neuroscience & Biobehavioral Reviews, 14,* 9–22.

Evans, T. D. (1989). *The art of encouragement.* Athens: University of Georgia.

Evans, T. D. (1995). The encouraging teacher. In G. M. Gazda, F. S. Asbury, F. M. Blazer, W. C. Childers, & R. P. Walters (Eds.)., *Human relations development.* 5th ed. Boston: Allyn & Bacon. Pp. 261–270.

Evans, T. D. (1996). Encouragement: The key to reforming classrooms. *Educational Leadership, 54,* 81–85.

Exline, R. (1972). Visual interaction: The glances of power and preference. In J. K. Cole (Ed.), *Nebraska symposium on motivation, 1971.* Vol. 19. Lincoln: University of Nebraska Press. Pp. 163–206.

Exline, R. V., Thibaut, J., Hickey, C. B., & Gumpert, P. (1970). Visual interaction in relation to Machiavellianism and an unethical act. In R. Christie & F. Geis, *Studies in Machiavellianism.* New York: Academic Press. Pp. 53–75.

Eysenck, H. J. (1967). *The biological basis of personality.* Springfield, IL: Charles C. Thomas.

Eysenck, M. W. (1984). Anxiety and the worry process. *Bulletin of the Psychonomic Society, 22,* 545–548.

Eysenck, M. W. (1987a). *A handbook of cognitive psychology.* Hillsdale, NJ: Erlbaum.

Eysenck, M. W. (1987b). Trait theories of anxiety. In J. Strelau & H. J. Eysenck (Eds.), *Personality dimensions and arousal.* New York: Plenum Press.

Eysenck, M. W. (1991). Trait anxiety and cognition. In C. D. Spielberger, I. G. Sarason, Z. Kulcsar, & G. L. Van Heck (Eds.), *Stress and emotion: Anxiety, anger, and curiosity.* Vol. 14. New York: Hemisphere. Pp. 77–84.

Eysenck, M. W. (1997). *Anxiety and cognition: A unified theory.* Hove, England: Psychology Press.

Fagot, B. I., & Leinbach, M. D. (1995). Gender knowledge in eqalitarian and traditional families. *Sex Roles, 32,* 513–526.

Fallon, A. E., & Rozin, P. (1985). Sex differences in perceptions of desirable body shape. *Journal of Abnormal Psychology, 94,* 102–105.

Fanselow, M. S. (1994). Neural organization of the defensive behavior system responsible for fear. *Psychonomic Bulletin and Review, 1,* 429–438.

Fanselow, M. S., DeCola, J. P., De Oca, B. M., & Landeira-Fernandez, J. (1995). Ventral and dorsolateral regions of the midbrain periaqueductal gray (PAG) control different stages of defensive behavior: Dorsolateral PAG lesions enhance the defensive freezing produced by massed and immediate shock. *Aggressive Behavior, 21,* 63–77.

Fanselow, M. S., Landeira-Fernandez, J., DeCola, J. P., & Kim, J. J. (1994). The immediate-shock deficit and postshock analgesis: Implications for the relationship between the analgesic CR and UR. *Animal Learning and Behavior, 22,* 72–76.

Fantino, E., Kasdon, D., & Stringer, N. (1970). The Yerkes-Dodson Law and alimentary motivation. *Canadian Journal of Psychology, 24,* 77–84.

Faris, P. L., Raymond, N. C., De Zwaan, M., Howard, L. A., Eckert, E. D., & Mitchell, J. E. (1992). Nociceptive, but not tactile, thresholds are elevated in bulimia nervosa. *Biological Psychiatry, 32,* 462–466.

Feather, N. T. (1961). The relationship of persistence at a task to expectation of success and achievement related motive. *Journal of Abnormal and Social Psychology, 63,* 552–561.

Feather, N. T. (1964). Level of aspiration behaviour in relation to payoffs and costs following success and failure. *Australian Journal of Psychology, 16,* 175–184.

Feather, N. T. (1965). The relationship of expectation of success to need achievement and test anxiety. *Journal of Personality and Social Psychology, 1,* 118–126.

Feather, N. T. (1988). From values to actions: Recent applications of the expectancy-value model. *Australian Journal of Psychology, 40,* 105–124.

Feather, N. T. (1991). Human values, global self-esteem, and belief in a just world. *Journal of Personality, 59,* 83–107.

Feather, N. T. (1992). Values, valences, expectations, and actions. *Journal of Social Issues, 48,* 109–124.

Feather, N. T. (1993). The rise and fall of political leaders: Attributions, deservingness, personality, and affect. *Australian Journal of Psychology, 45,* 61–68.

Feather, N. T. (1995). Values, valences, and choice: The influence of values on the perceived attractiveness and choice of alternatives. *Journal of Personality and Social Psychology, 68,* 1135–1151.

Feather, N. T., & Simon, J. G. (1971). Attribution of responsibility and valence of outcome in relation to initial confidence and success and failure of self and other. *Journal of Personality and Social Psychology, 18,* 173–188.

Feeney, J. A., & Noller, P. (1992). Attachment style and romantic love: Relationship dissolution. *Australian Journal of Psychology, 44,* 69–74.

Ferguson, E. D. (1957). An evaluation of two types of kindergarten attendance programs. *Journal of Educational Psychology, 48,* 287–301.

Ferguson, E. D. (1958). The effect of sibling competition and alliance on level of aspiration, expectation, and performance. *Journal of Abnormal and Social Psychology, 56,* 213–222.

Ferguson, E. D. (1962). Ego involvement: A critical examination of some methodological issues. *Journal of Abnormal and Social Psychology, 64,* 407–417.

Ferguson, E. D. (1982). *Motivation: An experimental approach.* Melbourne, FL: Krieger.

Ferguson, E. D. (1983a). Effect of motivation on position

and location judgments under lateral and foveal viewing. *Bulletin of the Psychonomic Society, 21,* 355 (Abstract).

Ferguson, E. D. (1983b). The effect of motivation and word characteristics on recognition. *American Journal of Psychology, 96,* 253–266.

Ferguson, E. D. (1984). Hemispheric asymmetry, field of viewing, and motivation affect word processing. Paper presented at the Psychonomic Society convention, November 10, 1984, Sant Antonio, TX.

Ferguson, E. D. (1987). Anxiety as avoidance: Defensive information processing as measured by decreased information intake in habituation to a tone. *Perceptual and Motor Skills, 65,* 301–302.

Ferguson, E. D. (1988). Motivational influences on word recognition: I. Foveal and parafoveal viewing. *Bulletin of the Psychonomic Society, 26,* 203–205.

Ferguson, E. D. (1989a). Adler's motivational theory: An historical perspective on belonging and the fundamental human striving. *Individual Psychology: The Journal of Adlerian Theory, Research & Practice, 45,* 354–361.

Ferguson, E. D. (1989b). Motivational influences on word recognition: II. Affective coding. *Bulletin of the Psychonomic Society, 27,* 307–310.

Ferguson, E. D. (1992a). Motivational influences on word recognition: III. Parafoveal processing differs from foveal processing. *Bulletin of the Psychonomic Society, 30,* 47–50.

Ferguson, E. D. (1992b). Parafoveal-foveal differences: Motivation and word characteristic effects. Paper presented at the XXV International Congress of Psychology, July 21, 1992, Brussels, Belgium.

Ferguson, E. D. (1993a). Motivational influences on word recognition: IV. Cortical magnification does not explain parafoveal versus foveal differences. *Bulletin of the Psychonomic Society, 31,* 602–604.

Ferguson, E. D. (1993b). Why do I drink? Am I thirsty? Is it me or my brain you're trying to explain? *Contemporary Psychology, 38,* 962–963.

Ferguson, E. D. (1995). *Adlerian theory: An introduction.* Chicago: Adler School of Professional Psychology.

Ferguson, E. D. (1996). Adlerian principles and methods apply to workplace problems. *Individual Psychology, 52,* 270–287.

Ferguson, E. D. (Ed.). (1989/1991). *Equality and social interest: A book of lectures from 1988 ICASSI in Greece.* Zurich: ICASSI. Chicago: Alfred Adler Institute.

Ferguson, E. D. & Schmitt, S. (1988). Gender-linked stereotypes and motivation affect performance in the Prisoner's Dilemma Game. *Perceptual and Motor Skills, 66,* 703–714.

Ferster, C. B., & DeMyer, M. K. (1962). A method for the experimental analysis of the behavior of autistic children. *The American Journal of Orthopsychiatry, 32,* 89–98.

Ferster, C. B., & Skinner, B. F. (1957). *Schedules of reinforcement.* New York: Appleton-Century-Crofts.

Festinger, L. (1942). Wish, expectation, and group standards as factors influencing level of aspiration. *Journal of Abnormal and Social Psychology, 37,* 184–200.

Fiedler, K., & Forgas, J. (1987). *Affect, cognition and social behavior.* Toronto: C. J. Hogrefe.

Field, T. (1996). Attachment and separation in young children. *Annual Review of Psychology, 47,* 541–561.

Finger, F. W., Reid, L. S., & Weasner, M. H. (1960). Activity changes as a function of reinforcement under low drive. *Journal of Comparative and Physiological Psychology, 53,* 385–387.

Finn, P. R., Sharkansky, E. J., Viken, R., West, T. L., Sandy, J., & Bufferd, G. M. (1997). Heterogeneity in the families of sons of alcoholics: The impact of familial vulnerability type on offspring characteristics. *Journal of Abnormal Psychology, 106,* 26–36.

Fischer, K. W., Shaver, P. R., & Carnochan, P. (1990). How emotions develop and how they organize development. *Cognition & Emotion, 4,* 81–127.

Fisher, E. B. Jr., Lichtenstein, E., & Haire-Joshu, D. (1993). Multiple determinants of tobacco use and cessation. In C. T. Orelans & J. Slade (Eds.), *Nicotine addiction: Principles and management.* New York: Oxford University Press. Pp. 59–88.

Fiske, S. T., & Glick, P. (1995). Ambivalence and stereotypes cause sexual harassment: A theory with implications for organizational change. *Journal of Social Issues, 51,* 97–115.

Fitzsimons, J. T. (1979). *The physiology of thirst and sodium appetite.* Cambridge: Cambridge University Press.

Fitzsimons, J. T. (1991). Evolution of physiological and behavioural mechanisms in vertebrate body fluid homeostasis. In D. J. Ramsay and D. A. Booth (Eds.), *Thirst: Physiological and psychological aspects.* New York: Springer. Pp. 3–22.

Flier, J. S., Cook, K. S., Usher, P., & Spiegelman, B. M. (1987). Severely impaired adipsin expression in genetic and acquired obesity. *Science, 237,* 405–408.

Flynn, J. P. (1967). The neural basis of aggression in cats. In D. C. Glass (Ed.), *Neurophysiology and emotion.* New York: Rockefeller University Press. Pp. 40–60.

Flynn, J. P. (1973). Patterning mechanisms, patterned reflexes, and attack behavior in cats. *Nebraska symposium on motivation, 1972.* Vol. 20. Lincoln: University of Nebraska Press. Pp. 125–153.

Folkard, S., Hume, K. I., Minors, D. S., Waterhouse, J. M., & Watson, F. L. (1985). Independence of the circadian rhythm in alertness from the sleep/wake cycle. *Nature, 313,* 678–679.

Folkard, S., Marks, M., & Froberg, J. E. (1986). Towards a causal nexus of human psychophysiological variables based on their circadian rhythmicity. *Revija za psihologiju, 16,* 1–9.

Folkard, S., Marks, M., Minors, D. S., & Waterhouse, J. M. (1985). Circadian rhythms in human performance and affective state. *Acta Psychiatrica Belgica, 85,* 568–581.

Folkard, S., Minors, D. S., & Waterhouse, J. M. (1985). Chronobiology and shift work: Current issues and trends. *Chronobiologia, 12,* 31–54.

Folkard, S., Wever, R. A., & Wildgruber, C. M. (1983). Multi-oscillatory control of circadian rhythms in human performance. *Nature, 305,* 223–226.

Folkman, S., & Lazarus, R. S. (1988). The relationship between coping and emotion: Implications for theory and research. *Social Science in Medicine, 26,* 309–317.

Folkman, S., & Lazarus, R. S. (1990). Coping and emotion. In N. Stein, B. Leventhal, & T. Trabasso (Eds.), *Psychological and biological approaches to emotion.* Hillsdale, NJ: Erlbaum. Pp. 313–332.

Forgas, J. P., & Bower, G. H. (1987). Mood effects on person perception judgments. *Journal of Personality and Social Psychology, 53,* 53–60.

Forgas, J. P., & Bower, G. H. (1988). Affect in social and personal judgments. In K. Fiedler & J. Forgas (Eds.), *Affect, cognition and social behavior: New evidence and integrative attempts.* Zurich: C. J. Hogrefe. Pp. 183–208.

Forgas, J. P., Bower, G. H., & Krantz, S. E. (1984). The influence of mood on the perception of social interaction. *Journal of Experimental Social Psychology, 20,* 497–513.

Foster, R. G. (1998). Shedding light on the biological clock. *Neuron, 20,* 829–832.

Fox, N. A., & Davidson, R. J. (1986). Taste-elicited changes in facial signs of emotion and the asymmetry of brain electrical activity in human newborns. *Neuropsychologia, 24,* 417–422.

Fox, N. A., & Davidson, R. J. (1988). Patterns of brain electrical activity during facial signs of emotion in ten month old infants. *Developmental Psychology, 24,* 230–236.

Frable, D. E. S. (1997). Gender, racial, ethnic, sexual, and class identities. *Annual Review of Psychology, 48,* 139–162.

Frank, L. G., Glickman, S. E., & Zabel, C. J. (1989). Ontogeny of female dominance in the spotted hyaena: Perspectives from nature and captivity. *Symposia of the Zoological Society of London, 61,* 127–146.

Franken, R. E. (1994). *Human motivation.* Pacific Grove, CA: Brooks/Cole.

Frankenhaeuser, M., Lundberg, U., & Fredrikson, M. (1989). Stress on and off the job as related to sex and occupational status in white-collar workers. *Journal of Organizational Behavior, 10,* 321–346.

Freeman, A., & Davison, M. R. (1997). Short-term therapy for the long-term patient. In L. VandeCreek, S. Knapp, & T. L. Jackson (Eds.), *Innovations in clinical practice: A source book.* Vol. 15. Sarasota, FL: Professional Resource Press. Pp. 5–24.

French, J. R. P., Jr., & Raven, B. H. (1959). The bases of social power. In D. Cartwright (Ed.), *Studies in social power.* Ann Arbor, MI: Institute for Social Research. Pp. 150–167.

Freud, S. (1901/1960). *The psychopathology of everyday life.* Vol. 6. London: Hogarth Press.

Freud, S. (1915/1959). *Instincts and their vicissitudes, collected papers* (Vol. 4, Pp. 60–83). New York: Basic Books.

Freud, S. (1920/1938). *A general introduction to psychoanalysis.* Garden City, NY: Garden City Publishing.

Freud, S. (1920/1975). *Beyond the pleasure principle.* New York: Norton.

Freud, S. (1926). *The problem of anxiety.* New York: W. W. Norton.

Freud, S. (1964). *Complete psychological works of Sigmund Freud.* London: Hogarth, 1964.

Friedman, M. I. (1990). Making sense out of calories. In E. M. Stricker (Ed.), *Neurobiology of food and fluid intake. Handbook of behavioral neurobiology.* Vol. 10. New York: Plenum Press. Pp. 513–529.

Friedman, M., & Rosenman, R. H. (1959). Association of specific overt behavior pattern with blood and cardiovascular findings. *Journal of the American Medical Association, 169,* 1286–1296.

Friedman, M., & Rosenman, R. H. (1974). *Type-A behavior and your heart.* New York: Knopf.

Friedman, M., Thoresen, C. E., Gill, J. J., Ulmer, D., Powell, L., Price, V., Brown, B., Thompson, L., Rabin, D. D., Breall, W. S., Gourg, E., Levy, R. A., & Dixon, T. (1986). Alteration of Type A behavior and its effect on cardiac recurrences in post myocardial infarction patients: Summary results of the Recurrent

Coronary Prevention Project. *American Heart Journal, 112,* 653–665.

Frijda, N. H. (1994). Universal antecedents exist, and are interesting. In P. Ekman & R. J. Davidson (Eds.), *The nature of emotion: Fundamental questions.* New York: Oxford University Press. Pp. 155–162.

Frijda, N. H., Mesquita, B., Sonnemans, J., & Van Goozen, S. (1991). The durations of affective phenomena or emotions, sentiments and passions. In K. T. Strongman (Ed.), *International review of studies on emotion.* Vol. 1. New York: Wiley. Pp. 187–225.

Frith, C. E., Dowdy, J., Ferrier, I. N., & Crow, T. J. (1985). Selective impairment of paired associate learning after administration of a centrally acting adrenergic agonist (clonidine). *Psychopharmacology, 87,* 490–493.

Funkenstein, D. H. (1955). The physiology of fear and anger. *Scientific American, 192* (No. 5), 74–80.

Fuoco, F. J., Lawrence, P. S., & Vernon, J. B. (1988). Post-reinforcement effects of token reinforcement, verbal praise, and self-monitoring in a residential psychiatric program. *Behavioral Residential Treatment, 3,* 267–286.

Fuster, J. M. (1958). Effects of stimulation of brain stem on tachistoscopic perception. *Science, 127,* 150.

Galef, B. G. (1970). Aggression and timidity: Response to novelty in feral Norway rats. *Journal of Comparative and Physiological Psychology, 70,* 370–381.

Galef, B. G. Jr., (1996). Social influences on food preferences and feeding behaviors of vertebrates. In E. D. Carpaldi (Ed.), *Why we eat what we eat: The psychology of eating.* Washington, DC: American Psychological Association. Pp. 207–231.

Galef, B. G., Jr. (1989). Socially-mediated attenuation of taste-aversion learning in Norway rats: Preventing development of food phobias. *Animal Learning and Behavior, 17,* 468–474.

Galef, B. G., Jr., & Beck, M. (1990). Diet selection and poison avoidance by mammals individually and in social groups. In E. M. Stricker (Ed.), *Neurobiology of food and fluid intake. Handbook of behavioral neurobiology. Vol. 10.* New York: Plenum Press. Pp. 329–349.

Garcia, J., & Rusiniak, K. W. (1979). What the nose learns from the mouth. Paper presented at the Symposium on Chemical Signals in Vertebrate and Aquatic Mammals, Syracuse University, New York.

Garcia, J., Ervin, F., & Koelling, R. (1966). Learning with prolonged delay of reinforcement. *Psychonomic Science, 5,* 121–122.

Garcia, J., Hankins, W. G., & Rusniak, K. W. (1974). Behavioral regulation of the milieu interne in man and rat. *Science, 185,* 824–831.

Garcia, J., Rusniak, K. W., & Brett, L. P. (1977). Conditioning food-illness aversions in wild animals: Caveant Cononici. In H. Davis & H. M. B. Hurwitz (Eds.), *Operant-Pavlovian interactions.* Hillsdale, NJ: Erlbaum.

Gardner, L., & Malmo, R. B. (1969). Effects of low-level septal stimulation on escape: Significance for limbic-midbrain interactions in pain. *Journal of Comparative and Physiological Psychology, 68,* 65–73.

Gatto, G. J., McBride, W. J., Murphy, J. M., Lumeng, L., & Li, T.-K. (1994). Ethanol self-infusion into the ventral tegmental area by alcohol-preferring rats. *Alcohol, 11,* 557–564.

Gazzaniga, M. S., & Sperry, R. W. (1967). Language after section of the cerebral commisures. *Brain, 90,* 131–148.

Geen, R. G. (1990). *Human aggression.* Pacific Grove, CA: Brooks/Cole.

Geen, R. G. (1991). Social motivation. *Annual Review of Psychology, 42,* 377–399.

Geen, R. G., & Thomas, S. L. (1986). The immediate effects of media violence on behavior. *Journal of Social Issues, 42,* 7–27.

Geisler, M. W., & Polich, J. (1992). P 300, food consumption, and memory performance. *Psychophysiology, 29,* 76–85.

Gerrard, C. K., Reznikoff, M., & Riklan, M. (1982). Level of aspiration, life satisfaction, and locus of control in older adults. *Experimental Aging Research, 8,* 119–121.

Getz, L. L., & Carter, C. S. (1996). Prairie-vole partnerships. *American Scientist, 84,* 56–62.

Gewirtz, J. L., & Pelaez-Nogueras, M. (1993). "Expectancy": sleight-of-hand mentalism, not mechanism or process. *American Psychologist, 48,* 1156–1157.

Gieselman, C. J., Martin, J. R., Vanderweele, D. A., & Novin, D. (1980). Analysis of meal patterning in intact and vagotomized rabbits. *Journal of Comparative and Physiological Psychology, 94,* 388–399.

Gilchrist, J. C., & Nesberg, L. S. (1952). Need and perceptual change in need-related objects. *Journal of Experimental Psychology, 44,* 369–376.

Gillette, M. U., & McArthur, A. J. (1996). Circadian actions of melatonin at the suprachiasmatic nucleus. *Behavioral Brain Research, 73,* 135–139.

Gilligan, S. G., & Bower, G. H. (1984). Cognitive consequences of emotional arousal. In C. E. Izard, J. Kagan, & & R. B. Zajonc (Eds.), *Emotions, cognition, and behavior.* New York: Cambridge University Press. Pp. 547–588.

Ginsburg, G. S., & Bronstein, P. (1993). Family factors related to children's intrinsic/extrinsic motivational orientation and academic performance. *Child Development, 64,* 1461–1474.

Glickman, S. E., Frank, L. G., Davidson, J. M., Smith, E. R., & Siiteri, P. K. (1987). Androstenedione may organize or activate sex reversed traits in female spotted hyenas. *Proceedings of the National Academy of Science, 84,* 3444–3447.

Glickman, S. E., Frank, L. G., Licht, P., Yalcinkaya, T., Siiteri, P. K., & Davidson, J. (1992). Sexual differentiation of the female spotted hyena: One of nature's experiments. *Annals of the New York Academy of Sciences, 662,* 135–159.

Glickman, W. E., & Schiff, B. B. (1967). A biological theory of reinforcement. *Psychological Review, 74,* 81–109.

Gold, G. J., & Raven, B. H. (1992). Interpersonal influence strategies in the Churchill-Roosevelt bases-for-destroyers exchange. *Journal of Social Behavior and Personality, 7,* 245–272.

Gold, P. E. (1991). An integrated memory regulation system: From blood to brain. In R. C. A. Frederickson, J. L. McGaugh, & D. L. Felten (Eds.), *Peripheral signaling of the brain: Role in neural-immune interactions and learning and memory.* Toronto: Hogrefe & Huber. Pp. 391–419.

Gold, P. E., & Stone, W. S. (1988). Neuroendocrine effects on memory in aged rodents and humans. *Neurobiology of Aging, 9,* 709–717.

Goodwin, D. W. (1994). *Alcoholism: The facts.* 2nd ed. New York: Oxford University Press.

Goodwin, D., Powell, B., & Brenner, D. (1969). Alcohol and recall: State-dependent effects in man. *Science, 163,* 1358–1360.

Gopnik, A., & Slaughter, V. (1991). Young children's understanding of changes in their mental states. *Child Development, 62,* 98–110.

Gottman, J. M., & Levenson, R. W. (1985). A valid procedure for obtaining self-report of affect in marital interaction. *Journal of Consulting and Clinical Psychology, 53,* 151–160.

Graeber, R. C. (1982). Alterations in performance following rapid transmeridian flight. In F. M. Brown & R. C. Graeber (Eds.), *Rhythmic aspects of behavior.* London: Lawrence Erlbaum Associates. Pp. 173–212.

Graeber, R. C. (1994). Jet lag and sleep disruption. In M. H. Kryger, T. Roth, & W. C. Dement (Eds.). *Principles and practice of sleep medicine.* Philadelphia: W. B. Saunders. Pp. 463–470.

Graham, F. K., & Clifton, R. K. (1966). Heart-rate change as a component of the orienting response. *Psychological Bulletin, 65,* 305–320.

Gray, J. A. (1991). *The psychology of fear and stress.* 2nd ed. New York: Cambridge University Press.

Green, D. M., & Swets, J. A. (1966). *Signal detection theory and psychophysics.* New York: Wiley.

Green, M. W., Elliman, N. A., & Rogers, P. J. (1996). Hunger, caloric preloading and the selective processing of food and body shape words. *British Journal of Clinical Psychology, 35,* 143–151.

Green, M. W., Rogers, P. J., & Hedderley, D. (1996). The time course of mood-induced decrements in colour-naming of threat-related words. *Current Psychology: Developmental, Learning, Personality, Social, 14,* 350–358.

Greenberg, J. (1985). Unattainable goal choice as a self-handicapping strategy. *Journal of Applied Social Psychology, 15,* 140–152.

Greenwood, C. R., Carta, J. J., Hart, B., Kamps, D., Terry, B., Arreaga-Mayer, C., Atwater, J., Walker, D., Risley, T., & Delquadri, J. C. (1992). Out of the laboratory and into the community: 26 years of applied behavior analysis at the Juniper Gardens children's project. *American Psychologist, 47,* 1464–1474.

Griggs, R. C., & Stunkard, A. (1964). The interpretation of gastric motility. II. Sensitivity and bias in the perception of gastric motility. *Archives of General Psychiatry, 11,* 82–89.

Grill, H. J., & Kaplan, J. M. (1990). Caudal brainstem participates in the distributed neural control of feeding. In E. M. Stricker (Ed.), *Neurobiology of food and fluid intake. Handbook of behavioral neurobiology. Vol. 10.* New York: Plenum Press. Pp. 125–150.

Grillon, C., & Ameli, R. (1993). Fear-potentiated startle: Relationship to the level of state/trait anxiety in healthy subjects. *Biological Psychiatry, 33,* 566–674.

Groebel, J., & Hinde, R. (1989). *Aggression and war.* New York: Cambridge University Press.

Grossman, S. P. (1990). *Thirst and sodium appetite: Physiological basis.* New York: Academic Press.

Guthrie, E. R. (1935). *The psychology of learning.* New York: Harper.

Haber, R. N. (1967). Repetition as a determinant of perceptual recognition processes. In W. Wathen-Dunn (Eds.), *Models for the perception of speech and visual form.* Cambridge, MA: MIT Press. Pp. 202–212.

Hadwin, J., & Perner, J. (1991). Pleased and surprised: Children's cognitive theory of emotion. *British Journal of Developmental Psychology, 9,* 215–234.

Haigler, V. F., Day, H. D., & Marshall, D. D. (1995). Parental attachment and gender-role identity. *Sex Roles, 33,* 203–220.

Halaas, J. L., Gajiwala, K. S., Maffei, M., Cohen, S. L.,

Chait, B. T., Rabinowitz, D., Lallone, R. L., Burley, S. K., & Friedman, J. M. (1995). Weight-reducing effects of the plasma protein encoded by the *obese* gene. *Science, 269,* 543–546.

Halberg, F., Engeli, M., Hamburger, C., & Hillman, D. (1965). Spectral resolution of low-frequency, small-amplitude rhythms in excreted 17-ketosteroids; probable androgen-induced circaseptan desynchronization. *Acta endocrinologica, 103,* 1–54.

Hall, D. F., & Latané, B. (1974). Acceptance and preference for inter- and intraspecies social contact in rats. Paper presented at the meeting of the American Psychological Association, New Orleans.

Hall, J. F. (1956). The relationship between external stimulation, food deprivation, and activity. *Journal of Comparative and Physiological Psychology, 49,* 339–341.

Hall, R. V., Lund, D., & Jackson, D. (1968). Effects of teacher attention on study behavior. *Journal of Applied Behavior Analysis, 1,* 1–12.

Halmi, K. A., Sunday, S., Puglisi, A., & Marchi, P. (1989). Hunger and satiety in anorexia and bulimia nervosa. In L. H. Schneider, S. J. Cooper, & K. A. Halmi (Eds.), *The psychology of human eating disorders: Preclinical and clinical perspectives.* Vol. 575. *Annals of the New York Academy of Sciences.* New York: New York Academy of Sciences. Pp. 431–444.

Halpern, D. F. (1992). *Sex differences in cognitive abilities.* 2nd ed. Hillsdale, NJ: Erlbaum.

Hamalainen, M., & Pulkkinen, L. (1995). Aggressive and non-prosocial behaviour as precursors of criminality. *Studies on Crime and Crime Prevention, 4,* 6–21.

Harlow, H. F. (1958). The nature of love. *American Psychologist, 13,* 673–685.

Harlow, H. F. (1971). *Learning to love.* San Francisco: Albion.

Harma, M. I., Ilmarinen, J., Knauth, P., Rutenfranz, J., & Hanninen, O. (1988a). Physical training intervention in female shift workers: I. The effects of intervention on firmness, fatigue, sleep, and psychosomatic symptoms. *Ergonomics, 31,* 39–50.

Harma, M. I., Ilmarinen, J., Knauth, P., Rutenfranz, J., & Hanninen, O. (1988b). Physical training intervention in female shift workers: The effects of intervention on the circadian rhythms of alertness, short-term memory, and body temperature. *Ergonomics, 31,* 51–63.

Harrington, M. E., Nance, D. M., & Rusak, B. (1987). Double-labeling of neuropeptide Y-immunoreactive neurons which project from the geniculate to the suprachiasmatic nuclei. *Brain Research, 410,* 275–282.

Harrington, M. E., & Rusak, B. (1986). Lesions of the thalamic intergeniculate leaflet alter hamster circadian rhythms. *Journal of Biological Rhythms, 1,* 309–325.

Harrington, M. E., & Rusak, B. (1988). Ablation of the geniculo-hypothalamic tract alters circadian activity rhythms of hamsters housed under constant light. *Physiology & Behavior, 42,* 183–189.

Harris, F. (1976). *Games.* Philadelphia: Frank Harris.

Harris, R. B. S. (1990). Role of set-point theory in the regulation of energy balance. *The Federation of American Societies for Experimental Biology Journal, 4,* 3310–3318.

Hartup, W. W. (1974). Aggression in childhood: Developmental perspectives. *American Psychologist, 29,* 336–341.

Hatsukami, D. K., Hughes, J. R., & Pickens, R. W. (1985). Blood nicotine, smoke exposure and tobacco withdrawal symptoms. *Addictive Behaviors, 10,* 413–417.

Hayamizu, T., & Weiner, B. (1991). A test of Dweck's model of achievement goals as related to perceptions of ability. *Journal of Experimental Education, 59,* 226–234.

Haynes, S. G., Levine, S., Scotch, N., Feinleib, M., & Kannel, W. B. (1978). The relationship of psychosocial factors to coronary heart disease in the Framingham Study: I. Methods and risk factors. *American Journal of Epidemiology, 107,* 362–383.

Hazan, C., & Shaver, P. R. (1987). Romantic love conceptualized as an attachment process. *Journal of Personality and Social Psychology, 52,* 511–524.

Heatherton, T. F., Mahamedi, F., Striepe, M., Field, A. E., & Keel, P. (1997). A 10-year longitudinal study of body weight, dieting, and eating disorder symptoms. *Journal of Abnormal Psychology, 106,* 117–125.

Heaton, A. W., & Kruglanski, A. W. (1991). Person perception by introverts and extraverts under time pressure: Effects of need for closure. *Personality and Social Psychology Bulletin, 17,* 161–165.

Hebb, D. O. (1955). Drives and the C. N. S. (conceptual nervous system). *Psychological Review, 62,* 243–254.

Heckhausen, H., & Gollwitzer, P. M. (1987). Thought content and cognitive functioning in motivational versus volitional states of mind. *Motivation and Emotion, 11,* 101–120.

Heckhausen, H., & Kuhl, J. (1985). From wishes to action: The dead ends and short cuts on the long way to action. In M. Frese and J. Sabini (Eds.), *Goal-directed behavior: Psychological theory and research on action.* Hillsdale, NJ: Erlbaum. Pp. 134–159.

Hedges, L. V., & Nowell, A. (1995). Sex differences in

mental test scores, variability, and numbers of high-scoring individuals. *Science, 269,* 41–45.

Hegland, S. M., & Rix, M. K. (1990). Aggression and assertiveness in kindergarten children differing in day care experiences. *Early Childhood Research Quarterly, 5,* 105–116.

Heider, F. (1958). *The psychology of interpersonal relationships.* New York: Wiley.

Heishman, S. J., Kozlowski, L. T., & Henningfield, J. E. (1997). Nicotine addiction: Implications for public health policy. *Journal of Social Issues, 53,* 13–32.

Helmers, K. F., Posluszny, D. M., & Krantz, D. S. (1994). Associations of hostility and coronary artery disease: A review of studies. In A. W. Siegman & T. W. Smith (Eds.), *Anger, hostility, and the heart.* Hillsdale, NJ: Erlbaum. Pp. 67–96.

Helmreich, R. L., & Spence, J. T. (1978). The Work and Family Orientation Questionnaire: An objective instrument to assess components of achievement motivation attitudes toward family and career. *JSAS Catalog of Selected Documents in Psychology, 8.*

Hendrick, C., & Hendrick, S. (1986). A theory and method of love. *Journal of Personality and Social Psychology, 50,* 392–402.

Hendrick, S., Hendrick, C., Slapion-Foote, M. J., & Foote, F. H. (1985). Gender differences in sexual attitudes. *Journal of Personality and Social Psychology, 48,* 1630–1642.

Hendrickson, A. E., Wagoner, N., & Cowan, W. M. (1972). An autoradiographic and electron microscopic study of retino-hypothalamic connections. *Zeitschrift fuer Zellforschung und Mikroscopische Anatomie, 135,* 1–26.

Henningfield, J. W., Cohen, C., & Pickworth, W. B. (1993). Psychopharmacology of nicotine. In C. T. Orelans & J. Slade (Eds.), *Nicotine addiction: Principles and management.* New York: Oxford University Press. Pp. 24–45.

Hergenhahn, B. R. (1997). *An introduction to the history of psychology.* 3rd ed. Pacific Grove, CA: Brooks/Cole.

Hess, E. H. (1959). Imprinting. *Science, 130,* 133–141.

Hess, W. R. (1957). *The functional organization of the diencephalon.* New York: Grune and Stratton.

Hetherington, M. M., & Macdiarmid, J. I. (1994). Pleasure and excess: Liking for and overconsumption of chocolate. *Physiology & Behavior, 57,* 27–35.

Hetherington, M., & Rolls, B. J. (1989). Sensory-specific satiety in anorexia and bulimia nervosa. In L. H. Schneider, S. J. Cooper, & K. A. Halmi (Eds.), *The psychology of human eating disorders: Preclinical and clinical perspectives.* Vol. 575. *Annals of the New York Academy of Sciences.* New York: New York Academy of Sciences. Pp. 387–398.

Hetherington, M. M., & Rolls, B. J. (1996). Sensory-specific satiety: Theoretical frameworks and central characteristics. In E. D. Capaldi (Ed.), *Why we eat what we eat: The psychology of eating.* Washington, DC: American Psychological Association. Pp. 267–290.

Heyman, G. D., & Dweck, C. S. (1992). Achievement goals and intrinsic motivation: Their relation and their role in adaptive motivation. *Motivation and Emotion, 16,* 231–247.

Heyman, G. M., & Tanz, L. (1995). How to teach a pigeon to maximize overall reinforcement rate. *Journal of the Experimental Analysis of Behavior, 64,* 277–298.

Hickey, T. L., & Spear, P. D. (1976). Retinogeniculate projections in hooded and albino rats: An autoradiographic study. *Experimental Brain Research, 24,* 523–529.

Higgins, E. T., Roney, C. J. R., Crowe, E., & Hymes, C. (1994). Ideal versus ought predilections for approach and avoidance: Distinct self-regulatory systems. *Journal of Personality and Social Psychology, 66,* 276–286.

Hilgard, E. R., & Marquis, D. G. (1940). *Conditioning and learning.* New York: Appleton-Century-Crofts.

Hill, A. J., & Blundell, J. E. (1989). Comparison of the action of macronutrients on the expression of appetite in lean and obese human subjects. In L. H. Schneider, S. J. Cooper, & K. A. Halmi (Eds.), *The psychology of human eating disorders: Preclinical and clinical perspectives.* Vol. 575. *Annals of the New York Academy of Sciences.* New York: New York Academy of Sciences. Pp. 529–531.

Hill, A. J., Oliver, S., & Rogers, P. J. (1992). Eating in the adult world: The rise of dieting in childhood and adolescence. *British Journal of Clinical Psychology, 31,* 95–105.

Hilliard, J. P., Fritz, G. K., & Lewiston, N. J. (1982). Goal-setting behavior of asthmatic, diabetic and healthy children. *Child Psychiatry and Human Development, 13,* 35–47.

Hilliard, J. P., Fritz, G. K., & Lewiston, N. J. (1985). Levels of aspiration of parents for their asthmatic, diabetic and healthy children. *Journal of Clinical Psychology, 41,* 587–597.

Himmelweit, H. T. (1947). A comparative study of the level of aspiration of normal and of neurotic persons. *British Journal of Psychology, 37,* 5–59.

Hine, D. W., Summers, C., Tilleczek, K., & Lewko, J. (1997). Expectancies and mental models as determinants of adolescents' smoking decisions. *Journal of Social Issues, 53,* 35–52.

Hinshaw, S. P. (1992). Externalizing behavior problems and academic underachievement in childhood and adolescence: Causal relationships and underlying mechanisms. *Psychological Bulletin, 111,* 127–155.

Hinz, L. D., & Williamson, D. A. (1987). Bulimia and depression: A review of the affective variant hypothesis. *Psychological Bulletin, 102,* 150–158.

Ho, M.-Y., Wogar, M. A., Bradshaw, C. M., & Szabadi, E. (1997). Choice between delayed reinforcers: Interaction between delay and deprivation level. *The Quarterly Journal of Experimental Psychology, 50B,* 193–202.

Hobfoll, S. E., Dunahoo, C. L., Ben-Porath, Y., & Monnier, J. (1994). Gender and coping: The dual-axis model of coping. *American Journal of Community Psychology, 22,* 49–82.

Hodapp, V. (1989). Anxiety, fear of failure, and achievement: Two path-analytical models. *Anxiety Research, 1,* 301–312.

Hoebel, B. G., Hernandez, L., Schwartz, D. H., Mark, G. P., & Hunter, G. A. (1989). Microdialysis studies of brain norepinephrine, serotonin, and dopamine release during ingestive behavior: Theoretical and clinical implications. In L. H. Schneider, S. J. Cooper, & K. A. Halmi (Eds.), *The psychology of human eating disorders: Preclinical and clinical perspectives.* Vol. 575. *Annals of the New York Academy of Sciences.* New York: New York Academy of Sciences. Pp. 171–191.

Hollenbeck, J. R., Williams, C. R., & Klein, H. J. (1989). An empirical examination of the antecedents of commitment to difficult goals. *Journal of Applied Psychology, 74,* 18–23.

Holt, R. R. (1989). College students' definitions and images of enemies. *Journal of Social Issues, 45,* 33–50.

Honma, K.-I., Honma, S., Nakamura, K., Sasaki, M., Endo, T., Takahashi, T. (1995). Differential effects of bright light and social cues on reentrainment of human circadian rhythms. *American Journal of Physiology, 268,* R528–R535.

Horne, J. A. (1988). *Why we sleep: The functions of sleep in humans and other mammals.* New York: Oxford University Press.

Horne, J. A., & Ostberg, O. (1976). A self-assessment questionnaire to determine morningness-eveningness in human circadian rhythms. *International Journal of Chronobiology, 4,* 97–110.

Horner, M. S. (1972). Toward an understanding of achievement-related conflicts in women. *Journal of Social Issues, 28,* 157–175.

Horney, K. (1937). *The neurotic personality of our time.* New York: W. W. Norton.

Horowitz, M. J., & Reidbord, S. P. (1992). Memory, emotion, and response to trauma. In S.-A. Christianson (Ed.), *The handbook of emotion and memory.* Hillsdale, NJ: Erlbaum. Pp. 343–357.

Horowitz, T., Wolfe, J., & Czeisler, C. (1998). A chronopsychological dissection of attention. Paper presented at the Psychonomic Society convention, Dallas, TX.

Houston, J. P. (1991). *Fundamentals of learning and memory.* 4th ed. New York: Harcourt, Brace, Jovanovich.

Hovland, C. I., & Riesen, A. H. (1940). Magnitude of galvanic and vasomotor response as a function of stimulus intensity. *Journal of General Psychology, 23,* 477–493.

Huebner, R. R., & Izard, C. E. (1988). Mothers' responses to infants' facial expressions of sadness, anger, and physical distress. *Motivation and Emotion, 12,* 185–196.

Hughes, R. J., Sack, R. L., & Lewy, A. J. (1998). The role of melatonin and circadian phase in age-related sleep-maintenance insomnia: Assessment in a clinical trial of melatonin replacement. *Sleep, 21,* 52–68.

Hull, C. L. (1932). The goal gradient hypothesis and maze learning. *Psychological Review, 39,* 25–43.

Hull, C. L. (1943). *Principles of behavior.* New York: Appleton-Century-Crofts.

Hull, C. L. (1951). *Essentials of behavior.* New Haven, CT: Yale University Press.

Humphrey, L. L. (1989). Observed family interactions among subtypes of eating disorders using structural analysis of social behavior. *Journal of Consulting and Clinical Psychology, 57,* 206–214.

Humphreys, M. S., & Revelle, W. (1984). Personality, motivation, and performance: A theory of the relationship between individual differences and information processing. *Psychological Review, 91,* 153–184.

Hunt, S. L. (1995). Task persistence and performance attainment as a function of praise, encouragement, and knowledge of results. Unpublished master's thesis, Southern Illinois University at Edwardsville.

Hunter, W. S. (1930). A further consideration of the sensory control of the maze habit in the white rat. *Journal of Genetic Psychology, 38,* 3–19.

Hupka, R. B., Zaleski, Z., Otto, J., Reidl, L., & Tarabrina, N. V. (1997). The colors of anger, envy, fear, and jealousy: A cross-cultural study. *Journal of Cross-Cultural Psychology, 28,* 156–170.

Hurt, R. D., Eberman, K. M., Slade, J., & Karan, L. (1993). Treating nicotine addiction in patients with other addictive disorders. In C. T. Orelans & J. Slade

(Eds.), *Nicotine addiction: Principles and management.* New York: Oxford University Press. Pp. 310–326.

Ickes, W. (1993). Traditional gender roles: Do they make, and then break, our relationships? *Journal of Social Issues, 49,* 71–85.

Isen, A. M. (1984). Toward understanding the role of affect in cognition. In R. S. Wyer, Jr., & T. K. Srull (Eds.), *Handbook of social cognition.* Vol. 3. Hillsdale, NJ: Erlbaum. Pp. 179–236.

Isen, A. M., & Gorgoglione, J. M. (1983). Some specific effects of four affect-induction procedures. *Personality and Social Psychology Bulletin, 9,* 136–143.

Ito, T. A., Miller, N., & Pollock, V. E. (1996). Alcohol and aggression: A meta-analysis on the moderating effects of inhibitory cues, triggering events, and self-focused attention. *Psychological Bulletin, 120,* 60–82.

Izard, C. E. (1971). *The face of emotion.* New York: Appleton-Century-Crofts.

Izard, C. E. (1977). *Human emotions.* New York: Plenum Press.

Izard, C. E. (1990). Facial expression and the regulation of emotions. *Journal of Personality and Social Psychology, 58,* 487–498.

Izard, C. E. (1994a). Innate and universal facial expressions: Evidence from developmental and cross-cultural research. *Psychological Bulletin, 115,* 228–299.

Izard, C. E. (1994b). Intersystem connections. In P. Ekman & R. J. Davidson (Eds.), *The nature of emotion:* Fundamental questions. New York: Oxford University Press. Pp. 356–361.

Jackson, L. A., Hodge, C. N., & Ingram, J. M. (1994). Gender and self-concept: A reexamination of stereotypic differences and the role of gender attitudes. *Sex Roles, 30,* 615–630.

James, W. (1884). What is an emotion? *Mind, 9,* 188–205.

James, W. (1890). *The principles of psychology, Vols. 1 and 2.* New York: Henry Holt.

Jarvik, M. E., & Henningfield, J. E. (1993). Pharmacological adjuncts for the treatment of tobacco dependence. In C. T. Orelans & J. Slade (Eds.), *Nicotine addiction: Principles and management.* New York: Oxford University Press. Pp. 245–261.

Jastrow, J. (1928). The place of emotion in modern psychology. In M. L. Reymert (Ed.), *The Wittenberg Symposium.* Worcester, MA: Clark University Press.

Jenkin, N. (1957). Affective processes in perception. *Psychological Bulletin, 54,* 100–127.

Jenkins, C. D., Zyzanski, S. J., & Rosenman, R. H. (1971). Progress toward validation of a computer scored test for the Type A coronary prone behavior pattern. *Psychosomatic Medicine, 33,* 193–202.

Jenks, S. M., Weldele, M., Frank, L. G., & Glickman, S. E. (1995). Acquisition of matrilineal rank in captive spotted hyenas (*Crocuta crocuta*): Emergence of a natural social system in peer-reared animals and their offspring. *Animal Behaviour, 50,* 893–904.

Jitsumori, M., & Yoshihara, M. (1997). Categorical discrimination of human facial expressions by pigeons: A test of the linear feature model. *The Quarterly Journal of Experimental Psychology, Section B, 50B,* 253–268.

John, O. P. (1990). The "big five" factor taxonomy: Dimensions of personality in the natural language and in questionnaires. In L. A. Pervin (Ed.), *Handbook of personality: Theory and research.* New York: Guilford Press.

Johnsen, B. H., Thayer, J. F., & Hugdahl, K. (1995). Affective judgment of the Ekman faces; A dimensional approach. *Journal of Psychophysiology, 9,* 193–202.

Johnson, R. F., Moore, R. Y., & Morin, L. P. (1989). Lateral geniculate lesions alter circadian activity rhythms in the hamster. *Brain Research Bulletin, 22,* 411–422.

Joiner, T. E., Jr., Heatherton, T. F., Rudd, M. D., & Schmidt, N. B. (1997). Perfectionism, perceived weight status, and bulimic symptoms: Two studies testing a diathesis-stress model. *Journal of Abnormal Psychology, 106,* 145–153.

Jones, D. C., & Costin, S. E. (1995). Friendship quality during preadolescence and adolescence: The contributions of relationship orientations, instrumentality, and expressivity. *Merrill Palmer Quarterly, 41,* 517–535.

Jordan, P. C. (1986). Effects of an extrinsic reward on intrinsic motivation: A field experiment. *Academy of Management Journal, 29,* 405–412.

Josephs, R., Larrick, R. P., Steele, C. M., & Nisbett, R. E. (1992). Protecting the self from the negative consequences of risky decisions. *Journal of Personality and Social Psychology, 62,* 26–37.

Juvonen, J., & Weiner, B. (1993). An attributional analysis of students' interactions: The social consequences of perceived responsibility. *Educational Psychology Review, 5,* 325–345.

Kalat, J. W. (1992). *Biological psychology.* 4th ed. Belmont, CA: Wadsworth.

Kanfer, R. (1994). Work motivation: New directions in theory and research. In C. L. Cooper & I. T. Robertson (Eds.), *Key reviews in managerial psychology: Concepts and research for practice.* New York: John Wiley. Pp. 1–53.

Kanfer R., & Ackerman, P. L. (1989). Motivation and

cognitive abilities: An integrative/aptitude-treatment interaction approach to skill acquisition. *Journal of Applied Psychology* (Monograph), *74*, 657–690.

Karli, P. (1956). The Norway rat's killing response to the white mouse: An experimental analysis. *Behaviour, 10*, 81–103.

Karniol, R., & Ross, M. (1996). The motivational impact of temporal focus: Thinking about the future and the past. *Annual Review of Psychology, 47*, 593–620.

Katkovsky, W., Crandall, V. C., & Good, S. (1967). Parental antecedents of children's beliefs in internal-external control of reinforcement in intellectual achievement situations. *Child Development, 38*, 765–776.

Keenleyside, M. C. (1937). Masculine protest by feminine methods. *International Journal of Individual Psychology, 3*, 171–178.

Keesey, R. E., & Powley, T. L. (1986). The regulation of body weight. *Annual Review of Psychology, 37*, 109–133.

Kelley, H. H. (1997). The "stimulus field" for interpersonal phenomena: The source of language and thought about interpersonal events. *Personality and Social Psychology Review, 1*, 140–169.

Kendler, H. H. (1946). The influence of simultaneous hunger and thirst drives upon the learning of two opposed spatial responses of the white rat. *Journal of Experimental Psychology, 36*, 212–220.

Kendler, H. H. (1987). *Historical foundations of modern psychology.* New York: Dorsey Press.

Kentridge, R. W., & Aggleton, J. P. (1990). Emotion: Sensory representation, reinforcement, and the temporal lobe. *Cognition and Emotion, 4*, 191–208.

Kimble, G. A. (1961). *Hilgard and Marquis' conditioning and learning.* 2nd ed. New York: Appleton-Century-Crofts.

Kinsey, A. C., Pomeroy, W. B., & Martin, C. E. (1948). *Sexual behavior in the human male.* Philadelphia: W. B. Saunders.

Kinsey, A. C., Pomeroy, W. B., Martin, C. E., & Gebhard, P. H. (1953). *Sexual behavior in the human female.* Philadelphia: W. B. Saunders.

Kintsch, W. (1962). Runway performance as a function of drive strength and magnitude of reinforcement. *Journal of Comparative and Physiological Psychology, 55*, 882–887.

Kintsch, W. (1977). *Memory and cognition.* 2nd ed. New York: Wiley.

Kissileff, H. R. (1989). Is there an eating disorder in the obese? In L. H. Schneider, S. J. Cooper, & K. A. Halmi (Eds.), *The psychology of human eating disorders: Preclinical and clinical perspectives.* Vol. 575.

Annals of the New York Academy of Sciences. New York: New York Academy of Sciences. Pp. 410–419.

Klein, D. C., & Moore, R. Y. (1979). Pineal N-acetyltransferase and hydroxyindole-O-methyltransferase: Control by the retinohypothalamic tract and the suprachiasmatic nucleus. *Brain Research, 174*, 245–262.

Klein, D. C., Moore, R. Y., & Reppert, S. M. (1991). *Suprachiasmatic nucleus: The mind's clock.* New York: Oxford University Press.

Klein, K. E., Wegmann, H. M., & Hunt, B. I. (1972). Desynchronization of body temperature and performance circadian rhythm as a result of outgoing and homegoing transmeridian flights. *Aerospace Medicine, 43*, 119–132.

Kleinmuntz, B., & Scucko, J. J. (1984). Lie detection in ancient and modern times. *American Psychologist, 39*, 766–776.

Klerman, E. B., Rimmer, D. W., Dijk, D. J., Kronauer, R. E., Rizzo, J. F., & Czeisler, C. A. (1998). Nonphotic entrainment of the human circadian pacemaker. *American Journal of Physiology, 274*, R991–R996.

Kling, J. W., & Schrier, A. M. (1972). Positive reinforcement. In J. W. Kling & L. A. Riggs (Eds.), *Woodworth & Schlosberg's experimental psychology.* Vol. II. 3rd ed. New York: Holt, Rinehart and Winston. Pp. 615–702.

Klinger, E. (1992). Motivation and imagination. *Psychologische Beitrage, 34*, 127–142.

Klinger, E., Barta, S. G., & Maxeiner, M. E. (1980). Motivational correlates of thought content frequency and commitment. *Journal of Personality and Social Psychology, 39*, 1222–1237.

Klotter, K. (1960). General properties of oscillating systems. *Cold Spring Harbor Symposia on Quantitative Biology, 25*, 185–187.

Klüver, H., & Bucy, P. C. (1939). Preliminary analysis of functions of the temporal lobes in monkeys. *Archives of Neurology and Psychiatry, 42*, 979–1000.

Knight, G. P., & Chao, C-C. (1991). Cooperative, competitive, and individualistic social values among 8- to 12-year-old siblings, friends, and acquaintances. *Personality and Social Psychology Bulletin, 17*, 201–211.

Knight, G. P., Fabes, R. A., & Higgins, D. A. (1996). Concerns about drawing causal inferences from meta-analyses: An example in the study of gender differences in aggression. *Psychological Bulletin, 119*, 410–421.

Knight, R. G., Ross, R. A., Collins, J. I., & Parmenter, S. A. (1985). Some norms, reliability and preliminary validity data for an S-R inventory of anger: The Subjective Anger Scale (SAS). *Personality and Individual Differences, 6,* 331–339.

Kobak, R. R., & Hazan, C. (1991). Attachment in marriage: Effects of security and accuracy of working models. *Journal of Personality and Social Psychology, 60,* 861–869.

Kocher, S. J., & Berry, L. L. (1982). Activating influences of rhythmic environmental stimuli and food deprivation. Unpublished student paper, Southern Illinois University at Edwardsville.

Koestner, R., & Zuckerman, M. (1994). Causality orientations, failure, and achievement. *Journal of Personality, 62,* 322–346.

Koestner, R., Zuckerman, M., & Koestner, J. (1987). Praise, involvement, and intrinsic motivation. *Journal of Personality and Social Psychology, 53,* 383–390.

Kogut, D., Langley, T., & O'Neal, E. C. (1992). Gender role masculinity and angry aggression in women. *Sex Roles, 26,* 355–368.

Kohn, A. (1986). *No contest: The case against competition.* Boston: Houghton Mifflin.

Kohn, A. (1993). *Punished by rewards: The trouble with gold stars, incentive plans, A's, praise, and other bribes.* New York: Houghton Mifflin.

Komorita, S. S., & Bass, A. R. (1967). Attitude differentiation and evaluative scales of the semantic differential. *Journal of Personality and Social Psychology, 6,* 241–244.

Komorita, S. S., & Ellis, A. L. (1988). Level of aspiration in coalition bargaining. *Journal of Personality and Social Psychology, 54,* 421–431.

Komorita, S. S., & Parks, C. D. (1995). Interpersonal relations: Mixed-motive interaction. *Annual Review of Psychology, 46,* 183–207.

Koob, G. F., & Le Moal, M. (1997). Drug abuse: Hedonic homeostatic dysregulation. *Science, 278,* 52–58.

Kopp, R. R. (1995). *Metaphor therapy: Using client-generated metaphors in psychotherapy.* New York: Brunner/Mazel.

Koss, M. P., Goodman, L. A., Browne, A., Fitzgerald, L. F., Keita, G. P., & Russo, N. P. (1994). *No safe haven: Male violence against women at home, at work, and in the community.* Washington, DC: American Psychological Association.

Koulack, D. (1997). Recognition memory, circadian rhythms, and sleep. *Perceptual and Motor Skills, 85,* 99–104.

Krantz, D. S., & Falconer, J. J. (1995). Measurement of cardiovascular responses. In S. Cohen, R. C. Kessler, & L. U. Gordon (Eds.), *Measuring stress: A guide for health and social scientists.* New York: Oxford University Press. Pp. 193–212.

Krantz, D. S., Glass, D. C., & Snyder, M. L. (1974). Helplessness, stress level, and the coronary prone behavior pattern. *Journal of Experimental Social Behavior, 10,* 284–300.

Kuhl, J., & Kazen, M. (1994). Self-discrimination and memory: State orientation and false self-ascription of assigned activities. *Journal of Personality and Social Psychology, 66,* 1103–1115.

Kuhl, J., & Kraska, K. (1989). Self-regulation and meta-motivation: Computational mechanisms, development, and assessment. In R. Kanfer, P. L. Ackerman, & R. Cudeck (Eds.), *Abilities, motivation, and methodology: The Minnesota symposium on learning and individual differences.* Hillsdale, NJ: Erlbaum. Pp. 343–374.

Kuo, Z. Y. (1938). Further study on the behavior of the cat towards the rat. *Journal of Comparative Psychology, 25,* 1–8.

Kuo, Z. Y. (1960). Studies on the basic factors in animal fighting: VII. Interspecies co-existence in mammals. *Journal of Genetic Psychology, 97,* 211–225.

Lacey, J. I. (1967). Somatic response patterning and stress: Some revisions of activation theory. In M. H. Appley and R. Trubull (Eds.), *Psychological stress: Issues in research.* New York: Appleton. Pp. 14–42.

Lacey, J. I., Kagan, J., Lacey, B. C., & Moss, H. A. (1963) The visceral level: Situational determinants and behavioral correlates of autonomic response patterns. In P. H. Knapp (Ed.), *Expression of the emotions in man.* New York: International Universities. Pp. 161–196.

Lacey, J. I., & Lacey, B. C. (1958). Verification and extension of the principle of autonomic response-stereotypy. *American Journal of Psychology, 71,* 50–73.

Ladish, C., & Polich, J. (1989). P300 and probability in children. *Journal of Experimental Child Psychology, 48,* 212–223.

Landis, C., & Hunt, W. A. (1932). Adrenaline and emotion. *Psychological Review, 39,* 467–485.

Lando, H. A. (1993). Formal quit smoking treatments. In C. T. Orelans & J. Slade (Eds.), *Nicotine addiction: Principles and management.* New York: Oxford University Press. Pp. 221–244.

Landreth, J. E., & Landreth, H. F. (1974). Effects of music on physiological response. *Journal of Research on Music Education, 22,* 4–12.

Lang, P. J. (1964). Experimental studies of desensitization psychotherapy. In J. Wolpe (Ed.), *The conditioning therapies.* New York: Holt, Rinehart, and Winston.

Lang, P. J. (1968). Fear reduction and fear behavior: Problems in treating a construct. In J. M. Shlien (Ed.), Research in psychotherapy. Vol. 3. Washington, DC: American Psychological Association. Pp. 90–103.

Lang, P. J. (1995). The emotion probe: Studies of motivation and attention. *American Psychologist, 50,* 372–385.

Lang, P. J., & Bradley, M. M. (1990). Emotion, attention, and the startle reflex. *Psychological Review, 97,* 377–395.

Lang, P. J., & Lazovik, A. D. (1963). Experimental desensitization of a phobia. *Journal of Abnormal and Social Psychology, 66,* 519–525.

Lang, P. J., Melamed, B. G., & Hart, J. D. (1970). A psychophysiological analysis of fear modification using an automated desensitization procedure. *Journal of Abnormal Psychology, 76,* 220–234.

Langevin, R. (Ed.). (1985). *Erotic preference, gender identity, and aggression in men: New research studies.* Hillsdale, NJ: Erlbaum.

Laplace, A. C., Chermack, S. T., & Taylor, S. P. (1994). Effects of alcohol and drinking experience on human physical aggression. *Personality and Social Psychology Bulletin, 20,* 439–444.

Larkin, K. T., Manuck, S. B., & Kasprowicz, A. L. (1989). Heart rate feedback-assisted reduction in cardiovascular reactivity to a videogame challenge. *The Psychological Record, 39,* 365–371.

Larson, R. W. (1987). On the independence of positive and negative affect within hour-to-hour experience. *Motivation and Emotion, 11,* 145–156.

Latané, B., & Schachter, S. (1962). Adrenaline and avoidance learning. *Journal of Comparative and Physiological Psychology, 55,* 369–372.

Latham, G. P., Erez, M., & Locke, E. A. (1988). Resolving scientific disputes by the joint design of crucial experiments by the antagonists: Application to the Erez-Latham dispute regarding participation in goal setting. *Journal of Applied Psychology* (Monograph), *73,* 753–772.

Lau, M. A., & Pihl, R. O. (1996). Cognitive performance, monetary incentive, and aggression. *Aggressive Behavior, 22,* 417–430.

Lavie, P. (1997). Melatonin: Role in gating nocturnal rise in sleep propensity. *Journal of Biological Rhythms, 12,* 657–665.

Lawson, N. O., Wee, B. E. F., Blask, D. E., Castles, C. G., Spriggs, L. L., & Hill, S. M. (1992). Melatonin decreases estrogen receptor expression in the medial preoptic area of inbred (LSH/SsLak) golden hamsters. *Biology of Reproduction, 47,* 1082–1090.

Lazarus, R., & Opton, E. M. Jr. (1966). The study of psychological stress: A summary of theoretical formulations and experimental findings. In C. D. Spielberger (Ed.), *Anxiety and behavior.* New York: Academic Press. Pp. 225–262.

Lazarus, R. S. (1966). *Psychological stress and the coping process.* New York: McGraw-Hill.

Lazarus, R. S. (1987). Emotion theory and psychotherapy. In J. D. Safran & L. S. Greenberg (Eds.), *Emotion, psychotherapy, and change.* New York: Guilford Press.

Lazarus, R. S. (1989). Constructs of the mind in health and psychotherapy. In A. Freeman, K. Simon, L. E. Beutler, & H. Arkowitz (Eds.), *Comprehensive handbook of cognitive therapy.* New York: Plenum Press. Pp. 99–121.

Lazarus, R. S. (1990). Stress, coping and illness. In H. S. Friedman (Ed.). *Personality and disease.* New York: Wiley. Pp. 97–120.

Lazarus, R. S. (1991a). Cognition and motivation in emotion. *American Psychologist, 46,* 352–367.

Lazarus, R. S. (1991b). *Emotion and adaptation.* New York: Oxford University Press.

Lazarus, R. S. (1991c). Progress on a cognitive-motivational-relational theory of emotion. *American Psychologist, 46,* 819–834.

Lazarus, R. S., & Folkman, S. (1984). *Stress, appraisal, and coping.* New York: Springer.

Lazarus, R. S., Yousem, H., & Arenberg, D. (1953). Hunger and perception. *Journal of Personality, 21,* 312–328.

Lazarus, R. W. (1991). *Emotion and adaptation.* New York: Oxford University Press.

Leak, G. K., & Gardner, L. E. (1990). Sexual attitudes, love attitudes, and social interest. *Individual Psychology: The Journal of Adlerian Theory, Research, and Practice, 46,* 55–60.

LeDoux, J. E. (1986). Sensory systems and emotions: A model of affective processing. *Integrative Psychiatry, 4,* 237–248.

LeDoux, J. E. (1989). Cognitive-emotional interactions in the brain. *Cognition and emotion, 3,* 267–289.

LeDoux, J. E. (1991). Emotion and the brain. *The Journal of NIH Research, 3,* 49–51.

LeDoux, J. E. (1995). Emotion: Clues from the brain. *Annual Review of Psychology, 46,* 209–35.

Lee, C., Bobko, P., Early, P. C., & Locke, E. A. (1991). An empirical analysis of a goal setting questionnaire. *Journal of Organizational Behavior, 12,* 467–482.

Lee, M. K., Graham, S. N., & Gold, P. E. (1988). Memory enhancement with posttraining intraventricular glucose injections in rats. *Behavioral Neuroscience, 102,* 591–595.

Lefcourt, H. M. (1992). Durability and impact of the locus of control construct. *Psychological Bulletin, 112,* 411–414.

Le Magnen, J. (1985). *Hunger.* New York: Cambridge University Press.

Lentz, T., & Cornelius, R. (1950). *All together: A manual of cooperative games.* St. Louis: Peace Research Laboratory.

Lepper, M. R., & Cordova, D. I. (1992). A desire to be taught: Instructional consequences of intrinsic motivation. *Motivation and Emotion, 16,* 187–208.

Lepper, M. R., & Green, D. (1978). Overjustification research and beyond: Toward a means-ends analysis of intrinsic and extrinsic motivation. In M. R. Lepper & D. Green (Eds.), *The hidden costs of reward: New perspectives on the psychology of human motivation.* Hillsdale, NJ: Erlbaum. Pp. 109–148.

Lerner, B. S., & Locke, E. A. (1995). The effects of goal setting, self-efficacy, competition, and personal traits on the performance of an endurance task. *Journal of Sport & Exercise Psychology, 17,* 138–152.

Levenson, H. (1972). Distinctions within the concept of internal-external control: Development of a new scale. *Proceedings of the American Psychological Association, 259–260.*

Levenson, H. (1974a). Activism and powerful others: Distinctions within the concept of internal-external control. *Journal of Personality Assessment, 38,* 377–383.

Levenson, H. (1974b). Multidimensional locus of control in prison inmates. Paper presented at the 82nd Annual Convention of the American Psychological Association, New Orleans.

Levenson, R. W. (1988). Emotion and the autonomic nervous system: A prospectus for research on autonomic specificity. In H. Wanger (Ed.), *Social psychophysiology and emotion: Theory and clinical applications.* London: Wiley. Pp. 17–42.

Levenson, R. W. (1992). Autonomic nervous system differences among emotions. *Psychological Science, 3,* 23–27.

Levenson, R. W. (1994). The search for autonomic specificity. In P. Ekman & R. J. Davidson (Eds.), *The nature of emotion.* New York: Oxford University Press. Pp. 252–257.

Levenson, R. W., Carstensen, L. L., Friesen, W. V., & Ekman, P. (1991). Emotion, physiology, and expression in old age. *Psychology and Aging, 6,* 28–35.

Levenson, R. W., Ekman, P., & Friesen, W. V. (1990). Voluntary facial action generates emotion-specific autonomic nervous system activity. *Psychophysiology, 27,* 363–384.

Levenson, R. W., Ekman, P., Heider, K., & Friesen, W. V. (1992). Emotion and autonomic nervous system activity in the Minangkabou of West Sumatra. *Journal of Personality and Social Psychology, 62,* 972–988.

Leventhal, H., & Tomarken, A. J. (1986). Emotion: Today's problems. In M. R. Rosenzweig & L. W. Porter (Eds.), *Annual review of psychology.* Vol. 37. Palo Alto, CA: Annual Reviews, Inc. Pp. 565–610.

Levine, D. S., & Leven, S. J. (Eds.). (1992). *Motivation, emotion, and goal direction in neural networks.* Hillsdale, NJ: Erlbaum.

Lewin, K. (1936). *Principles of topological psychology.* New York: McGraw-Hill.

Lewin, K., Dembo, T., Festinger, L., & Sears, P. S. (1944). Level of aspiration. In J. McV. Hunt (Ed.), *Personality and the behavior disorders.* New York: Ronald. Pp. 333–378.

Lewy, A. J., & Sack, R. L. (1996). The role of melatonin and light in the human circadian system. *Progress in Brain Research, 111,* 205–216.

Lewy, A. J., Wehr, T. A., Goodwin, F. K., Newsome, D. A., & Markey, S. P. (1980). Light suppresses melatonin in humans. *Science, 210,* 1267–1269.

Ley, R. G., & Bryden, M. P. (1979). Hemispheric differences in processing emotions and faces. *Brain and Language, 7,* 127–138.

Libby, M. N., & Aries, E. (1989). Gender differences in preschool children's narrative fantasy. *Psychology of Women Quarterly, 13,* 293–306.

Liberson, W. T. (1945). Problem of sleep and mental disease. *Digest of Neurology and Psychiatry, 13,* 93–108.

Lieberman, D. A., Davidson, F. H., & Thomas, G. V. (1985). Marking in pigeons: The role of memory in delayed reinforcement. *Journal of Experimental Psychology: Animal Behavior Processes, 11,* 611–624.

Lieberman, H. R., Wurtman, J. J., & Teicher, M. H. (1989). Circadian rhythms of activity in healthy young and elderly humans. *Neurobiology of Aging, 10,* 259–265.

Liebert, R. M., & Sprafkin, J. (1988). *The early window: Effects of television on children and youth.* 3rd ed. New York: Pergamon.

Light, K. C., & Obrist, P. A. (1983). Task difficulty, heart rate reactivity, and cardiovascular responses to an appetitive reaction time task. *Psychophysiology, 20,* 301–312.

Linden, S. E., Savage, L. M., & Overmier, J. B. (1997). General learned irrelevance: A Pavlovian analog to learned helplessness. *Learning and Motivation, 28,* 230–247.

Lindsley, D. B. (1951). Emotion. In S. S. Stevens (Ed.), *Handbook of experimental psychology.* New York: Wiley. Pp. 473–516.

Liu, C., Weaver, D. R., Jin, X., Shearman, L. P., Pieschl, R. L., Gribkoff, V. K., & Reppert, S. M. (1997). Molecular dissection of two distinct actions of melatonin on the suprachiasmatic circadian clock. *Neuron, 19,* 91–102.

Livingstone, M. S., & Hubel, D. H. (1981). Effects of sleep and arousal on the processing of visual information in the cat. *Nature, 291,* 554–561.

Locke, E. A. (1966). The relationship of intentions to level of performance. *Journal of Applied Psychology, 50,* 60–66.

Locke, E. A., & Bryan, J. F. (1968). Grade goals as determinants of academic achievement. *Journal of General Psychology, 79,* 217–228.

Locke, E. A., & Latham, G. P. (1990). *A theory of goal setting and task performance.* Englewood Cliffs, NJ: Prentice-Hall.

Locke, E. A., Latham, G. P., & Erez, M. (1988). The determinants of goal commitment. *Academy of Management Review, 13,* 23–39.

Loeber, R., & Hay, D. (1997). Key issues in the development of aggression and violence from childhood to early adulthood. *Annual Review of Psychology, 48,* 371–410.

Loftus, G. R., & Loftus, E. F. (1976). *Human memory.* Hillsdale, NJ: Erlbaum.

Lograno, D. E., Matteo, F., Trabucchi, M., Govoni, S., Cagiano, R., Lacomba, C., & Cuomo, V. (1993). Effects of chronic ethanol intake at a low dose on the rat brain dopaminergic system. *Alcohol, 10,* 45–49.

Logue, A. W., Forzano, L. B., & Tobin, H. (1992). Independence of reinforcer amount and delay: The generalized matching law and self-control in humans. *Learning and Motivation, 23,* 326–342.

Longstreth, L. E. (1972). A cognitive interpretation of secondary reinforcement. In J. K. Cole (Ed.), *Nebraska symposium on motivation, 1971.* Vol. 19. Lincoln: University of Nebraska Press. Pp. 33–80.

Lopes, L. L. (1987). Between hope and fear: The psychology of risk. In L. Berkowitz (Ed.), *Advances in experimental social psychology.* Vol. 20. New York: Academic Press. Pp. 255–295.

Lopez, M., Balleine, B., & Dickinson, A. (1992). Incentive learning and the motivational control of instrumental performance by thirst. *Animal Learning & Behavior, 20,* 322–328.

Lorenz, K. (1966). *On aggression.* New York: Harcourt.

Lubin, B. (1965). Adjective checklist for measurement of depression. *Archives of General Psychiatry, 12,* 57–62.

Lucion, A. B., & de Almeida, R. M. M. (1996). On the dual nature of maternal aggression in rats. *Aggressive Behavior, 22,* 365–373.

Lundin, R. W. (1967). *An objective psychology of music.* 2nd ed. New York: Ronald Press.

Lykken, D. T. (1980). *A tremor in the blood: Uses and abuses of the lie detector.* New York: McGraw-Hill.

Lykken, D. T. (1984). Polygraphic interrogation. *Nature, 307,* 361–373.

MacIntosh, A. (1942). Differential effect of the status of the competing group upon levels of aspiration. *American Journal of Psychology, 55,* 546–554.

MacLean, P. D., & Delgado, J. M. R. (1953). Electrical and chemical stimulation of frontotemporal portion of limbic system in the waking animal. *Electroencephalography and Clinical Neurophysiology, 5,* 91–100.

MacLeod, C., & Hagan, R. (1992). Individual differences in the selective processing of threatening information, and emotional responses to a stressful life event. *Behavior Research and Therapy, 30,* 151–161.

MacRae, J. R., Scoles, M. T., & Siegel, S. (1987). The contribution of Pavlovian conditioning to drug tolerance and dependence. Special issue: Psychology and addiction. *British Journal of Addiction, 82,* 371–380.

MacRae, J. R., & Siegel, S. (1987). Extinction of tolerance to the analgesic effect of morphine: Intracerebroventricular administration and effects of stress. *Behavioral Neuroscience, 101,* 790–796.

Magdol, L., Moffitt, T. E., Caspi, A., Newman, D. L., Fagan, J., & Silva, P. A. (1997). Gender differences in partner violence in a birth cohort of 21-year olds: Bridging the gap between clinical and epidemiological approaches. *Journal of Consulting and Clinical Psychology, 65,* 68–78.

Maier, S. F. (1991). Stressor controllability, cognition and fear. In J. Madden IV (Ed.), *Neurobiology of learning, emotion, and affect.* New York: Raven Press. Pp. 155–193.

Maier, S. F., Seligman, M. E. P., & Solomon, R. L. (1969). Pavlovian fear conditioning and learned helplessness. In B. A. Campbell & R. M. Church (Eds.), *Punishment and aversive behavior.* New York: Appleton. Pp. 299–342.

Maki, P., Overmier, J. B., Delos, S., & Gutmann, A. J. (1995). Expectancies as factors influencing conditional discrimination performance of children. *The Psychological Record, 45,* 45–71.

Malamuth, N. (1984). Aggression against women: Cultural and individual causes. In N. Malamuth & E. Donnerstein (Eds.), *Pornography and sexual aggression.* New York: Academic Press. Pp. 19–52.

Malmo, R. B. (1957). Anxiety and behavioral arousal. *Psychological Review, 64,* 276–287.

Malmo, R. B. (1959). Activation: A neuropsychological dimension. *Psychological Review, 66,* 367–386.

Malmo, R. B. (1965). Physiological gradients and behavior. *Psychological Bulletin, 64,* 225–234.

Malmo, R. B. (1966). Studies of anxiety: Some clinical origins of the activation concept. In C. D. Spielberger (Ed.), *Anxiety and behavior.* New York: Academic Press. Pp. 157–177.

Malmo, R. B. (1975). *On emotions, needs, and our archaic brain.* New York: Holt, Rinehart, and Winston.

Malmo, R. B., & Malmo, H. P. (1979). Responses of lateral preoptic nerons in the rat to hypertonic sucrose and NaCl. *Electroencephalography and Clinical Neurophysiology, 46,* 401–408.

Malmo, R. B., & Malmo, H. P. (1983). Experiments on the neuropsychology of thirst. *International Journal of Psychophysiology, 1,* 25–48.

Malmo, R. B., & Malmo, H. P. (1988). Effects of intracerebroventricular angiotensin II and olfactory stimuli on multiple unit activity in preoptic and anterior hypothalamic areas: Medial-lateral comparison. *Electroencephalography and Clinical Neurophysiology, 70,* 256–269.

Mandler, G. (1975). *Mind and emotion.* New York: Wiley.

Mandler, G. (1984). *Mind and body.* New York: W. W. Norton.

Mandler, G. (1992). Memory, arousal, and mood: A theoretical integration. In S.-A. Christianson (Ed.), *The handbook of emotion and memory.* Hillsdale, NJ: Erlbaum. Pp. 93–110.

Mandler, G., & Sarason, S. B. (1952). A study of anxiety and learning. *Journal of Abnormal and Social Psychology, 47,* 166–173.

Manning, C. A., Parsons, M. W., Cotter, E. M., & Gold, P. A. (1997). Glucose effects on declarative and nondeclarative memory in healthy elderly and young adults. *Psychobiology, 25,* 103–108.

Maren, S., Aharonov, G., Stote, D. L., & Fanselow, M. S. (1996). N-methyl-D-aspartate receptors in the basolateral amygdala are required for both acquisition and expression of conditional fear in rats. *Behavioral Neuroscience, 110,* 1365–1374.

Maren, S., DeCola, J. P., Swain, R. A., Fanselow, M. S., & Thompson, R. F. (1994). Parallel augmentation of hippocampal long-term potentiation, theta rhythm, and contextual fear conditioning in water-deprived rats. *Behavioral Neuroscience, 108,* 44–56.

Marshall, G., & Zimbardo, P. G. (1979). Affective consequences of inadequately explained physiological arousal. *Journal of Personality and Social Psychology, 37,* 970–988.

Martin C. L., & Ruble, D. N. (1997). A developmental perspective of self-construals and sex differences: Comment on Cross and Madson (1997). *Psychological Bulletin, 122,* 45–50.

Martin, R. J., White, B. D., & Hulsey, M. G. (1991). The regulation of body weight. *American Scientist, 79,* 528–541.

Maslach, C. (1979). Negative emotional biasing of unexplained arousal. *Journal of Personality and Social Psychology, 37,* 953–969.

Masters, W. V., & Johnson, V. E. (1966). *Human sexual response.* Boston: Little, Brown.

Masters, W. V., & Johnson, V. E. (1970). *Human sexual inadequacy.* Boston: Little, Brown.

Masters, W. V., & Johnson, V. E. (1975). *The pleasure bond.* Boston: Little, Brown.

Mathews, A., & MacLeod, C. (1985). Selective processing of threat cues in anxiety states. *Behaviour Research & Therapy, 31,* 563–569.

Matsumoto, D. (1987). The role of facial response in the experience of emotion: More methodological problems and a meta-analysis. *Journal of Personality and Social Psychology, 52,* 769–774.

Mattes, R. (1990). Hunger ratings are not a valid proxy measure of reported food intake in humans. *Appetite, 15,* 103–113.

Maude, D., Wertheim, E. H., Paxton, S., Gibbons, K., & Szmukler, G. (1993). Body dissatisfaction, weight loss behaviours, and bulimic tendencies in Australian adolescents with an estimate of female data representativeness. *Australian Psychologist, 28,* 128–132.

Mauro, R. (1988). Opponent processes in human emotions? An experimental investigation of hedonic contrast and affective interactions. *Motivation and Emotion, 12,* 333–351.

Mayer, J. (1952). The glucostatic theory of regulation of food intake. *Bulletin of the New England Medical Center, 14,* 43–49.

Mayer, J. (1953). Glucostatic mechanism of regulation of food intake. *New England Journal of Medicine, 249,* 13–16.

Mayhew, R., & Edelmann, R. J. (1989). Self esteem, irrational beliefs and coping strategies in relation to eating problems in a non-clinical population. *Personality and Individual Differences, 10,* 581–584.

Maywood, E. S., Smith, E., Hall, S. J., & Hastings, M. H. (1997). A thalamic contribution to arousal-induced, non-photic entrainment of the circadian clock of the Syrian hamster. *European Journal of Neuroscience, 9,* 1739–1747.

Mazur, J. E. (1995). Conditioned reinforcement and choice with delayed and uncertain primary reinforcers. *Journal of the Experimental Analysis of Behavior, 36,* 139–150.

McAllister, W. R., & McAllister, D. E. (1971). Behavioral measurement of conditioned fear. In F. R. Brush (Ed.), *Aversive conditioning and learning.* New York: Academic Press. Pp. 105–179.

McClelland, D. C. (Ed.). (1955). *Studies in motivation.* New York: Appleton.

McClelland, D. C. (1961). *The achieving society.* New York: Van Nostrand.

McClelland, D. C. (1973). The two faces of power. In D. C. McClelland & R. S. Steele (Eds.), *Human motivation: A book of readings.* Morristown, NJ: General Learning Press. Pp. 300–316.

McClelland, D. C., & Atkinson, J. W. (1948). The projective expression of needs: I. The effect of different intensitities of the hunger drive on perception. *Journal of Psychology, 25,* 205–222.

McClelland, D. C., Atkinson, J. W., Clark, R. A., & Lowell, E. L. (1953). The achievement motive. New York: Appleton-Century-Crofts.

McClelland, D. C., Clark, R. A., Roby, T. B., & Atkinson, J. W. (1949). The projective expression of need for achievement on thematic apperception. *Journal of Experimental Psychology, 39,* 242–255.

McClelland, D. C., Koestner, R., & Weinberger, J. (1989). How do self-attributed and implicit motives differ? *Psychological Review, 96,* 690–702.

McClelland, D. C., & Liberman, A. M. (1949). The effect of need for achievement on recognition of need-related words. *Journal of Personality, 18,* 236–251.

McClelland, D. C., Ross, G., & Patel, V. (1985). The effect of an academic examination on salivary norepinephrine and immunoglobulin levels. *Journal of Human Stress, 11,* 52–59.

McCord, P. R., & Wakefield, D. A. (1981). Arithmetic achievement as a function of introversion-extraversion and teacher-presented reward and punishment. *Personality and Individual Differences, 2,* 145–152.

McCullers, J. C., Fabes, R. A., & Moran, J. D. III. (1987). Does intrinsic motivation theory explain the adverse effects of rewards on immediate task performance? *Journal of Personality and Social Psychology, 52,* 1027–1033.

McDonald, R. J., & White, N. M. (1995). Hippocampal and nonhippocampal contributions to place learning in rats. *Behavioral Neuroscience, 109,* 579–593.

McDougall, W. (1923). *Outline of psychology.* New York: Scribner.

McHoskey, J. (1995). Narcissism and Machiavellianism. *Psychological Reports, 77,* 755–759.

McHugh, P. R. (1990). Clinical issues in food ingestion and body weight maintenance. In E. M. Stricker (Ed.), *Neurobiology of food and fluid intake. Handbook of behavioral neurobiology.* Vol. 10. New York: Plenum Press. Pp. 531–547.

McHugh, P. R., Moran, T. H., & Killilea, M. (1989). The approaches to the study of human disorders in food ingestion and body weight maintenance. In L. H. Schneider, S. J. Cooper, & K. A. Halmi (Eds.), *The psychology of human eating disorders: Preclinical and clinical perspectives.* Vol. 575. *Annals of the New York Academy of Sciences.* New York: New York Academy of Sciences. Pp. 1–11.

McNulty, J. A., & Noseworthy, W. J. (1966). Physiological response specificity, arousal, and task performance. *Perceptual and Motor Skills, 23,* 987–996.

Mednick, M. T. (1989). Fear of success. In H. Tierney (Ed.), *Women's studies encyclopedia.* Vol. 1. Westport, CT: Greenwood.

Meehl, P. E. (1954). *Clinical vs. statistical prediction.* Minneapolis: University of Minnesota Press.

Mehrabian, A. (1995). Theory and evidence bearing on a scale of trait arousability. *Current Psychology (New Brunswick): Developmental, -Learning, -Personality, -Social, 14,* 3–28.

Mehrabian, A., & Epstein, N. (1972). A measure of emotional empathy. *Journal of Personality, 40,* 525–543.

Meijer, J. H., & Rietveld, W. J. (1989). Neurophysiology of the suprachiasmatic circadian pacemaker in rodents. *Physiological Reviews, 69,* 671–707.

Meisel, R. L., & Sachs, B. D. (1994). The physiology of male sexual behavior. In E. Knobil & J. D. Neill (Eds.), *The physiology of reproduction.* New York: Raven Press. Pp. 3–105.

Mendolia, M., & Kleck, R. E. (1993). Effects of talking about a stressful event on arousal: Does what we talk about make a difference? *Journal of Personality and Social Psychology, 64,* 283–292.

Meredith, C. W., & Evans, T. (1990). Encouragement in the family. *Individual Psychology: The Journal of Adlerian Theory, Research, & Practice, 46,* 187–192.

Messer, M. H. (1996). Managing the angry employee: Anger-management skills build on disengagement, validation. *Employee Assistance,* July/August, 22–23.

Messer, M. H., Coronado-Bogdaniak, R., & Dillon, L. J. (1993). *Managing anger: A handbook of proven techniques.* Chicago: The Anger Clinic.

Messick, D. M., & Librand, W. B. G. (1995). Individual heuristics and the dynamics of cooperation in large groups. *Psychological Review, 102,* 131–145.

Meyer, D. E., Schvaneveldt, R. W., & Ruddy, M. G. (1974). Functions of graphemic and phonemic codes in visual word recognition. *Memory and Cognition, 2,* 309–321.

Meyer, W. U. (1992). Paradoxical effects of praise and criticism on perceived ability. In W. Stroebe & M. Hewstone (Eds.), *European review of social psychology.* Vol. 3. Chichester, England: Wiley. Pp. 259–283.

Meyer-Bernstein, E. L., & Morin, L. P. (1996). Differential serotonergic innervation of the suprachiasmatic nucleus and the intergeniculate leaflet and its role in circadian rhythm modulation. *Journal of Neuroscience, 16,* 2097–2111.

Miles, L. E., & Dement, W. C. (1980). Sleep and aging. *Sleep, 3,* 119–220.

Milgram, S. (1963). Behavioral study of obedience. *Journal of Abnormal and Social Psychology, 67,* 371–378.

Milgram, S. (1965). Some conditions of obedience and disobedience to authority. *Human Relations, 18,* 57–75.

Milgram, S. (1974). *Obedience to authority: An experimental view.* New York: Harper & Row.

Miller, A., & Hom, H. L. (1990). Influence of extrinsic and ego incentive value on persistence after failure and continuing motivation. *Journal of Educational Psychology, 82,* 539–545.

Miller, A. G., Collins, B. E., & Brief, D. E. (1995). Perspectives on obedience to authority: The legacy of the Milgram experiments. *Journal of Social Issues, 51,* 1–19.

Miller, N. E. (1948). Studies of fear as an acquirable drive: I. Fear as motivation and fear-reduction as reinforcement in learning of new responses. *Journal of Experimental Psychology, 38,* 89–106.

Mills, R. S., & Grusec, J. E. (1989). Cognitive, affective, and behavioral consequences of praising altruism. *Merrill Palmer Quarterly, 35,* 299–326.

Milner, J. S. (1974). Effects of food deprivation and competition in interspecies aggression in the rat. Paper presented at the meeting of the American Psychological Association, New Orleans.

Milner, J. S. (1993). Social information processing and physical child abuse. *Clinical Psychology Review, 13,* 275–294.

Mineka, S. (1992). Evolutionary memories, emotional processing, and emotional disorders. In D. Medin (Ed.), *The psychology of learning and motivation.* Vol. 28. New York: Academic Press. Pp. 161–206.

Mineka, S., & Sutton, S. K. (1992). Cognitive biases and the emotional disorders. *Psychological Science, 3,* 65–69.

Minors, D., Atkinson, G., Bent, N., Rabbitt, P., & Waterhouse, J. (1998). The effects of age upon some aspects of lifestyle and implications for studies on circadian rhythmicity. *Age and Ageing, 27,* 57–72.

Minors, D. S., Rabbitt, P. M. A., Worthington, H., & Waterhouse, J. M. (1989). Variation in meals and sleep-activity patterns in aged subjects; its relevance to circadian rhythm studies. *Chronobiology International, 6,* 139–146.

Mistlberger, R. E., Bergmann, B. M., Waldenar, W., & Rechtschaffen, A. (1983). Recovery sleep following sleep deprivation in intact and suprachiasmatic nuclei-lesioned rats. *Sleep, 6,* 217–233.

Mitler, M. M., Carskadon, M. A., Czeisler, C. A., Dement, W. C., Dinges, D. F., & Graeber, R. C. (1988). Catastrophes, sleep, and public policy: Consensus report. *Sleep, 11,* 100–109.

Mogg, K., & Marden, B. (1990). Processing of emotional information in anxious subjects. *British Journal of Clinical Psychology, 29,* 227–229.

Monaghan, E. P., & Glickman, S. E. (1993). Hormones and aggressive behavior. In J. B. Becker, S. M. Breedlove, & D. Crews (Eds.), *Behavioral endocrinology.* Cambridge, MA: MIT Press. Pp. 261–285.

Mone, M. A., & Baker, D. D. (1992). A social-cognitive, attributional model of personal goals: An empirical evaluation. *Motivation and Emotion, 16,* 297–321.

Money, J. (1961). Hermaphroditism. In A. Ellis & A. Abarbanel (Eds.), *The encyclopedia of sexual behavior.* New York: Hawthorn. Pp. 472–484.

Money, J., & Ehrhardt, A. A. (1972). *Man and woman, boy and girl.* Baltimore, MD: Johns Hopkins University Press.

Monk, T. H. (1986). Advantages and disadvantages of rapidly rotating shift schedules—a circadian viewpoint. *Human Factors, 28,* 553–557.

Monk, T. H. (1987). Subjective ratings of sleepiness—the underlying circadian mechanisms. *Sleep, 10,* 343–353.

Monk, T. H. (1989). A visual analogue scale technique to measure global vigor and affect. *Psychiatry Research, 27,* 89–99.

Monk, T. H. (1990). Shiftworker performance. *Occupational Medicine: State of the Art Reviews, 5,* 183–198.

Monk, T. H. (1991). Circadian aspects of subjective sleepiness: A behavioral messenger? In T. H. Monk (Ed.), *Sleep, sleepiness, and performance.* New York: Wiley. Pp. 39–63.

Monk, T. H., Buysse, D. J., Reynolds, C. F. III, Jarrett, D. B., & Kupfer, D. J. (1992). Rhythmic vs. homeostatic influences on mood, activation, and performance in young and old men. *Journal of Gerontology: Psychological Sciences, 47,* 221–227.

Monk, T. H., Buysse, D. J., Reynolds, C. F., Kupfer, D. J., & Houck, P. R. (1996). Subjective alertness rhythms in elderly people. *Journal of Biological Rhythms, 11,* 268–276.

Monk, T. H., & Embrey, D. E. (1981). A field study of circadian rhythms in actual and interpolated task performance. In A. Reinberg, N. Vieux, & P. Andlauer (Eds.), *Night and shift work: Biological and social aspects.* Oxford: Pergamon Press. Pp. 473–480.

Monk, T. H., Flaherty, J. F., Frank, E., Hoskinson, K., & Kupfer, D. J. (1990). The social rhythm metric: An instrument to quantify the daily rhythms of life. *The Journal of Nervous and Mental Disease, 178,* 120–126.

Monk, T. H., & Moline, M. L. (1989). The timing of bedtime and waketime decisions in free-running subjects. *Psychophysiology, 26,* 304–310.

Monk, T. H., Moline, M. L., Fookson, J. E., & Peetz, S. M. (1989). Circadian determinants of subjective alertness. *Journal of Biological Rhythms, 4,* 393–404.

Monk, T. H., Reynolds, C. F. III, Machen, M. A., & Kupfer, D. J. (1992). Daily social rhythms in the elderly and their relation to objectively recorded sleep. *Sleep, 15,* 322–329.

Montague, A. (Ed.). (1978). *Learning non-aggression.* New York: Oxford University Press.

Mook, D. G. (1990). Satiety, specifications and stop-rules: Feeding as voluntary action. In A. N. Epstein & A. R. Morrison (Eds.), *Progress in psychobiology and physiological psychology.* Vol. 14. New York: Academic Press. Pp. 1–65.

Moore, L. A., Hughes, J. N., & Robinson, M. (1992). A comparison of the social information-processing abilities of rejected and accepted hyperactive children. *Journal of Clinical Child Psychology, 21,* 123–131.

Moore, R. Y. (1978). Central neural control of circadian rhythms. In W. F. Ganong & L. Martini (Eds.), *Frontiers in Neuroendocrinology, 5,* New York: Raven Press. Pp. 185–206.

Moore, R. Y. (1995). Organization of the mammalian circadian system. In D. J. Derek & K. Ackrill (Eds.), *Circadian clocks and their adjustment* (Ciba Foundation Symposium, 183). Chichester: Wiley. Pp. 88–106.

Moore, R. Y. (1997). Circadian rhythms: Basic neurobiology and clinical applications. *Annual Review of Medicine, 48,* 253–266.

Moore, R. Y., & Lenn, N. J. (1972). A retinohypothalamic projection in the rat. *Journal of Comparative Neurology, 146,* 1–14.

Moore-Ede, M. C., Sulzman, F. M., & Fuller, C. A. (1982). *The clocks that time us.* Cambridge, MA: Harvard University Press.

Moos, R. H. (1992a). *Coping responses inventory: Adult form manual.* Palo Alto, CA: Center for Health Care Evaluation, Stanford University.

Moos, R. H. (1992b). Understanding individuals' life contexts: Implications for stress reduction and prevention. In M. Kessler, S. E. Godston, & J. Joffe (Eds.), *The present and future of prevention research.* Newbury Park, CA: Sage. Pp. 196–213.

Morehouse, R. E., Farley, F. H., & Youngquist, J. V. (1990). Type T personality and the Jungian classification system. *Journal of Personality Assessment, 54,* 231–235.

Morgenstern, J., Langenbucher, J., Labouvie, E., & Miller, K. J. (1997). The comorbidity of alcoholism and personality disorders in clinical population: Prevalence rates and relation to alcohol typology variables. *Journal of Abnormal Psychology, 106,* 74–84.

Morin, L. (1988). Age-related changes in hamster circadian period, entrainment, and rhythm splitting. *Journal of Biological Rhythms, 3,* 237–248.

Moruzzi, G., & Magoun, H. W. (1949). Brain stem reticular formation and activation of the EEG. *Electroencephalography and Clinical Neurophysiology, 1,* 455–473.

Mosak, H. H. (1977). *On purpose: Collected papers.* Chicago: Adler School of Professional Psychology.

Mosak, H. H., & Dreikurs, R. (1973). Adlerian psychotherapy. In R. J. Corsini (Ed.), *Current psychotherapies.* Itasca, IL: Peacock.

Motowidlo, S. J. (1979). Development of a measure of generalized expectancy of task success. *Educational Psychological Measurement, 39,* 69–80.

Moulton, R. W. (1965). Effects of success and failure on level of aspiration as related to achievement motives. *Journal of Personality and Social Psychology, 1,* 399–406.

Mowrer, O. H. (1940). Anxiety reduction and learning. *Journal of Experimental Psychology, 27,* 497–516.

Mowrer, O. H. (1950). *Learning theory and personality dynamics.* New York: Ronald.

Mowrer, O. H. (1951). Two-factor learning theory: Summary and comment. *Psychological Review, 58,* 350–354.

Mowrer, O. H. (1960). *Learning theory and behavior.* New York: Wiley.

Mowrer, O. H., & Aiken, E. G. (1954). Contiguity vs. drive-reduction in conditioned fear: Temporal variations in conditioned and unconditioned stimulus. *American Journal of Psychology, 67,* 26–38.

Moyer, K. E. (1976). *The psychology of aggression.* New York: Harper & Row.

Mrosovsky, N. (1996). Locomotor activity and non-photic influences on circadian clocks. *Biological Reviews, 71,* 343–372.

Muller, J. E., Stone, P. H., Turi, Z. G., Rutherford, J. D., Czeisler, C. A., Parker, C., Poole, W. K., Passamani, E., Roberts, R., Robertson, T., Sobel, B. E., Willerson, J. T., & Braunwald, E. (1985). Circadian variation in the frequency of onset of acute myocardial infarction. *New England Journal of Medicine, 313,* 1315–1322.

Munk, M. H. J., Roelfsema, P. R., Konig, P., Engel, A. K., & Singer, W. (1996). Role of reticular activation in the modulation of intracortical synchronization. *Science, 272* (12 April), 271–274.

Muris, P., & Steerneman, P. (1996). The role of parental fearfulness and modeling in children's fear. *Behaviour Research & Therapy, 34,* 265–268.

Murphy, C. M., & O'Farrell, T. J. (1996). Marital violence among alcoholics. *Current Directions in Psychological Science, 5,* 183–186.

Murray, H. A. (1938). *Explorations in personality.* New York: Oxford University Press.

Musty, R. E. (1976/1982). Homeostatic drives and consummatory behavior: Hunger and thirst. In E. D. Ferguson, *Motivation: An experimental approach.* Originally published in 1976. Reprinted Melbourne, FL: Krieger. Pp. 194–231.

Musty, R. E. (1982). Homeostatic drives and consummatory behavior: Hunger and thirst. In Ferguson, E. D. *Motivation: An experimental approach.* Melbourne, FL: Krieger.

Myers, B. L., & Badia, P. (1995). Changes in circadian rhythms and sleep quality with aging: Mechanisms and interventions. *Neuroscience and Biobehavioral Reviews, 19,* 553–571.

Nader K., & van der Kooy, D. (1994). The motivation produced by morphine and food is isomorphic: Approaches to specific motivational stimuli are learned. *Psychobiology, 22,* 68–76.

Neiss, R. (1988). Reconceptualizing arousal: Psychobiological states in motor performance. *Psychological Bulletin, 103,* 345–366.

Neiss, R. (1990). Ending arousal's reign of error: A reply to Anderson. *Psychological Bulletin, 107,* 101–105.

Nelson, J. G. (1992). Class clowns as a function of the Type T psychobiological personality. *Personality and Individual Differences, 13,* 1247–1248.

Nestler, E. J., & Aghajanian, G. K. (1997). Molecular and cellular basis of addiction. *Science, 278,* 58–63.

Netter, P. (1991). Do biochemical response patterns tell us anything about trait anxiety? In C. D. Spielberger, I. G. Sarason, Z. Kulcsar, & G. L. Van Heck (Eds.), *Stress and emotion: Anxiety, anger, and curiosity.* Vol. 14. New York: Hemisphere. Pp. 187–213.

Newell, A., & Simon, H. A. (1961). Computer simulation of human thinking. *Science, 134,* 2011–2017.

Niaura, R. S., Rohsenow, D. J., Binkoff, J. A., Monti, P. M., Pedraza, M., & Abrams, D. B. (1988). Relevance of cue reactivity to understanding alcohol and smoking relapse. *Journal of Abnormal Psychology, 97,* 133–152.

Nisbett, R. E. (1972). Eating behavior and obesity in men and animals. *Advances in Psychosomatic Medicine, 1,* 173–193.

Noel, M. B., & Wise, R. A. (1993). Ventral tegmental injections of morphine but not U-50,488H enhance feeding in food-deprived rats. *Brain Research, 632,* 68–73.

Nolen-Hoeksema, S., Girgus, J. S., & Seligman, M. E. P. (1986). Learned helplessness in children: A longitudinal study of depression, achievement, and explanatory style. *Journal of Personality and Social Psychology, 51,* 435–442.

Novaco, R. W. (1975). *Anger control: The development and evaluation of an experimental treatment.* Lexington, MA: Lexington Books.

Nowlis, V. (1965). Research with the Mood Adjective Check List. In S. S. Tomkins & C. E. Izard (Eds), *Affect, cognition, and personality.* New York: Springer. Pp. 352–389.

Nunez, J. F., & Ferre, P. (1995). Postnatal handling reduces emotionality ratings and accelerates two-way active avoidance in female rats. *Physiology & Behavior, 57,* 831–835.

Oakhill, J. (1988). Text memory and integration at different times of day. *Applied Cognitive Psychology, 2,* 203–212.

Obrist, P. A. (1981). *Cardiovascular psychophysiology: A perspective.* New York: Plenum.

Obrist, P. A., Webb, R. A., Sutterer, J. R., & Howard, J. L. (1970). Cardiac deceleration and reaction time: An evaluation of two hypotheses. *Psychophysiology, 6,* 695–706.

Oden, G. C. (1977). Fuzziness in semantic memory. Choosing exemplars of subjective categories. *Memory & Cognition, 5,* 198–204.

Ohman, A. (1996). Preferential preattentive processing of

threat in anxiety: Preparedness and attentional biases. In R. M. Rappee (Ed.), *Current controversies in the anxiety disorders.* New York: Guilford. Pp. 253–290.

Oldfield, B. J. (1991). Neurochemistry of the circuitry subserving thirst. In D. J. Ramsay and D. A. Booth (Eds.), *Thirst: Physiological and psychological aspects.* New York: Springer. Pp. 176–193.

Olds, J., & Milner, P. M. (1954). Positive reinforcement produced by electrical stimulation of septal area and other regions of rat brain. *Journal of Comparative and Physiological Psychology, 47,* 419–427.

Olmsted, M. P., Davis, R., Garner, D. M., Eagle, M., Rockert, W., & Irvine, M. J. (1991). Efficacy of a brief group psychoeducational intervention for bulimia nervosa. *Behaviour Research and Therapy, 29,* 71–84.

O'Neal, E. C. (1991). Violence and aggression. In R. M. Baron & W. G. Graziano (Eds.), *Social psychology.* Fort Worth, TX: Holt, Rinehart and Winston. Pp. 310–351.

O'Neal, E. C., Kipnis, D., & Craig, K. M. (1994). Effects on the persuader of employing a coercive influence technique. *Basic and Applied Social Psychology, 15,* 225–238.

O'Neal, E. C., Macdonald, P. J., Cloninger, C., & Levine, D. (1979). Coactor's behavior and imitative aggression. *Motivation and Emotion, 3,* 373–379.

Orbell, J., Dawes, R., & Schwartz-Shea, P. (1994). Trust, social categories, and individuals: The case of gender. *Motivation and Emotion, 18,* 109–128.

Orlick, T. (1978). *The cooperative sports and games book.* New York: Pantheon.

Osborne, S. R. (1978). A quantitative analysis of the effects of the amount of reinforcement on two response classes. *Journal of Experimental Psychology: Animal Behavior Processes, 4,* 297–317.

Ostmann, A. (1992). The interaction of aspiration levels and the social field in experimental bargaining. *Journal of Economic Psychology, 13,* 233–261.

O'Sullivan, J. T. (1993). Preschoolers' beliefs about effort, incentives, and recall. *Journal of Experimental Child Psychology, 55,* 396–414.

Ottaviani, R., & Beck, A. T. (1988). Cognitive theory of depression. In K. Fiedler & J. Forgas (Eds.), *Affect, cognition and social behavior: New evidence and integrative attempts.* Zurich: C. J. Hogrefe. Pp. 209–218.

Overmier, J. B., & Seligman, M. E. P. (1967). Effects of inescapable shock upon subsequent escape and avoidance responding. *Journal of Comparative and Physiological Psychology, 63,* 28–33.

Overmier, J. B., & Wielkiewicz, R. M. (1983). On unpredictability as a causal factor in "learned helplessness." *Learning and Motivation, 14,* 324–337.

Overskeid, G., & Svartdal, F. (1996). Effect of reward on subjective autonomy and interest when initial interest is low. *The Psychological Record, 46,* 319–322.

Oyster, C. K. (1992). Perceptions of power: Female executives' descriptions of power usage by "best" and "worst" bosses. *Psychology of Women Quarterly, 16,* 527–533.

Palanza, P., Parmigiani, S., & Vom Saal, F. S. (1995). Urine marking and maternal aggression of wild female mice in relation to anogenital distance at birth. *Physiology and Behavior, 58,* 827–835.

Panksnepp, J. (1986). The neurochemistry of behavior. In M. R. Rosenzweig & L. W. Porter (Eds.), *Annual review of psychology.* Vol. 37. Palo Alto, CA: Annual Reviews, Inc. Pp. 77–107.

Papez, J. W. (1937). A proposed mechanism of emotion. *Archives of Neurology and Psychiatry, 38,* 725–743.

Park, B., & Hahn, S. (1988). Sex-role identity and the perception of others. *Social Cognition, 6,* 61–87.

Parker, J. G., & Asher, S. R. (1993). Beyond group acceptance: Friendship and friendship quality as distinct dimensions of children's peer adjustment. In D. Perlman & W. H. Jones (Eds.), *Advances in personal relationships.* Vol. 4. Greenwich, CT: JAI Press, Jessica Kingsley. Pp. 261–294.

Parks, C. D., & Vu, A. D. (1994). Social dilemma behavior of individuals from highly individualist and collectivist cultures. *Journal of Conflict Resolution, 38,* 708–718.

Parsons, M. W., & Gold, P. E. (1992). Scopolamine-induced deficits in spontaneous alternation performance: Attenuation with lateral ventricle injections of glucose. *Behavioral and Neural Biology, 57,* 90–92.

Paulhus, D., & Christie, R. (1981). Spheres of control: An interactionist approach to assessment of perceived control. In H. M. Lefcourt (Ed.), *Research with the locus of control construct.* Vol. 1. New York: Academic Press. Pp. 161–188.

Pavlov (1928). *Lectures on conditioned reflexes.* New York: International.

Pavlov (1941). *Conditioned reflexes and psychiatry.* New York: International.

Pavlov, I. P. (1927). *Conditioned reflexes.* London: Oxford University Press.

Pedersen, J. M., Glickman, S. E., Frank, L. G., & Beach,

F. A. (1990). Sex differences in the play behavior of immature spotted hyenas, *Crocuta crocuta*. *Hormones and Behavior, 24,* 403–420.

Pelchat, M. L., Grill, H. J., Rozin, P., & Jacobs, J. (1983). Quality of acquired responses to tastes by *Rattus norvegicus* depends on type of associated discomfort. *Journal of Comparative Psychology, 97,* 140–153.

Pelleymounter, M. A., Cullen, M. J., Baker, M. B., Hecht, R., Winters, D., Boone, T., & Collins, F. (1995). Effects of the *obese* gene product on body weight regulation in *ob/ob* mice. *Science, 269,* 540–543.

Pellis, S. M., MacDonald, N. L., & Michener, G. R. (1996). Lateral display as a combat tactic in Richardson's ground squirrel *Spermophilus richardsonii*. *Aggressive Behavior, 22,* 119–134.

Pellis, S. M., Pellis, V. C., & Kolb, B. (1992). Neonatal testosterone augmentation increases juvenile play fighting but does not influence the adult cominance relationships of male rats. *Aggressive Behavior, 18,* 437–447.

Pellis, S. M., Pellis, V. C., & McKenna, M. M. (1993). Some subordinates are more equal than others: Play fighting amongst adult subordinate male rats. *Aggressive Behavior, 19,* 385–393.

Peplau, L. A., Hill, C. T., & Rubin, Z. (1993). Sex role attitudes in dating and marriage: A 15-year follow-up of the Boston couples study. *Journal of Social Issues, 49,* 31–52.

Pervin, L. A. (1992). The rational mind and the problem of volition. *Psychological Science, 3,* 162–164.

Peterson, C., & Barrett, L. C. (1987). Explanatory style and academic performance among university freshmen. *Journal of Personality and Social Psychology, 53,* 603–607.

Peterson, C., & Bossio, L. M. (1991). *Health and optimism.* New York: Free Press.

Peterson, C., Maier, S. F., & Seligman, M. E. P. (1993). *Learned helplessness: A theory for the age of personal control.* New York: Oxford University Press.

Pfefferbaum, B., & Wood, P. B. (1994). Self-report study of impulsive and delinquent behavior in college students. *Journal of Adolescent Health, 15,* 295–302.

Phillips, R. E. (1968). Comparison of direct and vicarious reinforcement and an investigation of methodological variables. *Journal of Experimental Psychology, 78,* 666–669.

Phillips, S. D., & Imhoff, A. R. (1997). Women and career development: A decade of research. *Annual Review of Psychology, 48,* 31–59.

Pickard, G. E. (1982). The afferent connections of the suprachiasmatic nucleus of the golden hamster with emphasis on the retinohypothalamic projection. *Journal of Comparative Neurology, 211,* 65–83.

Pickard, G. E., Ralph, M. R., & Menaker, M. (1987). The intergeniculate leaflet partially mediates effects of light on circadian rhythms. *Journal of Biological Rhythms, 2,* 35–56.

Piedmont, R. L. (1988). An interactional model of achievement motivation and fear of success. *Sex Roles, 19,* 467–490.

Piedmont, R. L. (1995). Another look at fear of success, fear of failure, and test anxiety: A motivational analysis using the five factor model. *Sex Roles, 32,* 139–158.

Pinel, J. P. J. (1990). *Biopsychology.* Boston: Allyn and Bacon.

Pitsounis, N. D., & Dixon, P. N. (1988). Encouragement versus praise: Improving productivity of the mentally regarded. *Individual Psychology: The Journal of Adlerian Theory, Research, & Practice, 44,* 507–512.

Pittendrigh, C. S. (1981a). Circadian systems: General perspective. In J. Aschoff (Ed.), *Handbook of behavioral neurobiology, Vol 4: Biological rhythms.* New York: Plenum Press. Pp. 57–80.

Pittendrigh, C. S. (1981b). Circadian systems: Entrainment. In J. Aschoff (Ed.), *Handbook of behavioral neurobiology, Vol 4: Biological rhythms.* New York: Plenum Press. Pp. 95–124.

Pittendrigh, C. S. (1993). Temporal organization: Reflections of a Darwinian clock-watcher. *Annual Review of Physiology, 55,* 17–54.

Pittendrigh, C. S., & Daan, S. (1974). Circadian oscillations in rodents: A systematic increase of their frequency with age. *Science, 186,* 548–550.

Pittendrigh, C. S., & Daan, S. (1976). A functional analysis of circadian pacemakers in nocturnal rodents. I. The stability and lability of spontaneous frequency. *Journal of Comparative Physiology, 106,* 223–252.

Placentini, A., Schell, A. M., & Vanderweele, D. A. (1993). Restrained and nonrestrained eaters' orienting responses to food and nonfood odors. *Physiology & Behavior, 53,* 133–138.

Pleck, J. H., Sonenstein, F. L., & Ku, L. C. (1993). Masculinity ideology: Its impact on adolescent males' heterosexual relationships. *Journal of Social Issues, 49,* 11–29.

Pliner, P. (1974). On the generalizability of the externality hypothesis. In S. Schachter & J. Rodin (Eds.), *Obese humans and rats.* New York: Wiley. Pp. 111–129.

Poothullil, J. M. (1992). Maltose: The primary signal of hunger and satiation in human beings. *Physiology & Behavior, 52,* 27–31.

Postman, L. (1947). The history and present status of the Law of Effect. *Psychological Bulletin, 44,* 489–563.

Postman, L. (1962). Rewards and punishments in human learning. In L. Postman (Ed.), *Psychology in the making.* New York: Knopf. Pp. 331–401.

Postman, L., & Crutchfield, R. C. (1952). The interaction of need, set and stimulus structure in a cognitive task. *American Journal of Psychology, 65,* 196–217.

Postman, L., & Schwartz, M. (1964). Studies of learning to learn: 1. Transfer as a function of method of practice and class of verbal materials. *Journal of Verbal Learning and Verbal Behavior, 3,* 37–49.

Preston, M. G., & Bayton, J. A. (1941). Differential effect of a social variable upon three levels of aspiration. *Journal of Experimental Psychology, 29,* 351–369.

Price, R. A., & Gottesman, I. I. (1991). Body fat in identical twins reared apart: Roles for genes and environment. *Behavior Genetics, 21,* 1–7.

Pubols, B. H., Jr. (1960). Incentive magnitude, learning and performance in animals. *Psychological Bulletin, 57,* 89–115.

Pulkkinen, L. (1996a). Female and male personality styles: A typological and developmental analysis. *Journal of Personality and Social Psychology, 70,* 1288–1306.

Pulkkinen, L. (1996b). Proactive and reactive aggression in early adolescence as precursors to anti- and prosocial behavior in young adults. *Aggressive Behavior, 22,* 241–257.

Pulkkinen, L., & Pitkanen, T. (1993). Continuities in aggressive behavior from childhood to adulthood. *Aggressive Behavior, 19,* 249–263.

Quiggle, N. L., Garber, J., Panak, W. F., & Dodge, K. A. (1993). Social information processing in aggressive and depressed children. *Child Development, 63,* 1305–1320.

Raccuglia, R. A., & Phaf, R. H. (1997). Asymmetric affective evaluation of words and faces. *British Journal of Psychology, 88,* 93–116.

Rachlin, H. (1997). Four teleological theories of addiction. *Psychonomic Bulletin & Review, 4,* 462–473.

Ragozzino, M. E., Unick, K. E., & Gold, P. E. (1996). Hippocampal acetylcholine release during memory testing in rats: Augmentation by glucose. *Proceedings of the National Academy of Sciences, 93,* 4693–4698.

Ramsay, D. J. (1991). Water: Distribution between compartments and its relationship to thirst. In D. J. Ramsay and D. A. Booth (Eds.), *Thirst: Physiological and psychological aspects.* New York: Springer. Pp. 23–34.

Ramsay, D. J., & Booth, D. A. (Eds.) (1991). *Thirst: Physiological and psychological aspects.* New York: Springer.

Ramsay, D. J., & Thrasher, T. N. (1990). Thirst and water balance. In E. M. Stricker (Ed.), *Neurobiology of food and fluid intake. Handbook of behavioral neurobiology.* Vol. 10. New York: Plenum Press. Pp. 353–387.

Ramsay, D. S., Seeley, R. J., Bolles, R. C., & Woods, S. C. (1996). Ingestive homeostasis: The primacy of learning. In E. D. Capaldi (Ed.), *Why we eat what we eat: The psychology of eating.* Washington, DC: American Psychological Association. Pp. 11–27.

Rapoport, A. (1970). Conflict resolution in the light of game theory and beyond. In P. Swingle (Ed.), *The structure of conflict.* New York: Academic Press. Pp. 1–43.

Ratcliff, R., & McKoon, G. (1981). Automatic and strategic priming in recognition. *Journal of Verbal Learning and Verbal Behavior, 20,* 204–215.

Raven, B. H. (1990). Political applications of the psychology of interpersonal influence and social power. *Political Psychology, 11,* 493–520.

Raven, B. H. (1992). A power/interaction model of interpersonal influence: French and Raven thirty years later. *Journal of Social Behavior and Personality, 7,* 217–244.

Raven, B. H. (1993). The bases of power: Origins and recent developments. *Journal of Social Issues, 49,* 227–251.

Raven, B. H., & Kruglanski, A. W. (1970). Conflict and power. In P. G. Swingle (Ed.), *The structure of conflict.* New York: Academic Press. Pp. 69–109.

Rawl, S. M. (1992). Perspectives on nursing care of Chinese Americans. *Journal of Holistic Nursing, 10,* 6–17.

Raynor, J. O. (1969). Future orientation and motivation in immediate activity: An elaboration of the theory of achievement motivation. *Psychological Review, 76,* 606–610.

Raynor, J. O. (1970). Relationships between achievement-related motives, future orientation, and academic performance. *Journal of Personality and Social Psychology, 15,* 28–33.

Rechtschaffen, A., Bergmann, B. M., Everson, C. A., Kushida, C. A., & Gilliland, M. A. (1989). Sleep deprivation in the rat: X. Integration and discussion of findings. *Sleep, 12,* 68–87.

Redd, M., & de Castro, J. M. (1992). Social facilitation of

eating: Effects of social instruction on food intake. *Physiology & Behavior, 52,* 749–754.

Redlin, U., & Mrosovsky, N. (1997). Exercise and human circadian rhythms: What we know and what we need to know. *Chronobiology International, 14,* 221–229.

Reebs, S. G., Lavery, R. J., & Mrosovsky, N. (1989). Running activity mediates the phase-advancing effects of dark pulses on hamster circadian rhythms. *Journal of Comparative Physiology A, 165,* 811–818.

Reeve, J., & Deci, E. L. (1996). Elements of the competitive situations that affect intrinsic motivation. *Personality and Social Psychology Bulletin, 22,* 24–33.

Reilly, T., Waterhouse, J., & Atkinson, G. (1997). Aging, rhythms of performance, and adjustments to changes in the sleep-activity cycle. *Occupational and Environmental Medicine, 54,* 812–816.

Reite, M., & Capitanio, J. P. (1985). On the nature of social separation and social attachment. In M. Reite & T. Field (Eds.), *Psychobiology of attachment and separation.* New York: Academic Press. Pp. 223–258.

Renfrew, J. W. (1997). *Aggression and its causes: A biopsychosocial approach.* New York: Oxford University Press.

Reppert, S. M., & Weaver, D. R. (1995). Melatonin madness. *Cell, 83,* 1059–1062.

Restoin, A., Montagner, H., Godard, D., Henry, J. C., Henrotte, J. G., Lombardot, M., Benedini, M., Pretet, M. T., & Prouteau, C. (1981). New data on circadian rhythms of corticosteroid hormones and magnesium in the young child in the day care centre and in the kindergarten. In A. Reinberg, N. Vieux, & P. Andlauer (Eds.), *Night and shift work: Biological and social aspects.* Oxford: Pergamon Press. Pp. 331–339.

Reuterman, N. A., & Burcky, W. D. (1989). Dating violence in high school: A profile of the victims. *Psychology: A Journal of Human Behavior, 26,* 1–5.

Revelle, W. (1989). Personality, motivation, and cognitive performance. In R. Kanfer, P. L. Ackerman, & R. Cudeck (Eds.), *Abilities, motivation, and methodology: The Minnesota Symposium on learning and individual differences.* Hillsdale, NJ: Erlbaum. Pp. 297–341.

Revelle, W., & Anderson, K. J. (1992). Models for the testing of theory. In A. Gale & M. W. Eysenck (Eds.), *Handbook of individual differences: Biological perspectives.* New York: Wiley.

Revelle, W., Anderson, K. J., & Humphreys, M. S. (1987). Empirical tests and theoretical extensions of arousal-based theories of personality. In J. Strelau & H. J. Eysenck (Eds.), *Personality dimensions and arousal.* London: Plenum. Pp. 17–36.

Revelle, W., Humphreys, M. S., Simon, L., & Gilliland, K. (1980). The interactive effect of personality, time of day, and caffeine: A test of the arousal model. *Journal of Experimental Psychology: General, 109,* 1–31.

Reynaert, C., Janne, P., Bosly, A., Staquet, P., Zdanowicz, N., Vause, M., Chatelain, B., & Lejeune, D. (1995). From health locus of control to immune control: Internal locus of control has a buffering effect on natural killer cell activity decrease in major depression. *Acta Psychiatrica Scandinavica, 92,* 294–300.

Richards, A., & Millwood, B. (1989). Color-identification of differentially valenced words in anxiety. *Cognition and Emotion, 3,* 171–176.

Richards, R. W., & Marcattilo, A. J. (1978). Simulus control and delayed reinforcement. *Learning and Motivation, 9,* 54–68.

Richardson, G. S., Carskadon, M. A., Orav, E. J., & Dement, W. C. (1982). Circadian variation of sleep tendency in elderly and young adult subjects. *Sleep, 5,* S82–S94.

Richardson, T. E. (1997). Conclusions from the study of gender differences in cognition. In P. J. Caplan, M. Crawford, J. S. Hyde, & T. E. Richardson (Eds.), *Gender differences in human cognition.* New York: Oxford University Press. Pp. 131–169.

Ritter, R. C., Brenner, L. A., & Tamura, C. S. (1994). Endogenous CCK and the peripheral neural substrates of intestinal satiety. In J. R. Reeve, Jr., V. Eysslelein, T. E. Solomon, & V. I. W. Go (Eds.), *Cholecystokinin.* Vol. 713. *Annals of the New York Academy of Sciences.* New York: New York Academy of Sciences. Pp. 255–267.

Robarchek, C. A., & Robarchek, C. J. (1992). Cultures of war and peace: A comparative study of Waorani and Semai. In J. Silverberg & J. P. Gray (Eds.), *Aggression and peacefulness in humans and other primates.* New York: Oxford University Press. Pp. 189–213.

Robbins, T. W. (1997). Arousal systems and attentional processes. *Biological Psychology, 45,* 57–71.

Roberts, G., Treasure, D. C., & Hall, H. K. (1994). Parental goal orientations and beliefs about the competitive-sport experience of their child. *Journal of Applied Social Psychology, 24,* 631–645.

Roberts, G. C., & Treasure, D. C. (1992). Children in sport. *Sport Science Review, 1,* 46–64.

Roberts, W. A. (1998). *Principles of animal cognition.* New York: McGraw-Hill.

Rodin, J., Elman, D., & Schachter, S. (1974). Emotionality and obesity. In S. Schachter & J. Rodin (Eds.), *Obese humans and rats.* New York: Wiley. Pp. 15–20.

Rolls, B. J. (1991). Physiological determinants of fluid intake in humans. In D. J. Ramsay and D. A. Booth (Eds.), *Thirst: Physiological and psychological aspects.* New York: Springer. Pp. 391–399.

Rolls, B. J., & Rolls, E. T. (1982). *Thirst.* Cambridge: Cambridge University Press.

Rolls, B. J., Rolls, E. T., Rowe, E. A., & Sweeney, K. (1981). Sensory specific satiety in man. *Physiology & Behavior, 27,* 137–142.

Rolls, B. J., Wood, R. J., Rolls, E. T., Lind, H., Lind, W., & Ledingham, J. G. G. (1980). Thirst following water deprivation in humans. *American Journal of Physiology, 239,* R476–482.

Rolls, E. T. (1990). A theory of emotion, and its application to understanding the neural basis of emotion. *Cognition and Emotion, 4,* 161–190.

Roney, C. J. R., & Sorrentino, R. M. (1995). Reducing self-discrepancies or maintaining self-congruence? Uncertainty orientation, self-regulation, and performance. *Journal of Personality and Social Psychology, 68,* 485–497.

Rosas, J. M., & Bouton, M. E. (1997). Renewal of a conditioned taste aversion upon return to the conditioning context after extinction in another one. *Learning and Motivation, 28,* 216–229.

Rosenman, R. H. (1978). The Interview method of assessment of the coronary-prone behavior pattern. In T. Dembroski, S. M. Weiss, J. Shields, S. Haynes, & M. Feinleib (Eds.), *Coronary-prone behavior.* New York: Springer Verlag. Pp. 55–69.

Rosenthal, N. E., Sack, D. A., Gillin, J. C., Lewy, A. J., Goodwin, F. K., Davenport, Y., Mueller, P. S., Newsome, D. A., & Wehr, T. A. (1984). Seasonal affective disorder: A description of the syndrome and preliminary findings with light therapy. *Archives of General Psychiatry, 41,* 72–80.

Rosenthal, N. E., Sack, D. A., Skwerer, R. G., Jacobsen, F. M., & Wehr, T. A. (1988). Phototherapy for seasonal affective disorder. *Journal of Biological Rhythms, 3,* 101–120.

Rosenwasser, A. M., & Adler, N. T. (1986). Structure and function in circadian timing systems: Evidence for multiple coupled circadian oscillators. *Neuroscience and Biobehavioral Reviews, 10,* 431–448.

Rosenwasser, A. M., Boulos, Z., & Terman, M. (1981). Circadian organization of food intake and meal patterns in the rat. *Physiology & Behavior, 27,* 32–39.

Rosenzweig, M. R., Leiman, A. L., & Breedlove, S. M. (1996). *Biological psychology.* Sunderland, MA: Sinauer.

Rotter, J. B. (1942). Level of aspiration as a method of studying personality: II. Development and evaluation of a controlled method. *Journal of Experimental Psychology, 31,* 410–421.

Rotter, J. B. (1966). Generalized expectancies for internal versus external control of reinforcement. *Psychological Monographs, 80* (1, Whole No. 609).

Rotter, J. B. (1990). Internal versus external control of reinforcement: A case history of a variable. *American Psychologist, 45,* 489–493.

Rotter, J. B. (1992). "Cognates of personal control: Locus of control, self-efficacy, and explanatory style": Comment. *Applied and Preventive Psychology, 1,* 127–129.

Rotter, J. B., Seeman, M., & Liverant, S. (1962). Internal versus external control of reinforcements: A major variable in behavior theory. In N. F. Washburne (Ed.), *Decisions, values, and groups.* New York: Pergamon. Pp. 473–516.

Routtenberg, A., & Lindy, J. (1965). Effects on the availability of rewarding septal and hypothalamic stimulation on bar pressing for food under conditions of deprivation. *Journal of Comparative and Physiological Psychology, 60,* 158–161.

Rowland, N. E., Li, B-H., & Morien, A. (1996). Brain mechanisms and the physiology of feeding. In E. D. Capaldi (Ed.), *Why we eat what we eat: The psychology of eating.* Washington, DC: American Psychological Association. Pp. 173–204.

Rozin, P. (1989). Disorders of food selection: The compromise of pleasure. In L. H. Schneider, S. J. Cooper, & K. A. Halmi (Eds.), *The psychology of human eating disorders: Preclinical and clinical perspectives.* Vol. 575. *Annals of the New York Academy of Sciences.* New York: New York Academy of Sciences. Pp. 376–386.

Rozin, P. (1996). Sociocultural influences on human food selection. In E. D. Capaldi (Ed.), *Why we eat what we eat: The psychology of eating.* Washington, DC: American Psychological Association. Pp. 233–263.

Rozin, P., & Fallon, A. E. (1987). A perspective on disgust. *Psychological Review, 94,* 23–41.

Rozin, P., & Fallon, A. (1988). Body image, attitudes to weight, and misperceptions of figure preferences of the opposite sex: A comparison of men and women in two generations. *Journal of Abnormal Psychology, 97,* 342–345.

Rozin, P. N., Millman, L., & Nemeroff, C. (1986). Operation of the laws of sympathetic magic in disgust and other domains. *Journal of Personality and Social Psychology, 50,* 703–712.

Rozin, P. N., & Shulkin, J. (1990). Food selection. In

E. M. Stricker (Ed.), *Neurobiology of food and fluid intake. Handbook of behavioral neurobiology.* Vol. 10. New York: Plenum Press. Pp. 297–327.

Rubin, Z. (1970). Measurement of romantic love. *Journal of Personality and Social Psychology, 16,* 265–273.

Rusak, B., & Zucker, I. (1979). Neural regulation of circadian rhythms. *Physiological Reviews, 59,* 449–526.

Russel, J. A. (1991). Culture and the categorization of emotions. *Psychological Bulletin, 110,* 426–450.

Sack, R. L., & Lewy, A. J. (1997). Melatonin as a chronobiotic: Treatment of circadian desynchrony in night workers and the blind. *Journal of Biological Rhythms, 12,* 595–603.

Sakai, L. M., Baker, L. A., Jacklin, C. N., & Shulman, I. (1995). Sex steroids at birth: Genetic and environmental variation and covariation. *Developmental Psychobiology, 24,* 559–570.

Saugstad. P. (1966). Effect of food deprivation on perception-cognition. *Psychological Bulletin, 65,* 80–90.

Sayette, M. A., Wilson, G. T., & Elias, M. J. (1993). Alcohol and aggression: A social information processing analysis. *Journal of Studies on Alcohol, 54,* 399–407.

Saylor, M., & Denham, G. (1993). Women's anger and self-esteem. In S. P. Thomas (Ed.), *Women and anger.* New York: Springer. Pp. 91–111.

Schachter, S. (1967). Cognitive effects on bodily functioning: Studies of obesity and eating. In D. C. Glass (Ed.), *Neurophysiology and emotion.* New York: Rockefeller University Press. Pp. 117–144.

Schachter, S. (1971). *Emotion, obesity and crime.* New York: Academic Press.

Schachter, S., & Singer, J. E. (1962). Cognitive, social, and physiological determinants of emotional state. *Psychological Review, 69,* 379–399.

Schallert, T. (1989). Preoperative intermittent feeding or drinking regimens enhance postlesion sensorimotor function. In J. Schulkin (Ed.), *Preoperative events: Their effects on behavior following brain damage.* Hillsdale, NJ: Erlbaum. Pp. 1–20.

Schallert, T. (1991). Neostriatal mechanisms affecting drinking. In D. J. Ramsay and D. A. Booth (Eds.), *Thirst: Physiological and psychological aspects.* New York: Springer. Pp. 232–239.

Schick, R. R., Schusdziarra, V., Yaksh, T. L., & Go, V. L. W. (1994). Brain regions where cholecystokinin exerts its effect on satiety. In J. R. Reeve, Jr., V. Eysslelein, T. E. Solomon, & V. I. W. Go (Eds.), *Cholecystokinin.* Vol. 713. *Annals of the New York Academy of Sciences.* New York: New York Academy of Sciences. Pp. 242–254.

Schmidt, H. O. (1945). Test profiles as a diagnostic aid: The Minnesota Multiphasic Inventory. *Journal of Applied Psychology, 29,* 115–131.

Schneider, S. L. (1992). Framing and conflict: Aspiration level contingency, the status quo, and current theories of risky choice. *Journal of Experimental Psychology: Learning, Memory, and Cognition, 18,* 1040–1057.

Schneider, T. (1976). *Everybody's a winner.* Boston: Little, Brown.

Schuster, B., Forsterling, F., & Weiner, B. (1989). Perceiving the causes of success and failure: A cross-cultural examination of attributional concepts. *Journal of Cross Cultural Psychology, 20,* 191–213.

Schwartz, G. E., & Johnson, H. J. (1969). Affective visual stimuli as operant reinforcers of the GSR. *Journal of Experimental Psychology, 80,* 28–32.

Schwarz, N., & Clore, G. L. (1988). How do I feel about it? The informative function of affective states. In K. Fiedler & J. Forgas (Eds.), *Affect, cognition and social behavior: New evidence and integrative attempts.* Zurich: C. J. Hogrefe. Pp. 44–62.

Scott, J. P. (1958). *Aggression.* Chicago: University of Chicago Press.

Sears, P. S. (1940). Levels of aspiration in academically successful and unsuccessful children. *Journal of Abnormal and Social Psychology, 35,* 498–536.

Segal, B., & Champion, R. A. (1966). The acquisition of activating and reinforcing properties by stimuli associated with food deprivation. *Australian Journal of Psychology, 18,* 57–62.

Seligman, M. E. P. (1975). *Helplessness: On depression, development, and death.* San Francisco: Freeman.

Seligman, M. E. P., & Groves, D. (1970). Non-transient learned helplessness. *Psychonomic Science, 19,* 191–192.

Seligman, M. E. P., & Maier, S. F. (1967). Failure to escape traumatic shock. *Journal of Experimental Psychology, 74,* 1–9.

Seligman, M. E. P., Maier, S. F., & Solomon, R. L. (1971). Unpredictable and uncontrollable aversive events. In F. R. Brush (Ed.), *Aversive conditioning and learning.* New York: Academic Press. Pp. 347–400.

Seligman, M. E. P., Nolen-Hoeksema, S., Thornton, N., & Thornton, K. M. (1990). Explanatory style as a mechanism of disappointing athletic performance. *Psychological Science, 1,* 143–146.

Seligman, M. E. P., & Schulman, P. (1986). Explanatory style as a predictor of performance as a life insurance sales agent. *Journal of Personality and Social Psychology, 50,* 832–838.

Selye, H. (1976). *The stress of life.* 2nd ed. New York: McGraw-Hill.

Sharma, M., Palacios-Bois, J., Schwartz, G., Iskandar, H., Thakur, M., Quirion, R., & Nair, N. P. V. (1989). Circadian rhythms of melatonin and cortisol in aging. *Biological Psychiatry, 25,* 305–319.

Sharp, S. (1995). How much does bullying hurt? The effects of bullying on the personal wellbeing and educational progress of secondary aged students. *Educational and Child Psychology, 12,* 81–88.

Shaver, P., Schwartz, J., Kirson, D., & O'Connor, C. (1987). Emotion knowledge: Further exploration of a prototype approach. *Journal of Personality and Social Psychology, 52,* 1061–1086.

Shaver, P. R., & Hazan, C. (1993). Adult romantic attachment: Theory and evidence. In D. Perlman & W. H. Jones (Eds.), *Advances in personal relationships.* Vol. 4. Greenwich, CT: JAI Press, Jessica Kingsley. Pp. 29–70.

Sheffield, F. D., & Roby, T. B. (1950). Reward value of a non-nutritive sweet taste. *Journal of Comparative and Physiological Psychology, 43,* 471–481.

Shiffman, S., Engberg, J. B., Paty, J. A., Perz, W. G., Gnys, M., Kassel, J. D., & Hickcox, M. (1997). A day at a time: Predicting smoking lapse from daily urge. *Journal of Abnormal Psychology, 106,* 104–116.

Shors, T. J., Seib, T. B., Levine, S., & Thompson, R. F. (1989). Inescapable versus escapable shock modulates long-term potentiation in the rat hippocampus. *Science, 244,* 224–226.

Shulman, B. (1968). *Essays in schizophrenia.* Baltimore, MD: Williams & Wilkins.

Shulman, B., & Mosak, H. H. (1967). Various purposes of symptoms. *Journal of Individual Psychology, 23,* 79–87.

Sidman, M. (1953). Avoidance conditioning with brief shock and no exteroceptive warning signal. *Science, 118,* 157–158.

Siegal, M. (1995). Becoming mindful of food and conversation. *Current Directions in Psychological Science, 4,* 177–181.

Siegel, J. M. (1985). The measurement of anger as a multidimensional construct. In M. A. Chesney & R. Rosenman (Eds.), *Anger and hostility in cardiovascular and behavioral disorders.* New York: Hemisphere. Pp. 59–81.

Siegel, P. S., & Stuckey, H. L. (1947). The diurnal course of water and food intake in the normal mature rat. *Journal of Comparative and Physiological Psychology, 40,* 365–370.

Siegel, R. K. (1989). *Intoxication: Life in pursuit of artificial paradise.* New York: Dutton.

Siegel, S. (1957). Level of aspiration and decision making. *Psychological Review, 64,* 253–262.

Siegel, S. (1988). State dependent learning and morphine tolerance. *Behavioral Neuroscience, 102,* 228–232.

Siegeltuch, M. B., & Baum, M. (1971). Extinction of well-established avoidance responses through response prevention (flooding). *Behavior Research and Therapy, 9,* 103–108.

Siegman, A. W. (1994a). Cardiovascular consequence of expressing and repressing anger. In A. W. Siegman & T. W. Smith (Eds.), *Anger, hostility, and the heart.* Hillsdale, NJ: Erlbaum. Pp. 173–197.

Siegman, A. W. (1994b). From Type A to hostility to anger: Reflections on the history of coronary-prone behavior. In A. W. Siegman & T. W. Smith (Eds.), *Anger, hostility, and the heart.* Hillsdale, NJ: Erlbaum. Pp. 1–21.

Siegman, A. W., & Smith, T. W. (1994). Introduction. In A. W. Siegman & T. W. Smith (Eds.), *Anger, hostility, and the heart.* Hillsdale, NJ: Erlbaum. Pp. vii–xv.

Simon, C. W., Wickens, D. D., Brown, U., & Pennock. L. (1951). Effect of the secondary reinforcing agents on the primary thirst drive. *Journal of Comparative and Physiological Psychology, 44,* 67–70.

Simon, H. A. (1978). Information-processing theory of human problem solving. In W. K. Estes (Ed.), *Handbook of learning and cognitive processes.* Hillsdale, NJ: Erlbaum. Pp. 271–295.

Simpson, C. (1951). *Adam in ochre: Inside aboriginal Australia.* Sydney: Angus and Robertson.

Simpson, J. A., & Gangestad, S. W. (1991). Individual differences in sociosexuality: Evidence for convergent and discriminant validity. *Journal of Personality and Social Psychology, 60,* 870–883.

Singh, D. (1973). Effects of preoperative training on food-motivated behavior of hypothalamic hyperphagic rats. *Journal of Comparative and Physiological Psychology, 84,* 47–52.

Singh, D. (1991). The nature and adaptive significance of female physical attractiveness. Unpublished manuscript. Austin: University of Texas.

Singh, D., & Sikes, S. (1974). Role of past experience on food-motivated behavior of obese humans. *Journal of Comparative and Physiological Psychology, 86,* 503–508.

Skinner, B. F. (1938). *The behavior of organisms: An experimental analysis.* New York: Appleton-Century.

Skinner, B. F. (1953). *Science and human behavior.* New York: Macmillan.

Skinner, B. F. (1962). Two synthetic social relations. *Journal of Experimental Analysis of Behavior, 5,* 531–533.

Skinner, B. F. (1969). *Contingencies of reinforcement.* Englewood Cliffs, NJ: Prentice-Hall.

Skinner, B. F. (1989). *Recent issues in the analysis of behavior.* Columbus, OH: Merrill.

Skinner, E. A. (1990). Age differences in the dimensions of perceived control during middle childhood: Implications for developmental conceptualizations and research. *Child Development, 61,* 1882–1890.

Skitka, L. J., & Maslach, C. (1996). Gender as schematic category: A role construct approach. *Social Behavior and Personality, 24,* 53–73.

Skwerer, R. G., Jacobsen, F. M., Duncan, C. C., Kelly, K. A., Sack, D. A., Tamarkin, L., Gaist, P. A., Kasper, S., & Rosenthal, N. E. (1988). Neurobiology of seasonal affective disorder and phototherapy. *Journal of Biological Rhythms, 3,* 135–154.

Slama, M., & Celuch, K. (1995). Self-presentation and consumer interaction styles. *Journal of Business and Psychology, 10,* 19–30.

Smale, L., & Holekamp, K. E. (1993). Growing up in the clan. *Natural History, 1,* 42–53.

Smith, G. P. (1974). Adrenal hormones and emotional behavior. In E. Stallar & J. M. Sprague (Eds.), *Progress in physiological psychology,* Vol. 5. New York: Academic Press. Pp. 299–352.

Smith, G. P., & Gibbs, J. (1994). Satiating effect of cholecystokinin. In J. R. Reeve, Jr., V. Eysslelein, T. E. Solomon, & V. I. W. Go (Eds.), *Cholecystokinin.* Vol. 713. *Annals of the New York Academy of Sciences.* New York: New York Academy of Sciences. Pp. 236–241.

Smith, G. T., Hohlstein, L. A., & Atlas, J. G. (1992). Accuracy of self-reported weight: Covariation with binger or restrainer status and eating disorder symptomatology. *Addictive Behaviors, 17,* 1–8.

Smith, H. L., & Dechter, A. (1991). No shift in locus of control among women during the 1970s. *Journal of Personality and Social Psychology, 60,* 638–640.

Smith, J. R., Karacan, I., & Yang, M. (1977). Ontogeny of delta activity during human sleep. *Electroencephalography and Clinical Neurophysiology, 43,* 229–237.

Smith, L. K., Field, E. F., Forgie, M. L., & Pellis, S. M. (1996). Dominance and age-related changes in the play fighting of intact and post-weaning castrated male rats (*Rattus norvegicus*). *Aggressive Behavior, 22,* 215–226.

Smith, P. B., Trompenaars, F., & Dugan, S. (1995). The Rotter locus of control scale in 43 countries: A test of cultural relativity. *International Journal of Psychology, 30,* 377–400.

Smith, P. K. (1988). Ethological approaches to the study of aggression in children. In J. Archer & K. Browne (Eds.), *Human aggression: Naturalistic approaches.* London: Routledge. Pp. 65–193.

Sobal, J., & Stunkard, A. J. (1989). Socioeconomic status and obesity: A review of the literature. *Psychological Bulletin, 105,* 260–275.

Sobel, J. (1983). *Everybody wins: Non-competitive games for young children.* New York: Walker.

Solomon, R., & Corbit, R. (1974). An opponent-process theory of motivation: Temporal dynamics of affect. *Psychological Review, 81,* 119–145.

Solomon, R. L. (1980). The opponent-process theory of acquired motivation: The costs of pleasure and the benefits of pain. *American Psychologist, 35,* 691–712.

Solomon, R. L. (1991). Acquired motivation and affective opponent-processes. In J. Madden IV (Ed.), *Neurobiology of learning, emotion and affect.* New York: Raven Press. Pp. 307–347.

Solomon, R. L., Kamin, L. J., & Wynne, L. C. (1953). Traumatic avoidance learning: The outcomes of several extinction procedures with dogs. *Journal of Abnormal and Social Psychology, 48,* 291–302.

Solomon, R. L., & Wynne, L. C. (1954). Traumatic avoidance learning: The principles of anxiety conservation and partial irreversibility. *Psychological Review, 61,* 353–385.

Sorenson, S. B., & White, J. W. (1992). Adult sexual assault: Overview of research. *Journal of Social Issues, 48,* 1–8.

Sorrentino, R. M., & Higgins, E. T. (1986). Motivation and cognition: Warming up to synergism. In R. M. Sorrentino & E. T. Higgins (Eds.), *Handbook of motivation and cognition: Foundations of social behavior.* New York: Guilford Press. Pp. 3–19.

Spence, J. T. (1974). The TAT and attitudes toward achievement in women: A new look at the motive to avoid success and a new method of measurement. *Journal of Consulting and Clinical Psychology, 42,* 427–437.

Spence, J. T. (1985). Gender identity and implications for concepts of masculinity and femininity. In T. B. Sonderegger (Ed.), *Nebraska Symposium on Motivation, 1984.* Vol. 32. Lincoln: University of Nebraska Press. Pp. 59–96.

Spence, J. T. (1993). Gender-related traits and gender ideology: Evidence for a multifactorial theory. *Journal of Personality and Social Psychology, 64,* 624–635.

Spence, J. T., & Helmreich, R. L. (1978). *Masculinity and femininity: Their psychological dimensions, correlates, and antecedents.* Austin, TX: University of Texas Press.

Spence, J. T., & Helmreich, R. L. (1983). Achievement-related motives and behaviors. In J. T. Spence (Ed.), *Achievement and achievement motivation.* San Fracisco: W. H. Freeman. Pp. 7–74.

Spence, J. T., Helmreich, R. L., & Pred, R. S. (1987). Impatience versus achievement strivings in the Type A pattern: Differential effects on students' health and academic achievement. *Journal of Applied Psychology, 72,* 522–528.

Spence, J. T., Helmreich, R. L., & Pred, R. S. (1988). Making it without losing it: Type A, achievement motivation, and scientific attainment revisited. *Personality and Social Psychology Bulletin, 14,* 495–504.

Spence, K. W. (1953). Learning and performance in eyelid conditioning as a function of the intensity of the UCS. *Journal of Experimental Psychology, 45,* 57–63.

Spence, K. W. (1956). *Behavior theory and conditioning.* New Haven, CT: Yale University Press.

Spence, K. W. (1958). A theory of emotionally based drive (D) and its relation to performance in simple learning situations. *American Psychologist, 13,* 131–141.

Spence, K. W. (1964). Anxiety (drive) level and performance in eyelid conditioning. *Psychological Bulletin, 61,* 129–139.

Spence, K. W., Farber, I. E., & McFann, H. H. (1956). The relation of anxiety (drive) level to performance in competitional and noncompetitional paired-associates learning. *Journal of Experimental Psychology, 52,* 296–305.

Spence, K. W., & Taylor, J. A. (1951). Anxiety and strength of the UCS as determiners of the amount of eyelid conditioning. *Journal of Experimental Psychology, 42,* 183–188.

Sperry, R. W. (1961). Cerebral organization and behavior. *Science, 133,* 1749–1757.

Spielberger, C. D. (1983). *Manual for the State-Trait Anxiety Inventory (Form Y).* Palo Alto, CA: Consulting Psychologists Press.

Spielberger, C. D. (1988). *State-Trait Anger Expression Inventory.* Odessa, FL: Psychological Assessment Resources.

Spielberger, C. D., Gorsuch, R. L., & Lushene, R. E. (1970). *Manual for the State-Trait Anxiety Inventory.* Palo Alto, CA: Consulting Psychologist Press.

Spielberger, C. D., Jacobs, G., Russell, S., & Crane, R. S. (1983). Assessment of anger: The state-trait anger scale. In J. N. Butcher & C. D. Spielberger (Eds.), *Advances in personality assessment.* Vol. 2. Hillsdale, NJ: Erlbaum.

Spielberger, C. D., Johnson, E., Russell, S., Crane, R., Jacobs, G., & Worden, T. (1985). The experience and expression of anger: Construction and validation of an anger expression scale. In M. A. Chesney & R. H. Rosenman (Eds.), *Anger and hostility in cardiovascular and behavioral disorder.* New York: McGraw-Hill. Pp. 5–30.

Spiteri, N. J. (1982). Circadian patterning of feeding, drinking and activity during food access in rats. *Physiology & Behavior, 28,* 139–147.

Spring, B., Chiodo, J., & Bowen, D. (1987). Carbohydrates, tryptophan, and behavior: A methodological review. *Psychological Bulletin, 102,* 234–256.

Stampfl, T. G., & Levis, D. J. (1968). Implosive therapy: A behavioral therapy? *Behavior Research and Therapy, 6,* 31–36.

Standing, L., Haber, R. N., Cataldo, M., & Sales, B. D. (1969). Two types of short-term visual storage. *Perception and Psychophysics, 5,* 193–196.

Stanley, B. G., & Gillard, E. R. (1994). Hypothalamic neuropeptide Y and the regulation of eating behavior and body weight. *Current Directions in Psychological Science, 3,* 9–15.

Staw, B. M. (1976). *Intrinsic and extrinsic motivation.* Morristown, NJ: General Learning Press.

Stefurak, T. L., & Van der Kooy, D. (1992). Saccarin's rewarding, conditioned reinforcing, and memory-improving properties: Mediation by isomorphic or independent processes? *Behavioral Neuroscience, 106,* 125–139.

Stein, A. H., & Bailey, M. M. (1973). The socialization of achievement orientation in females. *Psychological Bulletin, 80,* 345–366.

Stein, L. (1958). Secondary reinforcement established with subcortical stimulation. *Science, 127,* 466–467.

Stephan, F. K., Berkley, K. J., & Moss, R. L. (1981). Efferent connections of the rat suprachiasmatic nucleus. *Neuroscience, 6,* 2625–2641.

Steriade, M. (1996). Arousal: Revisiting the reticular activating system. *Science, 272* (12 April), 225–226.

Steriade, M., McCormick, D. A., & Sejnowski, T. J. (1993). Thalamocortical oscillations in the sleeping and aroused brain. *Science, 262* (29 October), 679–685.

Sternberg, R. J. (1986). A triangular theory of love. *Psychological Review, 93,* 119–135.

Sternberg, R. J. (1987). Liking versus loving: A comparative evaluation of theories. *Psychological Bulletin, 102,* 331–345.

Sternberg, R. J. (1988). *The triangle of love.* New York: Basic Books.

Sternberg, R. J. (1994). Love is a story. *The General Psychologist, 30,* 1–11.

Sternberg, R. J. (1995). Love as a story. *Journal of Social and Personal Relationships, 12,* 541–546.

Stone, W. S., Rudd, R. J., & Gold, P. E. (1990). Glucose and physostigmine effects on morphine- and amphetamine-induced increases in locomotor activity in mice. *Behavioral and Neural Biology, 54,* 146–155.

Stone, W. S., Rudd, R. J., & Gold, P. E. (1992). Glucose attenuation of scopolamine- and age-induced deficits in spontaneous alternation behavior in regional brain (-sup-3H) 2-deoxyglucose uptake in mice. *Psychobiology, 20,* 270–279.

Stoney, C. M., & Engebretson, T. O. (1994). Anger and hostility: Potential mediators of the gender difference in coronary heart disease. In A. W. Siegman & T. W. Smith (Eds.), *Anger, hostility, and the heart.* Hillsdale, NJ: Erlbaum. Pp. 215–237.

Stricker, E. M. (1991). Central control of water and sodium chloride intake in rats during hypovolaemia. In D. J. Ramsay & D. Booth (Eds.), *Thirst: Physiological and psychological aspects.* New York: Springer Verlag. Pp. 194–203.

Stricker, E. M., & Verbalis, J. G. (1990). Sodium appetite. In E. M. Stricker (Ed.), *Neurobiology of food and fluid intake. Handbook of behavioral neurobiology.* Vol. 10. New York: Plenum Press. Pp. 387–419.

Stricker, E. M., & Verbalis, J. G. (1993). Hormones and ingestive behaviors. In J. B. Becker, S. M. Breedlove, & D. Crews (Eds.), *Behavioral endocrinology.* Cambridge, MA: MIT Press.

Strier, K. B. (1990). New World primates, new frontiers: Insights from the woolly spider monkey, or muriqui (*Brachyteles arachnoides*). *International Journal of Primatology, 11,* 7–19.

Stromberg, M. F., Bersh, P. J., Whitehouse, W. G., Neuman, P., & Mongeluzzi, D. L. (1997). The effect of water deprivation on shock-escape impairment after exposure to inescapable shock. *The Psychological Record, 47,* 335–350.

Stroop, J. R. (1935). Studies of interference in serial verbal interactions. *Journal of Experimental Psychology, 18,* 643–662.

Studd, M. V. (1996). Sexual harassment. In D. M. Buss & N. M. Malamuth (Eds.), *Sex, power, conflict: Evolutionary and feminist perspectives.* New York: University Press. Pp. 54–89.

Stunkard, A. (1982). Anorectic agents lower a body weight set point. *Life Sciences, 30,* 2043–2055.

Stunkard, A., & Koch, C. (1964). The interpretation of gastric motility: I. Apparent bias in the reports of hunger by obese persons. *Archives of General Psychiatry, 11,* 74–82.

Stunkard, A. J., & Messick, S. (1985). The three-factor eating questionnaire to measure dietary restraint, disinhibition and hunger. *Journal of Psychosomatic Research, 29,* 71–83.

Suberi, M., & McKeever, W. F. (1977). Differential right hemispheric memory storage of emotional and nonemotional faces. *Neuropsychologia, 15,* 757–768.

Sullivan, B. F., & Schwebel, A. I. (1995). Relationship beliefs and expectations of satisfaction in marital relationships: Implications for family practitioners. *The Family Journal: Counseling and Therapy for Couples and Families, 3,* 298–305.

Sutcliffe, J. P. (1955). Task variability and the level of aspiration. *Australian Journal of Psychology,* Monograph Supplement, No. 2.

Sutton, S. K., & Davidson, R. J. (1997). Prefrontal brain asymmetry: A biological substrate of the behavioral approach and inhibition systems. *Psychological Science, 8,* 204–210.

Svartdal, F. (1993). Working harder for less: Effect of incentive value on force of instrumental response in humans. *Quarterly Journal of Experimental Psychology: A. Human Experimental Psychology, 46A,* 11–34.

Swaab, D. F., Fliers, E., & Partiman, T. S. (1985). The suprachiasmatic nucleus of the human brain in relation to sex, age, and senile dementia. *Brain Research, 342,* 37–44.

Swaab, D. F., Van Someren, E. J. W., Zhou, J. N., & Hofman, M. A. (1996). Biological rhythms in the human life cycle and thier relationship to functional changes in the suprachiasmatic nucleus. *Progress in Brain Research, 111,* 349–368.

Swanson, L. W., & Cowan, W. M. (1975). Efferent connections of the suprachiasmatic nucleus of the hypothalamus. *Journal of Comparative Neurology, 160,* 1–12.

Swanson, L. W., Cowan, W. M., & Jones, E. G. (1974). An autoradiographic study of the efferent connections of the ventral lateral geniculate nucleus in the albino rat and the cat. *Journal of Comparative Neurology, 156,* 143–164.

Symons, D. (1979). *The evolution of human sexuality.* New York: Oxford University Press.

Szczepanska-Sadowska, E. (1991). Hormonal inputs to thirst. In D. J. Ramsay & D. Booth (Eds.), *Thirst: Physiological and psychological aspects.* New York: Springer Verlag. Pp. 110–130.

Takahashi, J. S., & Menaker, M. (1984). Circadian rhythmicity: Regulation in the time domain. In R. F. Goldberger & K. R. Yamamoto (Eds.), *Biological regula-*

tion and development Vol 3B. New York: Plenum Press. Pp. 285–303.

Tamarkin, L., Baird, C. J., & Almeida, O. F. X. (1985). Melatonin: A coordinating signal for mammalian reproduction? *Science, 227,* 714–720.

Tan, N., Morimoto, K., Sugiura, T., Morimoto, A., & Murakami, N. (1992). Effects of running training on the blood glucose and lactate in rats during rest and swimming. *Physiology & Behavior, 51,* 927–931.

Tavris, C. (1989). *Anger: The misunderstood emotion.* Rev. ed. New York: Simon & Schuster.

Taylor, J. A. (1951). The relationship of anxiety to the conditioned eyelid response. *Journal of Experimental Psychology, 41,* 81–92.

Taylor, J. A. (1953). A personality scale of manifest anxiety. *Journal of Abnormal and Social Psychology, 48,* 285–290.

Taylor, J. A. (1956). Physiological need, set, and visual duration threshold. *Journal of Abnormal and Social Psychology, 62,* 96–99.

Taylor, S. L., O'Neal, E. C., Langley, T., & Butcher, A. H. (1991). Anger arousal, deindividuation, and aggression. *Aggressive Behavior, 17,* 193–206.

Taylor, S. P. (1993). Experimental investigation of alcohol-induced aggression in humans. *Alcohol Health and Research World, 17,* 108–112.

Taylor, S. P., & Chermack, S. T. (1993). Alcohol, drugs, and human physical aggression. *Journal of Studies on Alcohol,* Supplement (September), 78–88.

Taylor, S. P., & Gammon, C. B. (1974). The effects of type and dose of alcohol on human aggression. Paper presented at the meeting of the American Psychological Association, New Orleans.

Teasdale, J. D., & Russell, M. C. (1983). Differential effects of induced mood on the recall of positive, negative, and neutral words. *British Journal of Clinical Psychology, 22,* 163–171.

Teicher, M. H., Glod, C. A., Magnus, E., Harper, D., Benson, G., Krueger, K., & McGreenery, C. E. (1997). Circadian rest-activity disturbances in seasonal affective disorder. *Archives of General Psychiatry, 54,* 124–130.

Teitelbaum, P. (1955). Sensory control of hypothalamic hyperphagia. *Journal of Comparative and Physiological Psychology, 48,* 156–163.

Teitelbaum, P., & Campbell, B. A. (1958). Ingestion patterns in hyperphagic and normal rats. *Journal of Comparative and Physiological Psychology, 51,* 135–141.

Terman, M., Terman, J. S., Quitkin, F. M., McGrath, P. J., Stewart, J. W., & Rafferty, B. (1989). Light therapy for seasonal affective disorder: A review of efficacy. *Neuropsychopharmacology, 2,* 1–22.

Thayer, R. E. (1970). Activation states as assessed by verbal reports and four psychophysiological variables. *Psychophysiology, 7,* 86–94.

Thayer, R. E. (1978). Toward a psychological theory of multidimensional activation (arousal). *Motivation and Emotion, 2,* 1–34.

Thayer, R. E. (1985). Activation (arousal): The shift from a single to a multidimensional perspective. In J. Strelau, A. Gale, & F. H. Farley (Eds.), *The biological bases of personality and behavior.* Vol. 1. Pp. 115–127. Washington, DC: Hemisphere.

Thayer, R. E. (1987). Energy, tiredness, and tension effects of a sugar snack versus moderate exercise. *Journal of Personality and Social Psychology, 52,* 119–125.

Thayer, R. E. (1987). Problem perception, optimism, and related states as a function of time of day (diurnal rhythm) and moderate exercise: Two arousal systems in interaction. *Motivation and Emotion, 11,* 19–36.

Thayer, R. E. (1989). *The biopsychology of mood and arousal.* New York: Oxford University Press.

Thayer, R. E. (1996). *The origin of everyday moods: Managing energy, tension, and stress.* New York: Oxford University Press.

Thayer, R. E., & Cox, S. J. (1968). Activation, manifest anxiety, and verbal learning. *Journal of Experimental Psychology, 78,* 524–526.

Thayer, R. E., Takahashi, P. J., & Pauli, J. A. (1988). Multidimensional arousal states, diurnal rhythms, cognitive and social processes, and extraversion. *Personality and Individual Differences, 9,* 15–24.

Thibaut, J. W., & Kelley, H. H. (1959). *The social psychology of groups.* New York: Wiley.

Thomas, S. P. (1993). Anger and its manifestation in women. In S. P. Thomas (Ed.), *Women and anger.* New York: Springer. Pp. 40–67.

Thompson, E. H., Jr. (Ed.). (1994). *Older men's lives.* Thousand Oaks, CA: Sage.

Thorndike, E. L. (1898). Animal intelligence: An experimental study of the associative processes in animals. *Psychological Review Monogram Supplement, 2,* Number 8.

Thorndike, E. L. (1911). *Animal intelligence.* New York: Macmillan.

Thorndike, E. L. (1913). *Educational psychology: Vol. II. The psychology of learning.* New York: Teachers College.

Thorndike, E. L. (1933). A proof of the law of effect. *Science, 77,* 173–175.

Thorndike, E. L. (1935). *The psychology of wants, interests and attitudes.* New York: Appleton.

Thorndike, E. L., & Lorge, I. (1944). *The teacher's book*

of 30,000 words. New York: Columbia University Press.

Thorne, B., & Henley, T. (1997). *Connections in the history and systems of psychology.* New York: Houghton Mifflin.

Thrasher, T. N. (1991). Volume receptors and the stimulation of water intake. In D. J. Ramsay and D. A. Booth (Eds.), *Thirst: Physiological and psychological aspects.* New York: Springer. Pp. 93–107.

Thune, L. E. (1951). Warm-up effect as a function of level of practice in verbal learning. *Journal of Experimental Psychology, 42,* 250–256.

Tinbergen, N. (1952). The curious behavior of the stickleback. *Scientific American, 187,* 22–26.

Titchener, E. D. (1896/1921). *An outline of psychology* (new edition with additions). New York: Macmillan.

Tobin, H., Logue, A. W., Chelonis, J. J., Ackerman, K. T., & May, J. G., III. (1996). Self-control in the monkey *Macaca fascicularis. Animal Learning and Behavior, 24,* 168–174.

Tolman, E. C. (1922). A new formula for behaviorism. *Psychological Review, 29,* 44–53.

Tolman, E. C. (1932). *Purposive behavior in animals and man.* New York: Appleton-Century-Crofts.

Tolman, E. C. (1948). Cognitive maps in rats and men. *Psychological Review. 55,* 189–208.

Tolman, E. C., & Honzik, C. H. (1930). Introduction and removal of reward, and maze performance in rats. *University of California Publications in Psychology, 4,* 257–275.

Tomarken, A. J., Davidson, R. J., Wheeler, R. E., & Doss, R. C. (1992) Individual differences in anterior brain asymmetry and fundamental dimensions of emotion. *Journal of Personality and Social Psychology, 62,* 676–687.

Tomkins, S. S. (1982). Affect theory. In P. Ekman (Ed.), *Emotion in the human face.* New York: Cambridge University Press. Pp. 353–395.

Tosini, G., & Menaker, M. (1996). Circadian rhythms in cultured mammalian retina. *Science, 272,* 419–421.

Treasure, D. C., & Roberts, G. C. (1994). Cognitive and affective concomitants of task and ego goal orientations during the middle school years. *Journal of Sport & Exercise Psychology, 16,* 15–28.

Turek, F. W., Penev, P., Zhang, Y., Van Reeth, O., Takahashi, J. S., & Zee, P. (1995). Alterations in circadian system in advanced age. In D. J. Derek & K. Ackrill (Eds.), *Circadian clocks and their adjustment* (Ciba Foundation Symposium, 183). Chichester: Wiley. Pp. 212–234.

Turek, F. W., & Van Reeth, O. (1996). Circadian rhythms. In M. J. Fregly & C. M. Blatteis (Eds.), *Handbook of Physiology.* Oxford: Oxford University Press. Pp. 1329–1360.

Turkewitz, G., Moreau, T., Birch, H. G., & Davis, L. (1971). Relationships among responses in the human newborn: The non-association and non-equivalence among different indicators of responsiveness. *Psychophysiology, 7,* 233–247.

U.S. Congress, Office of Technology Assessment (1991). *Biological rhythms: Implication for the worker.* OTA-BA-463. Washington, DC: U.S. Government Printing Office.

U.S. Congress, Office of Technology Assessment (1993). *Biological components of substance abuse and addiction,* OTA-BP-BBS-117. Washington, DC: U.S. Government Printing Office.

Underwood, B. J. (1945). The effect of successive interpolations on retroactive and proactive inhibition. *Psychological Monographs, 59,* Number 3.

Underwood, B. J. (1948). Retroactive and proactive inhibition after five and forty-eight hours. *Journal of Experimental Psychology, 38,* 29–38.

Underwood, B. J. (1957). *Psychological research.* New York: Appleton.

Underwood, B. J., & Schultz, R. W. (1960). *Meaningfulness and verbal learning.* Philadelphia: Lippincott.

Vaccarino, F. J., Schiff, B. B., & Glickman, S. E. (1989). Biological view of reinforcement. In S. B. Klein & R. R. Mowrer (Eds.), *Contemporary learning theories.* Hillsdale, NJ: Erlbaum. Pp. 111–142.

Van Cauter, E. (1990). Diurnal and ultradian rhythms in human endocrine function: A minireview. *Hormone Research, 34,* 45–53.

Van Cauter, E., Plat, L., Leproult, R., & Copinschi, G. (1998). Alterations of circadian rhythmicity and sleep in aging: Endocrine consequences. *Hormone Research, 49,* 147–152.

Van Cauter, E., & Turek, F. W. (1990). Strategies for resetting the human circadian clock. *New England Journal of Medicine, 322,* 1306–1308.

Van Gool, W. A., & Mirmiran, M. (1986). Aging and circadian rhythms. *Progress in Brain Research, 70,* 255–277.

Van Ittalie, T. B., & Kissileff, H. R. (1990). Human obesity: A problem in body energy economics. In E. M. Stricker (Ed.), *Neurobiology of food and fluid intake. Handbook of behavioral neurobiology.* Vol. 10. New York: Plenum Press. Pp. 207–240.

Van Lange, P. A. M., Otten, W., De Bruin, E. M. N., & Joireman, J. A. (1997). Development of prosocial, individualistic, and competitive orientations: Theory and preliminary evidence. *Journal of Personality and Social Psychology, 73,* 733–746.

Van Reeth, O., & Turek, F. W. (1989a). Administering tri- azolam on a circadian basis entrains the activity rhythm of hamsters. *American Journal of Physiology, 256,* R639–R645.

Van Reeth, O., & Turek, F. W. (1989b). Stimulated activ- ity mediates phase shifts in the hamster circadian clock induced by dark pulses or benzodiazepines. *Na- ture, 339,* 49–51.

Van Reeth, O., Sturis, J., Byrne, M. M., Blackman, J. D., L'Hermite-Baleriaux, M., Leproult, R., Oliner, C., Refetoff, S., Turek, F. W., & Van Cauter, E. (1994). Nocturnal exercise phase delays circadian rhythms of melatonin and thyrotropin secretion in normal men. *American Journal of Physiology, 266,* E964–E974.

Velten, E. A. (1968). A laboratory task for induction of mood states. *Behavior Research and Therapy, 6,* 473– 482.

Verbalis, J. G. (1990). Clinical aspects of body fluid homeostasis in humans. In E. M. Stricker (Ed.), *Neu- robiology of food and fluid intake. Handbook of be- havioral neurobiology.* Vol. 10. New York: Plenum Press. Pp. 421–462.

Verney, E. B. (1947). The antidiuretic hormone and fac- tors which determine its release. *Proceedings of the Royal Society of London* (Biol.), *135,* 25–106.

Vidacek, S., Kaliterna, L., Radosevic-Vidacek, B., & Folkard, S. (1988). Personality differences in the phase of circadian rhythms: A comparison of morn- ingness and extraversion. *Ergonomics, 31,* 873–888.

Viemero, V., & Paajanen, S. (1992). The role of fantasies and dreams in the TV viewing-aggression relation- ship. *Aggressive Behavior, 18,* 109–116.

Vokac, Z., Gundersen, N., Magnus, P., Jebens, E., & Bakka, T. (1981). Circadian rhythm of urinary excre- tion of mercury. In A. Reinberg, N. Vieux, & P. And- lauer (Eds.), *Night and shift work: Biological and social aspects.* Oxford: Pergamon Press. Pp. 425– 431.

Volkmer, R. E., & Feather, N. T. (1991). Relations be- tween Type A scores, internal locus of control and test anxiety. *Personality and Individual Differences, 12,* 205–209.

Vrana, S. R., & Lang, P. J. (1990). Fear imagery and the startle-probe reflex. *Journal of Abnormal Psychology, 99,* 189–197.

Wade, C., (1993). The impact of gender and culture on our conception of psychology. *The General Psychol- ogist, 29,* 78–81.

Wade, G. N. (1975). Some effects of ovarian hormones on food intake and body weight in female rats. *Jour-*
nal of Comparative and Physiological Psychology, 88, 183–193.

Wall, J. E., & Holden, E. W. (1994). Aggressive, as- sertive, and submissive behaviors in disadvantaged, inner-city preschool children. *Journal of Clinical Child Psychology, 23,* 382–390.

Walton, D., & Latané, B. (1973). Visual vs. physical so- cial deprivation and affiliation in rats. *Psychonomic Science, 26,* 4–6.

Ward, K. D., Klesges, R. C., & Halpern, M. T. (1997). Predictors of smoking cessation and state-of-the-art smoking interventions. *Journal of Social Issues, 53,* 129–144.

Warwick, A. S., Costanzo, P. R., Gill, J. M., & Schiffman, S. S. (1989). Eating restraint, presentation order, and time of day are related to sweet taste preferences. In L. H. Schneider, S. J. Cooper, & K. A. Halmi (Eds.), *The psychology of human eating disorders: Preclini- cal and clinical perspectives. Annals of the New York Academy of Sciences, 575,* 236–243.

Wasman, M., & Flynn, J. P. (1962). Directed attack elicited from hypothalamus. *Archives of Neurology, 6,* 220–227.

Waterhouse, J. (1993). Circadian rhythms. *British Med- ical Journal, 306,* 448–451.

Watson, D. (1967). Relationship between locus of control and anxiety. *Journal of Personality and Social Psy- chology, 6,* 91–93.

Watson, D., & Baumal, E. (1967). Effect of locus of con- trol and expectation of future control upon present performance. *Journal of Personality and Social Psy- chology, 6,* 212–215.

Watson, D., & Clark, L. A. (1992). Affects separable and inseparable: On the hierarchial arrangement of the negative affects. *Journal of Personality and Social Psychology, 62,* 489–505.

Watson, D., Clark, L. A., & Tellegen, A. (1988). Devel- opment and validation of brief measures of positive and negative affect: The PANAS scales. *Journal of Personality and Social Psychology, 54,* 1063–1070.

Watson, J. B. (1925). *Behaviorism.* New York: Norton.

Watson, J. B., & Rayner, R. (1920). Conditioned emo- tional reactions. *Journal of Experimental Psychology, 3,* 1–14.

Watson, J. P., Gaind, R., & Marks, I. M. (1972). Physio- logical habituation to continuous phobic stimulation. *Behavior Research and Therapy, 10,* 269–278.

Watson, J. P., & Marks, I. M. (1971). Relevant and irrel- evant fear in flooding: A cross-over study of phobic patients. *Behavior Therapy, 2,* 275–293.

Watts, A. G., Swanson, L. W., & Sanchez-Watts, G. (1987). Efferent projections of the suprachiasmatic nucleus: I. Studies using anterograde transport of *Phaseolus vulgaris* leucoagglutinin in the rat. *Journal of Comparative Neurology, 258,* 204–229.

Watts, D. P. (1994). Agonistic relationships between female mountain gorillas *(Gorilla gorilla beringei). Behavioral Ecology and Sociobiology, 34,* 347–358.

Weaver, D. R. (1997). Reproductive safety of melatonin: A "wonder drug" to wonder about. *Journal of Biological Rhythms, 12,* 682–689.

Weaver, D. R., Rivkees, S. A., Carlson, L. L., & Reppert, S. M. (1991). Localization of melatonin receptors in mammalian brain. In D. C. Klein, R. Y. Moore, & S. M. Reppert (Eds.), *Suprachiasmatic nucleus: The mind's clock.* New York: Oxford University Press. Pp. 289–308.

Webb, W. B. (1974). Sleep as an adaptive response. *Perceptual and Motor Skills, 38,* 1023–1027.

Wee, B. E. F., Francis, T. J., Lee, C. Y., Lee, J. M., & Dohanich, G. P. (1995). Mate preference and avoidance in female rats following treatment with scopolamine. *Physiology & Behavior, 58,* 97–100.

Wee, B. E. F., & Turek, F. W. (1989). Midazolam, a short-acting benzodiazepine, resets the circadian clock of the hamster. *Pharmacology, Biochemistry, and Behavior, 32,* 901–906.

Wee, B. E. F., Weaver, D. R., & Clemens, L. G. (1988). Hormonal restoration of masculine sexual behavior in long-term castrated B6D2F1 mice. *Physiology & Behavior, 42,* 77–82.

Wehr, T. A. (1996). A "clock for all seasons" in the human brain. *Progress in Brain Research, 111,* 321–342.

Weinberg, M. S., Williams, C. J., & Pryor, D. W. (1994). *Dual attraction: Understanding bisexuality.* New York: Oxford University Press.

Weiner, B. (1985). An attributional theory of achievement motivation and emotion. *Psychological Review, 92,* 548–573.

Weiner, B. (1986). *An attribution theory of motivation and emotion.* New York: Springer-Verlag.

Weiner, B. (1991). Metaphors in motivation and attribution. *American Psychologist, 46,* 921–930.

Weiner, B. (1991). On perceiving the other as responsible. In R. Dienstbier (Ed.), *Nebraska symposium on motivation, 1990.* Vol. 38. Lincoln: University of Nebraska Press. Pp. 165–198.

Weiner, B. (1993). On sin versus sickness: A theory of perceived responsibility and social motivation. *American Psychologist, 48,* 957–965.

Weiner, B. (1994a). Ability versus effort revisited: The moral determinants of achievement evaluation and achievement as a moral system. *Educational Psychologist, 29,* 163–172.

Weiner, B. (1994b). Integrating social and personal theories of achievement striving. *Review of Educational Research, 64,* 557–573.

Weiner, B., Frieze, I., Kukla, A., Reed, L., Rest, S., & Rosenbaum, R. M. (1971). *Perceiving the causes of success and failure.* Morristown, NJ: General Learning Press.

Weiner, B., & Graham, S. (1989). Understanding the motivational role of affect: Life-span research from an attributional perspective. *Cognition and Emotion, 3,* 401–419.

Weiner, B., & Kukla, A. (1970). An attributional analysis of achievement motivation. *Journal of Personality and Social Psychology, 15,* 1–20.

Weiner, B., Perry, R. P., & Magnusson, J. (1988). An attributional analysis of reactions to stigmas. *Journal of Personality and Social Psychology, 55,* 738–748.

Weingarten, H. P. (1985). Stimulus control of eating: Implications for a two-factor theory of hunger. *Appetite, 6,* 387–401.

Weiss, R. S. (1990). *Staying the course: The emotional and social lives of men who do well at work.* New York: The Free Press.

Weitzman, E. D., Moline, M. L., Czeisler, C. A., & Zimmerman, J. C. (1982). Chronobiology of aging: Temperature, sleep-wake rhythms and entrainment. *Neurobiology of Aging, 3,* 299–309.

Welsh, D. K., Logothetis, D. E., Meister, M., & Reppert, S. M. (1995). Individual neurons dissociated from rat suprachiasmatic nucleus express independently phased circadian firing rhythms. *Neuron, 14,* 697–706.

Welsh, G. S., & Dahlstrom, W. G. (Eds.). (1956). *Basic readings on the MMPI in psychology and medicine.* Minneapolis: University of Minnesota Press.

Wenar, C. (1953). The effects of a motor handicap on personality: I. The effects on level of aspiration. *Child Development, 24,* 123–130.

Werner, H. (1940/1961). *Comparative psychology of mental development.* New York: Science Editions, Inc.

Werner, H. (1957). The concept of development from a comparative and organismic point of view. In D. B. Harris (Ed.), *The concept of development.* Minneapolis: University of Minnesota Press. Pp. 125–148.

Werner, H. D. (1982). *Cognitive therapy.* New York: Freeman.

Wertheim, E. H., Gaab, C., Coish, B. J., & Weiss, K.

(1989). Long-term follow-up of a group treatment program for bulimia. In P. Lovibond & P. Wilson (Eds.), *Clinical and abnormal psychology.* North-Holland: Elsevier. Pp. 199–206.

Wertheim, E. H., Paxton, S. J., Maude, D., Szmukler, G. I., Gibbons, K., & Hiller, L. (1992). Psychosocial predictors of weight loss behavior and binge eating in adolescent girls and boys. *International Journal of Eating Disorders, 12,* 151–160.

Wertheimer, M. (1987). *A brief history of psychology.* 3rd ed. New York: Holt, Rinehart, and Winston.

Wever, R. A. (1982). Behavioral aspects of circadian rhythmicity. In F. M. Brown & R. C. Graeber (Eds.), *Rhythmic aspects of behavior.* London: Lawrence Erlbaum Associates. Pp. 105–171.

Whalen, R. (1966). Sexual motivation. *Psychological Review, 73,* 151–163.

Whitaker, A., Davies, M., Shaffer, D., Johnson, J., Abrams, S., Walsh, B. T., & Kalikow, K. (1989). The struggle to be thin: A survey of anorexic and bulimic symptoms in a non-referred adolescent population. *Psychological Medicine, 19,* 143–163.

White, N. M. (1991). Peripheral and central memory enhancing actions of glucose. In R. C. A. Frederickson, J. L. McGaugh, & D. L. Felten (Eds.), *Peripheral signaling of the brain: Role in neural-immune interactions and learning and memory.* Toronto: Hogrefe & Huber. Pp. 421–441.

White, N. M. (1996). Beyond reward and dopamine to multiple causes and individual differences. *Addiction, 91,* 960–965.

White, P. H., Kjelgaard, M. M., & Harkins, S. G. (1995). Testing the contribution of self-evaluation to goal-setting effects. *Journal of Personality and Social Psychology, 69,* 69–79.

Wilfley, D. E., Agras, W. S., Telch, C. F., Rossiter, E. M., Schneider, J. A., Cole, A. G., Sifford, L., & Raeburn, S. D. (1993). Group cognitive-behavioral therapy and group interpersonal psychotherapy for the nonpurging bulimic: A controlled comparison. *Journal of Consulting and Clinical Psychology, 61,* 296–305.

Wilkinson, R. T. (1982). The relationship between body temperature and performance across circadian phase shifts. In F. M. Brown & R. C. Graeber (Eds.), *Rhythmic aspects of behavior.* London: Lawrence Erlbaum Associates. Pp. 213–240.

Williams, B. A. (1994a). Conditioned reinforcement: Experimental and theoretical issues. *Behavior Analyst, 17,* 261–285.

Williams, B. A. (1994b). Conditioned reinforcement: Ne-
glected or outmoded explanatory construct? *Psychonomic Bulletin & Review, 1,* 457–475.

Williams, J. H. (1983). *Psychology of women: Behavior in a biosocial context.* 2nd ed. New York: W. W. Norton.

Williams, J. M. G. (1992). Autobiographical memory and emotional disorders. In S.-A. Christianson (Ed.), *The handbook of emotion and memory.* Hillsdale, NJ: Erlbaum. Pp. 451–477.

Williams, J. M. G., Mathews, A., & MacLeod, C. (1996). The emotional Stroop task and psychopathology. *Psychological Bulletin, 120,* 3–24.

Williams, R., Karacan, I., & Hursch, C. (1970). *Electroencephalography of human sleep: Clinical applications.* New York: Wiley.

Wilson, A., Brooks, D. C., & Bouton, M. E. (1995). The role of the rat hippocampal system in several effects of context in extinction. *Behavioral Neuroscience, 109,* 828–836.

Wilson, D. S., Near, D., & Miller, R. R. (1996). Machiavellianism: A synthesis of the evolutionary and psychological literatures. *Psychological Bulletin, 119,* 285–299.

Wilson, E. O. (1979). *On human nature.* New York: Bantam.

Wilson, J. R. (1992). Bulimia nervosa: Occurrence with psychoactive substance use disorders. *Addictive Behaviors, 17,* 603–607.

Windle, M. (1994). Temperamental inhibition and activation: Hormonal and psychosocial correlates and associated psychiatric disorder. *Personality and Individual Differences, 17,* 61–70.

Winn, P. (1995). The lateral hypothalamus and motivated behavior: An old syndrome reassessed and a new perspective gained. *Current Directions in Psychological Science, 4,* 182–187.

Wise, P. M., Cohen, I. R., Weiland, N. G., & London, E. D. (1988). Aging alters the circadian rhythm of glucose utilization in the suprachiasmatic nucleus. *Proceedings of the National Academy of Science, 85,* 5305–5309.

Wise, R. A. (1996). Addictive drugs and brain stimulation reward. *Annual Review of Neuroscience, 19,* 319–340.

Wispé, L. G., & Drambarean, N. C. (1953). Physiological need, word frequency, and visual duration thresholds. *Journal of Experimental Psychology, 46,* 25–31.

Wollnik, F. (1989). Physiology and regulation of biological rhythms in laboratory animals: An overview. *Laboratory Animals, 23,* 107–125.

Wolpe, J. (1958). *Psychotherapy by reciprocal inhibition.* Stanford, CA: Stanford University Press.

Wolpe, J. (1963). Quantitative relationships in the systematic desensitization of phobias. *American Journal of Psychiatry, 119,* 1062.

Wolpe, J. (1997). From psychoanalytic to behavioral methods in anxiety disorders: A continuing evolution. In J. K. Zeig (Ed.), *The evolution of psychotherapy: The third conference.* New York: Brunner/Mazel. Pp. 107–116.

Wood, C. G., Jr., & Hokanson, J. E. (1965). Effects of induced muscular tension on performance and the inverted-U function. *Journal of Personality and Social Psychology, 1,* 506–510.

Woods, S. C., & Gibbs, J. (1989). The regulation of food intake by peptides. In L. H. Schneider, S. J. Cooper, & K. A. Halmi (Eds.), *The psychology of human eating disorders: Preclinical and clinical perspectives.* Vol. 575. *Annals of the New York Academy of Sciences,* New York: New York Academy of Sciences. Pp. 236–243.

Woodworth, R. S. (1918). *Dynamic psychology.* New York: Columbia University Press.

Woodworth, R. S., & Schlosberg, H. (1954). *Experimental psychology.* New York: Holt, Rinehart, and Winston.

Wright, R. A., Brehm, J. W., Crutcher, W., Evans, M. T., & Jones, A. (1990). Avoidant control difficulty and aversive incentive appraisals: Additional evidence of an energization effect. *Motivation and Emotion, 14,* 45–73.

Wright, R. A., & Gregorich, S. (1989). Difficulty and instrumentality of imminent behavior as determinants of cardiovascular response and self-reported energy. *Psychophysiology, 26,* 586–592.

Wright, R. A., Shaw, L. L., & Jones, C. R. (1990). Task demand and cardiovascular response magnitude: Further evidence of the mediating role of success importance. *Journal of Personality and Social Psychology, 59,* 1250–1260.

Wundt, W. (1902). *Outlines of psychology.* 2nd rev. English ed. London: Williams & Norgate.

Wundt, W. (1910). *Principles of physiological psychology* (Vol. 1). New York: Macmillan.

Yahne, C. E., & Long, V. O. (1988). The use of support groups to raise self-esteem for women clients. *College Health, 37,* 79–83.

Yamasaki, K. (1992). Type A personality and level of aspiration in preschool children: Some basic characteristics of aspiration levels and their modifications by introducing risk-taking and competitive situations. *Japanese Journal of Psychology, 63,* 51–54.

Yerkes, R. M., & Dodson, J. D. (1908). The relation of strength of stimulus to rapidity of habit-formation. *Journal of Comparative Neurology and Psychology, 18,* 159–482.

Young, P. T. (1948). Appetite, palatability and feeding habit: A critical review. *Psychological Bulletin, 45,* 289–320.

Young, P. T. (1949). Food-seeking drive, affective process, and learning. *Psychological Review, 56,* 98–121.

Young, P. T., & Chaplin, J. P. (1945). Studies of food preference, appetite and dietary habit: III. Palatability and appetite in relation to bodily need. *Comparative Psychology Monographs,* Serial Number 95, *18,* Number 3, 1–45.

Young, P. T., & Greene, J. T. (1953). Quantity of food ingested as a measure of relative acceptability. *Journal of Comparative and Physiological Psychology, 46,* 288–294.

Young, P. T., & Richey, H. W. (1952). Diurnal drinking patterns in the rat. *Journal of Comparative and Physiological Psychology, 45,* 80–89.

Young, S. L., Bohenek, D. L., & Fanselow, M. S. (1995). Scopolamine impairs acquisition and facilitates consolidation of fear conditioning: Differential effects for tone vs. context conditioning. *Neurobiology of Learning and Memory, 63,* 174–180.

Zabel, C. J., Glickman, S. E., Frank, L. D., Woodmansee, K. B., & Keppel, G. (1992). Coalition formation in a colony of prepubertal spotted hyenas. In A. H. Harcourt & F. B. M. De Waal (Eds.), *Coalitions and alliances in humans and other animals.* New York: Oxford University Press. Pp. 113–135.

Zajonc, R. B. (1985). Emotion and facial efference: A theory reclaimed. *Science, 228,* 15–21.

Zajonc, R. B., Murphy, S. T., & Inglehart, M. (1989). Feeling and facial efference: Implications of the vascular theory of emotion. *Psychological Review, 96,* 395–416.

Zeaman, D. (1949). Response latency as a function of the amount of reinforcement. *Journal of Experimental Psychology, 39,* 466–483.

Zeigler, H. P. (1991). Drinking in mammals: Functional morphology, orosensory modulation and motor control. In D. J. Ramsay & D. Booth (Eds.), *Thirst: Physiological and psychological aspects.* New York: Springer Verlag. Pp. 241–257.

Zellner, D. A., Harner, D. E., & Adler, R. L. (1989). Effects of eating abnormalities and gender on perceptions of desirable body shape. *Journal of Abnormal Psychology, 98,* 93–96.

Zhang, Y., Proenca, R., Maffei, M., Barone, M., Leopole, L., & Friedman, J. M. (1994). Positional cloning of the mouse *obese* gene and its human homologue. *Nature, 372,* 425–432.

Zigler, E., & Kanzer, P. (1962). The effectiveness of two classes of verbal reinforcers on the performance of middle and lower class children. *Journal of Personality, 30,* 157–163.

Zimbardo, P. G., & Weber, A. L. (1994). *Psychology.* New York: HarperCollins.

Zinbarg, R. E., Barlow, D. H., Brown, T. A., & Hertz, R. M. (1992). Cognitive-behavioral approaches to the nature and treatment of anxiety disorders. *Annual Review of Psychology, 43,* 235–267.

Author Index

Abbott, F., 313
Abramson, L. Y., 238
Abramson, Z., 308
Abrhams, L., 277
Achermann, P., 52
Ackerman, K. T., 190
Ackerman, P. L., 232
Ader, R., 301
Adler, A., 2, 11, 97–99, 104, 112, 200,
  215, 224, 226, 233, 269, 272, 308,
  316, 319, 324
Adler, K. A., 98, 121
Adler, N. T., 31, 41, 42
Adler, R. L., 164
Aggleton, J. P., 124, 287, 288
Aghajanian, G. K., 195
Aguilera, N., 244
Aharonov, G., 288
Aiken, E. G., 284
Ainsworth, M. D. S., 317–18, 322
Aks, D. J., 20–21
Albers, H. E., 53
Alexinsky, T., 17
Allgeier, E. R., 307
Almeida, O. F. X., 43
Alpert, R., 295
Amabile, T. M., 199, 200
Ameli, R., 294
Amsel, A., 254, 255, 279
Anagnostaras, S. G., 284, 288
Ancoli, S., 89
Anderson, C. A., 244
Anderson, D. E., 15
Anderson, J. R., 113, 114, 115
Anderson, K. J., 4, 29
Antonides, G., 267
Antony, M. M., 294
Appley, M. H., 2
Arankowsky, S. G., 178
Archer, J., 256
Arenberg, D., 174

Arendt, J., 43, 44, 48
Aries, E., 277
Aschoff, J., 31, 32, 33, 35, 37, 38, 50, 52
Ashbrook, P. W., 119, 120
Asher, S. R., 319
Astington, J. W., 108
Aston-Jones, G., 17
Atkinson, G., 55, 68, 70
Atkinson, J. W., 10, 123, 174, 209–10,
  211, 212, 216, 218, 226, 294
Atlas, J. G., 164
Austin, J. T., 217
Averill, J. R., 15, 22–23, 239, 244, 245,
  251, 281
Ax, A., 240
Azrin, N. H., 186, 256

Babkoff, H., 74
Bachmann, T., 109
Badia, P., 55, 56
Baell, W. K., 166
Baenninger, L. P., 260
Baenninger, R., 260
Bailey, D. S., 273
Bailey, M. M., 315
Baird, C. J., 43
Baker, D. D., 232
Baker, L. A., 302
Baker, M. B., 143
Bakka, T., 75
Baldeweg, T., 130
Balleine, B., 139, 165, 166, 189, 208
Bandura, A., 198, 199, 227, 231, 233,
  274
Bare, J. K., 30
Barefoot, J. C., 247
Barinaga, M., 143
Barlow, D. H., 99, 100, 293, 294, 295
Barrett, L. C., 238
Barta, S. G., 243
Barth, R., 276

Bartoshuk, L. M., 155
Bass, A. R., 187
Bates, F. C., 167
Bates, J. E., 275
Baum, A., 18
Baum, M., 286, 304
Baumal, E., 230
Baumeister, A., 18, 23
Baumeister, R. F., 186, 207, 301, 313
Bayton, J. A., 217, 219, 221
Beach, F. A., 305
Beall, A. E., 321
Beck, A. T., 99, 101, 111
Beck, M., 152–53
Becker, A. S., 114
Becker, J. B., 302
Beersma, D. G. M., 52
Belinger, C., 139
Bem, S. L., 311, 312
Bennett, J., 122
Ben-Porath, Y., 278
Bent, N., 55
Bergmann, B. M., 51, 53
Berk, M. L., 41
Berkley, K. J., 41
Berkowitz, L., 242, 243–44, 251, 252,
  253, 254, 262, 274
Berman, M., 263
Berndt, C. H., 1, 245
Berndt, R. M., 1, 245
Bernstein, I. L., 150
Berntson, G. G., 82
Berridge, K. C., 26
Berry, L. L., 167, 168
Bersh, P. J., 289
Bertenthal, B. I., 292
Betley, G., 277
Betsch, T., 274
Bettencourt, B. A., 272
Billis, R. E., 221
Birch, D., 210

Birch, H. G., 19
Birch, L. L., 165
Birenbaum, M., 314
Black, A. H., 285
Black, R. W., 184
Blalock, J. A., 272
Blanchard, D. C., 252, 253, 256, 258, 259, 279, 288
Blanchard, R. J., 252, 253, 256, 258, 259, 260, 264, 279, 288
Blankenship, V., 211
Blass, E. M., 163, 316
Blehar, M. C., 318
Block, S., 244
Blundell, J. E., 162
Bobko, P., 232
Bohenek, D. L., 284
Boivin, D. B., 70
Bolles, R. C., 9, 23, 132, 177, 288
Bonson, J. R., 264
Booth, D. A., 145, 169
Borbely, A., 52, 53, 68
Born, J., 130
Bossio, L. M., 121
Bottome, P., 272
Boulos, Z., 48, 58
Bouton, M. E., 286, 287
Bowen, D., 264
Bower, G. H., 11, 14, 66, 90, 100, 111–13, 114, 115–19, 120, 121, 125, 127, 243
Bowlby, J., 318
Bradley, M. M., 290
Bradshaw, C. M., 187
Brady, J. V., 15
Brazier, M. M., 169, 170, 171, 173
Breedlove, S. M., 159, 302, 303, 308, 309, 314
Brehm, J. W., 4, 25, 82
Brenner, D., 120
Brenner, L. A., 139
Brett, L. P., 150
Brewin, C. R., 292
Brief, D. E., 270
Broadbent, D. E., 126
Broadhurst, P. L., 28, 29
Brod, H., 313
Bronson, F. H., 142
Bronstein, P., 202
Brooks, D. C., 287
Brosschot, J. F., 229
Brown, J. L., 189
Brown, P. J., 164
Brown, T. A., 100, 294, 295
Brown, U., 131
Brownell, K. D., 166
Bryan, J. F., 218

Bryden, M. P., 114, 125
Buck, R., 88
Buckner, D. N., 19
Bucy, P. C., 261
Burcky, W. D., 322
Burger, J. M., 222
Burn, P., 143
Burns, D. D., 99
Bushman, B. J., 274
Buss, A. H., 248, 265
Buss, D. M., 165, 306, 307, 323
Butcher, A. H., 274
Buysse, D. J., 54, 66, 68, 70, 72
Byrne, D., 295

Cacciopo, J. T., 82
Cagnacci, A., 44
Cairns, K. J., 186
Campbell, B. A., 136, 167
Campbell, S. L., 285
Campbell, S. S., 41
Campfield, L. A., 139, 143
Campos, J. J., 292
Candland, D. K., 25
Cannon, W. B., 131, 132, 133, 167
Cantor, N., 225–26, 233
Cantrell, P. J., 319
Cantril, H., 90
Capaldi, E. D., 131, 170
Capitanio, J. P., 320
Caplan, P. J., 314
Card, J. P., 40
Carlson, L. L., 43
Carlson, N. R., 15, 19
Carnochan, P., 107
Carr, P. G., 315, 316
Carrier, J., 54
Carskadon, M. A., 55
Carstensen, L. L., 85
Carter, C. S., 304
Carton, J. S., 228
Cascio, 202
Cassel, P., 110, 200, 202, 239, 242
Casy, T., 74
Cataldo, M., 175
Cattell, R. B., 247, 295
Celuch, K., 278
Cervone, D., 227
Champion, R. A., 188
Chao, C.-C., 266
Chaplin, J. P., 153
Chapman, D. W., 221
Chelonis, J. J., 190
Cherek, D. R., 208
Chermack, S. T., 273
Chiodo, J., 264
Christianson, S. A., 121

Christie, R., 229, 276
Clark, L. A., 72, 73, 93, 101
Clark, M. S., 121
Clark, R. A., 209
Clemens, L. G., 303
Clifton, R. K., 19
Cloninger, C., 274
Clore, G. L., 109, 112
Cofer, C. N., 2
Cohen, C., 194
Cohen, I. R., 56
Cohen, L. D., 221
Cohen, N., 301
Cohen, O., 319
Cohen, R. A., 53
Cohen, S., 299, 301
Coish, B. J., 166
Coleman, L. M., 239
Coleman, R. M., 70
Collier, G., 148, 199
Collins, A. M., 114, 115
Collins, B., 229
Collins, B. E., 270
Collins, J. L., 246
Colombo, G., 192
Condry, J., 214
Cook, K. S., 142
Cook, W. W., 247
Copinschi, G., 52
Corban, C. M., 167
Corbett, W. W., 132
Corbit, R., 102
Cordova, D. I., 206
Coren, S., 20–21
Cornelius, R., 266
Coronado-Bogdaniak, R., 250
Costanzo, P. R., 58
Costin, S. E., 320
Cotter, E. M., 177
Courts, F. A., 4
Covington, M. V., 210, 211, 237, 299, 300
Cowan, W. M., 40, 41
Cox, S. J., 22
Craig, K. M., 272
Craik, F. I. M., 118
Crandall, V. C., 228
Crane, R. S., 101
Craske, M. G., 100, 293
Crawford, M., 314
Crespi, L. P., 169, 170, 184
Crews, D., 303
Crick, N. R., 275, 293
Cromwell, R. L., 18, 23
Cross, H. R., 167
Cross, S. E., 301, 313
Crow, T. J., 27

Crowe, E., 238, 296
Crutcher, W., 25
Crutchfield, R. C., 174
Cullen, M. J., 143
Czeisler, C. A., 31, 47, 52, 53, 55, 65, 68, 69, 70

Daan, S., 32, 37, 52, 53, 55
Dabbs, J. M., Jr., 261, 262
Dachowski, L., 173
Dahlstrom, W. G., 247
Dallert, K. M., 60
Danziger, R., 1
Darley, J. M., 26
Darwin, C., 2, 84, 96
Davidson, F. H., 190
Davidson, J., 87
Davidson, J. M., 305
Davidson, R. J., 86, 113, 114, 121, 122–23, 124, 126, 127, 128, 296
Davies, A., 139
Davis, L., 19
Davison, M. R., 99
Dawes, R., 267
Dawkins, R., 258
Dawson, G., 124, 125
Dawson, G. R., 166
Day, H. D., 319
Deacon, S., 48
De Almeida, R. M. M., 259
Deaux, K., 313
De Bruin, E. M. N., 301
De Castro, J. M., 58, 130, 133, 153, 158
DeCharms, R., 199
Dechter, A., 230
Deci, E. L., 199, 202–6, 215, 277, 278
DeCola, J. P., 173, 288
Deffenbacher, J. L., 242, 246
De Giorgio, R., 139
Delgado, J. M. R., 259, 260
Delos, S., 208
Dembo, T., 217
Dement, C., 53
Dement, W. C., 54, 55
DeMyer, M. K., 186
Denenberg, V. H., 318
Denham, G., 239–40
De Oca, B. M., 288
Derakshan, N., 297, 298
DeRoshia, 32
Derryberry, D., 207
Dess, N. K., 166, 289
DeToledo, L., 285
Deutsch, J. A., 139, 140
Deutsch, M., 267
DeVore, I., 257, 304

Devos, R., 143
Dickenberger, D., 274
Dickinson, A., 139, 165, 166, 189, 208
Dieter, E., 90, 92–93, 94, 102, 110, 225, 226, 299
Dijk, D. J., 52, 53
Dill, J. C., 244
Dillon, L. J., 250
Dimberg, U., 291
Dimmick, D., 201, 202, 224
Dinsmoor, J. A., 285
Dixon, D. N., 202
Dodge, K. A., 275
Dodson, J. D., 28, 29
Dohanich, G. P., 303
Dollard, J., 254, 255
Dominowski, R. L., 60
Domjan, M., 190, 307
Donnerstein, E., 275
Doob, L. W., 254
Doss, R. C., 123
Dougherty, D. M., 208
Douvan, E., 187
Dowdy, J., 27
Drambarean, N. C., 174, 175
Dreikurs, R., 11, 98, 99, 110, 121, 198, 199, 200–202, 203, 205, 208, 215, 224, 226, 232, 233, 239, 240, 242, 243, 247, 251, 269, 284, 293, 307
Drewnowski, A., 157, 158, 159, 162, 165
Driscoll, J. M., 277
Dryden, W., 99
Dudley, L. M., 18
Duffy, E., 4, 14, 27, 81, 99, 115
Duffy, V. B., 155
Dugan, S., 229
Dunahoo, C. L., 278
Dunne, M. P., 308
Durkee, A., 248, 265
Dweck, C. S., 212, 222–24, 227, 232

Eason, R. G., 18
Easterbrook, J. A., 15
Eastman, C. I., 40, 46, 69
Eber, H. W., 247
Eberman, K. M., 198
Eccles (Parsons), J., 225, 237
Eccles, J. S., 224, 225, 233, 314
Edelmann, R. J., 165
Edgar, D. M., 53
Edwards, J. M., 295
Eghrari, H., 203
Ehrenfreund, D., 170, 172, 173, 189
Ehrhardt, A. A., 307, 310
Eibl-Eibesfeldt, I., 96, 253, 255
Eisler, R. M., 272

Ekman, P., 10, 18, 84, 85, 86, 87, 88, 89, 90, 92, 93, 96, 99, 100, 101, 102, 104, 106, 107, 113, 239, 240, 241, 244, 245, 251
Ekstrand, B. R., 60
Elias, M. J., 275
Elliman, N. A., 177
Elliott, E. S., 223, 224
Ellis, A., 99
Ellis, A. L., 222
Ellis, H. C., 6, 114, 119, 120, 127
Ellison, G. D., 196
Ellsworth, P., 85, 107, 244
Elman, D., 156
Elmore, D. K., 133, 158
Elms, A. C., 270
Embrey, D. E., 63
Emery, R. E., 252
Emmons, R. A., 90, 93, 101, 110, 225, 226, 299
Endler, N. S., 295
Engebretson, T. O., 250
Engel, A. K., 4
Engel, B. T., 15
Engeli, M., 31
Enright, T. E., 35
Enzle, M. E., 267
Epstein, A. N., 132, 147
Epstein, L. H., 166
Epstein, N., 101
Erbaujh, J. K., 101
Erez, M., 232
Ervin, F., 150
Ervin, G. N., 139
Erwin, R. J., 7, 175, 176, 179
Estes, W. K., 282, 284
Esteves, F., 291, 292
Evans, K. R., 185
Evans, M. T., 25
Evans, T. B., 201
Evans, T. D., 224
Everson, C. A., 51
Exline, R., 257, 276
Eysenck, H. J., 76, 77, 78, 80, 295
Eysenck, M. W., 295, 297, 298, 299

Fabes, R. A., 206, 272
Fagot, B. I., 319
Falconer, J. J., 15
Fallon, A. E., 150, 151, 165
Fanselow, M. S., 173, 284, 288
Fantino, E., 28
Farber, I. E., 296
Faris, P. L., 163
Farley, F. H., 274
Feather, N. T., 212–13, 214, 216, 221, 229, 237

Feeney, J. A., 322, 323
Feham, H. L., 130
Feinlieb, M., 246
Ferguson, E. D., 7, 16, 18, 23, 98, 99,
    112, 123, 126, 130, 143, 175, 176,
    177, 179, 180, 200, 208, 218, 219,
    220, 226, 232, 252, 268, 270, 281,
    287, 295, 298, 318, 319, 320
Ferre, P., 318
Ferrier, I. N., 27
Ferster, C. B., 185, 186
Festinger, L., 217, 221
Fial, R. A., 259
Fiedler, K., 81
Field, A. E., 161
Field, E. F., 259
Field, T., 317, 318
Finger, F. W., 24, 25
Finkelstein, J. A., 41
Finn, P. R., 196
Fischer, K. W., 107, 108
Fisher, E. B., Jr., 197, 198
Fisher, J. A., 165
Fiske, S. T., 313
Fitzsimons, J. T., 143, 144
Flaherty, C. F., 173
Flaherty, J. F., 71
Fleeson, W., 225
Flier, J. S., 142
Fliers, E., 56
Fliess, W., 31–32
Flores, T., 258
Flynn, J. P., 113, 260
Folkard, S., 59, 60, 61, 62, 64, 65, 77–
    78, 79
Folkman, S., 96, 299
Fookson, J. E., 63
Foote, F. H., 308
Forgas, J., 81
Forgas, J. P., 111, 112
Forgie, M. L., 259
Forsterling, F., 239
Forzano, L. B., 190
Foster, R. G., 41
Fox, N. A., 113, 122, 124
Frable, D. E. S., 310
Francis, T. J., 303
Frank, E., 71
Frank, L. D., 305
Frank, L. G., 305
Franken, R. E., 10
Frankenhaeuser, M., 240
Fredrikson, M., 240
Freeman, A., 99
French, J. R. P., Jr., 271, 280
Freud, S., 2, 10, 82, 97, 98, 99, 101, 183,
    200, 281, 319

Friedman, M., 248
Friedman, M. I., 160
Friesen, W. V., 84, 85, 86, 87, 88, 89, 90,
    99, 107, 113, 240, 241, 244
Frijda, N. H., 11, 94, 100, 101, 105, 109
Frith, C. E., 27
Fritz, G. K., 221
Froberg, J. E., 64
Fujita, F., 93
Fuller, C. A., 33, 47, 53, 68
Funkenstein, D. H., 240
Fuoco, F. J., 186
Fuster, J. M., 18

Gaab, C., 166
Gainde, R., 15
Gajiwala, K. S., 143
Galef, B. G., 152, 259
Gammon, C. B., 196
Gangestad, S. W., 308
Garber, J., 275
Garcia, J., 150, 181, 291
Gardner, L., 290
Gardner, L. E., 308, 323, 324
Gatto, G. J., 192, 194
Gazzaniga, M. S., 113
Gebhard, P. H., 307
Gebhardt, W. A., 229
Geen, R. G., 242, 252, 274, 275, 294
Geis, F., 276
Geisler, M. W., 179, 180
Gerrard, C. K., 219, 221
Getz, L. L., 304
Gewirtz, J. L., 187
Gibbons, K., 160
Gibbs, J., 139, 141
Gieselman, C. J., 58
Gilchrist, J. C., 174
Gill, J. M., 58
Gillard, E. R., 136
Gillette, M. U., 43
Gilligan, S. C., 14
Gilligan, S. G., 100, 113, 114, 115–18,
    120
Gilliland, M. A., 51
Ginsberg, G. S., 202
Girgus, J. S., 237
Gladue, B., 263
Glass, D. C., 248
Glick, P., 313
Glickman, S. E., 185, 259, 263, 305
Glickman, W. E., 24
Glucksberg, S., 26
Go, V. L., 139
Godaert, G. L. R., 229
Gold, G. J., 271
Gold, P. E., 177–79

Goleman, D. J., 122
Gollwitzer, P. M., 232
Good, S., 228
Goodwin, D., 120
Goodwin, D. W., 197
Goodwin, F. K., 46
Gopnik, A., 108
Gorgoglione, J. M., 120
Gorsuch, R. L., 8, 101, 295
Gottesman, I. I., 142
Gottman, J. M., 85, 89, 100
Goumard, B. R., 167
Graeber, R. C., 47, 48
Graham, F. K., 19
Graham, S., 242, 243
Graham, S. N., 178
Gray, J. A., 286, 287, 288, 295–96
Green, D., 199
Green, M. W., 177, 297, 298
Greenberg, J., 218, 221
Greenberg, R. L., 99
Greene, J. T., 131, 154
Greenwood, C. R., 186
Gregorich, S., 15
Gregory, M., 126
Grey, L., 110, 201, 202, 269, 284
Griggs, R. C., 157, 158, 159, 167
Grill, H. J., 129, 136, 137, 150
Grillon, C., 294
Groebel, J., 255
Grossman, S. P., 143
Groves, D., 25, 285
Grunberg, N., 18
Grunwald, B. B., 99, 110, 200, 239, 269
Grusec, J. E., 186
Guisez, Y., 143
Gumpert, P., 276
Gundersen, N., 75
Guthrie, E. R., 184
Gutmann, A. J., 208

Haber, R. N., 175, 295
Hadwin, J., 108
Hagan, R., 298
Hahn, S., 312
Haigler, V. F., 319
Haire-Joshu, D., 197
Hake, D. F., 256
Halaas, J. L., 143
Halberg, F., 31
Halcomb, C. G., 167
Hall, D. F., 260
Hall, H. K., 266
Hall, J. F., 167
Hall, R. V., 186
Hall, S. J., 40
Halmi, K. A., 130

Halpern, D. F., 313, 314
Halpern, M. T., 198
Hamalainen, M., 276
Hamburger, C., 31
Hamlin, P. H., 199
Hankins, W. G., 150
Hanninen, O., 69
Hansen, R. D., 267
Harkins, S. G., 235
Harlow, H. F., 316–17, 318, 319–20
Harma, M. I., 69
Harner, D. E., 164
Harrington, M. E., 40
Harris, F., 266
Harris, R. B. S., 136, 140, 141, 160
Hart, J. D., 99, 290
Hartup, W. W., 276
Hastings, M. H., 40
Hatsukami, D. K., 197
Hawkins, W. F., 18, 23
Hay, D., 252
Hayamizu, T., 224
Hayes, S. G., 246
Hazan, C., 307, 318, 320, 322, 323
Heaton, A. W., 249
Hebb, D. J., 27, 28, 48
Heckhausen, H., 232, 233
Hedderley, D., 297
Hedges, L. V., 315
Hegland, S. M., 278
Heideman, P. D., 142
Heider, K., 84, 236, 244, 250
Heishman, S. J., 197
Helmers, K. F., 248
Helmreich, R. L., 237, 249, 250, 269, 311
Hendrick, C., 308, 323
Hendrick, S., 308, 323
Hendrickson, A. E., 40
Hendrie, C. A., 288
Henley, T., 1
Hennessey, B. A., 199, 200
Henningfield, J. W., 194, 197
Herbert, T. B., 299, 301
Hergenhahn, B. R., 1
Hernandez, L., 169
Hertz, R. M., 295
Hess, E. H., 317
Hess, W. R., 260
Hetherington, M. M., 154, 155, 158, 162, 163, 169
Hetherton, T. F., 161, 164
Heyman, G. D., 212, 224
Heyman, G. M., 187
Hickey, C. B., 276
Hickey, T. L., 40
Higgins, D. A., 272

Higgins, E. T., 110, 238, 296
Hilgard, E. R., 184
Hill, A. J., 162, 163
Hill, C. T., 312
Hill, D., 124
Hilliard, J. P., 221
Hillman, D., 31
Himmelweit, H. T., 221
Hinde, R., 255
Hine, D. W., 238
Hinshaw, S. P., 277
Hinz, L. D., 160
Hirsch, E., 199
Ho, M.-Y., 187
Hobfoll, S. E., 278
Hodapp, V., 222
Hodge, C. N., 313
Hoebel, B. G., 169
Hoese, E. K., 40, 69
Hofman, M. A., 56
Hohlstein, L. A., 164
Holden, E. W., 278
Holekamp, K. E., 305
Hollenbeck, J. R., 232
Holley, 32
Honma, K.-I., 31
Honzik, C. H., 184, 185
Hori, P., 252, 256, 288
Horn, H. L., 206, 212
Horne, J. A., 14, 49, 50, 51, 52, 53, 62, 75, 76
Horner, M. S., 315
Horney, K., 281–82
Horowitz, M. J., 121
Horowitz, T., 65
Horvath, T., 167
Hoskinson, K., 71
Houck, P. R., 54
Houston, J. P., 6, 167, 174
Hovland, C. I., 167
Howard, J. L., 15
Hubel, D. H., 74
Huebner, R. R., 293
Hugdahl, K., 244
Hughes, J. N., 275
Hughes, J. R., 197
Hughes, R. J., 55
Hull, C., 27
Hull, C. L., 3, 14, 131, 143, 157, 167, 183, 184, 185, 189
Hulsey, M. G., 132, 136
Hume, K. I., 62, 65
Humphrey, L. L., 161
Humphreys, M. S., 4, 29, 77, 80, 210
Hunt, B. I., 48
Hunt, R. R., 6
Hunt, S. L., 202

Hunt, W. A., 90
Hunter, G. A., 169
Hunter, W. S., 184
Hupka, R. B., 92
Hursch, C., 54
Hurt, R. D., 198
Hutchinson, R. R., 256
Hutton, D. G., 186
Hyde, J. S., 314
Hymes, C., 238, 296

Ickes, W., 312
Ilmarinen, J., 69
Imhoff, A. R., 316
Inglehart, M., 87
Ingram, J. M., 313
Isaac, J. L., 239
Isen, A. M., 120
Ito, T. A., 273
Izard, C. E., 10, 87, 96, 99, 113, 293

Jacklin, C. N., 302
Jackson, D., 186
Jackson, L. A., 313, 314
Jacobs, G., 101
Jacobs, J., 150
Jacobsen, F. M., 46
James, W., 2, 3, 10, 11, 13, 82, 84, 85, 104
Jarrett, D., 66, 71
Jarvick, M. E., 197
Jastrow, J., 101–2
Jebens, E., 75
Jenkin, N., 174
Jenkins, C. D., 248
Jenks, S. M., 305
Jitsumori, M., 92
Jiwani, N., 227
John, O. P., 101
Johnson, B. H., 244
Johnson, H. J., 186
Johnson, R. F., 40
Johnson, V. E., 307, 308
Joiner, T. E., Jr., 161
Joireman, J. A., 301
Jones, A., 25
Jones, C. R., 15
Jones, D. C., 320
Jones, E. G., 40
Jordan, P. C., 205
Josephs, R., 238
Jourden, F. J., 227
Jussim, L., 239
Juvonen, J., 237

Kagan, J., 19, 123
Kahle, J., 277

Kalat, J. W., 26, 246, 261, 264
Kaliterna, L., 78
Kamin, L. J., 284
Kanfer, R., 232
Kannel, W. B., 246
Kanzer, P., 187
Kaplan, J. M., 129, 136, 137
Karacan, I., 54
Karan, L., 198
Karli, P., 259
Karniol, R., 6, 235
Kasdon, D., 28
Kasprowicz, A. L., 249
Katkovsky, W., 228
Kazen, M., 232
Keel, P., 161
Keenleyside, M. C., 272
Keesey, R. E., 132, 136, 142, 159
Kelley, H. H., 267
Kendler, H. H., 2, 3, 166
Kentridge, R. W., 124, 287, 288
Keppel, G., 305
Kerbeshian, M. C., 142
Kermoian, R., 292
Killilea, M., 161
Kim, J. J., 288
Kimble, G. A., 11, 167, 189, 190
Kinchla, R. A., 26
King, L. A., 101
Kinsey, A. C., 307
Kintsch, W., 89, 118
Kipnis, D., 272
Kirson, D., 85
Kissileff, H. R., 159, 160, 162
Kjelgaard, M. M., 235
Kleck, R. E., 293
Klein, D., 40, 43
Klein, H. J., 232
Klein, K. E., 48
Kleinmuntz, B., 18
Klerman, E. B., 31
Klesges, R. C., 198
Kling, J. W., 191
Klinger, E., 232–33, 243
Klinger, L. G., 124
Klotter, K., 35
Klüver, H., 261
Knauth, P., 69
Knight, G. P., 266, 272
Knight, R. G., 246
Kobak, R. R., 307, 322
Koch, C., 157
Koch, S., 130
Kocher, S. J., 167, 168
Koelling, R., 150
Koestner, J., 205
Koestner, R., 205, 207, 210, 231
Kogut, D., 275

Kohn, A., 208, 269
Kolb, B., 261
Komorita, S. S., 187, 222, 266
Konig, P., 4
Konner, M., 164
Koob, G. F., 195
Kopp, R. R., 99
Koss, M. P., 293
Koulack, D., 59
Kozlowski, L. T., 197
Kraemer, R., 314
Krantz, D. S., 15, 248
Krantz, S. E., 111
Kraska, K., 4
Krauchi, K., 44
Kraus, R. M., 267
Kruglanski, A. W., 249, 267
Krusell, 202
Ku, L. C., 313
Kubiak, P., 17
Kuhl, J., 4, 232, 233
Kukla, A., 236
Kuo, Z. Y., 260
Kupfer, D. J., 54, 66, 71
Kushida, C. A., 51

Labouvie, E., 196
Lacey, B. C., 19, 123
Lacey, J. I., 15, 19, 123
Ladish, C., 179
Landeira-Fernandez, J., 288
Landis, C., 90
Lando, H. A., 197
Landreth, H. F., 167
Landreth, J. E., 167
Lang, P. J., 99, 290
Lange, C., 10, 13, 83
Langenbucher, J., 196
Langevin, R., 307
Langley, T., 274, 275
Laplace, A. C., 273
Larkin, K. T., 249
Larrick, R. P., 238
Larsen, R. J., 90, 110
Larson, R. W., 94
Latané, B., 90, 260
Latham, G. P., 217, 231, 232
Lau, M. A., 275
Laumann-Billings, L. L., 252
Lavery, R. J., 38
Lavie, P., 44, 55
Lawrence, P. S., 186
Lawson, N. O., 44
Lazarus, R. S., 4, 20, 81, 84, 85, 88, 90, 95–96, 97, 98, 99, 100, 101, 102, 104, 106, 107, 108, 109, 110, 174, 239, 240, 243, 247, 251, 281, 294, 299

Lazovik, A. D., 290
Leak, G. K., 308, 323, 324
LeDoux, J. E., 113, 287, 288
Lee, C., 232
Lee, C. Y., 303
Lee, J. M., 303
Lee, M. K., 177
Leeka, J., 72, 73
Lefcourt, H. M., 229
Leiberman, D. A., 190
Leiman, A. L., 159
Leinbach, M. D., 319
Le Magnen, J., 133, 134, 135, 136, 139, 140, 141, 142, 154
Lemeignan, M., 244
Le Moal, M., 195
Lenn, N. J., 40
Lentz, T., 266
Leone, D. R., 203
Lepper, M. R., 199, 206
Leproult, R., 52
Lerner, B. S., 227
Leven, S. J., 99, 114
Levenson, R. W., 18, 84, 85, 87, 88, 89, 90, 92, 93, 96–97, 98, 99, 100, 101, 104, 106, 107, 109, 113, 229, 240, 241, 244
Leventhal, H., 81, 120
Levine, D., 274
Levine, D. S., 99, 114
Levine, S., 90, 110, 246, 289
Levis, D. J., 286
Levitsky, D., 148
Lewin, K., 213, 217–18, 219, 225, 226, 233
Lewiston, N. J., 221
Lewko, J., 238
Lewy, A. J., 46, 47, 55, 68, 69
Ley, R. G., 114, 125
Li, B.-H., 58, 132
Li, T.-K., 192
Libby, M. N., 277
Liberman, A. M., 173
Liberson, W. T., 69
Librand, W. B. G., 267
Lichtenstein, E., 197
Lieberman, H. R., 54, 55
Liebert, R. M., 274
Light, K. C., 15
Linden, S. E., 289
Lindsley, D. B., 15, 18
Lindsley, O. R., 186
Lindy, J., 191
Lipkus, F. M., 247
Littwin, G. H., 123, 294
Liu, C., 43, 44
Liu, L., 40, 69
Liverant, S., 228

Livingstone, M. S., 74
Locke, E. A., 217, 218, 227, 230–31, 232, 234
Lockley, S. W., 48
Loeber, R., 252
Loftus, E. F., 114, 115, 121
Loftus, G. R., 114
Logothetis, D. E., 41
Lograno, D. E., 194
Logue, A. W., 190
London, E. D., 56
Long, V. O., 250
Longstreth, L. E., 208
Lopes, L. L., 222
Lopez, M., 189
Lorge, I., 176
Lowe, C. A., 267
Lowell, E. L., 209
Lubin, B., 101
Lucion, A. B., 259
Lumeng, L., 192
Lund, D., 186
Lundberg, U., 240
Lundin, R. W., 167
Lushene, R. E., 8, 101
Lykken, D. T., 18

Maccarini, M. R., 139
Macdiarmid, J. I., 155
MacDonald, N. L., 257
Macdonald, P. J., 274
Machen, M. A., 71
Machiavelli, N., 276
MacIntosh, A., 221
MacIntyre, D. I., 319
MacLan, P. D., 260
MacLean, P. D., 260
MacLeod, C., 297, 298
MacRae, J. R., 194
Madson, L., 301, 313
Maffei, M., 142, 143
Magdol, L., 252
Magee, L., 258
Magnus, P., 75
Magnusson, J., 236
Magoun, H. W., 15, 18
Mahamedi, F., 161
Maier, S. F., 25, 285, 289
Maki, P., 208
Malamuth, N., 275
Malmo, H. P., 145, 167
Malmo, R. B., 11, 14, 18, 27, 145, 167, 290
Malmo, R. G., 5, 10, 26
Mandler, G., 97, 104, 295
Manning, C. A., 177, 180
Manuck, S. B., 249
Marcattilo, A. J., 190
Marchi, P., 130

Marden, B., 297
Maren, S., 173, 177, 180, 284, 288
Mark, G. P., 169
Markey, S. P., 46
Marks, I. M., 15, 286
Marks, M., 60, 64
Marquis, D. G., 184
Marshall, D. D., 319
Marshall, G., 91
Martin, C. E., 307
Martin, C. L., 301
Martin, J. R., 58
Martin, R. J., 132, 136, 140, 141, 142
Maslach, C., 91, 92, 93, 106, 117, 310
Masters, W. V., 307, 308
Mathews, A., 297
Matter, W. W., 167
Mattes, R., 158
Maude, D., 160, 164, 165
Mauro, R., 102–3, 105
Maxeiner, M. E., 243
May, J. G., III, 190
Mayer, J., 132
Mayer, J. D., 121
Mayhew, R., 165
Maywood, E. S., 40
Mazur, J. E., 190
McAllister, D. E., 284
McAllister, W. R., 284
McArthur, A. J., 43
McBride, W. J., 192
McClelland, D. C., 174, 196, 197, 209–10, 211, 212, 216, 224, 273, 288, 315
McCord, P. R., 296, 297
McCormick, D. A., 4, 15, 75
McCormick, N. B., 307
McCullers, J. C., 206
McDonald, R. J., 180
McDougall, W., 3
McFann, H. H., 296
McGrath, J. J., 19
McHoskey, J., 276
McHugh, P. R., 161
McKeever, W. F., 114, 125, 126
McKenna, M. M., 259
McKoon, G., 60
McNulty, J. A., 19, 20
Medley, D. M., 247
Mednick, M. T., 315, 316
Meehl, P. E., 247
Mehrabian, A., 101, 249
Meijer, J. H., 40, 41
Meisel, R. L., 303
Meister, M., 41
Melamed, B. G., 99, 290
Menaker, M., 40, 41
Mendelsohn, M., 101

Mendolia, M., 293
Meredith, C. W., 201
Mesquita, B., 94, 109
Messer, M. H., 250
Messick, D. M., 267
Messick, S., 133, 158
Meyer, D. E., 60
Meyer, W. U., 207
Meyer-Bernstein, E. L., 40–41
Michener, G. R., 257
Middleton, B., 48
Mikulineer, M., 74
Milberg, S., 121
Miles, L. E., 54
Milgram, S., 270–71, 274, 280
Miller, A., 206, 212
Miller, A. G., 270, 271
Miller, K. J., 196
Miller, N., 272, 273
Miller, N. E., 254, 282
Miller, R. R., 276
Millman, L., 151
Mills, R. S., 186
Millwood, B., 297
Milner, J. S., 259, 260, 275
Milner, P. M., 191
Mineka, S., 291, 295
Minors, D., 54, 55
Minors, D. S., 60, 61, 62
Mir, D., 259
Mirmiran, M., 55, 56
Mistlberger, R. E., 53
Mitler, M. M., 68, 69
Mock, J. E., 101
Mogg, K., 297
Moline, M. L., 55, 63, 64
Monaghan, E. P., 259, 263
Mone, M. A., 232
Money, J., 307, 309
Mongeluzzi, D. L., 289
Monk, T. H., 37, 54, 55, 62, 64, 65–66, 67, 68, 70, 71, 72, 74, 76, 77, 79
Monnier, J., 278
Montague, A., 268
Monteiro, K. P., 14, 117, 120
Mook, D. G., 148
Moore, B. A., 114
Moore, L. A., 275
Moore, R. Y., 40, 41, 42, 43
Moore-Ede, M. C., 33, 47, 48, 68, 69, 70
Moos, R. H., 299, 300
Moran, J. D., III, 206
Moran, T. H., 161
Moreau, T., 19
Morehouse, R. E., 274
Morgenstern, J., 196
Morien, A., 58, 132
Morimoto, A., 159

Morimoto, K., 159
Morin, L. P., 40, 41, 55
Moruzzi, G., 15, 18
Mosak, H. H., 99, 121, 226
Moss, H. A., 19, 123
Moss, R. L., 41
Motowidlo, S. J., 226–27
Moulton, R. W., 222
Mowrer, O. H., 254, 283, 284
Moyer, K. E., 256, 261, 263, 271
Mrosovsky, N., 38, 40
Muller, J. E., 45
Muller, T., 42
Munk, M. H. J., 4
Murakami, N., 159
Muris, P., 292
Murphy, C. M., 273
Murphy, J. M., 192
Murphy, P. J., 41
Murphy, S. T., 87
Murray, H., 209
Musty, R. E., 30, 132, 137, 146, 147, 148
Myers, B. L., 55, 56

Nader, K., 196
Nagy, Z. M., 25
Nance, D. M., 40
Near, D., 276
Neiss, R., 26
Nelson, J. G., 274
Nemeroff, C., 151
Nesberg, L. S., 174
Nestler, E. J., 195
Netter, P., 288, 289
Neuman, P., 289
Newell, A., 114
Newsome, D. A., 46
Ngo-Muller, V., 36
Niaura, R. S., 197
Noel, M. B., 196
Nolen-Hoeksema, S., 237
Noller, P., 323
Noseworthy, W. J., 19, 20
Novaco, R. W., 242
Novin, D., 58
Nowell, A., 315
Nowicki, S., 228
Nowlis, V., 91, 101
Nunez, J. F., 318

Oakhill, J., 66
Obrist, P. A., 15
O'Connor, C., 85
O'Connor, P. A., 211
Oden, G. C., 174

O'Farrell, T. J., 273
Ohman, A., 290–91
Oldfield, B. J., 145
Olds, J., 191
O'Leary, T. A., 100
Oliver, S., 163
Olmsted, M. P., 166
Omelich, C. L., 210, 211, 237
O'Neal, E. C., 252, 272, 274, 275
O'Neil, P. M., 166
Opton, E. M., Jr., 20
Orav, E. J., 55
Orbeell, J., 267
Orlick, T., 266
Osborne, S. R., 170, 189
Ostberg, O., 75, 76
Ostmann, A., 222
O'Sullivan, J. T., 206
Ottaviani, R., 111
Ottaway, S. A., 114
Otten, W., 301
Otto, J., 92
Overmier, J. B., 25, 208, 285, 289
Overskeid, G., 204, 206
Owens, J., 170

Paajanen, S., 275
Palanza, P., 263
Palmer, K. A., 170
Panagiotides, H., 124
Panak, W. F., 275
Panksnepp, J., 26
Papez, J. W., 260
Park, B., 312
Parker, J. D. A., 295
Parker, J. G., 319
Parks, C. D., 266, 269
Parmenter, S. A., 246
Parmigiani, S., 263
Parra, C., 291
Parsons, M. W., 178
Partiman, T. S., 56
Patel, V., 288
Patrick, B. C., 203
Paulhus, D., 229
Pauli, J. A., 25, 75, 76
Pavlov, I., 102, 282
Paxton, S., 160
Pedersen, J. M., 305
Peetz, S. M., 63
Pelaez-Nogueras, M., 187
Pelchat, M. L., 150
Pelleymounter, M. A., 143
Pellis, S. M., 257, 258, 259, 261
Pellis, V. C., 259, 261
Pennock, L., 131
Peplau, L. A., 312

Pepper, F. C., 99, 110, 200, 239, 269
Perner, J., 108
Perry, M., 265
Perry, R. P., 236
Pervin, L. A., 219
Peterson, C., 121, 238, 289, 299, 300
Pettit, G. S., 275
Pfefferbaum, B., 274
Phaf, R. H., 114
Phillips, R. E., 186
Phillips, S. D., 316
Pickard, G. E., 40, 41
Pickens, R. W., 197
Pickworth, W. B., 194
Piedmont, R. L., 315
Pietrowsky, R., 130
Pihl, R. O., 275
Pinel, J. P. J., 133, 140, 141, 146, 148
Pitkanen, T., 276
Pitsounis, N. D., 202
Pittendrigh, C. S., 32, 37, 41, 55
Placentini, A., 130
Plat, L., 52
Pleck, J. H., 313
Pliner, P., 156
Pohl, H., 35
Polich, J., 179, 180
Pollock, V. E., 273
Pomeroy, W. B., 307
Poothullil, J. M., 155
Porac, J., 277
Posluszny, D. M., 248
Postman, L., 60, 174, 184
Potthoff, A. D., 196
Powell, B., 120
Powley, T. L., 132, 136, 142, 159
Pred, R. S., 249
Preston, M. G., 217, 219
Price, R. A., 142
Proneca, R., 142
Pryor, D. W., 306
Pubols, B. H., Jr., 170
Puglisi, A., 130
Pulkkinen, L., 276

Quiggle, N. L., 275
Quillian, M. R., 114

Rabbit, P., 54, 55
Raccuglia, R. A., 114
Rachlin, H., 187
Radosevic-Vidacek, B., 78
Ragozzino, M. E., 178
Rajkowski, J., 17
Ralph, M. R., 40
Ramsay, D. J., 145, 146
Ramsay, D. S., 132, 141, 144

Rapoport, A., 267
Ratcliff, R., 60
Raven, B. H., 267, 271–72, 280
Rawl, S. M., 245
Rayner, R., 83, 84, 99, 108, 282
Raynor, J. O., 211
Rechtschaffen, A., 51, 53
Redd, M., 153
Redlin, U., 40
Reebs, S. G., 38
Reeve, J., 278
Reid, L. S., 24, 25
Reidbord, S. P., 121
Reidl, L., 92
Reilly, T., 55, 68, 70
Reite, M., 320
Renfrew, J. W., 260
Reppert, S. M., 40, 41, 43, 44
Restoin, A., 75
Reuterman, N. A., 322
Revelle, W., 4, 29, 77, 80, 210
Reynaert, C., 229
Reynolds, C. F., III, 54, 66, 71, 79
Reznikoff, M., 219
Richards, A., 297
Richards, R. W., 190
Richardson, G. S., 55
Richardson, T. E., 314
Richey, H. W., 58, 131
Riesen, A. H., 167
Rietveld, W. J., 40, 41
Riklan, M., 219
Ritter, R. C., 139
Rivkees, S. A., 43
Rix, M. K., 278
Robarchek, C. A., 269
Robarchek, C. J., 269
Robbins, T. W., 19
Roberts, G. C., 266, 277
Roberts, W. A., 167, 190
Robinson, M., 275
Robinson, T. E., 26
Roby, T. B., 186, 209
Rodgers, R. J., 288
Rodin, J., 156
Rodriguez, I. A., 119
Roelfsema, P. R., 4
Rogers, P. J., 163, 177, 297
Rolls, B. J., 143, 144, 145, 148, 154,
    158, 162, 163, 169, 181, 287
Rolls, E. T., 123–24, 143, 144, 145, 154
Roney, C. J. R., 238, 296
Rosas, J. M., 286
Roseman, R. H., 248
Rosenthal, N. E., 45, 46
Rosenwasser, A. M., 31, 41, 42, 58
Rosenzweig, M. R., 159

Ross, D., 274
Ross, G., 288
Ross, J., 121
Ross, M., 6, 235
Ross, R. A., 246
Ross, S. A., 274
Rotter, J. B., 212, 221, 227–28, 229,
    230, 233, 236
Routtenberg, A., 191
Rowe, E. A., 154
Rowland, N. E., 58, 132, 140, 142
Rozin, P., 149, 150, 151, 152, 165, 181
Rubin, H. B., 256
Rubin, Z., 312, 324
Ruble, D. N., 301
Rudd, M. D., 161
Rudd, R. J., 178
Ruddy, M. G., 60
Rusak, B., 40, 42
Rusniak, K. W., 150, 291
Russel, J. A., 245
Russell, M. C., 118
Russell, S., 101
Rutenfranz, J., 69
Ryan, R. M., 202, 203, 205

Sachs, B. D., 303
Sack, D. A., 46, 47
Sack, R. L., 55, 68, 69
Sakai, L. M., 302
Sales, B. D., 175
Sallery, R. D., 256
Sanchez-Watts, G., 41
Sarason, S. B., 295
Saron, C., 122
Saron, D., 87
Saugstad, P., 173
Savage, L. M., 289
Sayette, M. A., 275
Saylor, M., 239–40
Schachter, S., 90–91, 102, 104, 106, 156
Schallert, T., 169, 177
Schell, A. M., 130
Schick, R. R., 139
Schiff, B. B., 24
Schiffman, S. S., 58
Schlosberg, H., 2
Schmidt, H. O., 247
Schmidt, N. B., 161
Schmitt, S., 208, 268
Schneider, T., 266
Schrier, A. M., 191
Schulman, P., 237
Schulz, R. W., 176
Schusdziarra, V., 139
Schuster, B., 239
Schvaneveldt, R. W., 60

Schwartz, D. H., 169
Schwartz, G. E., 122, 186
Schwartz, J., 85
Schwartz, M., 60
Schwartz-Shea, P., 267
Schwarz, N., 109, 112
Schwebel, A. I., 324
Scoles, M. T., 194
Scotch, N., 246
Scott, J. P., 255
Scucko, J. J., 18
Sears, P. S., 217, 221
Sears, R. R., 254
Seeley, R. J., 132
Seeman, M., 228
Seeney, K., 154
Segal, B., 188
Seib, T. B., 289
Sejnowski, T. J., 4, 15, 75
Self, E. A., 4, 25, 82
Seligman, M. E. P., 25, 237, 251, 285,
    289
Selye, H., 96, 98, 239
Senulis, A., 87
Sharkey, K. J., 319
Sharma, M., 55
Sharp, S., 278
Shaver, P., 85, 107
Shaver, P. R., 318, 320, 322, 323
Shaw, L. L., 15
Sheffield, F. D., 167, 186
Shide, D. J., 163
Shiff, B. B., 185
Shiffman, S., 194
Shors, T. J., 289
Showers, C. J., 207
Shulkin, J., 149, 150, 152
Shulman, B., 99, 121
Shulman, I., 302
Sidman, M., 283
Siegal, M., 151
Siegel, J. M., 246
Siegel, P. S., 58
Siegel, R. K., 191, 194, 197
Siegel, S., 194, 218
Siegeltuch, M. B., 286
Siegman, A. W., 249, 250
Siiteri, P. K., 305
Sikes, S., 156
Simon, C. W., 131
Simon, H. A., 114
Simon, J. G., 213
Simpson, C., 1, 245
Simpson, J. A., 308
Singer, J. E., 90–91, 102, 104, 106
Singer, W., 4
Singh, D., 156, 165

Skene, D. J., 48
Skinner, B. F., 183, 184, 185, 186, 214, 282
Skinner, E. A., 228
Skitka, L. J., 310
Skwerer, R. G., 45, 46
Slade, J., 198
Slama, M., 278
Slapion-Foote, M. J., 308
Slaughter, V., 108
Smale, L., 305
Smith, E., 40
Smith, E. R., 305
Smith, F. J., 139, 143
Smith, G. P., 139, 240
Smith, G. T., 164
Smith, H., 93
Smith, H. L., 230
Smith, J. R., 54
Smith, L. K., 259
Smith, P. B., 229
Smith, P. K., 275
Smith, T. W., 250
Snyder, M. L., 248
Sobal, J., 164
Sobel, J., 266
Solomon, R., 102, 103, 105, 196, 240, 242, 251, 284, 285
Soltz, V., 110, 201, 239, 242, 293
Sommer, K. L., 301, 313
Sonenstein, F. L., 313
Sonnemans, J., 94, 109
Sorenson, S. B., 307
Sorrentino, R. M., 110, 238
Spear, P. D., 40
Spence, J. T., 167, 237, 249, 250, 269, 310, 311, 315, 324
Spence, J. W., 282
Spence, K. W., 27, 184, 189, 295–96, 299
Sperry, R. W., 113
Spiegelman, B. M., 142
Spieker, S., 124
Spielberger, C. D., 8, 101, 246, 247, 295, 297
Spiteri, N. J., 58
Sprafkin, J., 274
Spring, B., 264
Stampfl, T. G., 286
Standing, L., 175
Stanghellini, V., 139
Stanley, B. G., 136
Staw, B. M., 199
Steele, C. M., 238
Steerneman, P., 292
Stefurak, T. L., 189–90

Stein, A. H., 315
Stein, L., 191
Stephan, F. K., 41
Steriade, M., 4, 15, 18, 75
Sternberg, R. J., 320, 321–22, 323
Stokker, L. G., 214
Stone, W. S., 178
Stoney, C. M., 250
Stote, D. L., 288
Stricker, E. M., 58, 140, 141, 147
Striepe, 161
Strier, K. B., 259
Stringer, N., 28
Stromberg, M. F., 289
Stroop, J. R., 297
Stuckey, H. L., 58
Studd, M. V., 313
Stunkard, A., 130, 133, 157, 158, 159, 164, 167
Suberi, M., 114, 125, 126
Sugiura, T., 159
Sullivan, B. F., 324
Sulzman, F. M., 33, 47, 68
Summers, C., 238
Sunday, S., 130
Sutcliffe, J. P., 221
Sutterer, J. R., 15
Sutton, S. K., 113, 295, 296
Svartdal, F., 204, 206
Swabb, D. F., 56
Swain, R. A., 173
Swanson, L. W., 40, 41
Symons, D., 306
Szabadi, E., 187
Szczepanska-Sadowska, E., 144, 145
Szmukler, G., 160

Takahashi, J. S., 40
Takahashi, P. J., 25, 75, 76
Tamarkin, L., 43
Tamura, C. S., 139
Tan, N., 159
Tanz, L., 187
Tarabrina, N. V., 92
Tatsuoka, M. M., 247
Tavris, C., 245
Taylor, J. A., 174, 282, 294, 296
Taylor, S., 263
Taylor, S. L., 274, 275
Taylor, S. P., 196, 273
Teasdale, J. D., 118, 238
Teicher, M. H., 45, 54
Teitelbaum, P., 132, 136
Tellegen, A., 101
Terman, M., 46, 47, 58
Thayer, J. F., 244

Thayer, R. E., 4, 20, 21, 22, 23, 25, 62, 65, 72, 73, 74, 75, 76, 77, 92, 97, 123, 140, 299
Thibaut, J., 267, 276
Thomas, C. G., 316
Thomas, G. V., 190
Thomas, R. L., 119
Thomas, S. L., 275
Thomas, S. P., 245, 246, 247, 249
Thompson, E. H., Jr., 313
Thompson, R. F., 173, 289
Thompson, V., 319
Thorndike, E. L., 176, 183, 184, 214
Thorne, B., 1
Thornton, K. M., 237
Thornton, N., 237
Thrasher, T. N., 144, 145, 146
Thune, L. E., 60
Tilleczek, K., 238
Tinbergen, N., 3, 258
Titchener, E. D., 2
Tobin, H., 190
Tolman, E. C., 3, 183, 185
Tomarken, A. J., 81, 113, 120, 122, 123
Tomkins, S. S., 87, 96
Tosini, G., 41
Treasure, D. C., 266, 277
Trompenaars, F., 229
Tulving, E., 118
Turek, F. W., 35, 38, 39, 40, 41, 55, 70
Turkewitz, G., 19

Ullsperger, P., 130
Underwood, B. J., 7, 9, 121, 176
Unick, K. E., 178
Usher, P., 142

Vaccarino, F. J., 185
Valente, E., 275
Van Cauter, E., 52, 55, 70
Vancouver, J. B., 217
Van der Kooy, D., 189–90, 196
Vanderweele, D. A., 58, 130
Van Gool, W. A., 55, 56
Van Goozen, S., 94, 109
Van Itallie, T. B., 159, 160
Van Lange, P. A. M., 301, 324
Van Reeth, O., 35, 38, 40, 41, 55, 69, 70
Van Someren, E. J. W., 56
Varner, L. J., 114
Velten, E. A., 119, 121
Venier, I. L., 26
Verbalis, J. G., 140, 141, 143, 144, 146, 147
Verney, E. B., 145
Vernon, J. B., 186

Vidacek, S., 78
Viemero, V., 275
Vitelli, R., 295
Vokac, Z., 75
Volkman, J., 221
Volkmer, R. E., 229
Volpe, A., 44
Vom Saal, F. S., 263
Vrana, S. R., 290
Vu, A. D., 269

Wade, C., 313
Wade, G. N., 147
Wagoner, N., 40
Wakefield, D. A., 296, 297
Waldenar, W., 53
Wall, J. E., 278
Wall, S., 318
Walton, D., 260
Ward, C. H., 101
Ward, K. D., 198
Warwick, A. S., 58
Washburn, A. L., 167
Wasman, M., 260
Waterhouse, J., 52, 54, 55, 60, 61, 62, 68, 70
Waters, E., 318
Watson, D., 72, 73, 93, 101, 229, 230
Watson, F. L., 62
Watson, J. B., 83–84, 85, 99, 104, 108, 282
Watson, J. P., 15, 286
Watts, A. G., 41
Watts, D. P., 259
Weasner, M. H., 24, 25
Weaver, D. R., 43, 44, 303
Webb, R. A., 15
Webb, W. B., 51
Weber, A. L., 10
Wee, B. E. F., 17, 30, 36, 38, 39, 42, 43, 135, 138, 193, 262, 303
Wegman, H. M., 48
Wehr, T. A., 38, 46
Weiland, N. G., 56
Weinberg, M. S., 306, 307
Weinberger, J., 210
Weiner, B., 212, 224, 236–37, 239, 242, 243, 244, 250, 251

Weingarten, H. P., 157
Weiss, K., 166
Weiss, R. S., 313
Weiss, S., 258
Weitzman, E. D., 55
Weldele, M., 305
Weller, A., 163
Welsh, D. K., 41
Welsh, G. S., 247
Wenar, C., 221
Werner, H., 108, 109
Werner, H. D., 99
Wertheim, E. H., 160, 165, 166
Wertheimer, M., 2, 183
Wever, R., 38, 52
Wever, R. A., 31, 59, 62, 65
Whalen, R., 307
Wheeler, R. E., 123
Whitaker, A., 164
White, B. D., 132, 136
White, J. W., 307
White, N. M., 178, 180, 185, 194, 196
White, P. H., 235
Whitehouse, W. G., 289
Whyte, E. C., 221
Wickens, D. D., 131
Wielkiewicz, R. M., 289
Wigfield, A., 224, 225
Wildgruber, C. M., 59, 62, 65
Wilfley, D. E., 166
Wilkinson, R. T., 66
Williams, B. A., 189
Williams, C. J., 306
Williams, C. R., 232
Williams, J. H., 307
Williams, J. M. G., 121, 297, 298
Williams, R., 54
Williamson, D. A., 160
Wilson, A., 287
Wilson, D. S., 276
Wilson, E. O., 265, 269
Wilson, G. T., 275
Wilson, J. R., 160
Windle, M., 272
Wing, R. R., 166
Winget, 32
Winn, P., 136
Winter, J. C., 264

Wirz-Justice, A., 44
Wise, R. A., 191, 192, 194, 196
Wispé, L. G., 174, 175
Wogar, M. A., 187
Wolfe, J., 65
Wollnik, F., 34
Wolpe, J., 99, 100, 290
Wood, P. B., 274
Wood, R., 227
Woodmansee, K. B., 305
Woods, S. C., 132, 141
Woodworth, R. S., 2, 3
Worthington, H., 54
Wright, R. A., 15, 25
Wundt, W., 2, 83, 84, 85, 90, 101, 104
Wurtman, J. J., 54
Wynne, L. C., 284, 285

Yahne, C. E., 250
Yaksh, T. L., 139
Yamasaki, K., 222
Yang, M., 54
Yankeelov, P. A., 277
Yerkes, R. M., 28, 29
Yoshihara, M., 92
Young, J. E., 99
Young, P. T., 58, 131, 153, 154, 155, 181
Young, S. L., 284
Youngquist, J. V., 274
Youngstedt, S. D., 40, 69
Yousem, H., 174

Zabel, C. J., 305
Zajonc, R. B., 87, 96
Zaleski, Z., 92
Zeaman, D., 170
Zeigler, H. P., 148
Zellner, D. A., 164, 165
Zhang, Y., 142
Zhou, J. N,, 56
Zigler, E., 187
Zimbardo, P. G., 10, 91
Zimmerman, J. C., 55
Zinbarg, R. E., 295
Zucker, I., 40, 42
Zuckerman, M., 205, 231
Zyzanski, S. J., 248

Subject Index

Ability, self-assessment of, 225
Absorptive phase, 133
Acetylcholine (ACh), 17, 18, 178, 194, 303
Achievement, 235–39, 250
Achievement motive/motivation, 8–9, 123, 216
  achievement performance, beliefs and, 211–12
  goal setting and, 222
  incentives and, 208–14
Achievement performance, 211–12
Acquisitive self-presentation style, 278
Action, motivation in, 10–11
Activation, 4, 6, 116
Activational processes, 263
Activation-Deactivation Adjective Check List (AD ACL), 21–22, 62, 72, 76
Active avoidance conditioning, 283, 287
Activity (running) wheels, 23–25, 29, 32, 33, 38–40, 41
AD ACL. *See* Activation-Deactivation Adjective Check List
Adaptation, 96–97
Adaptive theory of sleep, 51
Addiction, 102, 192–98. *See also* Substance dependence
Adipocytes, 141
Adipsin, 142
Adlerian theory, 113
  on anger, 247, 250
  on competition, 269, 270
  on goals, 220, 232
  on incentives, 202, 203, 205
  on love, 323, 324
Ad libitum feeding, 133
Adrenal cortex, 240
Adrenal gland, 240

Adrenalin. *See* Epinephrine
Adrenocorticotropic hormone (ACTH), 18, 52, 57
Aerobic metabolism, 22
Affect
  cognition and, 113
  emotion and, 100–101, 105
  global, 71, 72
Affective aggression, 252, 274
Affiliative motivation, 5, 8, 196
African Americans, 245, 315
Agape, 323
Agentic characteristics, 311, 320, 324
Aggression, 235–51, 252–80. *See also* Anger
  affective, 252, 274
  alcohol and, 196–97, 258, 273–74, 275, 280
  in animals, 255–60
  assertiveness distinguished from, 277–79, 280
  childhood experiences and, 275–76, 280
  conspecific, 255–58, 279
  culture and, 268–70, 279
  defensive, 252–53, 260
  fear-induced, 256
  instrumental, 252, 256, 271, 274, 278
  intermale, 256
  interspecies, 259–60, 279
  irritable, 256
  Machiavellianism and, 276–77, 280
  mastery distinguished from, 252, 277, 290
  maternal, 256, 259
  in media, 274–75, 280
  motivational aspects of, 252–54
  power and, 252, 270–74, 280
  predatory, 256, 279
  self-interest versus collective interest in, 264–70, 279

sex-related, 256
  situational variables in, 258–59
Aging
  biological rhythms and sleep and, 54–56
  memory and, 178–79
  mood and, 70–72
Agonistic behavior, 255, 257, 258, 263, 279
AIDS, 306, 313
Albert (child), 83–84, 188
Alcohol, 158, 192–94, 195, 198, 209
  aggression and, 196–97, 258, 273–74, 275, 280
  learning and, 120
  power and, 196, 197, 272–73
Aldosterone, 146–47
Alertness, 64–65
Alertness-sleepiness rhythms, 62–64, 72, 79
Alpha animals, 256, 257, 258, 259, 263, 279
Alpha waves, 50
Alzheimer's disease, 56, 178
Amazon Waorani, 269
Amenorrhea, 160
Amount of motivation, 4, 6
Amphetamine, 178, 194
Amplitude, of biological rhythms, 35–37, 50, 54, 55
Amplitude disorders, 45
Amygdala
  aggression and, 260, 261, 279
  anger and, 246
  emotion and, 113, 123–24
  fear and anxiety and, 287, 288, 300
  hunger and, 180
  sexual motivation/behavior and, 304
  substance abuse and, 192
Anaerobic metabolism, 22
Androgens, 263, 302, 305–6, 313, 324

Androgyny, 311, 312, 319, 324
Anger, 109, 122–23, 239–50, 251, 254
    aggression distinguished from, 252
    expression versus experience of, 250
    hostility distinguished from, 247–48,
        251
    measurement of, 246–47
    rules for expressing, 245–46
    situations giving rise to, 242–44
Anger Expression Scale, 246
Angiotensin, 147
Angiotensin I, 144
Angiotensin II, 144, 145, 147, 167, 181
Angiotensin III, 145
Animism, 2
Annoyance/irritation, 242, 243
Anorexia nervosa, 130, 160–63, 164,
    181–82
Antecedent conditions, 1
Anticipatory satiety, 141
Antidiuretic hormone (ADH), 145
Anxiety, 6, 10, 123, 281–300. See also
        State anxiety; Trait anxiety
    avoidance conditioning and, 282–84,
        285–86, 287, 300
    construct of, 8
    coping with, 297–300
    escape conditioning and, 282–84, 300
    fear distinguished from, 294
    flooding and, 286, 290, 300
    hunger and, 177
    individual differences in, 293–301
    learned helplessness and, 285–86,
        289–90, 300
    learning, 284
    locus of control and, 229
    psychobiological findings, 286–90
    punishment and, 282, 284–85, 300
    test-taking, 210, 211, 213, 216
Anxiolytic drugs, 287, 288
Anxious/ambivalent attachment style,
    318, 322
Appetite, 149–55, 181
Appetitive responses, 129–30
Appetizingness, 152–55, 181
Appraisal
    of consequences, 97, 98
    emotion and, 95, 96, 99, 104
    secondary, 97
Approach, 121–28
Approach reward strategy, 297
APS. See Arousal Predisposition Scale
Arab students, 314
Argentina, 271
Arginine vasopressin (AVP), 145, 146
Arousability, 20–21
Arousal, 4, 6, 14–29, 64

aggression and, 274–76
cognitive, 20, 21
construct of, 14–19
defining and measuring, 14–15
of emotion, 89, 90–91, 97
energetic, 21–23, 29, 76–77
memory and, 179
motor activity and, 23–26
performance and, 23–29
situational specificity and response
    stereotypy of, 19–20, 29
somatic, 20, 21
state versus trait, 20–21, 29
tense, 21–23, 29, 76–77
Arousal Predisposition Scale (APS),
    20–21
Artificial insemination, 306
Aspiration. See Level of aspiration
ASQ. See Attributional Style Question-
    naire
Assertiveness, 277–79, 280
Associative memory, 289
Associative network formulation, 113,
    114–19, 120, 127
Asthmatic children, 221–22
Attachment styles, 308, 318–19, 322–23
Attainment discrepancy, 219, 232
Attention capacity, 119–20
Attributional Style Questionnaire (ASQ),
    238
Attribution theory, 212, 235–39, 250–51
Australia, 308
Australian aboriginals, 245
Autistic children, 186
Autobiographical memory, 118, 121
Autonomic nervous system
    arousal and, 15, 29
    emotion and, 88–90, 113
    hunger and, 138–39
    schematic representation of, 16
Autonomy, 231
Avoidance conditioning, 282–84, 285–
    86, 287, 300
    active and passive, 283, 287
Avoidant attachment style, 308, 318, 322
Avoid punishment strategy, 297

Bait shyness, 150, 151–52
Basal metabolic rate, 159, 182
Bases of power, 271–72
Basic emotions, 85–87, 89, 96. See also
        Pure emotions
Behavior
    aggression as, 252
    hostility and, 248
    motivation as an explanation for,
        1–2

Behaviorism, 2, 3, 14, 184
Behavior modification, 186, 214
Beliefs
    on achievement, 211–12
    as cold cognitions, 110–11
    emotion and, 98
    on locus of control, 227–30
    on self-efficacy, 226–27
    taste aversions and, 150–51
Bem Sex-Role Inventory (BSRI), 311,
    319
Benzodiazepines, 38, 40
Beta waves, 50
Binge eating, 160, 164, 165
Biologically preprogrammed tenden-
    cies, 4
Biological rhythms, 30–57. See also Cir-
        cadian rhythms; Sleep
    advantages of timekeeping, 44–45
    aging and, 54–56
    biorhythms versus, 31–32
    circannual, 31
    control of, 40–44
    defined, 30
    effects of disrupting, 45–48
    motivation and, 30
    seasonal, 38, 56
    ultradian, 31
*Biopsychology of Mood and Arousal,
    The* (Thayer), 21
Blended emotions, 107–8
Blood pressure, 15, 249, 250
Body mass index (BMI), 161
Body temperature, 68
    alertness-sleepiness rhythms and,
        62–64
    biological rhythms and, 45, 55
    circadian rhythms and, 32
    mood and, 71
    performance and, 65
    sleep and, 51, 52, 53, 54
    time of day and, 66, 75, 76, 78
Body temperature rhythms, 61–62
Body weight
    ideal, 163–66
    instability in, 158–60
    maintenance of, 142, 155–60
    short- versus long-term regulation of,
        132–33
Bombesin, 140
Bonding, 317, 320, 321
Brain. See also specific regions
    aggression and, 258–59, 260–61, 262,
        279
    arousal and, 15, 19, 29
    emotion and, 113, 121–25
    fear and anxiety and, 286–88, 300

Brain (*continued*)
  gender differences and, 314
  hunger and, 132
  rewards and, 185
  sexual dimorphism and, 302
  sexual motivation/behavior and, 304, 305
Brain lesions
  aggression and, 258–59, 261
  emotion and, 122
  hunger and, 134, 136
Brain stimulation. *See also* Intracranial self-stimulation
  aggression and, 258–59, 261
  hunger and, 134
BSRI. *See* Bem Sex-Role Inventory
Bulimia nervosa, 130, 160–63, 164, 182
Buss-Durkee Hostility Inventory, 248

Cafeteria feeding experiments, 152
Caffeine, 77, 194, 197
Calories, 133, 159
Carbohydrates, 141, 148, 159, 264
Casein, 153–54
Castration, 303
Catatoxic response, 235, 239
Catharsis, 241–42
Caudal brainstem, 136–37
Causal belongingness hypothesis, 118–19
Cellular dehydration, 143–44, 145, 148, 181
Central nervous system (CNS)
  arousal and, 15
  hunger and, 132, 133–37
  sex-related hormones and, 302
Cerebral asymmetry, 121–25
Chance orientation, 230
Chernobyl nuclear power plant, 69
Cholecystokinin (CCK), 139, 140, 165, 181
Circadian rhythms, 44–48, 58
  aggression and, 261
  aging and, 54–56
  defined, 31
  effects of disrupting, 45–48
  measurement of, 32–38
  melatonin and, 43, 44
  nonphotic factors influencing, 38–40
  oscillators in, 41–42
  sleep and, 52–54, 57
Circannual rhythms, 31
Circumstances, variation in, 5, 6
Classical (Pavlovian) conditioning, 27, 188
  emotion and, 83–84, 99

fear and anxiety and, 283
hunger and, 131
substance abuse and, 194
taste aversions and, 150, 151
Clocks. *See* Pacemakers
Cocaine, 194
Coercive power, 271, 272, 280
Cognition, 3, 10
  anger and, 240–42, 251
  anxiety and, 297–300
  cold, 110–11, 127
  emotion and, 83, 84–85, 95, 106–14
  hostility and, 248
  hot, 110–11, 127
  mood and, 110–13
  self-generated, 298
Cognitive abilities, 313–15, 325
Cognitive arousal, 20, 21
Cognitive distortions, 111
Cognitive evaluation theory, 203, 215
Cognitive-neoassociationist theory, 243, 251
Cognitive-physiological formulation of emotion, 90
Cognitive restructuring, 242, 251
Cognitive revolution, 3
Cognitive tasks, 297–99
Cognitive therapy, 99
Cold cognitions, 110–11, 127
Collective interest, 264–70, 279
Commitment
  goal, 231, 232, 234
  in love, 320, 321
Communal traits, 311, 320, 324
Competence, 222–24, 225, 227, 233
Competition, 237, 251
  aggression and, 264–70, 278–79
  intentional, 269
  intergroup, 269
  intragroup, 269
  structural, 269
Concepts, 114, 115
Conceptual clarity, 10
Conditioned emotional response (CER), 284
Conditioned response (CR), 84
Conditioned (secondary) rewards, 131, 187–89
Conditioned stimuli (CS)
  emotion and, 83
  fear and anxiety and, 283, 286, 289, 291
  hunger and, 157, 167
  taste aversions and, 150
  thirst and, 167

Conditioning
  avoidance, 282–84, 285–86, 287, 300
  classical. *See* Classical (Pavlovian) conditioning
  escape, 282–84, 300
  of fear and anxiety, 290–92
  instrumental, 183–86, 283
  operant, 99, 183–86, 283
Consequences, 4, 201
  appraisal of, 97, 98
Conspecifics
  aggression in, 255–58, 279
  demonstrator, 152
Constructs
  of arousal, 14–19
  defining, 7–9, 12
  of motivation, 2–3, 6, 7–9, 12
Consummate love, 321
Consummatory responses, 129–30, 134, 157, 170, 173
Contact comfort, 316, 325
Contrast effects, 169–70, 182
Controllability, 236–37, 239, 250
Control-optimism, 214
Cook-Medley Ho scale, 247
Coordination situation, 267
Coping, 96–97
Core sleep, 52, 53
Coronary heart disease (CHD), 248–50, 251
Cortex, 15, 19, 29, 113
Corticosteroids, 18
Corticotropin-releasing hormone (CRH), 140
Cortisol, 52, 54, 55, 57, 70, 240
Critical period, 317
Cues
  anger and, 243
  arousal and, 27
  external, 155–57
  hunger and, 155–60, 166–69
  internal, 155–57, 166–67
  social, 31
  thirst and, 166–69
Culture
  aggression and, 268–70, 279
  anger and, 245, 251
  father's role and, 319
  gender differences and, 313–14, 316
  hunger and, 149–50, 181
  locus of control beliefs and, 229–30
  love and, 321
  mastery and, 277
  praise and, 187
  sexual motivation/behavior and, 306
Current concerns, 243

Defection, 267
Defensive aggression, 252–53, 260
Defensive denial, 20
Definitions
  of arousal, 14–15
  of biological rhythms, 30
  of circadian rhythms, 31
  of constructs, 7–9, 12
  of emotion, 82–85
  of hunger, 7–9, 129–30
  of motivation, 1, 7–10
  operational, 9–10, 13
  response, 7–9, 12
  stimulus, 7, 8, 12
  stimulus-response, 9, 12–13
  of thirst, 143–45
Delayed recall, 66
Delay-of-reinforcement gradient, 190, 215
Delta waves, 50, 54, 320
Democratization, 309–10
Demonstrator conspecifics, 152
Dependent variables, 7, 12, 230, 234
Depression, 122, 124–25
  arousal and, 22–23
  cognition and, 111
  eating disorders and, 165
  hunger and, 158, 160
  information processing and, 119–20
  locus of control and, 229
Desynchronization
  external, 47
  internal, 47, 48, 69
Diabetic children, 221–22
Diastolic blood pressure, 15, 249
Directional fractionation, 19
Directionality
  hunger and thirst in, 166–77
  of motivation, 4, 5, 6, 10, 14
Discrimination learning, 28
Disease, 96, 98, 247
Disinhibition, 158
Diuresis, 145
Diurnal creatures, 30, 31, 35, 44
Domestic violence, 252, 270, 319, 322
Dominance, 293
Dominican Republic, 308
Dopamine, 26, 185, 192, 194, 195, 215, 303
Drive, 1, 2, 3, 6
  aggression as, 255
  fear and anxiety as, 282
  hunger as, 157
Drive reduction, 185
Drive stimuli, 157, 166
Drive theory, 27, 28, 296

Drug abuse. *See* Substance abuse
Duchenne smile, 86
Duration
  of emotion, 81–82, 94
  of melatonin release, 43
Dynamic characteristics, 6
Dynamogenic tension, 4

Eating disorders, 130, 149, 160–63, 164, 165, 181–82. *See also specific types*
Eating restraint, 58–59, 133, 158, 163, 181
Ecological perspective, 108–9
Effect, Law of. *See* Law of Effect
Effort, 120, 206, 216, 218
Ego involvement, 205–6, 207, 219, 220
EI$_R$, 219–20
Elaboration, 118
Electrocardiogram (EKG) measures, 15, 18, 29
Electroencephalogram (EEG) measures
  of arousal, 15, 18
  of circadian rhythms, 32
  of emotion, 113, 122, 124–25
  of nicotine effects, 194
  of sleep, 48–50, 51, 53, 54, 57
  of thirst, 173
Electromyogram (EMG) measures, 18, 29, 122
Emotion, 2, 4, 81–105, 106–28
  affect and, 100–101, 105
  approach and withdrawal, 121–28
  as associative network formulation, 113, 114–19, 120, 127
  basic, 85–87, 89, 96
  blended, 107–8
  categories of, 84, 85–90, 101–2
  cerebral asymmetry and, 121–25
  changing of, 99–100
  classification of, 85–90
  cognition and, 83, 84–85, 95, 106–14
  cognitive-physiological formulation of, 90
  definitions of, 82–85
  developmental factors in, 107–8
  dimensions of, 84, 92–95, 101–2
  duration of, 81–82, 94
  ecological perspective on, 108–9
  facial expression and, 87–88, 96
  historical considerations, 83–85
  hostility and, 248
  information processing and, 113–21
  James-Lange theory of, 10, 13, 83, 88, 104
  long- versus short-term targets of, 109–10

mood and, 82, 100–101, 104–5
motivation and, 10–11, 81–82
multiple targets of, 106–7
opponent processes and, 102–3, 105
person-environment relationships in, 95–99, 104
phasic, 109–10
pure, 107–8
resource allocation and, 119–20, 127
Schachter-Singer hypothesis of, 90–91, 92, 104
tonic, 109–10
visual recognition of stimuli, 125–27
Emotional faces, 125
Emotional Stroop test, 297, 298, 300
Emotional tone, 100
Emotion intensity effect, 116
Empty love, 321
Encoding, 66, 119, 120
Encouragement, 201–2, 224, 233
Energetic arousal, 21–23, 29, 76–77
Energizing aspect of motivation, 4, 5, 6, 10, 14. *See also* Arousal
Energy
  mood and, 72–75
  regulation of, in hunger, 129–43
Energy mobilization, 4, 6
Entrainment, 31, 35, 37, 40, 43, 44, 320
Epinephrine (adrenaline)
  anger and, 240
  arousal and, 18
  emotion and, 90–91
  fear and anxiety and, 288, 300
  memory and, 179
  mood and, 75
  time of day and, 65
Eros, 323
Erotic stimuli, 307
Escape conditioning, 282–84, 300
Eskimos, 314
Estimate of Self-Competence scale, 226–27
Estradiol, 302, 324
Estrogen receptors, 44
Estrogens, 261, 263, 302, 303, 304, 324
Estrous cycle/estrus, 31, 303, 304, 305
Ethoexperimental observations, 256
Eveningness, 54–55, 68, 75–79, 80
Event-related brain potentials (ERPs), 179–80
Evolutionary factors
  in emotion, 106
  in fear and anxiety, 288, 291–92, 293
  in love, 323
  in sexual motivation/behavior, 306, 307

Exchange situation, 267
Excitement, 308
Exercise, 40, 69, 142, 182
Expectancy-value theory, 212–14
Expectations. *See also* Level of expecta-
    tion
  fear and anxiety and, 285
  goals and, 224–26
  obesity and, 156–57
Expert power, 271
Explanatory styles, 121, 237–38, 251
Expressive movements, 84
Expressive traits, 311, 320, 324
External beliefs, 229
External control of reinforcement belief,
    228–30, 234, 236, 250
External cues, 155–57
External desynchronization, 47
External rewards, 199–206, 216
External variables, 4
Extinction, 99, 285, 286, 291, 300
Extracellular dehydration, 143, 144–45,
    181
Extraversion, 76–79, 80, 295, 297
Extrinsic incentives, 211–12
Extrinsic motivation, 215

Face muscles, 87–88
Face validity, 10
Facial expression, 87–88, 96, 124, 125,
    244
Facilitation, 59, 60
Factor L, 247–48
Failure
  attributions for, 236
  expectancy-value theory and, 212–14
  fear of, 316
  incentives and achievement motive,
    208–14, 216
  locus of control and, 227–30
  performance versus learning goals
    and, 224
  self-efficacy beliefs and, 226–27
Failure acceptors, 211
Failure-avoiding, 210–11
False smiles, 85
Fat, 142, 159
Fathers, 319
Fatigue, 59–60, 65
Fear, 281–93
  anger compared with, 240
  anxiety distinguished from, 294
  avoidance conditioning and, 282–84,
    285–86, 287, 300
  escape conditioning and, 282–84, 300
  flooding and, 286, 290, 300

learned helplessness and, 285–86,
    289–90, 300
  learning without awareness, 290–92
  occurrence versus disposition of, 281
  psychobiological findings in, 286–90
  punishment and, 282, 284–85, 300
  social variables involved in learning,
    292–93
  taste aversions and, 150
Fear-induced aggression, 256
Feedback hypothesis of emotion, 87
Feedforward regulation, 131–32, 141,
    181
Feelings, 2
Fertility value, 306
Field studies, 7, 12
Fight or flight response, 96, 240, 244,
    288
Fixed interval (FI) reinforcement sched-
    ules, 185
Fixed ratio (FR) reinforcement sched-
    ules, 185
Flooding, 286, 290, 300
Fractional desynchronization technique,
    61–62, 63
Framingham scale, 246, 247
Free fatty acids, 141–42
Free recall, 118
Free-running rhythms (τ), 32–38, 55, 56
Freudian theory, 254
Friendship, 319–21, 325
Fructose, 178
Frustration, 244, 251
Frustration-aggression hypothesis, 254–
    55, 261, 279
Frustrative nonreward, 254, 287
Functionalism, 2

Galanin, 140
Galvanic skin response (GSR), 18, 19,
    29, 186
Games, 265–68, 279
Game theory, 266
Gastric motility, 157, 167, 181
Gender, 301, 309–16
  aggression and, 280
  anger and, 250
  arousal and, 21
  assertiveness and, 278, 279
  ideal weight preferences and, 164, 165
  importance of, 309–10
  love and, 320
  mastery and, 277
  thirst and, 147
Gender differences, 313–16, 325
Gender identity, 310–11, 324–25

Gender roles, 272–73, 309–10, 312
Gender schemas, 309–10, 311–13, 315,
    325
Gender stereotypes, 310, 311, 324
Genetic factors
  in eating disorders, 161
  in obesity, 142–43, 157
  in sexual motivation/behavior, 308
  in substance abuse, 195
Geniculohypothalamic tract, 40
Global affect, 71, 72
Global-specific dimension of attribu-
    tions, 237–38, 251
Global vigor, 71, 72
Glucocorticoids, 18
Glucose, 135, 136, 139–40, 159, 181
  biological rhythms and, 56
  interaction with insulin, 140–41
  memory and, 177–80, 182, 190
Glucostatic hypothesis, 140
Glycogen, 141
Glycoproteins, 142
Goal attainment, 225
Goal boxes, 11
Goal commitment, 231, 232, 234
Goal directedness, 97–99
Goal discrepancy, 219, 221, 227
Goal importance, 225
Goal intensity, 231
Goal level, 230, 231, 234
Goals, 1, 13, 217–34
  content of, 217
  emotion and, 10–11, 82
  factors influencing, 243
  incentives distinguished from, 198
  intentions (volitions) and, 232
  learning, 212, 222–24, 233
  levels of aspiration and expectation
    and, 217–22, 233
  performance, 212, 217–18, 222–24,
    233
  performance and, 219, 230–33, 234
  planning for, 217
  preset, 230–31
  self-set, 230–31, 232, 234
  speed versus accuracy in, 231
  stimulation and, 60–61, 79
  structure of, 217
Goal setting
  individual differences in, 222–26
  theories of, 230–31
Goal specificity, 231
Goal striving, 217, 231–33
Gonadal steroid hormones. *See* Sex-
    related hormones
Growth hormone, 52, 55, 57

Habit, 2, 192
Head hunting, 244
Heart rate
anger and, 244
arousal and, 15, 18, 19
of bonded peers, 320
fear and anxiety and, 290
Type A personality and, 249, 250
Hedonic factors
in affect, 101
in emotion, 82, 98, 102–3, 123
in hunger, 153–55, 160, 170, 182
in rewards, 185, 187, 214
Hedonic ratings, 58
Heightened sensitivity hypothesis, 167
Helplessness, 212, 223–24, 226, 232, 233. See also Learned helplessness
Hendrick, Hendrick, Slapion-Foote, and Foote sexual attitude scale, 308
Hermaphrodites, 303, 309
Heroin, 197
5–HIAA. See 5–Hydroxy-indole-acetic acid
Hippocampus
aggression and, 259, 260, 261, 279
fear and anxiety and, 287, 300
hunger and, 180
substance abuse and, 192, 194
thirst and, 173, 178
Homeostasis, 131–32, 141, 180–81
Homosexuals, 309
Hormones. See also Sex-related hormones
aggression and, 261–64, 279
sexual motivation/behavior and, 302–4, 308, 324
thirst and, 147
Hostility, 247–48, 251
Hot cognitions, 110–11, 127
5HT. See Serotonin
Hunger, 149–82, 188, 214
aggression and, 259–60
appetitive responses in, 129–30
as arousal state, 23–25, 26
biological processes and energy regulation in, 129–43
biological rhythms and, 30
cholecystokinin and, 139, 140, 165, 181
concepts of, 130–33
consummatory responses and, 129–30, 134, 157, 170, 173
cues and, 155–60, 166–69
culture and, 149–50, 181
definitions of, 7–9, 129–30
directional effects of, 166–78

food deprivation and desirability in, 169–70
group differences in, 161–63
instrumental responses in, 129–30, 170–73
interactive effects of food and, 169–73
lipids and, 141–43
morphine and, 185, 196
onset and cessation of eating in, 133–39
short- versus long-term regulation in, 132–33
social enhancement and, 152–53
subjective reports of, 157–58
terms in, 133
time of day and, 58–59
validity of measurements, 10
5–Hydroxy-indole-acetic acid (5–HIAA), 264
Hyenas, spotted, 304–6, 324
Hyperphagia, 133
Hypersominia, 54
Hypertonic condition, 144
Hypnosis, 91, 102–3, 111, 117
Hypophagia, 133
Hypothalamic-pituitary-adrenocortical (HPA) system, 18
Hypothalamic-pituitary-gonadal axis, 43–44
Hypothalamus, 191
aggression and, 260
aging and, 56
emotion and, 113, 124
hunger and, 132, 137, 138, 139, 180
lateral. See Lateral hypothalamus
medial, 139
paraventricular, 136
periformical, 136
sexual dimorphism and, 302
sexual motivation/behavior and, 304
thirst and, 181
ventromedial, 134, 136, 140, 156
Hypotonic condition, 144
Hypovolemia, 144–45, 146, 147, 181

Ideal self-guides, 296
Ideational beliefs, 150–51
Ilongot, 244
Immediate recall, 66
Immune system activity, 229, 299
Implosive therapy, 286, 290
Imprinting, 317
Impulsivity, 76–79, 80
Incentive motivation, 11–12, 13, 188, 198–208, 215

Incentives, 13, 198–214, 215–16. See also Rewards
achievement motivation and, 208–14
extrinsic, 211–12
intrinsic, 212
motivation-performance relationship and, 206–7
negative, 11, 198
positive, 11, 198
Incentive value learning, 208
Incentive value of food, 152, 154
Independent variables, 7, 12, 230, 234
Individual Psychology, 97–98. See also Adlerian theory
Individual variation, 5, 6
Informational influence, 271
Information processing
aggression and, 275
computer-based perspectives on, 114
emotion and, 113–21
hunger and thirst and, 173–78
time pressure and, 249
Information purchasing, 175
Infradian rhythms, 31
Instinct, 3, 6
Instrumental aggression, 252, 256, 271, 274, 278
Instrumental characteristics, 311, 320, 324
Instrumental conditioning, 183–86, 283
Instrumental responses, 129–30, 170–73
Insulin, 140–41, 154, 159, 179, 181
cephalic phase of release, 133, 141
Intensity. See also Arousal
of emotion, 90–91, 93, 94, 116, 119, 121
goal, 231
information processing and, 116
of motivation, 4, 6
Intentional competition, 269
Intentions (volitions), 10–11, 232, 236
Interference, 59–60
Intergeniculate leaflet (IGL), 40, 41
Intergroup competition, 269
Intermale aggression, 256
Internal control of reinforcement belief, 228–30, 233–34, 236, 250, 293
Internal cues, 155–57, 166–67
Internal desynchronization, 47, 48, 69
Internal-External Locus of Control scale, 228
Internal motivation, 317
Interspecies aggression, 259–60, 279
Intervening variables, 3–4, 5, 6, 7, 8, 12
Intimacy, 320, 321

Intracranial self-stimulation. *See also* Brain stimulation
  hunger and, 134–35, 136
  in substance abuse studies, 191–95, 215
Intragroup competition, 269
Intrinsic incentives, 212
Intrinsic motivation, 199–206, 215, 224
Introversion
  morningness-eveningness and, 76–79, 80
  trait anxiety and, 295–97
Inuit society, 268–69
Inverted-U hypothesis, 26–29
IPAT scale, 295
Irritable aggression, 256
Italy, 271

James-Lange theory, 10, 13, 83, 88, 104
Japan, 271
JAS. *See* Jenkins Activity Survey for Health Predictions
Jealousy, 323
Jenkins Activity Survey for Health Predictions (JAS), 248–49
Jet lag, 47–48, 53, 55

K complexes, 50
Klüver-Bucy syndrome, 261
Knowledge, 95

Laboratory studies, 7, 12
Lateral geniculate body, 74
Lateral hypothalamus (LH)
  hunger and, 26, 133–36, 139, 140
  thirst and, 145–46
Law of Effect, 184, 214
Law of sympathetic magic, 151
Learned helplessness, 25, 238, 285–86, 289–90, 300
Learned irrelevance, 289
Learning, 3–4
  aggression and, 274–76
  arousal and, 28
  discrimination, 28
  emotion and, 84, 116–21, 124
  hunger and, 173
  incentive value, 208
  motivation distinguished from, 6
  nicotine effects and, 197
  rewards and, 184, 185, 186, 187–90, 214, 215
  thirst and, 173
  vicarious, 186
Learning anxiety, 284
Learning goals, 212, 222–24, 233

Learning history, 292
Learning-to-learn, 59, 60
Left brain hemisphere
  emotion and, 113–14, 122, 124, 126, 128
  sexual dimorphism and, 302
Legitimate power, 271, 272
Level of aspiration (LA), 217–22, 233
Level of expectation (LE), 217–22, 233
Lie detectors, 18
Lifestyle, 226
Life tasks, 226, 233
Light-dark cycle, 31, 32–35, 37, 43, 47, 61
Limbic system, 113
Links, 115
Lipids, 141–43
Lipogenesis, 142
Lipolysis, 142
Lipostatic hypothesis, 141, 142
Liver, 139, 142, 160, 178, 181
Locomotor activity. *See* Motor activity
Locus ceruleus, 194
Locus of causality, 203
Locus of control of reinforcement, 212, 227–30, 233–34, 237
  external, 228–30, 234, 236, 250
  internal, 228–30, 233–34, 236, 250, 293
Long-term memory (LTM), 6, 64, 66, 179, 180
Long-term potentiation (LTP), 289
Lordosis, 303
Love, 109, 110, 301, 316–24
  consummate, 321
  empty, 321
  parent-child, 316–19, 325
  peer relationships and friendship, 319–21, 325
  romantic, 321–24, 325
  as a story, 321–22, 323
  triangular theory of, 320, 321
Love acts, 323
Love styles, 323
Ludus, 323
Luteinizing hormone (LH), 56

Machiavellianism, 276–77, 280
Male gender role, 272–73
Maltose, 155
Mania (love style), 323
Manifest Anxiety Scale (MAS), 294
Marijuana, 194
MAS. *See* Manifest Anxiety Scale
Masculine gender role stress (MGRS), 272

Masculine protest, 272
Masking factors, 60–61
Masking smiles, 85
Mastery, 212, 223, 226, 233, 237, 250–51, 252, 277, 280
Mastery motivation, 277
Maternal aggression, 256, 259
Measurement
  of anger, 246–47
  of arousal, 14–15
  of circadian rhythms, 32–38
  of gender identity, 311
Media, aggression in, 274–75, 280
Medial hypothalamus, 139
Medulla, 240
Melatonin, 41, 42–44, 46, 48, 55, 56, 69
Memory, 3–4, 6
  associative, 289
  autobiographical, 118, 121
  emotion and, 93–95, 116–21, 124
  event-related brain potentials and, 179–80
  glucose and, 178–80, 182, 190
  incentives and, 206
  long-term, 6, 64, 66, 179, 180
  rewards and, 185, 189–90, 214
  saccharin and, 189–90
  short-term. *See* Short-term memory
  time of day and, 65–66, 67, 80
Men's movement, 313
Menstrual cycle, 31, 320
MEQ. *See* Morningness-eveningness questionnaire
Mesocorticolimbic pathway (MCLP), 192, 193, 215
Mesolimbic system, 185
Microsleeps, 54, 69
Midazolam, 38, 39
Minangkabou, 85
Minnesota Multiphasic Personality Inventory (MMPI), 247
Mixed-motive games, 266–67, 279
MMPI. *See* Minnesota Multiphasic Personality Inventory
Modeling, 12, 13, 274–75, 292
Monoamine, 55
Mood, 116
  cognition and, 110–13
  emotion and, 82, 100–101, 104–5
  time of day and, 66, 70–75
Mood Adjective Check List, 91
Mood-congruent effect, 116, 117–19, 127, 173
Mood form, 92–93
Morningness, 54–55, 68, 75–79, 80

Morningness-eveningness questionnaire (MEQ), 75–76, 78
Morphine, 178, 185, 194, 196
Motivation
    achievment. *See* Achievement motive/motivation
    affiliative, 5, 8, 196
    amount of, 4, 6
    behavior and, 1–2
    biological rhythms and, 30
    constructs of, 2–3, 6, 7–9, 12
    definitions of, 1, 7–10
    directionality of, 4, 5, 6, 10, 14
    emotion and, 10–11, 81–82
    energizing aspect of, 4, 5, 6, 10, 14
    extrinsic, 215
    historical considerations, 1–6
    incentive, 11–12, 13, 188, 198–208, 215
    intensity of, 4, 6
    intrinsic, 199–206, 215, 224
    learning distinguished from, 6
    mastery, 277
    performance and, 206–7
    phasic, 5–6
    primary, 130–31, 180, 187, 188
    rewards as, 11–12
    secondary. *See* Secondary motivation
    sexual. *See* Sexual motivation/behavior
    social, 98, 304
    stability of, 5–6
    tonic, 5–6
    variability of, 4–5, 6
Motivational states, 4, 5, 6, 129–30
Motivational traits, 4, 6
Motor activity
    arousal and, 23–26
    circadian rhythms and, 32–38
Multidimensional Anger Inventory, 246
Mutual behavior control, 267
Mutual fate control, 267

nAch, 209–10, 211, 212, 214, 222, 228, 232, 276
Naps, 52
National Association of Female Executives, 271
Natural killer (NK) cells, 229
Negative contrast effect (NCE), 169–70, 173
Negative feedback, 131–32
Negative incentives, 11, 198
Negative palatability shifts, 150
Negative reinforcement, 196, 198, 214, 215, 282, 300

Negative transfer, 59
Neurochemistry of anger, 240
Neuropeptide Y (NPY), 136, 140, 181
Neurotic hostility, 248
Neuroticism, 76–77, 295–97
Neurotransmitters. *See also specific types*
    anger and, 240
    arousal and, 15–18, 19
    fear and anxiety and, 288–89
    substance abuse and, 192
    time of day and, 58
New Look studies, 173–75, 177
New Zealand tribal groups, 314
Nicotine, 194–95, 197–98, 238
Nigrostriatal system, 185
Nocturnal creatures, 30, 31, 35
Nodes, 114–19
Norepinephrine (noradrenaline)
    anger and, 240
    arousal and, 17–18, 27–28
    fear and anxiety and, 288–89, 300
    hunger and, 140
    memory and, 178
    sexual motivation/behavior, 303–4
    sleep and, 51
    time of day and, 58, 65
N-person games, 267
Nucleus accumbens, 192

Obedience studies, 270–71, 274, 280
Obesity, 130, 134, 136, 141, 181–82
    cues and, 155–60
    eating disorders and, 160–63
    expectations and, 156–57
    genetic factors in, 142–43, 157
    socioeconomic status and, 164
    working for food and, 156–57
ob gene, 142–43
Offset Aggression System, 261
Onset Aggression System, 260–61
Open field, 25–26
Operant conditioning, 99, 183–86, 283
Operational definitions, 9–10, 13
Opiates, 157, 185
Opponent processes, 102–3, 105, 196, 241, 242, 251
Optimism, 300
    control-, 214
Optimistic explanatory style, 238
Optional sleep, 52, 53
Organisms, 2, 3
Organizational processes, 263
Organum vasculosum laminae terminalis (OVLT), 145, 146
Orgasm, 308

Oscillators, 41–42, 65. *See also* Pacemakers
Osmolality, 143–44, 146
Osmole, 143
Osmoreceptors, 145–46, 181
Osmosis, 143
Osmotic pressure, 143, 145
Ought self-guides, 296
Overstrivers, 211
Ovulation, 302
Oxytocin, 140, 147

Pacemakers (clocks), 37, 38, 40–41, 53, 55, 56, 61. *See also* Oscillators
Pain thresholds, 163
Palatability, 150, 153, 154, 155, 181
Pancreas, 140, 141
PAQ. *See* Personal Attributes Questionnaire
Parasympathetic nervous system, 15
Paraventricular hypothalamus, 136
Paraventricular nucleus, 136
Parent-child love, 316–19, 325
Passion, 320, 321
Passive avoidance conditioning, 283, 287
Pavlovian conditioning. *See* Classical (Pavlovian) conditioning
Peer relationships, 319–21, 325
Perception effects, 174, 177, 182
Perch hopping behavior, 32
Performance
    achievement, 211–12
    arousal and, 23–29
    goals and, 219, 230–33, 234
    incentives and, 206–7
    motivation and, 206–7
    quantity versus quality of, 26–27
    rewards and, 187–90, 215, 217
    time of day and, 64–68, 79
Performance discrepancy, 219
Performance goals, 212, 217–18, 222–24, 233
Periformical hypothalamus, 136
Period, of biological rhythms, 30, 35, 55
Period disorders, 45
Peripheral nervous system (PNS)
    arousal and, 15
    emotion and, 87
    hunger and, 132, 138–39
Permissiveness, 308
Persistence, 254
Personal Attributes Questionnaire (PAQ), 311
Personality characteristics, 75–79
Personal power, 196, 197

Person-environment relationships, 95–99, 104
Pessimism, 299, 300
Pessimistic explanatory style, 238, 251
Phase, of biological rhythms, 37, 55
Phase advance of biological rhythms, 37, 47, 48, 55, 70
Phase delay of biological rhythms, 37, 47, 48, 70
Phase disorders, 45
Phase reference point of biological rhythms, 37
Phase relationships of biological rhythms, 37
Phase-shifting hypothesis, 46
Phase shifts in biological rhythms, 37, 38, 40, 44, 68, 69
Phasic emotions, 109–10
Phasic motivation, 5–6
Pheromones, 31, 263, 304
Photoperiods, 38, 42
Phototherapy, 45–47, 48, 69–70
Physiological processes
  in anger, 240
  in arousal, 18–19
  in emotion, 84, 89, 90–91, 113–14
Pineal gland, 42, 43, 56
Pituitary gland, 302
Plateau, 308
Pleasantness-unpleasantness dimension, 101–2, 105, 110
Positive contrast effect (PCE), 169–70, 173
Positive incentives, 11, 198
Positive reinforcement, 185–86, 196, 214
Positive transfer, 60
Postabsorptive phase, 133, 141
Postprandial interval, 133
Power, 209, 289
  aggression and, 252, 270–74, 280
  alcohol and, 196, 197, 272–73
  anger and, 239–40, 242, 251
  bases of, 271–72
  coercive, 271, 272, 280
  expert, 271
  informational influence and, 271
  legitimate, 271, 272
  male gender role and, 272–73
  personal, 196, 197
  referent, 271, 272
  reward, 271
  social, 196, 197
Pragma, 323
Prairie voles, 304–6, 324
Praise, 201–3, 214, 216
  ego versus task involvement and, 205–6

variety of meanings, 207–8
  as a verbal reinforcer, 186–87
Preabsorption phase, 133
Predatory aggression, 256, 279
Preparedness, 291–92
Preprandial interval, 133
Primary motivation, 130–31, 180, 187, 188
Primary rewards, 131, 187, 189
Primary thirst, 143
Priming, 59, 60, 118, 174
Prince, The (Machiavelli), 276
Prisoner's Dilemma Game (PDG), 266–68, 269
Private logic, 98
Procedural clarity, 10
Process C, 52, 53
Processing capacity, 120
Process S, 52–53
Progesterone, 261, 302–3
Progestins, 302, 324
Projection, 174
Propositions, 114, 115
Psychodynamic theorists, 2
Psychogalvanic response (PGR). See Galvanic skin response
Punishment, 184, 214, 282, 284–85, 296, 297, 300
Pure emotions, 107–8. See also Basic emotions
Puzzle boxes, 184, 185

Questionnaires, 8

Race, 245, 250, 315
Rape, 306, 307
Raphe nuclei, 40–41
Rapid eye movement (REM) sleep, 31, 50, 51, 52, 53, 54, 55, 61
Reaction time (RT), 65, 78–79
Reactive (expressive) hostility, 248
Reality testing, 286
Referent power, 271, 272
Reinforcement, 185
  locus of control of. See Locus of control of reinforcement
  negative, 196, 198, 214, 215, 282, 300
  positive, 185–86, 196, 214
  schedules of, 185
Relaxation training, 242, 251, 290
Reliability, 9, 13
Religion, 149, 151
Renin, 144, 181
Replicability, 9
Repression-sensitization, 295
Reproduction, 38, 306–7

Resolution, 308
Resource allocation, 119–20, 127
Response, 2
  appetitive, 129–30
  conditioned, 84
  conditioned emotional, 284
  consummatory, 129–30, 134, 157, 170, 173
  instrumental, 129–30, 170–73
Response definitions, 7–9, 12
Response generation, 174, 177
Response production, 174
Response stereotyping, 19–20, 29, 258
Restrained eaters. See Eating restraint
Reticular activating system (RAS), 15–18, 29
Reticular formation, 15, 29, 137
Retinohypothalamic tract, 40, 42
Retrieval, 66, 119, 120, 178, 179
Retroactive inhibition, 121
Reward power, 271
Rewards, 4, 13, 183–98, 214, 217. See also Incentives
  associative aspects of, 185, 214
  conditioned (secondary), 131, 187–89
  controlling aspect of, 203
  delay of, 190, 215
  external, 199–206, 216
  informational aspect of, 187, 203
  magnitude of, 170–73, 189–90, 192, 215
  as motivation, 11–12
  primary, 131, 187, 189
  studies of, 183–87
  substance abuse and, 190–98, 215
  unlearned, 187–89
Reward systems, 191–92
Right brain hemisphere
  emotion and, 113–14, 122, 124, 125, 126, 128
  sexual dimorphism and, 302
Risk-taking behavior, 210–11, 238
Romantic love, 321–24, 325
Rotter Form Board, 221–22, 225
Running wheels. See Activity (running wheels) wheels

Saccharin, 140, 154, 189–90, 215
Sadness, 123
Salt appetite, 146–47. See also Sodium
Satietin, 140, 142
Schachter-Singer hypothesis, 90–91, 92, 104
Scopolamine, 303
Search tasks, 66
Seasonal affective disorder (SAD), 45–47, 56, 165–66

Seasonal rhythms, 38, 56
Secondary appraisal, 97
Secondary motivation, 188
   in fear and anxiety, 283–84
   in hunger, 130–31
Secondary rewards. *See* Conditioned
   (secondary) rewards
Secondary thirst, 143
Secure attachment style, 318, 322,
   323–24
Selective sensitivity, 167
Self-concept, 121, 224, 233, 238, 314
Self-determination, 203, 215
Self-efficacy, 226–27, 231, 233, 293
Self-esteem, 238, 242, 247, 250,
   299–300
Self-generated cognition, 298
Self-interest, 264–70, 279
Self-report ratings
   of arousal, 20–21
   of attachment styles, 322
   of emotion, 93–95
   of hostility, 247–48
Self-stimulation studies, 191–94
Semai, 269
Semantic differential test, 187
Sensitivity-activation hypothesis,
   167–69
Sensory-affective beliefs, 150, 151
Sensory-specific satiety, 154, 155–56,
   162
Sentiment, 110
Septum, 191, 261, 279, 287
Serotonin (5HT), 17, 18, 140, 264, 279,
   304
Set-point theory, 142, 159–60, 180
Sex-related aggression, 256
Sex-related hormones
   aggression and, 261–64
   melatonin and, 43
   sexual motivation/behavior and,
      302–4, 308, 324
   thirst and, 147
Sex-role socialization, 315
Sex-typing, 311–12, 313, 324–25
Sexual arousability, 307–8, 324
Sexual arousal, 307–8, 324
Sexual dimorphism, 302–3, 305, 308,
   310, 324
Sexual instrumentality, 308
Sexual motivation/behavior, 301, 302–9,
   324
   for reproduction, 306–7
   substance abuse and, 196
Shift work, 37, 40, 53, 55, 68–70, 79–80
Short-term memory (STM)
   emotion and, 118

glucose and, 179–80
   time of day and, 64–65, 66, 77–78, 79
Shuttle boxes, 191, 283–85
Sibling relationships, 220–21, 319,
   320–21
Sidman avoidance conditioning procedure, 283
Single cell activity, recording of, 135
Sinusoidal waves, 35, 36
Situational specificity, 19–20, 29
Situational variables
   in aggression, 258–59
   in emotion, 82
16 PF test, 247
Skill, 218
Skill orientation, 230
Skinner boxes, 184, 189, 191–92, 282,
   284
Sleep, 48–56, 79
   adaptive theory of, 51
   aging and, 54–56
   arousal and, 14, 20
   circadian rhythms and, 52–54, 57
   core, 52, 53
   jet lag and, 47, 48
   micro, 54, 69
   optional, 52, 53
   rapid eye movement, 31, 50, 51, 52,
      53, 54, 55, 61
   reasons for, 51–52
   repair and restorative function of, 51,
      52
   stages of, 48–50
   time since, 59
   two-process model of, 52, 53
Sleep apnea, 54
Sleep debt/deficit, 61, 69, 70
Sleep deprivation, 51, 52, 57, 66, 69,
   70–71, 74
Sleep disturbances, 71–72, 178
Sleep latencies, 53
Sleep rhythms, 61–62
Sleep spindles, 50
Sleep-wake cycle, 44, 45, 57, 59, 61–62,
   68, 72, 181
Slow wave sleep (SWS), 50, 52, 54, 55,
   61
Smiles
   Duchenne, 86
   false, 85
   masking, 85
   muscles in, 122
Smoking. *See* Nicotine
Snakes, fear of, 290, 291
Social animals, 304–6, 324
Social cues, 31
Social dilemmas, 267

Social enhancement, 152–53
Social interest, 200, 201, 308. *See also*
   Adlerian theory
Socially acquired introjects, 203
Social motivation, 98, 304
Social power, 196, 197
Social Rhythm Metric, 71–72
Socioeconomic status, 164
Sodium, 143, 144, 145. *See also* Salt ap-
   petite
Somatic arousal, 20, 21
Species-specific variation, 5, 6
Spheres of Control scale, 229
Sports, 265–68, 279
Spreading activation, 115
Stability of motivation, 5–6
Stable-unstable dimension of attribu-
   tions, 236, 237–38, 250
STAI. *See* State-Trait Anxiety Inventory
Startle reflex, 95, 290
State anxiety, 5, 294–95, 297–98,
   299–300
State-dependent effect, 117, 118,
   120–21, 127
States
   arousal as, 20–21, 29
   emotion as, 81, 109
   motivational, 4, 5, 6, 129–30
State-Trait Anxiety Inventory (STAI),
   295
Stimulation, 60–61, 79
Stimuli, 2, 4
   conditioned. *See* Conditioned stimuli
   drive, 157, 166
   erotic, 307
   unconditioned. *See* Unconditioned
      stimuli
Stimulus definitions, 7, 8, 12
Stimulus-intensity dynamism, 167
Stimulus-organism-response (S-O-R)
   model, 2
Stimulus-response definitions, 9, 12–13
Stomach, 139, 140
Storage, 66, 178, 179
Storge, 323
Strange situation, 317–18
Stress, 96, 198, 250
Stroop test, 297. *See also* Emotional
   Stroop test
Structural competition, 269
Structure of goals, 217
Subfornical organ (SFO), 145
Subjective Anger Scale, 246
Submission, 293
Substance abuse, 190–98, 215
Substance dependence, 195, 215. *See*
   also Addiction

Substance use, 195, 215
Success
    attributions for, 236
    expectancy-value theory and, 212–14
    fear of, 315–16, 325
    incentives and achievement motive, 208–14, 216
    locus of control and, 227–30
    self-efficacy beliefs and, 226–27
    valence and, 225
Success-seeking, 210–11
Sucrose, 58, 131, 140, 316
Sugar, 177–79. *See also specific types*
Suprachiasmatic nucleus (SCN), 40–41, 42, 43, 53, 56
Sweetness, 58, 170
Sympathetic magic, law of, 151
Sympathetic nervous system, 15, 113, 240
Syntoxic response, 235, 239
Systematic desensitization, 290
Systolic blood pressure, 15

Tachistoscope, 125, 174
Tahitian society, 268–69
Task assessment, 225
Task involvement, 205–6
Task mastery, 266, 277
Tasks
    belief about success or failure in, 226–27
    cognitive, 297–99
    goals and, 224–26, 233
    life, 226, 233
    search, 66
    time of day and, 65–68
Task values, 225, 233
Task variables, 120
Taste, 149–55
    group differences in, 161–63
    time of day and, 58–59
Taste aversions, 150–52, 181
TAT. *See* Thematic Apperception Test
Temporal lobe, 124, 261
Tense arousal, 21–23, 29, 76–77
Tension
    dynamogenic, 4
    mood and, 72–75
Testosterone
    aggression and, 261–64, 279
    male gender role and, 273

sexual motivation/behavior and, 302–3, 309, 324
    Type A personality and, 249–50
Test-taking anxiety, 210, 211, 213, 216
Thalamus, 15, 29, 113
Thematic Apperception Test (TAT), 209
Theta waves, 50
Thirst, 180–81, 182
    biological processes and fluid regulation in, 143–49
    cellular dehydration in, 143–44, 145, 148, 181
    cues and, 166–69
    definitions of, 143–45
    directional effects of, 166–78
    extracellular dehydration in, 143, 144–45, 181
    onset and cessation of drinking in, 147–49
    primary, 143
    salt appetite and, 146–47
    secondary, 143
Three Mile Island nuclear power plant, 69
Thrill seeking, 274
Thyroxine, 51
Time of day, 58–80
    mood and, 66, 70–75
    performance and, 64–68, 79
    personality characteristics and, 75–79
    variables of importance in addition to, 59–61
Time pressure, 249
Tonic emotions, 109–10
Tonic motivation, 5–6
Touch thresholds, 163
Trait Anger Expression Inventory, 246
Trait anxiety, 5, 294–98, 299–300
Trait Arousability Scale, 249
Traits
    arousal as, 20–21, 29
    emotion as, 81, 109
    motivational, 4, 6
Triangular theory of love, 320, 321
Triglycerides, 141–42
Tryptophan, 264
12-step programs, 198
Twin studies, 302, 308
Two-process model of sleep, 52, 53
Type A personality, 248–50, 251
Type B personality, 248, 251
Type T personality, 274

Ultradian rhythms, 31
Unconditioned stimuli (US), 27
    emotion and, 83
    fear and anxiety and, 283, 286, 288, 289
    hunger and, 167
    taste aversions and, 150
    thirst and, 167
Undifferentiated persons, 311, 325
Unlearned rewards, 187–89
Urges, 194–95

Vagus nerve, 139
Valence, 213–14, 216, 218, 225
Validity, 9–10, 13
Variability of motivation, 4–5, 6
Variable interval (VI) reinforcement schedules, 185
Variable ratio (VR) reinforcement schedules, 185
Variables
    dependent, 7, 12, 230, 234
    external, 4
    independent, 7, 12, 230, 234
    intervening, 3–4, 5, 6, 7, 8, 12
Vasopressin, 145–46, 147, 181
Velten mood-induction procedure, 119
Ventral tegmental area, 192
Ventromedial hypothalamus (VMH), 134, 136, 140, 156
Vicarious learning, 186
Vigilance, 65, 78, 79
Visual cortex, 74
Vitalism, 2

Wake after sleep onset (WASO), 54
Warm-up, 59, 60
Will, 2, 3, 6, 10
Wishes, 10
Withdrawal
    from drugs, 195, 197, 198
    emotional, 121–28
Work and Family Orientation (WOFO) Questionnaire, 237, 249
World beliefs, 229
Worry, 299

Yerkes-Dodson law, 26–29
Yo-yo effect, 159
Yugoslavia, 306

Zeitgebers, 31, 35, 37, 40, 47, 56, 62, 63